Current Progress in Hepatology Research

Current Progress in Hepatology Research

Editor: Tucker Banks

AMERICAN
MEDICAL PUBLISHERS
www.americanmedicalpublishers.com

AMERICAN
MEDICAL PUBLISHERS
www.americanmedicalpublishers.com

Cataloging-in-Publication Data

Current progress in hepatology research / edited by Tucker Banks.
p. cm.
Includes bibliographical references and index.
ISBN 979-8-88740-036-5
1. Hepatology. 2. Hepatology--Research. 3. Gastroenterology. 4. Digestive organs--Diseases.
5. Gastrointestinal system. 6. Gastrointestinal system--Diseases. I. Banks, Tucker.
RC845 .C87 2023
616.362--dc23

American Medical Publishers,
41 Flatbush Avenue,
1st Floor, New York,
NY 11217, USA

ISBN 979-8-88740-036-5 (Hardback)

Contents

Preface

Hepatology is the branch of medicine that is concerned with the study of liver, gallbladder, biliary tree, and pancreas. It also deals with the treatment of disorders associated with these organs. There are several types of hepatologic diseases including acute liver failure, alcoholic liver disease, hepatitis B and C, autoimmune liver diseases, primary biliary cholangitis, cirrhosis, non-alcoholic fatty liver disease, etc. In recent years, there has been significant clinical research on the development of novel therapies, improving diagnostic modalities, and predictors of outcome for liver and related disorders. Breakthrough has been achieved in the introduction and application of biomarkers for the early diagnosis of hepatocellular carcinoma, drug-induced liver injury, hepatitis B and hepatitis C. A number of latest researches have been included to keep the readers up-to-date with the global concepts in hepatology. Researchers and students in this field will be greatly assisted by it.

After months of intensive research and writing, this book is the end result of all who devoted their time and efforts in the initiation and progress of this book. It will surely be a source of reference in enhancing the required knowledge of the new developments in the area. During the course of developing this book, certain measures such as accuracy, authenticity and research focused analytical studies were given preference in order to produce a comprehensive book in the area of study.

This book would not have been possible without the efforts of the authors and the publisher. I extend my sincere thanks to them. Secondly, I express my gratitude to my family and well-wishers. And most importantly, I thank my students for constantly expressing their willingness and curiosity in enhancing their knowledge in the field, which encourages me to take up further research projects for the advancement of the area.

Editor

1

Targeting of Hepatic Macrophages by Therapeutic Nanoparticles

Clara I. Colino [1,2], *José M. Lanao* [1,2*] *and Carmen Gutierrez-Millan* [1,2]

[1] *Area of Pharmacy and Pharmaceutical Technology, Department of Pharmaceutical Sciences, University of Salamanca, Salamanca, Spain,* [2] *The Institute for Biomedical Research of Salamanca (IBSAL), Salamanca, Spain*

***Correspondence:**
José M. Lanao
jmlanao@usal.es

Hepatic macrophage populations include different types of cells with plastic properties that can differentiate into diverse phenotypes to modulate their properties in response to different stimuli. They often regulate the activity of other cells and play an important role in many hepatic diseases. In response to those pathological situations, they are activated, releasing cytokines and chemokines; they may attract circulating monocytes and exert functions that can aggravate the symptoms or drive reparation processes. As a result, liver macrophages are potential therapeutic targets that can be oriented toward a variety of aims, with emergent nanotechnology platforms potentially offering new perspectives for macrophage vectorization. Macrophages play an essential role in the final destination of nanoparticles (NPs) in the organism, as they are involved in their uptake and trafficking *in vivo*. Different types of delivery nanosystems for macrophage recognition and targeting, such as liposomes, solid-lipid, polymeric, or metallic nanoparticles, have been developed. Passive targeting promotes the accumulation of the NPs in the liver due to their anatomical and physiological features. This process is modulated by NP characteristics such as size, charge, and surface modifications. Active targeting approaches with specific ligands may also be used to reach liver macrophages. In order to design new systems, the NP recognition mechanism of macrophages must be understood, taking into account that variations in local microenvironment may change the phenotype of macrophages in a way that will affect the uptake and toxicity of NPs. This kind of information may be applied to diseases where macrophages play a pathogenic role, such as metabolic disorders, infections, or cancer. The kinetics of nanoparticles strongly affects their therapeutic efficacy when administered *in vivo*. Release kinetics could predict the behavior of nanosystems targeting macrophages and be applied to improve their characteristics. PBPK models have been developed to characterize nanoparticle biodistribution in organs of the reticuloendothelial system (RES) such as liver or spleen. Another controversial issue is the possible toxicity of non-degradable nanoparticles, which in many cases accumulate in high percentages in macrophage clearance organs such as the liver, spleen, and kidney.

Keywords: hepatic macrophages, nanoparticles, drug delivery, biodistribution, Kupffer cells, toxicity

INTRODUCTION

The use of particles as carriers of therapeutic agents for liver targeting is not a new idea. Hepatic nanoparticle uptake and distribution was initially studied as a drawback to be avoided because it entails a lack of specific selective distribution to other desired targets as well as toxicity and safety concerns. Nevertheless, from another point of view, strategies of selective delivery to different kinds of hepatic cells have also been explored in the search for specific targets of drugs included in nanoparticulated systems, such as hepatocytes, hepatic stellar cells, endothelial cells, and also the Kupffer cells (KC), the resident liver macrophages.

The liver is a very complex organ with many cells that are different in both morphology and functionality but which are nonetheless strongly inter-related. Although there are some other hepatic cells with phagocytic activity, KCs are undoubtedly the main ones responsible for phagocytosis in the liver. Moreover, it is estimated that they constitute 80–90% of all the macrophages present in the body (1).

Kupffer cells are the liver-resident macrophages, considered professional phagocytes to distinguish them from facultative ones. They are the largest mononuclear phagocyte population in the body and constitute approximately 20% of non-parenchymal liver cells. They present functional heterogeneity, likely due to their different origins and intrinsic plasticity (2).

They have an evident role in monitoring the blood entering the zone in order to endocytose debris, degenerated cells and any potentially harmful materials from the gut and circulation stream. Their strategic location at the luminal side of the hepatic sinusoidal endothelium allows them to act as sentinels that capture and process particles. They are involved in antigen presentation and processing and in the modulation of some hepatocyte functions.

Activation of Kupffer cells can induce a series of events to inhibit pathogen replication, recruit other immune cells into the liver, and activate them. On the other hand, interaction derived from infiltration immune cells leads to KC regulation (2). These complex and multiple inter-relationships with other hepatic cells and their concomitant role in immunological processes provide KCs with a wide variety of receptors that can be harnessed for their specific targeting (3, 4).

Due to the involvement of KCs in the evolution of many liver diseases, modulation of their activity may be used for therapeutic ends and nanosystems constitute promising alternatives for achieve this goal. In the present work, we will focus on the proposed nanosystems for targeting hepatic macrophages in order to improve pathological processes in the liver. The role of macrophages in liver diseases, the types of nanovehicles used, their characteristics, and the influence of the phenotype will be revised. Also, pharmacokinetic models for characterizing the biodistribution of NPs in the liver are addressed.

MONOCYTE–MACROPHAGE SYSTEM (MPS)

Macrophages have been considered to be a part of different body systems throughout history. Previously considered as reticulo-endothelial system (RES) cells, nowadays, macrophages are generally considered to belong to the monocyte mononuclear phagocyte or monocyte macrophage system (MPS), originally defined as a cell lineage of promonocytes that give rise to monocytes that finally becomes macrophages in tissues. This concept was later reformulated to include dendritic cells (5), and recently also the concept of the MPS has been questioned, based on evidence that tissue resident macrophages may be a separate lineage seeded during embryonic development and capable of self-renewal. The newly proposed nomenclature classifies mononuclear phagocytes according to their ontogeny, location, and/or morphology (6). Regarding the phagocytic cells in liver, the main difference of the newly proposed nomenclature is that macrophages and derived monocyte cells are considered to be separate entities (7).

Macrophages

Macrophages are specialized phagocytic cells strategically distributed in the body and specifically adapted to each tissue once they are settled. They are non-migratory cells that monitor their surrounding environment and process the material they engulf. They also recruit other immune cells, playing an important role in immune defense and homeostatic processes (8). To fulfill their functions, macrophages possess a wide range of sensing molecules specialized according to the tissue in which they are nested in each case.

Due to their central role in homeostasis, inflammation, and immunity, macrophages have arisen as interesting targets for therapeutic intervention (9).

Tissue macrophages are a very heterogeneous group of cells due to their different origins and their adaptation to the local environment. The contributions of embryonic origins and adult bone marrow cells vary depending on the tissues, with even tissue-resident macrophages of prenatal origin deriving from different hematopoietic stem cells.

In view of the new evidence that questions the previous MPS model, it is postulated that there are two groups of macrophages in tissues: one coming from prenatally established populations and a second one originating from infiltrated monocytes that are more related to inflammatory conditions. **Figure 1** illustrates the different origins and development processes of tissue-resident macrophages.

It has been demonstrated in mice that there are also several monocyte-derived tissue macrophage populations whose phenotypes reflect different origins. One such population is made up of macrophages originating from Ly-6C high expressing monocytes (classical monocytes), mainly coming from bone marrow, that express inflammatory chemokine receptors (like CCR2), pattern-recognition receptors, and cytokines. Another population is made up of macrophages derived from Ly-6C low expressing monocytes (non-classical monocytes), mainly coming from the spleen, that present a patrolling behavior and express more scavenging receptors. In the steady state, classical ones can leave the bloodstream and patrol extravascular tissues. They can be converted in some proportion into Ly-6C low expressing monocytes and transport antigens to lymph nodes. Non-classical monocytes patrol the intravascular spaces to clear

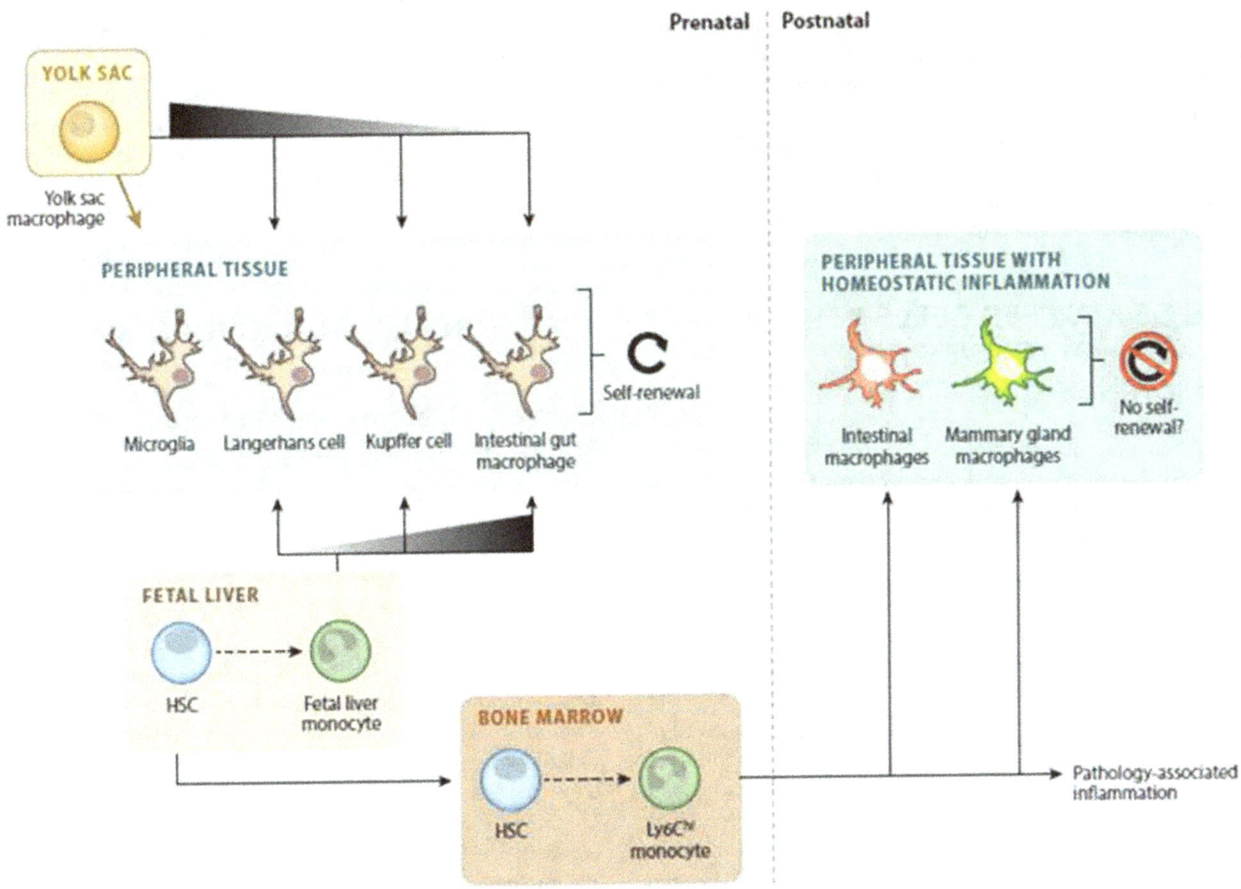

FIGURE 1 | Tissue-resident macrophages development. Adapted with permission (9).

dying endothelial cells. Under inflammation, classical monocytes differentiate to macrophages that are capable of self-renewal (10).

Despite the differences between mice and humans, genetic expression studies have demonstrated that these two subsets of monocytes are also present in humans, together with another intermediate subset between the classical and the non-classical (11, 12).

With respect to the macrophages that are present in the liver, although traditionally the term hepatic macrophages and Kupffer cells (KC) are used almost interchangeably, modifications to the MPS model mentioned above have also affected this assumption. After injury, heterogeneous hepatic macrophages populations can be observed, such as liver-resident macrophages or KCs and two subsets of bone marrow monocyte-derived macrophages (MoMFs), as well as peritoneal macrophages for subcapsular regions of the liver (13).

Classification

It is well-established in mice that macrophages can undergo two different activation states: M1 or classically activated and M2 or alternatively activated. M1 macrophages can produce pro-inflammatory cytokines and chemokines, high levels of reactive nitrogen and oxygen intermediates. They can also facilitate Th1 response and strong antimicrobial and antineoplastic effect. M2 ones are suppressive, involved in cellular repair and characterized by efficient phagocytic activity and high expression of scavenger, galactose, and mannose-type receptors. M1 and M2 even present different iron, glucose, and amino acid metabolism (2, 4). Although not much information is available regarding human beings, there is evidence to suggest a similar behavior in human macrophages (14). This traditional dichotomic classification seems to be too simplistic in view of recent increases in our knowledge of this area due to new sophisticated characterization techniques. Regarding Kupffer cells, their great flexibility and plasticity allow them to adopt a range of multiple intermediate phenotypes depending on the signals, which can lead to a broad spectrum of activation states (13, 15). Nevertheless, this simple classification into two possible extreme activation states is still used as a reference for KC behavior.

Differences not only in activation but also in origin have a great impact on the different subsets that can be defined for liver macrophages. The ontogeny and maintenance of resident hepatic macrophages have been the objects of many studies by important research groups, which have demonstrated that, besides the existence of self-renewal processes from prenatally settled local precursor cells, Kupffer cell populations are maintained by the infiltration of circulating bone-derived monocytes that differentiate into Kupffer cells in the liver (16, 17). Murine models have provided evidence that MoMF can contribute to regenerating the resident liver macrophage population when KC are massively depleted (18).

On the other hand, even some studies with models of sterile liver injury have shown phagocytes with an expression of the transcription factor GATA-6, suggesting macrophage infiltration from the peritoneal cavity (19).

ROLE OF KUPFFER CELLS IN HEPATIC DISEASES: CYTOKINES AND CHEMOKINES

Due to their physiological functions, Kupffer cells are involved in local cell communication and homeostasis maintenance. The prominent role of KCs in immune processes, particle engulfment, antigen presentation, and the attraction and stimulation of T cells is well-known. They recruit other immune cells in the liver and release mediators to initiate response in other liver cells (2, 13).

Regarding other types of hepatic macrophages, it is known that bone marrow-derived macrophages participate in liver repair and regeneration but functional differences with Kupffer cells have not been clearly established. Following their activation, they produce cytokines that trigger a cascade of responses in other cells. If we accept the classical M1/M2 classification, it can be said that M1 KCs release proinflammatory cytokines, including tumor necrosis factor (TNF)-a, IL-6 and IL-1β, while M2 KCs release IL-4, IL-10, IL-13, and transforming growth factor-β. Consequently, the balance between these two phenotypes can ultimately lead to many different effects such as liver damage and wound repair (20).

The complex roles and expression of different KC phenotypes can lead to both protective and harmful responses (2, 21), and since it is required that their activation be precise, timely and localized, any KC dysregulation can lead to significant pathology (15). However, the results of some studies and hypotheses regarding these opposing effects are disputed. In some cases, KC depletion can be beneficial because of the reduction of inflammation or fibrosis but, on the other hand, the suppression of KC's role against pathogen invasion can clearly be harmful. Further studies must be done in order to conclude if KC depletion could prevent or exacerbate liver damage.

Thus, liver macrophages play an essential role in many pathogenic stages such as acute liver injury, fatty liver disease, fibrosis, cirrhosis, and liver tumors (22), constituting potential therapeutic targets for liver disease treatments. However, the pathogenesis of the disease treated and the phenotype of the macrophages targeted are points to consider when targeting macrophages (23).

In response to liver injuries such as alcoholic liver and non-alcoholic fatty liver disease (NAFLD) diseases, Kupffer cells are activated and a polarization to an M1-like phenotype is promoted in resident as well as monocyte-derived macrophages (24, 25). When injury ends, there is a switch to M2 restorative macrophages that release anti-inflammatory cytokines, regenerative growth factors, and matrix degrading metalloproteinase (MMP) expression, which promote tissue repair (26).

Macrophage polarization also has an important role in the growth and development of tumoral tissues. Macrophages in tumor tissues (TAMs) are mostly M2-like cells that produce tumor-promoting cytokines and growth factors that promote tumor expansion, angiogenesis, metastasis, and immune cell evasion. TAMs also contribute to drug resistance (27, 28).

TARGETING LIVER MACROPHAGES WITH NPs

Delivery Systems for Macrophages Recognition and Targeting

Liver macrophages are specialized in the internalization of foreign nanoparticles, playing an essential role in its destination in the organism, since they are involved in their uptake and trafficking *in vivo*. Therapeutic capacity and clearance mechanisms in clinically relevant nanomedicines have been linked to macrophage activity. However, due to their pathophysiological roles in diseases (29), liver macrophages are also potential therapeutic targets for a variety of aims, from cell activation to monocyte recruitment or macrophage differentiation (30). Emerging nanotechnology systems may offer new perspectives for macrophage vectorization. After intravenous administration, nanoparticles are opsonized in the bloodstream before being phagocytized by macrophages and accumulated in the RES organs. This passive targeting promotes the accumulation of the NPs in the liver, a process that increases within tumors due to the EPR (enhanced permeability and retention) effect (31).

Kupffer cells internalize NPs through multiple scavenger, toll-like, mannose, and Fc receptors (23). The mechanisms involved are macropinocytosis, clathrin-mediated endocytosis, caveolin-mediated endocytosis, and additional endocytotic pathways (1, 32, 33). Clathrin-mediated endocytosis has been pointed out as responsible for the internalization of size ranges of approximately 100–350 nm, while caveolin-mediated mechanism is responsible for the endocytosis of 20–100 nm particles (34–36). Macropynocitosis allows for large volume extracellular internalization of 0.5–5 μm nanosystems (23). The internalization process is then modulated by the size of the NPs as well as other characteristics such as charge. Larger nanoparticles generally show more efficient hepatic uptake: a diameter >200 nm is preferred for liver deposition (1, 37–39). Charged NPs, especially those with a positive charge, are taken up to a greater extent than those with a neutral charge (23, 39). Shape also has a great impact on NP uptake and elongated NPs are taken up less by macrophages than spherical ones (40). However, cylindrical silica NPs showed the highest accumulation in the liver compared to other shapes (41). Moreover, surface hydrophobic NPs tend to be opsonized by proteins that make them attractive to the phagocytic cells of the MPS (42–44).

Therefore, the success of therapeutic strategies targeting liver macrophages involves the use of different NP types with appropriate properties to allow them to be preferentially taken up by the liver. Incorporation of ligands to the surface of NPs increases specificity through active targeting (21, 31).

Liposomes

Liposomes are biodegradable vesicles with an aqueous core and a phospholipidic membrane that can carry hydrophilic as well as hydrophobic compounds. They have the advantage of being both biocompatible and biodegradable, whereas their instability is one of their main drawbacks. Macrophages, especially KCs, readily phagocytose circulating liposomes (45), causing them to accumulate in the liver (46). The liposomes proposed for the vectorization to hepatic macrophages have mainly sizes of ~100 nm due to restrictions on parenteral formulations. This passive targeting has been exploited for the administration of anti-infective drugs that have an effect on liver macrophages, some examples of which are shown in **Table 1**. For instance, commercial liposomal formulations of amphotericin B (Ambisome) allow the drug to accumulate in spleen and liver macrophages that constitute a reservoir of *Leishmania*, reducing the drug's nephrotoxicity (54, 55). Besides, the encapsulation of vancomycin in liposomes improves its poor penetration into cells, allowing its targeting to Kupffer cells. In a mouse model, such formulations reduced the intracellular Methicillin-resistant *Staphylococcus aureus* (MRSA) reservoir where the bacteria can survive and proliferate, significantly increasing the survival rate of infected mice over those treated with the drug solution (48, 49).

Liposomes are also suitable vehicles for the targeting of anti-inflammatory compounds such as dexamethasone, curcumin, or calcitriol to the liver. They show improved results over the free drug in the treatment of acute and chronic liver disease models in mice. Pharmacokinetic studies show the preferential uptake of the liposomes by the liver although they accumulate not only in Kupffer cells but also in monocytes, infiltrating macrophages and, to a lesser extent, T cells. Liposomes also induce a repolarization of macrophages to a regulatory phenotype (50, 51).

Pathological conditions may influence the liposomes behavior, and recently, changes in spatial distribution and a decrease in the liposomes uptake by macrophages has been described in liver fibrosis (56).

Liposomes can be decorated for active vectorization with surface modifiers, such as mannose that has been proposed for the treatment of liver tumors in order to increase liposome uptake by macrophages via receptor-mediated endocytosis. The increase in mannose ligand concentration leads to a higher accumulation percentage in the livers of mice. Also, active targeting of an immunomodulator to liver by mannose-decorated liposomes resulted in more effective inhibition of metastasis than when delivered by liposomes without mannose (53, 57).

Substances attached to liposome surface may produce other effects. Some arginine-like ligands may switch macrophages to the M1 phenotype in order to achieve an antitumor effect. In a study with a library of this kind of ligands, nitroarginine, and acetylglutamine DOPE:DOPC liposomes were the most effective for the redirection of macrophage phenotypes (52).

In summary, preferentially uptake of liposomes by liver macrophages make them suitable vehicles for the vectorization of anti-inflammatory, anti-infective or other drugs for the treatment of liver diseases. When associated with anti-inflammatory compounds, they are able to promote the macrophages' regulatory state and reduce the dose for the treatment of acute and chronic liver injury. The decoration of the surface of liposomes with arginine-like and mannose ligands may be useful for anti-tumor treatments.

Lipoplexes

Inhibition of regulatory pathways triggered by macrophages via the use of gene therapies is another strategy for the treatment of macrophage-associated diseases. Lipid-based NPs are the most successful non-viral vehicles for targeting RNAi to Kupffer cells and can reach a high efficiency of transfection. Although they are sometimes referred to as liposomes, lipoplexes are usually different in both structure and composition. They are based on cationic lipids that are able to both bind and condense negatively charged iRNA through electrostatic interactions and to deliver the payload into the cytoplasm

TABLE 1 | Characteristics of some liposomes proposed for liver macrophages targeting.

Composition	Size/nm	Active	Effect	References
HSPC, CHOL, DSPG	80	Amphotericin B	Leishmanicide	(47)
DCP, DMPG, CHOL	527.6 ± 58.2	Vancomycin	Improvement of MRSA infection	(48, 49)
DPPC: PEG-(2000)-DSPE: NBD-PE:CHOL	100	Dexamethasone	Switch to M2 phenotype Liver injury and liver fibrosis reduction	(50)
EPC:CHOL	100–150	Curcumin 1,25-dihydroxy-vitamin D3 (calcitriol)	Switch to M2 phenotype Reduction in liver inflammation, fibrosis and fat accumulation	(51)
DOPC: DOPE	83.5–108.8	Arginin-like ligands	Switch to M1 phenotype Antitumor	(52)
DSPC: CHOL: Mannose	~95	Muramyl dipeptide (MDP)	Increase of Kupffer cells tumoricidal activity	(53)

HSPC, hydrogenated soy phosphatidylcholine; CHOL, cholesterol; DSPG, distearoyl phosphatidylglycerol; DSPC, distearoyl 3 phosphatidylcholine; DCP, dicethylphosphate; DMPG, dimyristoylphoshatidylglycerol; DPPC, dipalmitoyl phosphatidylcholine; PEG-(2000)-DSPE, polyethyleneglycol-(2000)-distearoyl phosphatidylethanolamine; NBD-PE, N-(7-Nitrobenz-2-oxa-1,3-diazol-4-yl)-1,2-dihexadecanoyl-sn-glycero-3-phosphoethanolamine, triethyl-ammonium salt); EPC, egg phosphatidylcholine; DOPC, 1,2-dioleoyl-sn-glycero-3-phosphocholine; DOPE, 1,2-dioleoyl-sn-glycero-3-phosphoethanolamine.

of target cells (58). They also incorporate neutral lipids in order to attenuate the toxicity of cationic lipids. Besides cell selectivity, the success of these kinds of therapies depends on transfection efficacy. Lipoplexes are engulfed by Kupffer cells through macropinocytosis and clathrin-mediated mechanisms after IV administration, but RNAi escape from endosomes is a rate-limiting step for these therapies (59). Proper lipid design allows RNAi to reach the cellular cytoplasm where it exerts its action. In this way, cationic lipid C12-200 eposide would prevent RNAi lysosomal degradation (58) through a micropinocytosis internalization mechanism as macropinosomes do not follow the endosomic degradation pathway (23). It was applied to inhibit the PD-1/PD-L1 pathway that contributes to the persistence of viral liver infections. Lipid NPs of 70–80 nm size were efficiently internalized (66.5%) and expressed by Kupffer cells after *in vivo* IV administration in viral-infected mice. This led to an enhanced antiviral effect. This promising antiviral immunotherapy may be applicable to vaccine development, to treat diverse viral liver infections and other diseases such as hepatocarcinome (60).

However, cationic lipids are used as vehicles for RNAi forming lipoplexes. A high transfection efficacy in Kupffer cells can be achieved with proper lipid selection, showing promising results in immunotherapy.

Inorganic Nanoparticles

Inorganic NPs are a broad group of metallic and non-metallic nanomaterials. Some of them are non-biodegradable, which constitutes a pitfall for their use. However, they possess excellent properties such as small size, high surface area, and easy functionalization and may induce *per se* responses in macrophages with different therapeutic applications as shown in **Table 2**.

Inorganic NPs have been used in the diagnostic and treatment of liver fibrosis and recently this topic has been reviewed in depth (65). For instance, the reduction of inflammatory macrophage activity caused by ceriumoxide NPs has been proposed to prevent hepatic dysfunction in septic rats. The NPs attenuate the expression of a number of different inflammatory macrophage mediators that are associated with sepsis, improving rat survival (61). This downregulation of Kupffer cell activity was also reported for gold nanoparticles (GNPs) in two rat liver-injury models causing antioxidant and antifibrotic effects (62).

Inflammatory diseases may also be treated by the switch of macrophages from an inflammatory ("M1") to an anti-inflammatory ("M2") phenotype. Carbohydrates are able to induce phenotypic changes promoting one or other activation state depending on their physical and chemical characteristics (66). As an example, glucomannan carbohydrate-decorated silicon oxide nanoparticles promote M2 polarization in macrophages by inducing clustering of mannose receptors (MR) on the cell surface. Although this was assayed in a murine inflammatory bowel disease model, it may be applied to other inflammatory diseases (63).

Conversely, induction of an immune response was the aim of calcium phosphate polyetilenimine/SiO_2 nanoparticles used as carriers of a Toll-like-3 ligand. The NPs targeted the liver with 30–40% NP-positive cells when administered intravenously to mice and could be applied to vaccination (67).

Another group of inorganic NPs with applications in liver macrophage vectorization is superparamagnetic iron oxide nanoparticles (SPIONs), which are promising nanomaterials as diagnostic, iron supplement, and drug carrier agents. Surface modifications can render a high biocompatibility (64). They are phagocytized by macrophages and induce a pro-inflammatory response (68–70) through the activation of the Toll-like receptor 4 (71). Recently, they have been proposed for the reeducation of M2 tumor-associated macrophages to an antitumor M1 state in cancer treatment. This effect was studied for carboxymethyldextran-coated iron oxide NPs (Ferumoxytol®), which are approved by the FDA for the treatment of iron deficiency and other clinical uses. In a mouse *in vivo* model, these NPs inhibited tumor growth and prevented metastasis development. This activity was associated with the increase of M1 macrophages that may have been promoted by iron overload (72, 73). The uptake mechanism of carboxy-dextran coated SPIONs by human macrophages is a clathrin-mediated and scavenger receptor endocytosis although macropinocytosis may also contribute to internalization (74). The recognition of SPIONs by macrophages depends on the particle size and surface modifier, and it is better for positively

TABLE 2 | Some examples of inorganic nanoparticles for liver macrophage targeting.

NPs type	Size/nm	Model	Effect	References
CeO_2	53.36 ± 7.04	Lipopolysaccharide induced severe sepsis in rats	Reduced expression of inflammatory macrophage mediators	(61)
Au	7.4 ± 1.6	Rat liver injury with ethanol and methamphetamine	Downregulation of Kupffer cells activity	(62)
Glucomannan-silica	27.6 ± 0.6 −28.89 ± 1.60	Murine inflammatory bowel disease	M2 polarization	(63)
SPIONs				
Dimercaptosuccinic acid	65	Murine and human M2 cells	Modification of M2 activation profile	(64)
3-Aminopropyl-triethoxysilane	54			
Aminodextran	150			

charged particles and for a size of ~60 nm of size, although such SPIONs show cytotoxicity (71, 74, 75).

The efficient SPION uptake by macrophages allows its use for labeling macrophages in a cellular therapy for the treatment of liver cirrhosis. The labeled cells were tracked *in vivo* by magnetic resonance and no effects on phagocytic activity or cell viability were observed (75). AuNPs have also been used to this end and 50 nm was proposed as the optimal size for labeling without toxicity concerns for both NPs types (76).

In summary, inorganic nanoparticles are able to stimulate and also inhibit the activity of macrophages. Moreover, they can promote a switch to a specific macrophage state. The desired effect depends on the disease to be treated. The interaction of SPIONs with macrophages has been well-characterized and a mathematical model for the prediction of NPs uptake has even been developed (74). However, further insights are needed to clarify the relationship between the characteristics of NPs and their therapeutic and toxic effects.

Polymeric NPs

Polymeric NPs are colloid systems made of natural or synthetic polymers. They consist of a matrix in which the drug is homogeneously distributed or may be structured in a nucleus and a polymeric shell (nanocapsules) (54). They display great versatility. A fundamental feature of these nanosystems is their biodegradability, which is essential for intravenous administration.

Polymers of polylactic–glycolic acids (PLGA) are the most used for drug delivery as they are compatible and biodegradable compounds, and are excipients approved by the FDA. NPs of these polyesthers show excellent properties as drug carriers for liver macrophages vectorization (77) in order to improve efficacy or reduce side effects. PLGA NPs have been proposed as carriers of an inhibitor of the spleen tyrosine kinase SYK. This enzyme is overexpressed in M1 macrophages and shows a positive correlation with the pathogenesis of NASH and alcoholic hepatitis in patients. Although the bare inhibitor was more effective *in vitro*, its incorporation to 160 nm PLGA nanoparticles improved its intrahepatic delivery and therapeutic efficacy *in vivo*. This ameliorated fibrosis, inflammation, and steatosis in mice after IV administration (**Figure 2**) (78).

The objective pursued for rosiglitazone NP incorporation was to reduce their serious side effects such as the increased risk of fatal cardiac arrhythmia. Rosiglitazone vectorization to macrophages using 200 nm PLGA/polyvinylic acid (PVA) nanospheres allows for its selective delivery to circulating

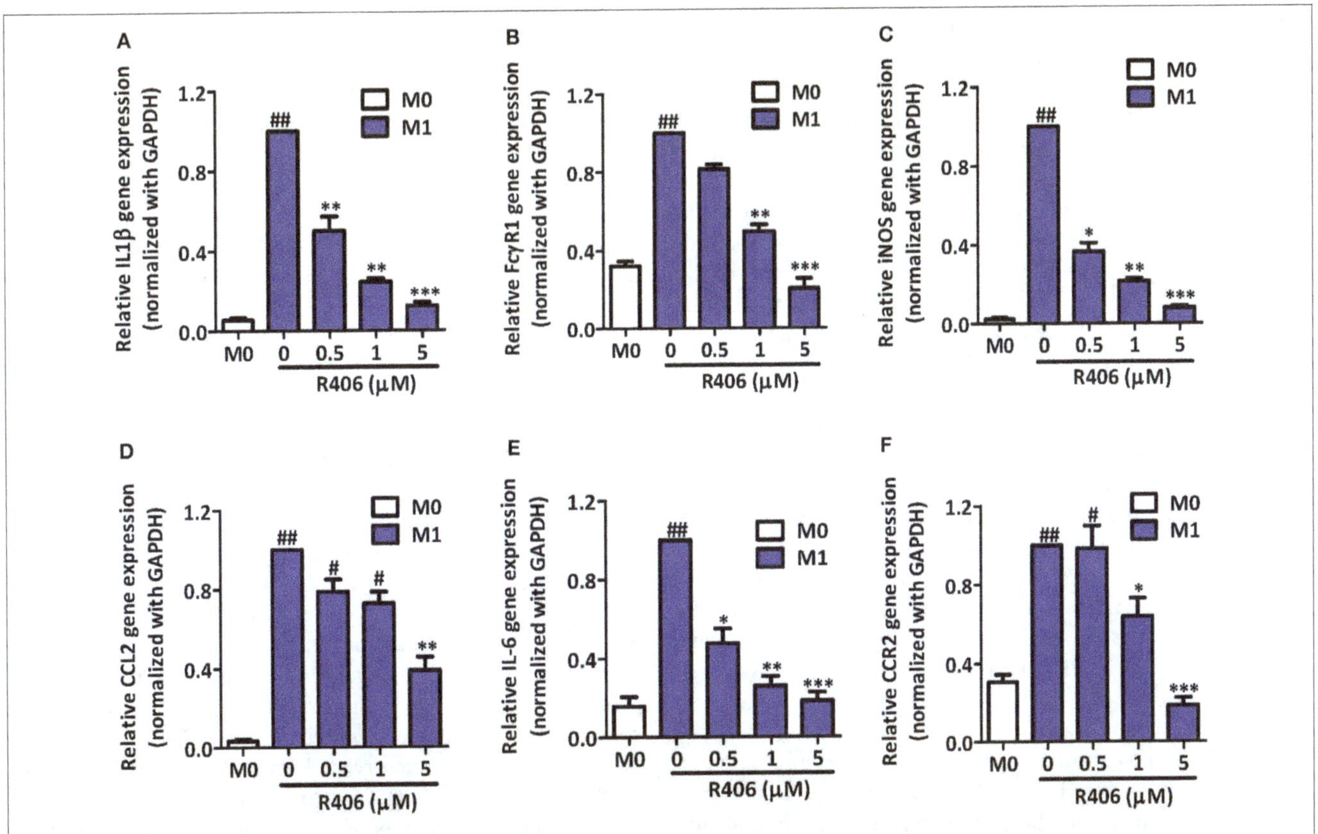

FIGURE 2 | Inhibition of M1-specific differentiation and inflammatory markers by R406 in RAW macrophages. Gene expression of M1 markers IL-1β **(A)**; FcγR1 **(B)**; iNOS **(C)**; CCL2 **(D)**; IL-6 **(E)**; and CCR2 **(F)** in RAW 264.7 cells after incubation with medium alone (M0) or M1 stimulus with R406 (0, 0.5, 1, and 5 μM). Expression values for the respective genes in untreated M1 macrophages were set at 1.0 to calculate the relative gene expression. Data are presented as mean + SEM. #$p < 0.05$, ##$p < 0.01$ denotes significance versus control M0 macrophages. *$p < 0.05$, **$p < 0.01$, and ***$p < 0.001$ denotes significance versus M1-differentiated macrophages. Reproduced with permission (78).

monocytes and Kupffer cells, reducing obesity-related inflammatory reaction in the white adipose tissue and liver and mitigating undesired effects (79).

Cationic polymers have been proposed as carriers of genetic material to reduce the expression of proteins related to liver diseases. This was the objective of RNAi for protein NOGOB encapsulation in [poly(amine-co-ester) (PACE) terpolymers] NPs. NOGOB promotes M1 polarization, stimulating the progression of alcoholic liver disease and liver fibrosis. The *in vivo* spleen administration of the NPs with a size of 240–300 nm allowed up to 60% Nogo-B protein suppression (80). This is a high transfection efficacy although alternative administration routes adequate for clinical use should be assayed. High transfection efficacy was also achieved by PLAcore/PVAshell NPs loaded with PEI-CD98 siRNA. The objective was the downregulation of CD98, a factor that is overexpressed in the livers of non alcoholic fatty liver disease (NAFLD) patients playing as a key inducer in this disease. The IV administration of CD98siRNA NPs with a size of 273.1 $\pm$ 19.3 nm effectively targeted liver hepatocytes and Kupffer cells, leading to a significant decrease of major proinflammatory cytokines and markers of NAFLD (81).

Chitosan, a biodegradable, positively charged polymer of natural origin is also widely used as a vehicle of RNAi. Quaternary chitosan NPs were designed for vectorization to macrophages of the RNAi of proinflammatory cytokine tumor necrosis factor TNFα. The NPs with sizes between 210 and 279 nm and zeta potentials from 14 to 22 mV achieved a high cellular uptake efficiency near 100% by RAW-274-7 macrophages. NPs cross-linking with TPP reduced their size and zeta potential, resulting in better transfection abilities (82). Polyethylenimine (PEI) is another cationic polymer with high transfection efficacy due to the proton–sponge phenomenon. In order to increase the chitosan's ability to transfect and reduce the PEI cytotoxicity, both components are mixed. NPs of sizes from 150 to 200 nm with both polymers achieved high macrophages transfection *in vitro* with non-cell toxicity (83). Functionalization of chitosan and other polymers, such as dendrimers with mannose, allows for active vectorization with a better selectivity for macrophage vectorization of RNAi and drugs (84–86).

The applications of polymeric NPs extend to HIV infections, where macrophages play a central role as virus reservoirs. Kutscher et al. designed GLU-decorated chitosan (CS) shell and polylactic-co-glycolic acid (PLGA) core nanoparticles (GLU-CS-PLGA) that recognize special receptors expressed in infected macrophages for the delivery of the antiretroviral drug nevirapine (87). Also, polymeric NPs modified with folic acid may target atazanavir/ritonavir to activated macrophages that overexpress folate receptor at an elevated level (88).

Polyesthers and chitosan are the polymers most often used in order to target drugs and RNAi to liver macrophages. To this end, NPs sizes of 150 to 300 nm have been prepared. Decoration with mannose and other ligands allow NPs to be selectively uptaken.

Other Nanosystems

Exosomes are phospholipidic nanoparticles of endosomal origin that are secreted by cells. They display similar advantages to synthetic nanoparticles, but they usually show higher biocompatibility and physiological activity. Like the majority of nano-sized vesicles, they also accumulate in the liver and may target Kupffer cells. Exosomes derived from mesenchymal stem cells reduce the levels of proinflammatory factors in murine macrophages *in vitro* with a decrease in biochemical and histological damage (89). These effects were also observed in an *in vivo* experimental lethal hepatic injury mouse model. The beneficial effect of these vesicles on reducing mortality implies modulation of the inflammatory response and activation of protective mechanisms to limit cell death (90).

Mesenchymal stem cell exosomes are then new types of nanovehicles with anti-inflammatory and protective effect in liver injury that constitute promising strategies for liver disease treatments.

IMPACT OF MACROPHAGE PHENOTYPE IN NPs UPTAKE AND TOXICITY

Nanosystems that specifically target and deliver therapeutics to polarized macrophages are of interest due to the role that they play in liver diseases. In order to improve the design of those drug delivery systems, the interaction of nanoparticles with macrophages of different phenotypes must be understood, which is why it has been the subject of several studies. Increased NP sequestration by M1 phenotypes has been reported as they are involved in biological processing of foreign materials. Thus, incorporation of phagocytosis promoters in lipid-latex nanoparticles allowed them to target inflammatory M1 macrophages (91). Also, a higher sequestration by inflammatory phenotype was found *in vitro* and *in vivo* for spherical silica nanoparticles. This was attributed to the silanol terminal groups that would attach to the receptors of anionic groups that are overexpressed in M1 macrophages (92).

However, M2 macrophages show increased expression of mannose and galactose receptors (93). This makes it possible to target specifically anti-inflammatory phenotypes with mannose–decorated nanoparticles (94). Pluronic and chitosan-based NPs of 150 to 265 nm, decorated with mannose, with positive and negative zeta potentials, respectively, can selectively target M2 macrophages to treat inflammatory diseases and HIV infections. The charge of the NPs and their degree of internalization are dependent on mannose density (84, 94).

Recently, a comparative study on gold nanoparticle uptake by human monocyte-derived macrophages of different phenotypic polarization showed, in general, higher internalization of gold nanoparticles by M2-polarized human macrophages in comparison with the M1-polarized cells. The extent of the uptake was positively correlated with the expression of M2 markers CD163 and CD206. Further investigation in human Kupffer cells showed comparable internalization of nanoparticles by those unstimulated Kupffer cells with a mixed M1/M2 phenotype and the M2-polarized cells, both of which ingested more nanoparticles than the M1-polarized cells did (28).

In short, various types of nanosystems have been designed for targeting polarized macrophages, although further research is necessary to define the NP characteristics necessary for promoting preferential M1 or M2 uptake.

HEPATIC BIODISTRIBUTION OF NANOPARTICLES

The kinetics of nanoparticles when administered *in vivo* strongly affects their therapeutic efficacy. Nanoparticular systems are recognized by macrophages of the mononuclear phagocyte system and tend to accumulate mainly in organs such as the liver, the spleen, or the lungs (95). The selective distribution of nanoparticular systems in these types of organs facilitates their use for the diagnosis and treatment of different types of pathologies.

Experimental studies conducted with cell lines and animals have brought about a clarification of the mechanisms of penetration into macrophages and hepatocytes using chitosan nanoparticles (96).

Figure 3 shows the arrangement of chitosan nanoparticles in Kupffer cells, hepatocytes, and in whole animals.

As shown in **Figure 3**, *in vivo* studies in mice demonstrate that, at the level of Kupffer cells, the cellular uptake of chitosan nanoparticles is produced via mechanisms of phagocytosis and clathrin- and caveolin-mediated endocytosis and their release through the lysosomal and multivesicular pathways. In addition, nanoparticles penetrate intracellularly into hepatocytes. The renal and hepatobiliary excretion pathways constitute the main routes of elimination *in vivo*, observing a slow elimination with a nanoparticle half-life of >60 days (96). In addition, *in vitro* studies conducted with murine macrophage cell lines show that chitosan nanoparticle uptake was clathrin-mediated endocytosis as a primary mechanism and also via phagocytosis as a secondary mechanism. After internalization, a large proportion of the nanoparticles may be excreted from the cells by lysosome-mediated and multivesicular body-mediated exocytosis (97).

Short-term biodistribution of silica nanoparticles in mice demonstrates their high accumulation in organs of the reticulo-endothelial system such as liver and spleen. At the same time, the animals in the experiment showed a clear increase in the number of hepatic macrophages over time. Aggregates of macrophages or microgranulomes increased between 6 and 24 h after silica nanoparticle administration. Clearance of silica nanoparticles

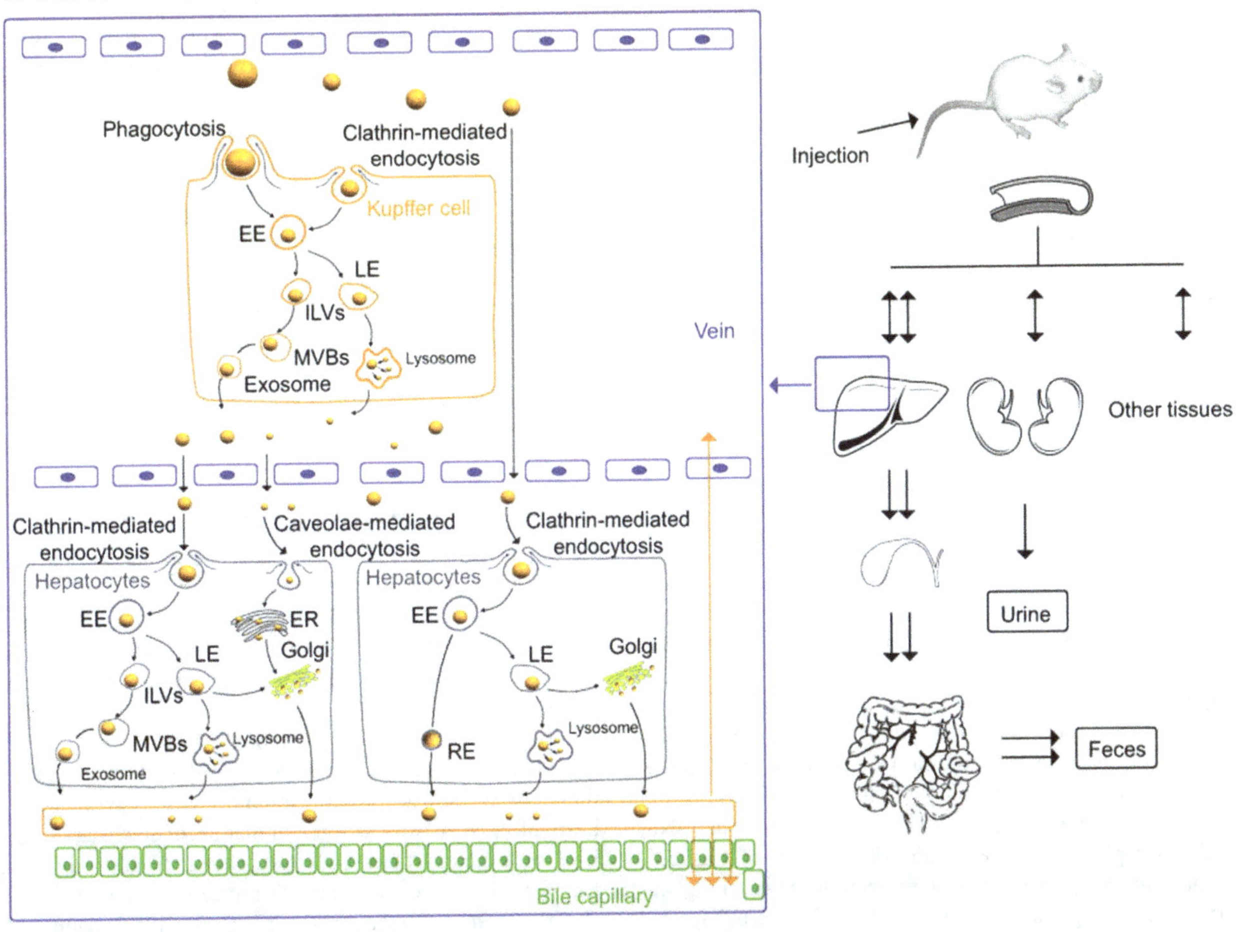

FIGURE 3 | *In vivo* distribution and elimination of chitosan nanoparticles in Kupffer cells and rat hepatocytes (96). International Journal of Nanomedicine. Reproduced with permission from Dove Medical Press Ltd.

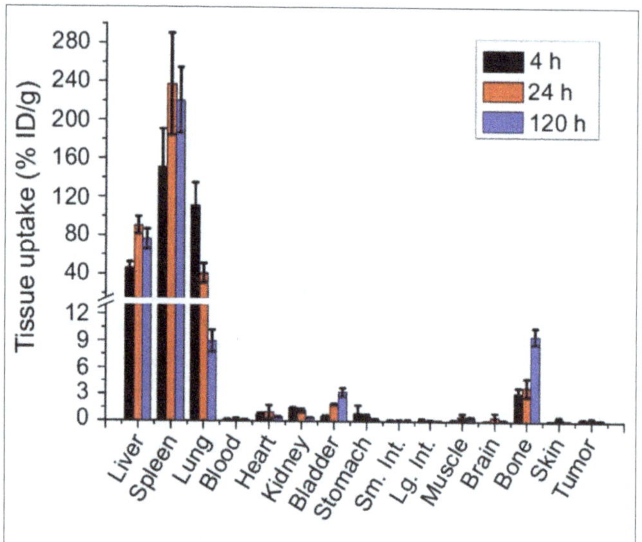

FIGURE 4 | Biodistribution of GNS-labeled macrophage cells at different times after IV administration in mice (102). International Journal of Nanomedicine. Reproduced with permission from Dove Medical Press Ltd.

from the liver appears to be slower than from the spleen, probably due to hepatic processing and biliary excretion (98).

Other authors also describe the retention of silica nanoparticles and the development of fibrosis in rat livers up to 60 days after IV administration (99).

Iron oxide nanoparticles are a type of system increasingly used for magnetic resonance imaging in diagnostic techniques (100). The administration of polyacrylic acid-coated iron oxide nanoparticles is associated with a selective distribution in the liver that produces proinflammatory activation and liver toxicity in mice. A high accumulation of iron was also observed by macrophages phagocytosis in the periportal zone of the hepatic acinus of the liver and in the splenic red pulp of the spleen which demonstrates the specific uptake of this type of nanoparticles by the monocyte–macrophage system (101).

Nanosystems are currently being combined with cell-based platforms with interesting biodistribution properties and with different therapeutic objectives.

As an example, plasmonic gold nanostars (GNS) were incorporated into immune system cells such as dendritic cells or macrophages obtained from bone marrow in order to investigate the biodistribution of these types of cells in a murine lymphoma model (102).

Figure 4 shows biodistribution in organs and tissues at different times in mice after IV administration of GNS-labeled macrophage cells. The quantification of gold in the different tissues was performed using an ICP-MS technique (102).

As shown in **Figure 4**, after IV administration of GNS-labeled macrophage cells, a specific distribution of this cell-based nanosystem preferably in the spleen, liver, and lung was observed, indicating that these organs had high macrophage cell accumulation. This type of cell-based delivery system presents interesting applications for cell-tracking studies (102).

Stabilin (-1 and -2) are specific receptors for the cellular uptake of different substances such as antisense oligonucleotides in the liver through clathrin-mediated endocytosis (103). Recent studies have been conducted to determine the mechanisms involved in the uptake of nanoparticles by hepatic macrophages. For this reason, an embryonic zebrafish model has been used to evaluate the interaction of nanoparticles with macrophages and endothelial cells using liposomes as nanoparticles. This research has demonstrated the role of the stabilin-2 receptor in the uptake of nanoparticles by endothelial cells. The nanoparticle uptake proved to be independent of the type of material and the functional properties of the nanoparticles but was influenced by the surface charge of the nanoparticle. In addition, the interaction between endothelial cells and nanoparticles can be blocked by competitive inhibitors of stabilin-2 such as dextran sulfate (104).

In another work about the mechanisms involved in the anti-inflammatory activity and in the recognition of crystals and nanomaterials by macrophages, cell-surface receptors or membrane cholesterol have been described as mechanisms involved in crystal nanoparticle recognition although other phagocytosis mechanisms are still unknown (105).

Pathological conditions may also influence NPs uptake. Liver fibrosis profoundly changes the myeloid compartment in the liver, with decreasing numbers of Kupffer cells and increasing numbers of MoMF. With the aim of investigating the changes in the targeting properties of different nanosystems in hepatic fibrosis, Ergen et al. studied the biodistribution of three intravenously injected carrier material, i.e., 10 nm poly(N-(2-hydroxypropyl)methacrylamide) polymers, 100-nm PEGylated liposomes, and 2,000 nm poly(butyl cyanoacrylate) microbubbles, in two fibrosis mice models. They found a decreased uptake of polymers and microbubbles by almost all myeloid cells of the fibrotic liver. However, liposomes had an overall higher targeting efficiency for endothelial and myeloid cells, which remained high even in fibrotic livers with around 60% carrier positive cells in healthy livers and after induction of liver fibrosis, although with a low specificity for the various cell populations. In all cases, Kupffer cells and monocyte-derived macrophages were the cells with increased percentage of carrier-positive cells (56).

Pharmacokinetic Models

Different pharmacokinetic models such as compartmental and especially physiologically based pharmacokinetic (PBPK) models have been developed to characterize the disposition of drugs in different organs and tissues, and especially in the liver, when they are administered in different types of nanoparticles (98, 106–112).

Classic pharmacokinetic models, such as the two-compartmental model, have been proposed to characterize the accumulation in the reticulo-endothelial system and in the livers of mice, as well as the elimination of superparamagnetic iron oxide nanoparticles (SPIONs). The model allows binding to Kupffer cells and extrahepatic clearance of nanoparticles to be characterized using dynamic magnetic resonance imaging (MRI) as seen in **Figure 5** (106). The constants K_{in} and K_{out} describe the kinetics of nanoparticles associated with and dissociated from

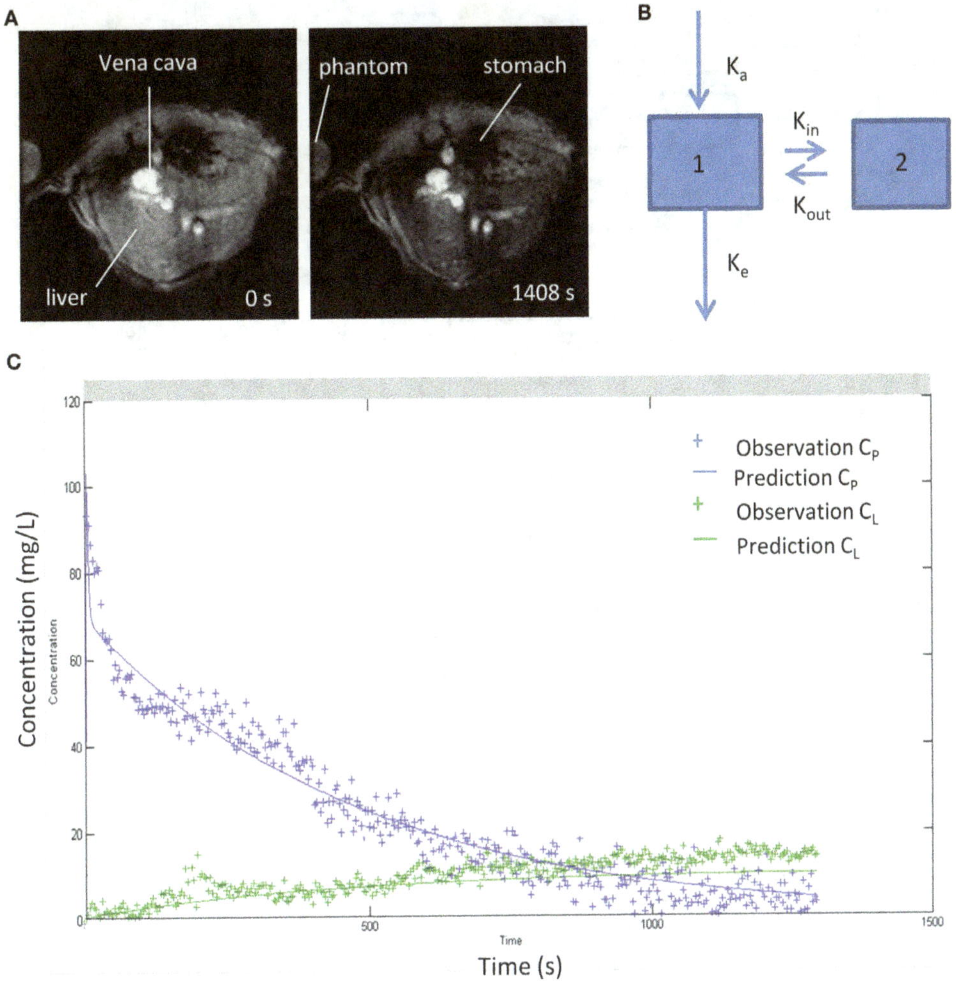

FIGURE 5 | (A) MR images of liver before and after 20 min of intravenous injection of iron oxide nanoparticles **(B)** Two-compartment kinetic model used to characterize blood pharmacokinetics and distribution in liver tissue of superparamagnetic iron oxide nanoparticle (SPIO). Compartments 1 and 2 represent blood and liver. **(C)** Pharmacokinetic profiles of nanoparticles in blood and liver fitted to the two-compartment model (106). Reproduced with permission.

the macrophage, and the constant K_e describes the elimination of nanoparticles from the blood compartment by the extrahepatic RES (97).

The kinetic parameters of distribution in the liver K_{in} and K_{out} are related to Kupffer cell numbers, allowing the function of the reticulo-endothelial system to be evaluated in different situations and presents therapeutic applications in liver disease, allowing the chronic liver injury to be evaluated, taking into account that the macrophages are integrated in different stages of the inflammatory process (106).

Physiologically Based Pharmacokinetic (PBPK) Models

PBPK models have been developed to characterize nanoparticle biodistribution in organs of the reticuloendothelial system (RES) such as the liver or the spleen.

PBPK models constitute an interesting strategy for modeling and simulation that allow the kinetic behavior of drugs in animals and humans to be predicted with a physiological basis. These models are based on grouping the body into different compartments that are assimilated to different organs and tissues. These compartments are defined by the volume of tissue and the blood flow that irrigates it. The mass balance of the drug throughout the body is defined through first-order differential equations. The distribution of the drug in each of the tissues can be perfusion-limited or diffusion-limited (112–114). Perfusion rate-limited kinetics occurs when blood flow limits tissue distribution. In the steady state, the concentration of drug in the tissue is in balance with the concentration of drug in the blood through a specific partition coefficient for each tissue. This type of distribution occurs in lipid molecules that easily penetrate the tissue. Permeability rate-limited kinetics occurs when permeability across the membrane constitutes the limiting process of intratisular distribution and occurs mostly in more polar or hydrophilic molecules (112, 113).

Specific PBPK models that consider the specific disposition properties of nanoparticles have been developed to characterize the biodistribution and elimination of nanoparticulate systems

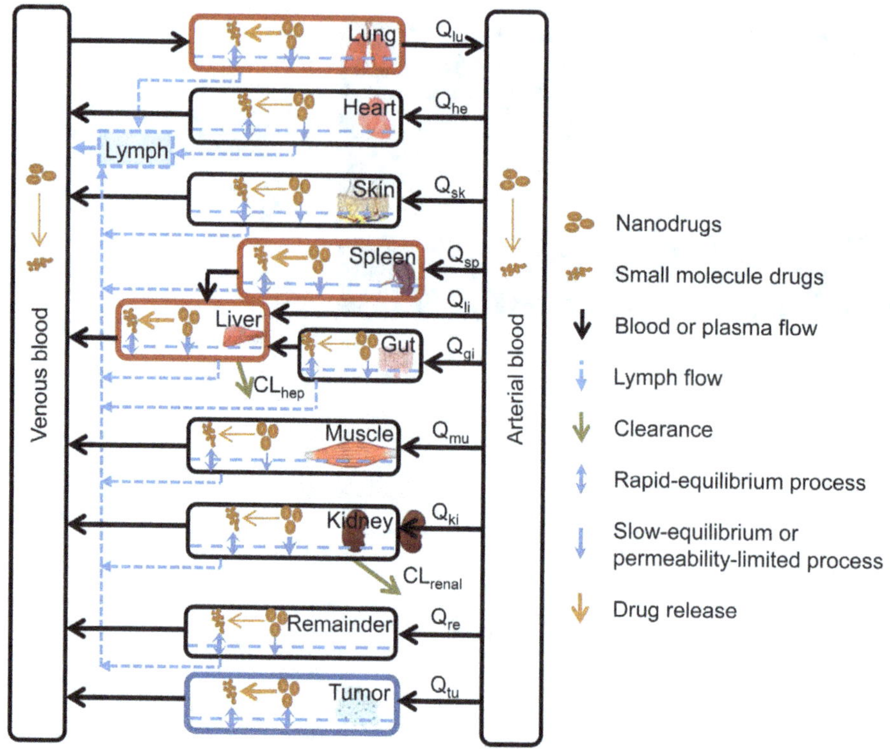

FIGURE 6 | Specific PBPK model to characterize the biodistribution of nanoparticles (112). Reproduced with permission.

in the whole body. This model assumes the existence of two PBPK submodels: one to characterize the disposition of the nanoparticles and another to characterize the disposition of the free drug as shown in **Figure 6**. This model predicts a greater accumulation of nanoparticles in the liver, spleen, and lungs due to the vascular structure of these tissues and the uptake of nanoparticles by the mononuclear phagocytic system. On the other hand, this type of model has some limitations, given that certain processes, such as aggregation or degradation of nanoparticles, among others, can change the properties of nanoparticles and their arrangement in different organs and tissue. In addition, this type of model allows the interaction between the drug, the nanoparticle, and the complex physiology of the organism to be modeled and simulated (112).

Some of these PBPK models have been designed to characterize the role of macrophages in drug tissue concentrations by combining the data from clinical studies with *in vitro* data. The model allows the concentration of the antibiotic moxifloxacin in tissues from biopsies to be predicted, including those from interstitial fluid, intracellular fluid, vascular space, and macrophages. The study showed that macrophages contribute to the accumulation of the drug in tissues from biopsies (109).

This same type of PBPK model has also been used to predict behavior in liver diseases such as liver cirrhosis. This model allows changes in the plasma concentrations of different drugs, such as alfentanil or lidocaine among others associated with Child-Pugh class A, B, and C liver cirrhosis, to be predicted (115).

Previously, general PBPK models that allow the distribution of drugs incorporated in different types of nanoparticles to be simulated have been described (111). The model was tested with different kinds of nanoparticles with differences in drug dose, size, charge, shape, or surface properties. This model also considers saturable phagocytosis of the nanoparticles. This model is based on another previously published model to characterize the biodistribution of PAA-PEG (116).

This model considers 10 anatomical compartments and each compartment is divided into three subcompartments that represent blood, tissue, and phagocytic cells.

Bigger nanoparticles are better recognized by the macrophages than smaller ones. On the other hand, cationic nanoparticles are better recognized by macrophages than anionic or neutral ones (112, 117). Based on this model, when nanoparticles are injected into the blood, they are captured by phagocytic cells of organs of the reticulo-endothelial system (RES) such as the liver and the spleen depending on their electric charge, size, and agglomeration state, among other factors (111).

In the field of toxicokinetics, PBPK models have been applied to characterize the biodistribution of silver nanoparticles compared to ionic silver. The PBPK model predicts a higher accumulation of silver in the liver as silver nanoparticles in comparison with ionic silver (118).

NANOPARTICLE TOXICITY

The toxicity of nanosystems is an important issue that may limit its applicability. Once in the organism, the processing and final fate of nanoparticles is dependent on their composition.

Liposomes are biodegradable phospholipidic-based nanosystems, and once administered, they are degraded by serum proteins in the blood circulation or by intracellular lipases. The degradation products of liposomes are their constituent lipid molecules that can be further metabolized by the body. This also holds for other lipids forming solid lipid nanoparticles. However, positively charged lipids show limited compatibility as they may induce cytokine activation and cellular toxicity with apoptosis (119).

Polymeric nanoparticles are modified in the organism, giving rise to constituent monomeric units or modified polymer chains. For biodegradable polymers, degradation products are smaller than the renal molecular weight cutoff size and can follow renal elimination (120, 121). For non-biodegradable components, the larger molecules may be cleared by hepatobiliary or the mononuclear phagocyte system, but their biotransformation in hepatocytes and macrophages may cause toxicity (122, 123). As their lipidic counterparts, cationic polymers such as PEI show high cellular toxicity (1).

The non-biodegradability of some inorganic NPs is a factor that leads to liver toxicity (124) and limits their applicability in humans. When NPs are not decomposed by the phagocytosis process, they will remain within the cell and be sequestered in the spleen and liver for long periods of time (122, 125–127). Once the nanoparticle-filled phagocyte dies, those nanoparticles are taken up again by other phagocytes of the same organ, resulting in a similar total amount of nanoparticles accumulated (128). NPs accumulate in the liver and especially in Kupffer cells (129) and could cause fibrosis and other histological tissue changes. They produce oxidative stress that in turn modulates the autophagic process in the liver, disrupting liver metabolism and homeostasis (65). This hepatic oxidative damage has been reported in both *in vitro* and *in vivo* models for AuNPs, SiO_2NPs, and AgNPs, with differences among the NP compositions (130–134). However, long-term effects need to be further characterized (65).

Tunable properties of NPs, such as shape, surface charge, and size, may affect their toxicity (135, 136). For instance, cerium oxide (CeO_2) NPs with rod-like shape showed higher and dose-dependently enhanced macrophage cytotoxicity responses with respect to cubic/octahedral NPs (137). The surface charge is also an important parameter that affects NP clearance rate. One study with mesoporous silica NPs (MSNs) showed that positively charged NPs were rapidly excreted from the liver into the gastrointestinal tract while negatively charged NPs remained sequestered in the liver (138). Also, the degradation of silica NPs to silicic acid for their renal excretion depends on the characteristics of the NPs, such as porosity, size, and surface chemistry (139–141).

Toxicity also depends greatly on the dose of the NPs, with cytotoxicity reported over certain doses for inorganic nanoparticles such as cerium oxide and gold NPs (61, 142, 143).

Therefore, tailoring the characteristics of NPs and controlling the doses of inorganic NPs used could overcome the toxicity problems in the liver and allow for their clinical application (65).

Biodegradable SPIONs or SiNPs offer a safer alternative. For instance, SPION administration is well-tolerated, and long-term *in vivo* biodistribution studies have shown that they can be transformed to non-superparamagnetic iron forms and eliminated with no signs of toxicity (64). However, in another study, toxicity of SPIONs and ultrasmall superparamagnetic iron oxide nanoparticles (USPIO) in human macrophages has been described (144).

CONCLUSIONS

Different types of NPs such as liposomes, solid lipid nanoparticles, inorganic NPs, or exosomes have been proposed for targeting liver macrophages in order to treat liver diseases. They are used as delivery systems but may also induce changes in macrophage phenotypes with influence in the progression of the illness. Lipids and polymeric NPs as vectors of RNAi may exert therapeutic effects by inhibiting regulatory pathways triggered by macrophages. Moreover, the interaction of NPs with macrophages depends on their phenotype, although this issue must be studied in more depth. The physiological-based pharmacokinetic models have been mainly used to describe and simulate NPs destination in the organism. Although strategies to vectorize liver macrophages with NPs are promising, compatibility issues, especially long-term toxicity, are drawbacks for certain systems, especially non-biodegradable ones.

AUTHOR CONTRIBUTIONS

All authors have equally contributed to the manuscript conception and preparation. JL and CC elaborated an abstract and an index and then all the three authors organized a well-balanced distribution of the different items. For their part of the work, the responsible person looked for the references, redacted the text and selected the images. CG-M was responsible of references database organization. CG-M and CC adapted the format to the journal template. JL, CG-M, and CC revised the whole content and approved the submitted version.

REFERENCES

1. Zhang YN, Poon W, Tavares AJ, McGilvray ID, Chan WCW. Nanoparticle-liver interactions: cellular uptake and hepatobiliary elimination. *J Control Release.* (2016) 240:332–48. doi: 10.1016/j.jconrel.2016.01.020
2. Ma Y, Yang M, He Z, Wei Q, Li J. The biological function of kupffer cells in liver disease. In: Ghosh A, editor. *Biology of Myelomonocytic Cells.* London: IntechOpen (2017).
3. Meijer DK, Molema G. Targeting of drugs to the liver. *Semin Liver Dis.* (1995) 15:202–56. doi: 10.1055/s-2007-1007278

4. Li P, He K, Li J, Liu Z, Gong J. The role of Kupffer cells in hepatic diseases. *Mol Immunol.* (2017) 85:222–9. doi: 10.1016/j.molimm.2017.02.018
5. Yona S, Gordon S. From the reticuloendothelial to mononuclear phagocyte system—the unaccounted years. *Front Immunol.* (2015) 6:328. doi: 10.3389/fimmu.2015.00328
6. Guilliams M, Ginhoux F, Jakubzick C, Naik SH, Onai N, Schraml BU, et al. Dendritic cells, monocytes and macrophages: a unified nomenclature based on ontogeny. *Nat Rev Immunol.* (2014) 14:571–8. doi: 10.1038/nri3712
7. Hume DA, Irvine KM, Pridans C. The mononuclear phagocyte system: the relationship between monocytes and macrophages. *Trends Immunol.* (2019) 40:98–112. doi: 10.1016/j.it.2018.11.007
8. Mildner A, Yona S, Jung S. A close encounter of the third kind: monocyte-derived cells. *Adv Immunol.* (2013) 120:69–103. doi: 10.1016/B978-0-12-417028-5.00003-X
9. Varol C, Mildner A, Jung S. Macrophages: development and tissue specialization. *Annu Rev Immunol.* (2015) 33:643–75. doi: 10.1146/annurev-immunol-032414-112220
10. Epelman S, Lavine KJ, Randolph GJ. Origin and functions of tissue macrophages. *Immunity.* (2014) 41:21–35. doi: 10.1016/j.immuni.2014.06.013
11. Ingersoll MA, Spanbroek R, Lottaz C, Gautier EL, Frankenberger M, Hoffmann R, et al. Comparison of gene expression profiles between human and mouse monocyte subsets. *Blood.* (2010) 115:e10–9. doi: 10.1182/blood-2009-07-235028
12. Schmidl C, Renner K, Peter K, Eder R, Lassmann T, Balwierz PJ, et al. Transcription and enhancer profiling in human monocyte subsets. *Blood.* (2014) 123:e90–9. doi: 10.1182/blood-2013-02-484188
13. Guillot A, Tacke F. Liver macrophages: old dogmas and new insights. *Hepatol Commun.* (2019) 3:730–43. doi: 10.1002/hep4.1356
14. Martinez FO, Helming L, Milde R, Varin A, Melgert BN, Draijer C, et al. Genetic programs expressed in resting and IL-4 alternatively activated mouse and human macrophages: similarities and differences. *Blood.* (2013) 121:e57–69. doi: 10.1182/blood-2012-06-436212
15. Dixon LJ, Barnes M, Tang H, Pritchard MT, Nagy LE. Kupffer cells in the liver. *Compr Physiol.* (2013) 3:785–97. doi: 10.1002/cphy.c120026
16. Klein I, Cornejo JC, Polakos NK, John B, Wuensch SA, Topham DJ, et al. Kupffer cell heterogeneity: functional properties of bone marrow derived and sessile hepatic macrophages. *Blood.* (2007) 110:4077–85. doi: 10.1182/blood-2007-02-073841
17. Zigmond E, Samia-Grinberg S, Pasmanik-Chor M, Brazowski E, Shibolet O, Halpern Z, et al. Infiltrating monocyte-derived macrophages and resident kupffer cells display different ontogeny and functions in acute liver injury. *J Immunol.* (2014) 193:344–53. doi: 10.4049/jimmunol.1400574
18. Scott CL, Zheng F, De Baetselier P, Martens L, Saeys Y, De Prijck S, et al. Bone marrow-derived monocytes give rise to self-renewing and fully differentiated Kupffer cells. *Nat Commun.* (2016) 7:10321. doi: 10.1038/ncomms10321
19. Wang J, Kubes P. A reservoir of mature cavity macrophages that can rapidly invade visceral organs to affect tissue repair. *Cell.* (2016) 165:668–78. doi: 10.1016/j.cell.2016.03.009
20. Sato K, Hall C, Glaser S, Francis H, Meng F, Alpini G. Pathogenesis of Kupffer cells in cholestatic liver injury. *Am J Pathol.* (2016) 186:2238–47. doi: 10.1016/j.ajpath.2016.06.003
21. Peterson KR, Cottam MA, Kennedy AJ, Hasty AH. Macrophage-targeted therapeutics for metabolic disease. *Trends Pharmacol Sci.* (2018) 39:536–46. doi: 10.1016/j.tips.2018.03.001
22. Ritz T, Krenkel O, Tacke F. Dynamic plasticity of macrophage functions in diseased liver. *Cell Immunol.* (2018) 330:175–82. doi: 10.1016/j.cellimm.2017.12.007
23. Gustafson HH, Holt-Casper D, Grainger DW, Ghandehari H. Nanoparticle uptake: the phagocyte problem. *Nano Today.* (2015) 10:487–510. doi: 10.1016/j.nantod.2015.06.006
24. Obstfeld AE, Sugaru E, Thearle M, Francisco AM, Gayet C, Ginsberg HN, et al. C-C chemokine receptor 2 (CCR2) regulates the hepatic recruitment of myeloid cells that promote obesity-induced hepatic steatosis. *Diabetes.* (2010) 59:916–25. doi: 10.2337/db09-1403
25. Krenkel O, Puengel T, Govaere O, Abdallah AT, Mossanen JC, Kohlhepp M, et al. Therapeutic inhibition of inflammatory monocyte recruitment reduces steatohepatitis and liver fibrosis. *Hepatology.* (2018) 67:1270–83. doi: 10.1002/hep.29544
26. Parola M, Pinzani M. Liver fibrosis: pathophysiology, pathogenetic targets and clinical issues. *Mol Aspects Med.* (2019) 65:37–55. doi: 10.1016/j.mam.2018.09.002
27. He H, Ghosh S, Yang H. Nanomedicines for dysfunctional macrophage-associated diseases. *J Control Release.* (2017) 247:106–26. doi: 10.1016/j.jconrel.2016.12.032
28. MacParland SA, Tsoi KM, Ouyang B, Ma XZ, Manuel J, Fawaz A, et al. Phenotype determines nanoparticle uptake by human macrophages from liver and blood. *ACS Nano.* (2017) 11:2428–43. doi: 10.1021/acsnano.6b06245
29. He C, Hu Y, Yin L, Tang C, Yin C. Effects of particle size and surface charge on cellular uptake and biodistribution of polymeric nanoparticles. *Biomaterials.* (2010) 31:3657–66. doi: 10.1016/j.biomaterials.2010.01.065
30. Tacke F. Targeting hepatic macrophages to treat liver diseases. *J Hepatol.* (2017) 66:1300–12. doi: 10.1016/j.jhep.2017.02.026
31. Li L, Wang H, Ong ZY, Xu K, Ee PLR, Zheng S, et al. Polymer- and lipid-based nanoparticle therapeutics for the treatment of liver diseases. *Nano Today.* (2010) 5:296–312. doi: 10.1016/j.nantod.2010.06.007
32. Dobrovolskaia MA, McNeil SE. Immunological properties of engineered nanomaterials. *Nat Nanotechnol.* (2007) 2:469–78. doi: 10.1038/nnano.2007.223
33. Xiao K, Li Y, Luo J, Lee JS, Xiao W, Gonik AM, et al. The effect of surface charge on *in vivo* biodistribution of PEG-oligocholic acid based micellar nanoparticles. *Biomaterials.* (2011) 32:3435–46. doi: 10.1016/j.biomaterials.2011.01.021
34. Parton RG. Caveolae meet endosomes: a stable relationship? *Dev Cell.* (2004) 7:458–60. doi: 10.1016/j.devcel.2004.09.009
35. Pelkmans L, Burli T, Zerial M, Helenius A. Caveolin-stabilized membrane domains as multifunctional transport and sorting devices in endocytic membrane traffic. *Cell.* (2004) 118:767–80. doi: 10.1016/j.cell.2004.09.003
36. Gratton SE, Ropp PA, Pohlhaus PD, Luft JC, Madden VJ, Napier ME, et al. The effect of particle design on cellular internalization pathways. *Proc Natl Acad Sci USA.* (2008) 105:11613–8. doi: 10.1073/pnas.0801763105
37. Hoshyar N, Gray S, Han H, Bao G. The effect of nanoparticle size on *in vivo* pharmacokinetics and cellular interaction. *Nanomedicine.* (2016) 11:673–92. doi: 10.2217/nnm.16.5
38. Kulkarni SA, Feng SS. Effects of particle size and surface modification on cellular uptake and biodistribution of polymeric nanoparticles for drug delivery. *Pharm Res.* (2013) 30:2512–22. doi: 10.1007/s11095-012-0958-3
39. Faraji AH, Wipf P. Nanoparticles in cellular drug delivery. *Bioorg Med Chem.* (2009) 17:2950–62. doi: 10.1016/j.bmc.2009.02.043
40. Arnida, Janat-Amsbury MM, Ray A, Peterson CM, Ghandehari H. Geometry and surface characteristics of gold nanoparticles influence their biodistribution and uptake by macrophages. *Eur J Pharm Biopharm.* (2011) 77:417–23. doi: 10.1016/j.ejpb.2010.11.010
41. Decuzzi P, Godin B, Tanaka T, Lee SY, Chiappini C, Liu X, et al. Size and shape effects in the biodistribution of intravascularly injected particles. *J Control Release.* (2010) 141:320–7. doi: 10.1016/j.jconrel.2009.10.014
42. Duan X, Li Y. Physicochemical characteristics of nanoparticles affect circulation, biodistribution, cellular internalization, and trafficking. *Small.* (2013) 9:1521–32. doi: 10.1002/smll.201201390
43. Esmaeili F, Ghahremani MH, Esmaeili B, Khoshayand MR, Atyabi F, Dinarvand R. PLGA nanoparticles of different surface properties: preparation and evaluation of their body distribution. *Int J Pharm.* (2008) 349:249–55. doi: 10.1016/j.ijpharm.2007.07.038
44. Hassan R, Tammam SN, Safy SE, Abdel-Halim M, Asimakopoulou A, Weiskirchen R, et al. Prevention of hepatic stellate cell activation using JQ1- and atorvastatin-loaded chitosan nanoparticles as a promising approach in therapy of liver fibrosis. *Eur J Pharm Biopharm.* (2019) 134:96–106. doi: 10.1016/j.ejpb.2018.11.018
45. Lefere S, Tacke F. Macrophages in obesity and non-alcoholic fatty liver disease: crosstalk with metabolism. *JHEP Reports.* (2019) 1:30–43. doi: 10.1016/j.jhepr.2019.02.004

46. Samuelsson E, Shen H, Blanco E, Ferrari M, Wolfram J. Contribution of Kupffer cells to liposome accumulation in the liver. *Colloids Surf B Biointerfaces.* (2017) 158:356–62. doi: 10.1016/j.colsurfb.2017.07.014
47. Stone NR, Bicanic T, Salim R, Hope W. Liposomal amphotericin B (AmBisome((R))): a review of the pharmacokinetics, pharmacodynamics, clinical experience and future directions. *Drugs.* (2016) 76:485–500. doi: 10.1007/s40265-016-0538-7
48. Sande L, Sanchez M, Montes J, Wolf AJ, Morgan MA, Omri A, et al. Liposomal encapsulation of vancomycin improves killing of methicillin-resistant Staphylococcus aureus in a murine infection model. *J Antimicrob Chemother.* (2012) 67:2191–4. doi: 10.1093/jac/dks212
49. Surewaard BG, Deniset JF, Zemp FJ, Amrein M, Otto M, Conly J, et al. Correction: identification and treatment of the Staphylococcus aureus reservoir *in vivo. J Exp Med.* (2016) 213:3087. doi: 10.1084/jem.2016033411032016c
50. Bartneck M, Scheyda KM, Warzecha KT, Rizzo LY, Hittatiya K, Luedde T, et al. Fluorescent cell-traceable dexamethasone-loaded liposomes for the treatment of inflammatory liver diseases. *Biomaterials.* (2015) 37:367–82. doi: 10.1016/j.biomaterials.2014.10.030
51. Maradana MR, Yekollu SK, Zeng B, Ellis J, Clouston A, Miller G, et al. Immunomodulatory liposomes targeting liver macrophages arrest progression of non-alcoholic steatohepatitis. *Metabolism.* (2018) 78:80–94. doi: 10.1016/j.metabol.2017.09.002
52. Bygd HC, Ma L, Bratlie KM. Physicochemical properties of liposomal modifiers that shift macrophage phenotype. *Mater Sci Eng C Mater Biol Appl.* (2017) 79:237–44. doi: 10.1016/j.msec.2017.05.032
53. Opanasopit P, Sakai M, Nishikawa M, Kawakami S, Yamashita F, Hashida M. Inhibition of liver metastasis by targeting of immunomodulators using mannosylated liposome carriers. *J Control Release.* (2002) 80:283–94. doi: 10.1016/S0168-3659(02)00006-8
54. Pei Y, Yeo Y. Drug delivery to macrophages: challenges and opportunities. *J Control Release.* (2016) 240:202–11. doi: 10.1016/j.jconrel.2015.12.014
55. Torrado JJ, Espada R, Ballesteros MP, Torrado-Santiago S. Amphotericin B formulations and drug targeting. *J Pharm Sci.* (2008) 97:2405–25. doi: 10.1002/jps.21179
56. Ergen C, Niemietz PM, Heymann F, Baues M, Gremse F, Pola R, et al. Liver fibrosis affects the targeting properties of drug delivery systems to macrophage subsets *in vivo. Biomaterials.* (2019) 206:49–60. doi: 10.1016/j.biomaterials.2019.03.025
57. Hagimori M, Chinda Y, Suga T, Yamanami K, Kato N, Inamine T, et al. Synthesis of high functionality and quality mannose-grafted lipids to produce macrophage-targeted liposomes. *Eur J Pharm Sci.* (2018) 123:153–61. doi: 10.1016/j.ejps.2018.07.036
58. Love KT, Mahon KP, Levins CG, Whitehead KA, Querbes W, Dorkin JR, et al. Lipid-like materials for low-dose, *in vivo* gene silencing. *Proc Natl Acad Sci USA.* (2010) 107:1864–9. doi: 10.1073/pnas.0910603106
59. Gilleron J, Querbes W, Zeigerer A, Borodovsky A, Marsico G, Schubert U, et al. Image-based analysis of lipid nanoparticle-mediated siRNA delivery, intracellular trafficking and endosomal escape. *Nat Biotechnol.* (2013) 31:638–46. doi: 10.1038/nbt.2612
60. Dolina JS, Sung SS, Novobrantseva TI, Nguyen TM, Hahn YS. Lipidoid nanoparticles containing PD-L1 siRNA delivered *in vivo* enter Kupffer cells and enhance NK and CD8(+) T cell-mediated hepatic antiviral immunity. *Mol Ther Nucleic Acids.* (2013) 2:e72. doi: 10.1038/mtna.2012.63
61. Selvaraj V, Nepal N, Rogers S, Manne ND, Arvapalli R, Rice KM, et al. Inhibition of MAP kinase/NF-kB mediated signaling and attenuation of lipopolysaccharide induced severe sepsis by cerium oxide nanoparticles. *Biomaterials.* (2015) 59:160–71. doi: 10.1016/j.biomaterials.2015.04.025
62. de Carvalho TG, Garcia VB, de Araujo AA, da Silva Gasparotto LH, Silva H, Guerra GCB, et al. Spherical neutral gold nanoparticles improve anti-inflammatory response, oxidative stress and fibrosis in alcohol-methamphetamine-induced liver injury in rats. *Int J Pharm.* (2018) 548:1–14. doi: 10.1016/j.ijpharm.2018.06.008
63. Gan J, Dou Y, Li Y, Wang Z, Wang L, Liu S, et al. Producing anti-inflammatory macrophages by nanoparticle-triggered clustering of mannose receptors. *Biomaterials.* (2018) 178:95–108. doi: 10.1016/j.biomaterials.2018.06.015
64. Rojas JM, Sanz-Ortega L, Mulens-Arias V, Gutierrez L, Perez-Yague S, Barber DF. Superparamagnetic iron oxide nanoparticle uptake alters M2 macrophage phenotype, iron metabolism, migration and invasion. *Nanomedicine.* (2016) 12:1127–38. doi: 10.1016/j.nano.2015.11.020
65. Tee JK, Peng F, Ho HK. Effects of inorganic nanoparticles on liver fibrosis: optimizing a double-edged sword for therapeutics. *Biochem Pharmacol.* (2019) 160:24–33. doi: 10.1016/j.bcp.2018.12.003
66. Lundahl MLE, Scanlan EM, Lavelle EC. Therapeutic potential of carbohydrates as regulators of macrophage activation. *Biochem Pharmacol.* (2017) 146:23–41. doi: 10.1016/j.bcp.2017.09.003
67. Sokolova V, Shi Z, Huang S, Du Y, Kopp M, Frede A, et al. Delivery of the TLR ligand poly(I:C) to liver cells *in vitro* and *in vivo* by calcium phosphate nanoparticles leads to a pronounced immunostimulation. *Acta Biomater.* (2017) 64:401–10. doi: 10.1016/j.actbio.2017.09.037
68. Mulens-Arias V, Rojas JM, Perez-Yague S, Morales MP, Barber DF. Polyethylenimine-coated SPIONs trigger macrophage activation through TLR-4 signaling and ROS production and modulate podosome dynamics. *Biomaterials.* (2015) 52:494–506. doi: 10.1016/j.biomaterials.2015.02.068
69. Laskar A, Eilertsen J, Li W, Yuan XM. SPION primes THP1 derived M2 macrophages toward M1-like macrophages. *Biochem Biophys Res Commun.* (2013) 441:737–42. doi: 10.1016/j.bbrc.2013.10.115
70. Kodali V, Littke MH, Tilton SC, Teeguarden JG, Shi L, Frevert CW, et al. Dysregulation of macrophage activation profiles by engineered nanoparticles. *ACS Nano.* (2013) 7:6997–7010. doi: 10.1021/nn402145t
71. Jin R, Liu L, Zhu W, Li D, Yang L, Duan J, et al. Iron oxide nanoparticles promote macrophage autophagy and inflammatory response through activation of toll-like Receptor-4 signaling. *Biomaterials.* (2019) 203:23–30. doi: 10.1016/j.biomaterials.2019.02.026
72. Zanganeh S, Hutter G, Spitler R, Lenkov O, Mahmoudi M, Shaw A, et al. Iron oxide nanoparticles inhibit tumor growth by inducing pro-inflammatory macrophage polarization in tumor tissues. *Nat Nanotechnol.* (2016) 11:986–94. doi: 10.1038/nnano.2016.168
73. Sindrilaru A, Peters T, Wieschalka S, Baican C, Baican A, Peter H, et al. An unrestrained proinflammatory M1 macrophage population induced by iron impairs wound healing in humans and mice. *J Clin Invest.* (2011) 121:985–97. doi: 10.1172/JCI44490
74. Lunov O, Zablotskii V, Syrovets T, Rocker C, Tron K, Nienhaus GU, et al. Modeling receptor-mediated endocytosis of polymer-functionalized iron oxide nanoparticles by human macrophages. *Biomaterials.* (2011) 32:547–55. doi: 10.1016/j.biomaterials.2010.08.111
75. Sharkey J, Starkey Lewis PJ, Barrow M, Alwahsh SM, Noble J, Livingstone E, et al. Functionalized superparamagnetic iron oxide nanoparticles provide highly efficient iron-labeling in macrophages for magnetic resonance-based detection *in vivo. Cytotherapy.* (2017) 19:555–69. doi: 10.1016/j.jcyt.2017.01.003
76. Sun X, Gamal M, Nold P, Said A, Chakraborty I, Pelaz B, et al. Tracking stem cells and macrophages with gold and iron oxide nanoparticles – the choice of the best suited particles. *Appl Mater Today.* (2019) 15:267–79. doi: 10.1016/j.apmt.2018.12.006
77. Park JK, Utsumi T, Seo YE, Deng Y, Satoh A, Saltzman WM, et al. Cellular distribution of injected PLGA-nanoparticles in the liver. *Nanomedicine.* (2016) 12:1365–74. doi: 10.1016/j.nano.2016.01.013
78. Kurniawan DW, Jajoriya AK, Dhawan G, Mishra D, Argemi J, Bataller R, et al. Therapeutic inhibition of spleen tyrosine kinase in inflammatory macrophages using PLGA nanoparticles for the treatment of non-alcoholic steatohepatitis. *J Control Release.* (2018) 288:227–38. doi: 10.1016/j.jconrel.2018.09.004
79. Di Mascolo D, C JL, Aryal S, Ramirez MR, Wang J, Candeloro P, et al. Rosiglitazone-loaded nanospheres for modulating macrophage-specific inflammation in obesity. *J Control Release.* (2013) 170:460–8. doi: 10.1016/j.jconrel.2013.06.012
80. Cui J, Piotrowski-Daspit AS, Zhang J, Shao M, Bracaglia LG, Utsumi T, et al. Poly(amine-co-ester) nanoparticles for effective Nogo-B knockdown in the liver. *J Control Release.* (2019) 304:259–67. doi: 10.1016/j.jconrel.2019.04.044
81. Canup BS, Song H, Le Ngo V, Meng X, Denning TL, Garg P, et al. CD98 siRNA-loaded nanoparticles decrease hepatic steatosis in mice. *Dig Liver Dis.* (2017) 49:188–96. doi: 10.1016/j.dld.2016.11.008

82. Xiao B, Ma P, Ma L, Chen Q, Si X, Walter L, et al. Effects of tripolyphosphate on cellular uptake and RNA interference efficiency of chitosan-based nanoparticles in Raw 264.7 macrophages. *J Colloid Interface Sci.* (2017) 490:520–8. doi: 10.1016/j.jcis.2016.11.088
83. Iranpur Mobarakeh V, Modarressi MH, Rahimi P, Bolhassani A, Arefian E, Atyabi F, et al. Optimization of chitosan nanoparticles as an anti-HIV siRNA delivery vehicle. *Int J Biol Macromol.* (2019) 129:305–15. doi: 10.1016/j.ijbiomac.2019.02.036
84. Chu S, Tang C, Yin C. Effects of mannose density on *in vitro* and *in vivo* cellular uptake and RNAi efficiency of polymeric nanoparticles. *Biomaterials.* (2015) 52:229–39. doi: 10.1016/j.biomaterials.2015.02.044
85. Jain K, Verma AK, Mishra PR, Jain NK. Surface-engineered dendrimeric nanoconjugates for macrophage-targeted delivery of amphotericin B: formulation development and *in vitro* and *in vivo* evaluation. *Antimicrob Agents Chemother.* (2015) 59:2479–87. doi: 10.1128/AAC.04213-14
86. Xiao B, Laroui H, Ayyadurai S, Viennois E, Charania MA, Zhang Y, et al. Mannosylated bioreducible nanoparticle-mediated macrophage-specific TNF-alpha RNA interference for IBD therapy. *Biomaterials.* (2013) 34:7471–82. doi: 10.1016/j.biomaterials.2013.06.008
87. Xavier RJ, Podolsky DK. Unraveling the pathogenesis of inflammatory bowel disease. *Nature.* (2007) 448:427–34. doi: 10.1038/nature06005
88. Puligujja P, McMillan J, Kendrick L, Li T, Balkundi S, Smith N, et al. Macrophage folate receptor-targeted antiretroviral therapy facilitates drug entry, retention, antiretroviral activities, and biodistribution for reduction of human immunodeficiency virus infections. *Nanomedicine.* (2013) 9:1263–73. doi: 10.1016/j.nano.2013.05.003
89. Jiang L, Zhang S, Hu H, Yang J, Wang X, Ma Y, et al. Exosomes derived from human umbilical cord mesenchymal stem cells alleviate acute liver failure by reducing the activity of the NLRP3 inflammasome in macrophages. *Biochem Biophys Res Commun.* (2019) 508:735–41. doi: 10.1016/j.bbrc.2018.11.189
90. Haga H, Yan IK, Takahashi K, Matsuda A, Patel T. Extracellular vesicles from bone marrow-derived mesenchymal stem cells improve survival from lethal hepatic failure in mice. *Stem Cells Transl Med.* (2017) 6:1262–72. doi: 10.1002/sctm.16-0226
91. Bagalkot V, Badgeley MA, Kampfrath T, Deiuliis JA, Rajagopalan S, Maiseyeu A. Hybrid nanoparticles improve targeting to inflammatory macrophages through phagocytic signals. *J Control Release.* (2015) 217:243–55. doi: 10.1016/j.jconrel.2015.09.027
92. Herd HL, Bartlett KT, Gustafson JA, McGill LD, Ghandehari H. Macrophage silica nanoparticle response is phenotypically dependent. *Biomaterials.* (2015) 53:574–82. doi: 10.1016/j.biomaterials.2015.02.070
93. Shrivastava R, Shukla N. Attributes of alternatively activated (M2) macrophages. *Life Sci.* (2019) 224:222–31. doi: 10.1016/j.lfs.2019.03.062
94. Hatami E, Mu Y, Shields DN, Chauhan SC, Kumar S, Cory TJ, et al. Mannose-decorated hybrid nanoparticles for enhanced macrophage targeting. *Biochem Biophys Rep.* (2019) 17:197–207. doi: 10.1016/j.bbrep.2019.01.007
95. Walkey CD, Olsen JB, Guo H, Emili A, Chan WC. Nanoparticle size and surface chemistry determine serum protein adsorption and macrophage uptake. *J Am Chem Soc.* (2012) 134:2139–47. doi: 10.1021/ja2084338
96. Jiang LQ, Wang TY, Wang Y, Wang ZY, Bai YT. Co-disposition of chitosan nanoparticles by multi types of hepatic cells and their subsequent biological elimination: the mechanism and kinetic studies at the cellular and animal levels. *Int J Nanomedicine.* (2019) 14:6035–60. doi: 10.2147/IJN.S208496
97. Jiang LQ, Wang TY, Webster TJ, Duan HJ, Qiu JY, Zhao ZM, et al. Intracellular disposition of chitosan nanoparticles in macrophages: intracellular uptake, exocytosis, and intercellular transport. *Int J Nanomedicine.* (2017) 12:6383–98. doi: 10.2147/IJN.S142060
98. Waegeneers N, Brasseur A, Van Doren E, Van der Heyden S, Serreyn PJ, Pussemier L, et al. Short-term biodistribution and clearance of intravenously administered silica nanoparticles. *Toxicol Rep.* (2018) 5:632–8. doi: 10.1016/j.toxrep.2018.05.004
99. Zhuravskii S, Yukina G, Kulikova O, Panevin A, Tomson V, Korolev D, et al. Mast cell accumulation precedes tissue fibrosis induced by intravenously administered amorphous silica nanoparticles. *Toxicol Mech Methods.* (2016) 26:260–9. doi: 10.3109/15376516.2016.1169341
100. Farrell BT, Hamilton BE, Dósa E, Rimely E, Nasseri M, Gahramanov S, et al. Using iron oxide nanoparticles to diagnose CNS inflammatory diseases and PCNSL. *Neurology.* (2013) 81:256–63. doi: 10.1212/WNL.0b013e31829bfd8f
101. Couto D, Freitas M, Costa VM, Chisté RC, Almeida A, Lopez-Quintela MA, et al. Biodistribution of polyacrylic acid-coated iron oxide nanoparticles is associated with proinflammatory activation and liver toxicity. *J Appl Toxicol.* (2016) 36:1321–31. doi: 10.1002/jat.3323
102. Liu Y, Huang W, Xiong C, Huang Y, Chen BJ, Racioppi L, et al. Biodistribution and sensitive tracking of immune cells with plasmonic gold nanostars. *Int J Nanomedicine.* (2019) 14:3403–11. doi: 10.2147/IJN.S192189
103. Miller CM, Donner AJ, Blank EE, Egger AW, Kellar BM, Ostergaard ME, et al. Stabilin-1 and stabilin-2 are specific receptors for the cellular internalization of phosphorothioate-modified antisense oligonucleotides (ASOs) in the liver. *Nucleic Acids Res.* (2016) 44:2782–94. doi: 10.1093/nar/gkw112
104. Campbell F, Bos FL, Sieber S, Arias-Alpizar G, Koch BE, Huwyler J, et al. Directing nanoparticle biodistribution through evasion and exploitation of stab2-dependent nanoparticle uptake. *ACS Nano.* (2018) 12:2138–50. doi: 10.1021/acsnano.7b06995
105. Nakayama M. Macrophage recognition of crystals and nanoparticles. *Front Immunol.* (2018) 9:103. doi: 10.3389/fimmu.2018.00103
106. Liu T, Choi H, Zhou R, Chen IW. Quantitative evaluation of the reticuloendothelial system function with dynamic MRI. *PLoS ONE.* (2014) 9:e103576. doi: 10.1371/journal.pone.0103576
107. Sweeney LM, MacCalman L, Haber LT, Kuempel ED, Tran CL. Bayesian evaluation of a physiologically-based pharmacokinetic (PBPK) model of long-term kinetics of metal nanoparticles in rats. *Regul Toxicol Pharmacol.* (2015) 73:151–63. doi: 10.1016/j.yrtph.2015.06.019
108. Cheng YH, Riviere JE, Monteiro-Riviere NA, Lin Z. Probabilistic risk assessment of gold nanoparticles after intravenous administration by integrating *in vitro* and *in vivo* toxicity with physiologically based pharmacokinetic modeling. *Nanotoxicology.* (2018) 12:453–69. doi: 10.1080/17435390.2018.1459922
109. Edginton AN, Ahr G, Willmann S, Stass H. Defining the role of macrophages in local moxifloxacin tissue concentrations using biopsy data and whole-body physiologically based pharmacokinetic modeling. *Clin Pharmacokinet.* (2009) 48:181–7. doi: 10.2165/00003088-200948030-00004
110. Aborig M, Malik PRV, Nambiar S, Chelle P, Darko J, Mutsaers A, et al. Biodistribution and physiologically-based pharmacokinetic modeling of gold nanoparticles in mice with interspecies extrapolation. *Pharmaceutics.* (2019) 11:E179. doi: 10.3390/pharmaceutics11040179
111. Carlander U, Li D, Jolliet O, Emond C, Johanson G. Toward a general physiologically-based pharmacokinetic model for intravenously injected nanoparticles. *Int J Nanomedicine.* (2016) 11:625–40. doi: 10.2147/IJN.S94370
112. Yuan D, He H, Wu Y, Fan J, Cao Y. Physiologically based pharmacokinetic modeling of nanoparticles. *J Pharm Sci.* (2019) 108:58–72. doi: 10.1016/j.xphs.2018.10.037
113. Jones H, Rowland-Yeo K. Basic concepts in physiologically based pharmacokinetic modeling in drug discovery and development. *CPT Pharmacomet Syst Pharmacol.* (2013) 2:e63. doi: 10.1038/psp.2013.41
114. Zhuang X, Lu C. PBPK modeling and simulation in drug research and development. *Acta Pharm Sin B.* (2016) 6:430–40. doi: 10.1016/j.apsb.2016.04.004
115. Edginton AN, Willmann S. Physiology-based simulations of a pathological condition: prediction of pharmacokinetics in patients with liver cirrhosis. *Clin Pharmacokinet.* (2008) 47:743–52. doi: 10.2165/00003088-200847110-00005
116. Li M, Al-Jamal KT, Kostarelos K, Reineke J. Physiologically based pharmacokinetic modeling of nanoparticles. *ACS Nano.* (2010) 4:6303–17. doi: 10.1021/nn1018818
117. Wilhelm S, Tavares AJ, Dai Q, Ohta S, Audet J, Dvorak HF, et al. Analysis of nanoparticle delivery to tumors. *Nat Rev Mater.* (2016) 1:16014. doi: 10.1038/natrevmats.2016.14
118. Bachler G, von Goetz N, Hungerbuhler K. A physiologically based pharmacokinetic model for ionic silver and silver nanoparticles. *Int J Nanomedicine.* (2013) 8:3365–82. doi: 10.2147/IJN.S46624
119. Epstein-Barash H, Gutman D, Markovsky E, Mishan-Eisenberg G, Koroukhov N, Szebeni J, et al. Physicochemical parameters

affecting liposomal bisphosphonates bioactivity for restenosis therapy: internalization, cell inhibition, activation of cytokines and complement, and mechanism of cell death. *J Control Release.* (2010) 146:182–95. doi: 10.1016/j.jconrel.2010.03.011

120. Choi HS, Liu W, Misra P, Tanaka E, Zimmer JP, Itty Ipe B, et al. Renal clearance of quantum dots. *Nat Biotechnol.* (2007) 25:1165–70. doi: 10.1038/nbt1340
121. Elsabahy M, Wooley KL. Design of polymeric nanoparticles for biomedical delivery applications. *Chem Soc Rev.* (2012) 41:2545–61. doi: 10.1039/c2cs15327k
122. Longmire M, Choyke PL, Kobayashi H. Clearance properties of nano-sized particles and molecules as imaging agents: considerations and caveats. *Nanomedicine.* (2008) 3:703–17. doi: 10.2217/17435889.3.5.703
123. Zamboni WC, Szebeni J, Kozlov SV, Lucas AT, Piscitelli JA, Dobrovolskaia MA. Animal models for analysis of immunological responses to nanomaterials: challenges and considerations. *Adv Drug Deliv Rev.* (2018) 136–137:82–96. doi: 10.1016/j.addr.2018.09.012
124. Cornu R, Beduneau A, Martin H. Influence of nanoparticles on liver tissue and hepatic functions: a review. *Toxicology.* (2020) 430:152344. doi: 10.1016/j.tox.2019.152344
125. Balasubramanian SK, Jittiwat J, Manikandan J, Ong CN, Yu LE, Ong WY. Biodistribution of gold nanoparticles and gene expression changes in the liver and spleen after intravenous administration in rats. *Biomaterials.* (2010) 31:2034–42. doi: 10.1016/j.biomaterials.2009.11.079
126. Karmali PP, Simberg D. Interactions of nanoparticles with plasma proteins: implication on clearance and toxicity of drug delivery systems. *Expert Opin Drug Deliv.* (2011) 8:343–57. doi: 10.1517/17425247.2011.554818
127. Desai N. Challenges in development of nanoparticle-based therapeutics. *AAPS J.* (2012) 14:282–95. doi: 10.1208/s12248-012-9339-4
128. Sadauskas E, Danscher G, Stoltenberg M, Vogel U, Larsen A, Wallin H. Protracted elimination of gold nanoparticles from mouse liver. *Nanomedicine.* (2009) 5:162–9. doi: 10.1016/j.nano.2008.11.002
129. Fraga S, Brandao A, Soares ME, Morais T, Duarte JA, Pereira L, et al. Short- and long-term distribution and toxicity of gold nanoparticles in the rat after a single-dose intravenous administration. *Nanomedicine.* (2014) 10:1757–66. doi: 10.1016/j.nano.2014.06.005
130. Abdelhalim MAK, Moussa SAA, Qaid HAY. The protective role of quercetin and arginine on gold nanoparticles induced hepatotoxicity in rats. *Int J Nanomedicine.* (2018) 13:2821–5. doi: 10.2147/IJN.S160995
131. Yu Y, Duan J, Li Y, Jing L, Yang M, Wang J, et al. Silica nanoparticles induce liver fibrosis via TGF-beta1/Smad3 pathway in ICR mice. *Int J Nanomedicine.* (2017) 12:6045–57. doi: 10.2147/IJN.S132304
132. Piao MJ, Kang KA, Lee IK, Kim HS, Kim S, Choi JY, et al. Silver nanoparticles induce oxidative cell damage in human liver cells through inhibition of reduced glutathione and induction of mitochondria-involved apoptosis. *Toxicol Lett.* (2011) 201:92–100. doi: 10.1016/j.toxlet.2010.12.010
133. Ramadi KB, Mohamed YA, Al-Sbiei A, Almarzooqi S, Bashir G, Al Dhanhani A, et al. Acute systemic exposure to silver-based nanoparticles induces hepatotoxicity and NLRP3-dependent inflammation. *Nanotoxicology.* (2016) 10:1061–74. doi: 10.3109/17435390.2016.1163743
134. Gaiser BK, Hirn S, Kermanizadeh A, Kanase N, Fytianos K, Wenk A, et al. Effects of silver nanoparticles on the liver and hepatocytes *in vitro. Toxicol Sci.* (2013) 131:537–47. doi: 10.1093/toxsci/kfs306
135. Hu Q, Zhao F, Fan M, He C, Yang X, Huang Z, et al. The influence of titanium dioxide nanoparticles on their cellular response to macrophage cells. *Comp Biochem Physiol C Toxicol Pharmacol.* (2019) 223:42–52. doi: 10.1016/j.cbpc.2019.05.006
136. Mohammadpour R, Yazdimamaghani M, Cheney DL, Jedrzkiewicz J, Ghandehari H. Subchronic toxicity of silica nanoparticles as a function of size and porosity. *J Control Release.* (2019) 304:216–32. doi: 10.1016/j.jconrel.2019.04.041
137. Forest V, Leclerc L, Hochepied JF, Trouve A, Sarry G, Pourchez J. Impact of cerium oxide nanoparticles shape on their *in vitro* cellular toxicity. *Toxicol In Vitro.* (2017) 38:136–41. doi: 10.1016/j.tiv.2016.09.022
138. Souris JS, Lee CH, Cheng SH, Chen CT, Yang CS, Ho JA, et al. Surface charge-mediated rapid hepatobiliary excretion of mesoporous silica nanoparticles. *Biomaterials.* (2010) 31:5564–74. doi: 10.1016/j.biomaterials.2010.03.048
139. King EJ, McGeorge M. The biochemistry of silicic acid: the solution and excretion of silica. *Biochem J.* (1938) 32:426–33. doi: 10.1042/bj0320426
140. Yu T, Hubbard D, Ray A, Ghandehari H. *In vivo* biodistribution and pharmacokinetics of silica nanoparticles as a function of geometry, porosity, and surface characteristics. *J Control Release.* (2012) 163:46–54. doi: 10.1016/j.jconrel.2012.05.046
141. He Q, Zhang Z, Gao Y, Shi J, Li Y. Intracellular localization and cytotoxicity of spherical mesoporous silica nano- and microparticles. *Small.* (2009) 5:2722–9. doi: 10.1002/smll.200900923
142. de Araujo RFJ, de Araujo AA, Pessoa JB, Freire Neto FP, da Silva GR, Leitao Oliveira AL, et al. Anti-inflammatory, analgesic and anti-tumor properties of gold nanoparticles. *Pharmacol Rep.* (2017) 69:119–29. doi: 10.1016/j.pharep.2016.09.017
143. Zhang N, Chen H, Liu AY, Shen JJ, Shah V, Zhang C, et al. Gold conjugate-based liposomes with hybrid cluster bomb structure for liver cancer therapy. *Biomaterials.* (2016) 74:280–91. doi: 10.1016/j.biomaterials.2015.10.004
144. Lunov O, Syrovets T, Buchele B, Jiang X, Rocker C, Tron K, et al. The effect of carboxydextran-coated superparamagnetic iron oxide nanoparticles on c-Jun N-terminal kinase-mediated apoptosis in human macrophages. *Biomaterials.* (2010) 31:5063–71. doi: 10.1016/j.biomaterials.2010.03.023

2

Hepatocyte-Derived Lipotoxic Extracellular Vesicle Sphingosine 1-Phosphate Induces Macrophage Chemotaxis

*Chieh-Yu Liao [1], Myeong Jun Song [1], Yandong Gao [2], Amy S. Mauer [1], Alexander Revzin [2] and Harmeet Malhi [1]**

[1] *Division of Gastroenterology and Hepatology, Mayo Clinic, Rochester, MN, United States,* [2] *Department of Physiology and Biomedical Engineering, Mayo Clinic, Rochester, MN, United States*

Correspondence:
Harmeet Malhi
Malhi.harmeet@mayo.edu

Background: The pathophysiology of non-alcoholic steatohepatitis involves hepatocyte lipotoxicity due to excess saturated free fatty acids and concomitant proinflammatory macrophage effector responses. These include the infiltration of macrophages into hepatic cords in response to incompletely understood stimuli. Stressed hepatocytes release an increased number of extracellular vesicles (EVs), which are known to participate in intercellular signaling and coordination of the behavior of immune cell populations via their cargo. We hypothesized that hepatocyte-derived lipotoxic EVs that are enriched in sphingosine 1-phosphate (S1P) are effectors of macrophage infiltration in the hepatic microenvironment.

Methods: Lipotoxic EVs were isolated from palmitate treated immortalized mouse hepatocytes and characterized by nanoparticle tracking analysis. Lipotoxic EV sphingolipids were quantified using tandem mass spectrometry. Wildtype and $S1P_1$ receptor knockout bone marrow-derived macrophages were exposed to lipotoxic EV gradients in a microfluidic gradient generator. Macrophage migration toward EV gradients was captured by time-lapse microscopy and analyzed to determine directional migration. Fluorescence-activated cell sorting along with quantitative PCR and immunohistochemistry were utilized to characterize the cell surface expression of $S1P_1$ receptor on intrahepatic leukocytes and hepatic expression of $S1P_1$ receptor, respectively.

Results: Palmitate treatment induced the release of EVs. These EVs were enriched in S1P. Palmitate-induced S1P enriched EVs were chemoattractive to macrophages. EV S1P enrichment depended on the activity of sphingosine kinases 1 and 2, such that, pharmacological inhibition of sphingosine kinases 1 and 2 resulted in a significant reduction in EV S1P cargo without affecting the number of EVs released. When exposed to EVs derived from cells treated with palmitate in the presence of a pharmacologic inhibitor of sphingosine kinases 1 and 2, macrophages displayed diminished chemotactic behavior. To determine receptor-ligand specificity, we tested the migration responses of macrophages genetically deleted in the $S1P_1$ receptor toward lipotoxic EVs. $S1P_1$ receptor knockout macrophages displayed a marked reduction in their chemotactic responses toward lipotoxic palmitate-induced EVs.

Conclusions: Palmitate-induced lipotoxic EVs are enriched in S1P through sphingosine kinases 1 and 2. S1P-enriched EVs activate persistent and directional macrophage chemotaxis mediated by the $S1P_1$ receptor, a potential signaling axis for macrophage infiltration during hepatic lipotoxicity, and a potential therapeutic target for non-alcoholic steatohepatitis.

Keywords: non-alcoholic steatohepatitis, palmitic acid, sphingosine kinase, sphingolipid signaling, ceramide

INTRODUCTION

Non-alcoholic fatty liver disease (NAFLD), the most frequent chronic liver disease worldwide, is characterized by hepatic steatosis (1). The vast majority of NAFLD patients have hepatic steatosis alone, termed non-alcoholic fatty liver (NAFL). Up to 20% of NAFLD patients develop non-alcoholic steatohepatitis (NASH) characterized by hepatocellular injury including ballooning, inflammation and the potential to develop hepatic fibrosis. The underlying importance of inflammation in NASH progression is well-recognized. In natural history studies with paired liver biopsies over time, it was noted that inflammation was the best predictor of future fibrosis risk (2). Mechanistically, preclinical and human data suggest that hepatocyte lipotoxicity, caused by the presence of excessive saturated free fatty acids (FFAs) and other toxic lipid moieties, is involved in provoking or perpetuating inflammation in NASH (3). While pathologic hepatocyte lipoapoptosis has been shown to contribute to proinflammatory responses in the liver (4), recent studies have focused on signaling events arising from damaged or stressed cells before the onset of cell death, such as extracellular vesicles (EVs) in mediating proinflammatory responses in the injured liver (5, 6).

Two notable features of inflammation in NASH are an increase in infiltrating immune cells and an increase in proinflammatory activation of immune cells (7). Enhanced lobular inflammation due to accumulation of a mixed inflammatory infiltrate that includes proinflammatory macrophages within hepatocyte cords is a diagnostic histologic feature of NASH (8). Many patterns of macrophage accumulation are recognized in NASH including clusters termed microgranulomas, fat droplet containing lipogranulomas, and surrounding ballooned hepatocytes termed "satellitosis" (8). Other cell types including lymphocytes, eosinophils, and neutrophils have also been observed in lobular inflammation. More recent studies have implicated other cells of the innate and adaptive immune system in portal inflammation (CD68, CD3, CD8, CD4, CD20, and neutrophil elastase) (9). The links between lipotoxic hepatocytes and immune cells, specifically, hepatocyte-originating signals that direct inflammatory cell infiltration, are not well-defined. Previous studies have defined the role of soluble mediators, such as the chemokine C-C motif chemokine ligand 2/monocyte chemoattractant protein 1 (CCL2/MCP1) and the receptors C-C motif chemokine receptor (CCR) 2 and 5 in NASH (10). In experimental mouse NASH, pharmacologic inhibition of CCR2 and 5 diminishes the recruitment of proinflammatory macrophages leading to amelioration of liver injury and inflammation (11). In a phase 2b human NASH trial of a dual CCR2/5 inhibitor, improvements in liver histology and fibrosis were reported (12). However, complete resolution of macrophage accumulation and inflammation has not been reported highlighting the need to understand additional macrophage recruitment signals. EVs are important cell-derived mediators of intercellular communication (6, 13, 14). These nanometer-sized vesicles participate in short and long-range signaling under normal and stressed conditions (13, 15, 16). The ability of macrophages to migrate through tissues to sites of injury is fundamental to their function as a part of the host innate immunity and inflammation (17). Whether hepatocyte-derived lipotoxic EVs contribute to macrophage infiltration in the hepatic microenvironment and the signaling mechanisms by which macrophages are recruited under lipotoxic stress conditions, still remains incompletely understood.

Palmitic acid (PA), the most abundant saturated FFA found in humans, which is elevated further in NASH, is a well-defined lipotoxic stressor (18). Hepatocytes treated with PA release an increased number of EVs (6, 19), which is in accordance with current evidence suggesting that circulating EVs are increased in NASH and correlate with macrophage accumulation in the liver (5, 20, 21). We have previously demonstrated that PA induces the release of ceramide-enriched EVs via the *do novo* synthesis of ceramide in the endoplasmic reticulum. Further, these EVs contain elevated levels of sphingosine 1-phosphate (S1P), which others have demonstrated to be important for the formation of a subtype of EVs known as exosomes (5, 22). S1P is a potent, bioactive sphingolipid known to regulate immune cell trafficking; and implicated in liver inflammation in NASH (23–25). However, the role of EV S1P cargo in macrophage recruitment is not well-understood. Formation of S1P occurs through the phosphorylation of sphingosine, a ceramide derivative, by sphingosine kinases (SphK) 1 and 2 (24, 26, 27). Our objective was to determine whether SphK-mediated production of S1P in EVs promotes macrophage recruitment via stimulation of the $S1P_1$ receptor. We demonstrate that SphK1 and SphK2 mediate the formation of S1P in PA-induced EVs, such that resulting EVs are enriched in S1P cargo to stimulate

Abbreviations: BMDM, bone marrow-derived macrophages; EVs, extracellular vesicles; FFA, free fatty acids; HPRT, Hypoxanthine-guanine phosphoribosyl transferase; IMH, immortalized mouse hepatocytes; IRE1α, inositol-requiring enzyme 1 α; LCM, L929 cell-conditioned medium; Non-alcoholic Fatty Liver; NAFLD, Non-alcoholic Fatty Liver Disease; NAFL, NASH, Non-alcoholic Steatohepatitis; PA, Palmitic acid; SphK, sphingosine kinase; SphK1, sphingosine kinase 1; SphK2, sphingosine kinase 2; S1P, sphingosine 1-phosphate; $S1P_1$, sphingosine 1-phosphate receptor 1.

macrophage migration. Furthermore, macrophages express the $S1P_1$ receptor needed for stimulation through the S1P signaling axis. When SphK1 and 2 are inhibited, EV S1P cargo is attenuated and macrophage chemotaxis toward these EVs is reduced. Thus, S1P is an important effector of macrophage chemotaxis, and likely important in this phenomenon *in vivo*. In support of this, the hepatic expression of $S1P_1$ receptor is increased in a murine dietary model of NASH. Our observations provide a potential mechanism for the observed macrophage infiltration in NASH, and identify a potential novel therapeutic target.

MATERIALS AND METHODS

Bone Marrow-Derived Macrophages (BMDM)

This study was carried out in accordance with the recommendations of the public health policy on the humane use and care of laboratory animals. The protocol was approved by the Institutional Care and Animal Use Committee (IACUC) of the Mayo Clinic. Bone marrow-derived macrophages (BMDM) were isolated from hind legs of wild type C57BL/6 mice as previously described by us (28). Once euthanized, the mouse was sprayed with 70% ethanol and the skin was cut open using sterile scissors to expose the hind legs. Cuts were made through the hip and ankle joints to remove each leg. The legs were placed in 70% ethanol for 2–3 min, then placed in phosphate-buffered saline (PBS) on ice. In the tissue culture hood, the leg muscle and epiphyses were removed and bone marrow flushed out onto a petri dish using a syringe and 25 gauge needle containing BMDM media. The BMDM media used for bone marrow differentiation consists of Roswell Park Memorial Institute (RPMI)-1640 supplemented with 20% L929 cell-conditioned medium (LCM), 10% fetal bovine serum (FBS), penicillin (100 units/mL) and streptomycin (100 μg/mL). The flushed media containing bone marrow was drawn through a 23 gauge needle 4–5 times to remove clumps. Bone marrow cells were plated onto 150 mm petri dishes (BD Falcon, Oxford, UK) and incubated at 37°C, 5% CO_2. BMDM media was changed every 2 days on Day 3 and Day 5, and BMDMs were dissociated with Accutase and used in experiments on Day 7.

Immunohistochemistry for $S1P_1$ Receptor

Diet-induced obesity and insulin resistance with concomitant NASH in mice fed a diet high in fat, fructose and cholesterol (FFC) has been well-characterized by us (29, 30). We utilized available archived formalin fixed paraffin embedded liver tissue samples from a previously published, IACUC approved, study where male mice had been fed the FFC diet for 20 weeks for $S1P_1$ receptor immunohistochemistry (30). Diet-induced NASH, liver injury and macrophage-mediated inflammation in this cohort have been previously published. Five μM liver sections were dewaxed and rehydrated through graded alcohols. Antigen retrieval was performed by heating in Tris-EDTA buffer (10 mM Tris 1 mM EDTA, pH 9.0) for 10 min at 95°C. After blocking endogenous peroxidase with 3% H_2O_2 in distilled water for 10 min, the sections were incubated in blocking buffer provided in the Vectastain ABC staining kit (Vector Laboratories), followed by anti-$S1P_1$ receptor antibody (1:100 dilution, Product # 55133-1-1AP, Proteintech) at 4°C in a humidified chamber, overnight. After washing in PBS, slides were incubated with biotin-conjugated secondary antibody, streptavidin conjugated to horseradish peroxidase, and lastly chromogenic substrate per the manufactures instructions (ABC, Vector Laboratories). Sections were dehydrated through graded alcohols and mounted using Permount mounting media (Sigma). Microscopy was performed using the Nikon NIS-Elements advanced research imaging software attached to a Nikon Eclipse TE300 microscope (Nikon, Japan), and the positive areas were captured at 20 × magnification with uniform settings of magnification, light, and exposure time for quantitative image analysis.

$S1P_1$ Receptor Knockout Bone Marrow-Derived Macrophages

Myeloid cell specific knockout mice (KO) mice were generated by crossing mice that express Cre recombinase under the lysozyme 2 promoter (lyzMcre) with mice having the $S1P_1$ exon 2 flanked by loxP recombination sites (The Jackson Laboratory Stock # 019141). The $S1P_1^{loxp}$ mice were generated by Richard Prolia and have been previously described (31). KOs were confirmed by genotyping and quantitative real time PCR (qPCR). BMDM were generated as described above.

Cell Culture

Immortalized mouse hepatocyte (IMH) cell-line has been previously described by us (5). Cells were cultured in Dulbecco's Modified Eagles Media (DMEM, Life Technologies) supplemented with 10% fetal bovine serum (FBS), glucose (4.5 g/L), penicillin (100 units/mL), and streptomycin (100 μg/mL).

Extracellular Vesicle Isolation

IMH cells were grown to 90% confluency in 150 mm tissue culture treated dishes. Cells were washed with PBS twice and treated with treatment media containing 400 μM palmitic acid (PA), 400 μM PA + 2 μM of MP-A08 inhibitor, or vehicle control for 20 h. Treatment media consisted of DMEM supplemented with 5% FBS (exosome-free), prepared by overnight ultracentrifugation at 100,000 × g for 16 h, and 1% bovine serum albumin (fatty acid free). Following the 20-h treatment, the cell culture supernatant was collected and centrifuged at 2,000 × g for 20 min to remove cells and cellular debris. Subsequently, the supernatant was extracted and ultracentrifuged at 10,000 × g for 40 min. Supernatant was again removed and further ultracentrifuged at 100,000 × g for 90 min to pellet EVs. The EV pellet was re-suspended in PBS and spun at 100,000 × g for 90 min again to wash the EVs. Pellets were re-suspended in PBS and characterized by nanoparticle tracking analysis or stored at −80°C until further use.

Caspase 3/7 Assay

IMH cells were plated at a density of 80,000/cm^2, attached for 24 h, and treated as above for 20 h. Following treatment, caspase 3/7 activity was measured using the Apo-ONE homogeneous caspase-3/7 assay (Promega) according to the manufacturer's instructions and previously described by us (32).

Morphologic Assessment of Apoptosis

IMH cells were plated in 6 well plates at a density of 80,000/cm^2, attached for 24 h and treated as above. Nuclear staining with 4′,6-diamidino-2-phenylindole (DAPI) and fluorescence microscopy were used to count total and apoptotic cells; at least 200 cells were counted per condition. Nuclear changes of chromatin condensation and nuclear fragmentation were considered apoptotic (32).

Sphingosine Kinase Activity

The activity of sphingosine kinases 1 and 2 in cells treated with palmitate with and without the pharmacologic inhibitor, MP-A08, was measured by utilizing a commercially available sphingosine kinase activity assay (Echelon Biosciences). Briefly, IMH cells were plated and treated as described above. Cell lysates were prepared in the provided buffer by freeze thaw followed by sonication. The assay was set up per manufacturer instructions and luminescence normalized to protein content.

Nanoparticle Tracking Analysis

The Nanosight NTA NS300 (Malvern Instruments, UK) was used to characterize EVs through the analysis of light scatter and Brownian motion of each sample (33). EV samples were diluted with PBS accordingly to maintain a concentration of 2E+08 to 8E+08 particles/mL, and a frame rate in between 10 and 40 particles/frame. Each sample was pumped through the observation chamber by a syringe pump at a constant rate of 25 μL/min. For each sample, 3 videos of 30 s were captured and analyzed by the nanoparticle tracking (NTA) software to obtain the concentration of particles (particles/mL) and size (nanometers). The EV concentration is normalized to the number of cells.

Lipidomics

EV sphingolipids were quantified by tandem mass spectrometry at the Mayo Clinic Metabolomics Core Laboratory, as described previously (34). EVs isolated from equal number of cells treated with vehicle, PA, or PA plus MP-A08 were analyzed to quantify changes in sphingolipid content.

CRISPR/Cas9 Gene Editing

SphK2 and SphK1 knockout cell lines for IMH cells were created using the Guide-it CRISPR/Cas9 system (TaKaRa Biotechnology Inc. Japan). The online tool (http://crispr.mit.edu) was used to determine the sgRNA target sequence for mouse SphK2 (5′-TGCGTGCACGCTGCGTCGTCCGG-3′) and mouse SphK1 (5′-ATATATTGCAGTGACGCGTG-3′). Oligonucleotides were annealed and cloned into the pGuide-it Vector (Clontech, Palo Alto, CA), plasmids isolated, then transfected onto HEK293T cells using Lenti-X Packaging Single Shots (VSV-G) following manufacturer's instructions (Clontech). Virus was harvested at 48 h and filtered through a 0.45 μM pore cellulose acetate filter (Millipore). Virus potency was verified by using Lenti-X GoStix (Clontech), then transferred onto wild type IMH cells for infection. Individual infected cells were flow-sorted into 96-well plates by green and red fluorescence for SphK2 and SphK1, respectively.

RNA Purification, Reverse Transcription-PCR, and Quantitative Real Time PCR

IMH or BMDM cells were washed with PBS, centrifuged, and pellets were suspended in Trizol. Flash-frozen cryo-preserved liver tissue from our previously published study described above was homogenized in Trizol (30). Total RNA was extracted using the Quick-RNA MiniPrep kit (Zymo Research. Irvine, CA), and the RNA yield was assessed by NanoDrop ND1000 (ThermoScientific, Waltham, MA). Reverse transcription of RNA into cDNA was performed with the iScript cDNA synthesis kit (Bio-Rad Laboratories, Hercules, CA). PCR amplification was run using the EmeraldAmp MAX Master Mix (TaKaRa) on the Tetrad Thermal Cycler (MJ Research Inc. Watertown, MA). Amplified products were analyzed by QIAxcel Advanced System (Qiagen). Quantitative real time PCR was carried out using the LightCycler 480 SYBR Green I Master Mix (Roche), and run on LightCycler 480 (Roche). Primers used for mouse SphK2 include: forward 5′-TTTACGAGGTGCTGAATGGG-3′ and reverse 5′-ACCGACAACCTGCTCAAAC-3′. Primers for mouse SphK1 include: forward 5′-TGAATGGGCTAATGG AACGG-3′ and reverse 5′-GTCTTCATTAGTCACCTGCT CG-3′. HPRT was used as the house keeping gene for qPCR using primers: forward 5′- TCAGTCAACGGGGGACATAAA-3′ and reverse 5′- GGGGCTGTACTGCTTAACCAG-3′. For $S1P_1$ receptor 5′-ATGGTGTCCACTAGCATCCC-3′ and 5′-CGATGTTCAACTTGCCTGTGTAG-3′ primers were utilized for both qPCR and standard reverse transcription PCR. For standard reverse transcription PCR primers for mouse $S1P_2$: forward 5′-ATGGGCGGCTTATACTCAGAG-3′ and reverse 5′-GCGCAGCACAAGATGATGAT-3′; $S1P_3$: forward 5′-ACTCTCCGGGAACATTACGAT-3′ and reverse 5′-CAAGACGATGAAGCTACAGGTG-3′; $S1P_4$: forward 5′-GTCAGGGACTCGTACCTTCCA-3′ and reverse 5′-GATGCAGCCATACACACGG-3′; $S1P_5$: forward 5′-GCTTTGGTTTGCGCGTGAG-3′ and reverse 5′-GGCGTCCTAAGCAGTTCCAG-3′; and 18S: forward 5′-CGCTTCCTTACCTGGTTGAT-3′ and reverse 5′-GAGCGACCAAAGGAACCATA-3′. PCR products were resolved by capillary electrophoresis using the QIAxcel Advanced System (Qiagen).

Microfluidic 2D Cell Migration Chamber

The microfluidic gradient generator is a 2D cell migration chamber that allows for a passive generation of a stable gradient in space and time. The device itself consists of a piece of PDMS bonded to a glass coverslip, and a network of micro-channels embedded in between (**Supplementary Figure 1**). The microfluidic devices were fabricated using standard soft lithography approaches. The design of the gradient generator was adapted from previous reports (35). The two circular wells on top are inlets for the chemoattractant (RPMI-1640 + EVs) and chemoattractant-free media (RPMI-1640). Immediately after the inlets is a sequence of balance and equilibrium channels, then a network of microchannels that combines and mixes the chemoattractant as they flow through. Each resulting channel at the end of the network contains a different proportion of the chemoattractant such that the gradient will be established in the cell chamber perpendicular to the direction of flow (34). BMDMs were dissociated with Accutase on Day 7 and reconstituted in complete BMDM media to give a concentration of 1E6 cells/mL. The cells were then seeded into the cell chamber of the gradient generator by backflow through the bottom port. Once the cells were spread throughout the chamber, the device was incubated at 37°C, 5% CO_2 for 1 h to allow the cells to adhere. Subsequently, 200 μL of serum free RPMI-1640 or serum free RPMI-1640+EVs was added to the left and right inlets at the top, respectively. The device was allowed to sit for 10 min for the media to flow through the micro-channels before image capture was begun.

Time-Lapse Microscopy

Following cell seeding and generation of the EV gradient, the microfluidic gradient generator was placed in the stage incubator. Images of macrophage migration in the cell chamber were captured every 15 s for 4 h using the 5x objective, Definite Focus (Zeiss) and the ZEN 2.3 lite software (Zeiss).

Cell Tracking and Analysis

All time-lapse images acquired through the Zen Pro imaging software (Zeiss) were exported as time-lapse videos (100 frames/second). The resulting video file was imported into ImageJ (National Institutes of Health, Bethesda, USA), and cells were tracked using the Manual Tracking plugin (Fabrice Cordelières, Institut Curie, Orsay, France). The resulting cell tracks were analyzed using the Chemotaxis and Migration Tool 2.0 (Ibidi GmbH, Munich, Germany). In each experiment, random migrating cells within frame were manually tracked (10–50 cells). The software was also used to plot cell tracks and calculate measured values, including the migratory persistence (forward migration index), angle of migration relative to the gradient axis, velocity, Euclidean and accumulated distances.

Fluorescence-Activated Cell Sorting (FACS)

Mouse liver was dissociated with the liver dissociation kit, mouse (Miltenyi Biotec, Germany), using the gentleMACS Dissociator (Miltenyi Biotec) following manufacturer's protocols. The liver digest was passed through a 40 μm filter (Falcon 352340; BD Biosciences) to remove large debris and cell clusters. The filtered dissociate was centrifuged at 300 × g for 5 min. The cells were re-suspended in 7 ml 25% Percoll in a 15 ml falcon tube, and 2 ml of 50 % Percoll was slowly laid on the bottom of the same tube with a glass Pasteur pipet. The tube was spun at 2,000 rpm, brakes removed, for 20 min at 4°C. After the tube was carefully removed from the centrifuge, 2–3 ml of debris was removed from the top of the gradient. Using a glass Pasteur pipet, cells from the band in between the middle colored interface and transparent interface below were removed without disturbing the RBC pellet at the bottom. To dilute out the Percoll, cells were transferred to a 50 ml falcon tube, the volume was brought up to 40 ml with SF-RPMI, and spun at 400 × g for 10 min. The supernatant was removed and cells re-suspended in PEB buffer, containing PBS, 0.5% bovine serum albumin (BSA) and 2 mM EDTA. Viable cells were counted on a hemocytometer using Trypan Blue (Gibco). Cells were then incubated with FcR Blocking Reagent (Miltenyi Biotec) for 5 min at 4°C, followed by CD45 conjugated to VioBlue (Miltenyi Biotec), F4/80 conjugated to APC-Cy7 (Biolegend), and mouse $S1P_1$-phycoerythrin (PE) conjugated antibody (RandD Systems) for 10 min at room temperature in the dark. Cells were centrifuged at 400 × g for 6 min at room temperature. Cells were washed once with PEB buffer, and centrifuged for 5 min at 400 × g. The supernatant was removed and cells were re-suspended in 1% paraformaldehyde. Flow cytometry was performed with the MACSQuant Analyzer 10 (Miltenyi Biotec). The stained population was acquired by gating side scattered light and forward scattered light to exclude the dead cell population, gated on CD45 positive and fluorescence minus one controls were used to identify and gate the cell population expressing both F4/80 and $S1P_1$ receptor. F4/80 and $S1P_1$ receptor expressing population is expressed as a percentage of CD45 high intrahepatic leukocytes. Graphs were made in Flowlogic software (Miltenyi Biotec).

Statistical Analysis

Statistical analysis and graphs were made in GraphPad Prism version 6.00 for Windows (GraphPad Software, La Jolla, CA). Mean ± S.E.M. are presented in each graph. The two-tailed student's t-test was used to compare groups, and the results were statistically significant when the p-value was <0.05. The Rayleigh Test of Uniformity was used to test a circular distribution of cell end points, and was performed using the Chemotaxis and Migration Tool 2.0. Rejection ($p < 0.05$) of the null hypothesis, which states that the distribution of cell end points is uniform, showed that there is sample mean direction of migration.

RESULTS

Macrophages Migrate Directionally and Persistently Toward PA-Induced EVs

Hepatic lipotoxicity, caused by the presence of excessive saturated free fatty acids (FFAs), and its related macrophage recruitment is implicated in NASH pathogenesis (19, 36). Previously, we found that PA promotes stress-induced release of EVs through the ER stress sensor IRE1α (5). To understand recipient cell responses, we asked whether PA-induced lipotoxic EVs could be a mediator of macrophage recruitment into the liver. Proinflammatory intrahepatic macrophages in NASH are derived from bone marrow-derived monocytes; therefore, we used BMDMs in these experiments as a surrogate for monocyte-derived macrophages. BMDMs were exposed to a Veh-EV or PA-EV gradient (EVs isolated from the same number of hepatocytes treated with vehicle or PA) through the microfluidic gradient generator for 4 h. BMDMs migrated directionally (Rayleigh Test $P < 0.05$) when exposed to PA-EVs but not when exposed to Veh-EVs (**Figure 1A**). BMDMs migrated at a higher velocity when exposed to PA-EVs throughout the duration of exposure, and at more acute angles toward PA-EVs (**Figures 1B,C**). A positive

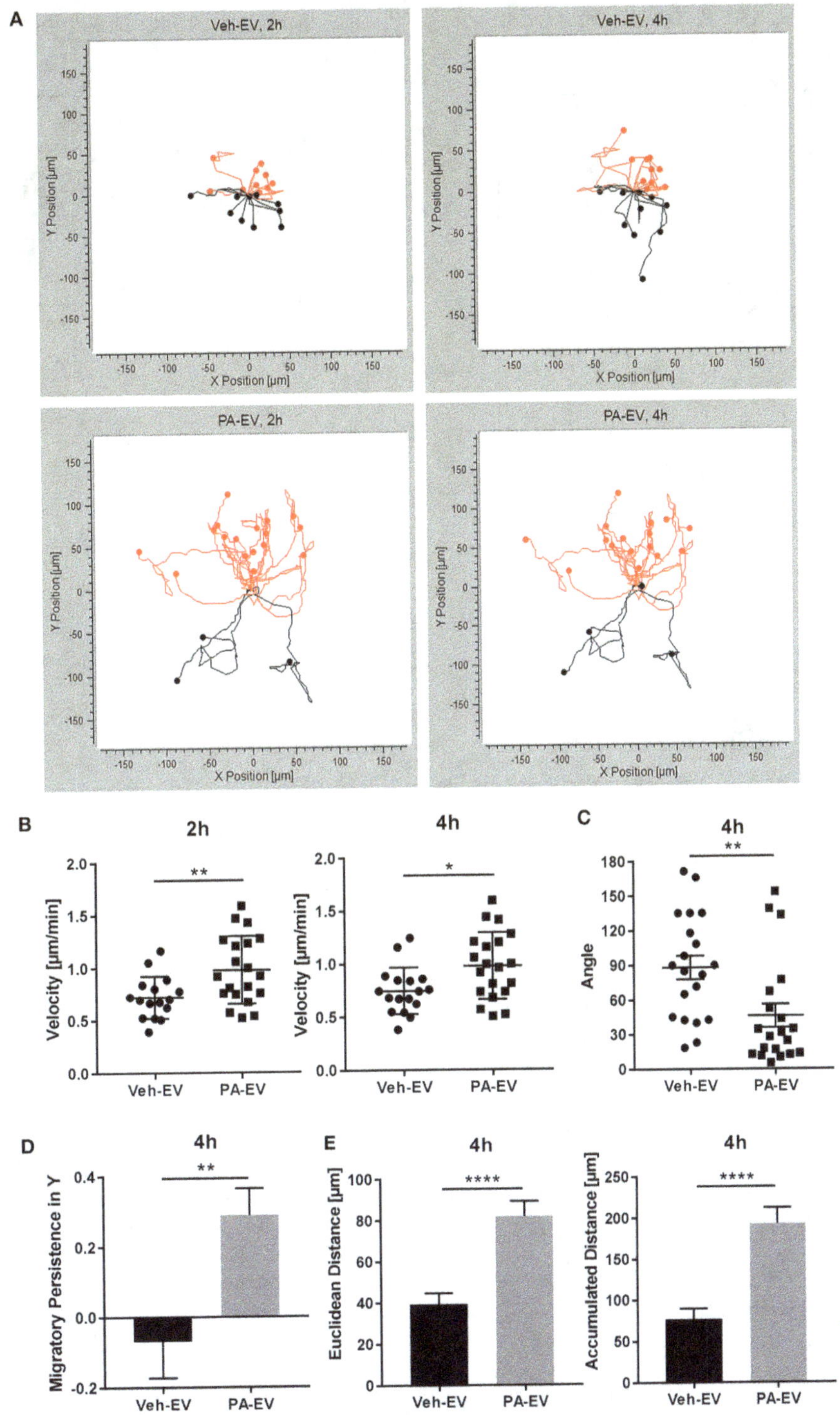

FIGURE 1 | PA-EVs are chemoattractive to macrophages. **(A)** Representative migration plots for 2D chemotaxis assay, showing BMDM migration trajectories of 20 randomly selected cells at 2 and 4 h ($n = 3$). BMDMs were seeded in the microfluidic gradient generator for 1 h, exposed to a Veh-EV or PA-EV gradient for 4 h, and captured by time-lapse microscopy. EVs were isolated from the same number of IMH cells treated with 400 µM PA or vehicle for 20 h. Cells highlighted in red are migrating up toward the positive end of the gradient. The Rayleigh test for uniformity was used to test whether the cell distribution was uniform. **(B)** Migration velocity when BMDMs were exposed to a Veh-EV vs. PA-EV gradient at 2 and 4 h ($n = 3$). **(C)** Angle between the cell's leading edge and gradient axis at 4 h in a Veh-EV vs. PA-EV gradient ($n = 3$). A more acute angle indicates that migration was more consistent with the gradient axis. **(D)** Migratory persistence in Y of BMDMs treated with Veh-EV vs. PA-EV gradient at 4 h ($n = 3$). Strong chemotaxis effects are characterized by higher migratory persistence in Y. **(E)** Euclidean distance (shortest distance between the start and end points) and accumulated distance (total path length) between BMDMs migrating in a Veh-EV or PA-EV gradient for 4 h ($n = 3$). $^*p < 0.05$, $^{**}p < 0.01$, $^{****}p < 0.0001$. All error bars are SEM.

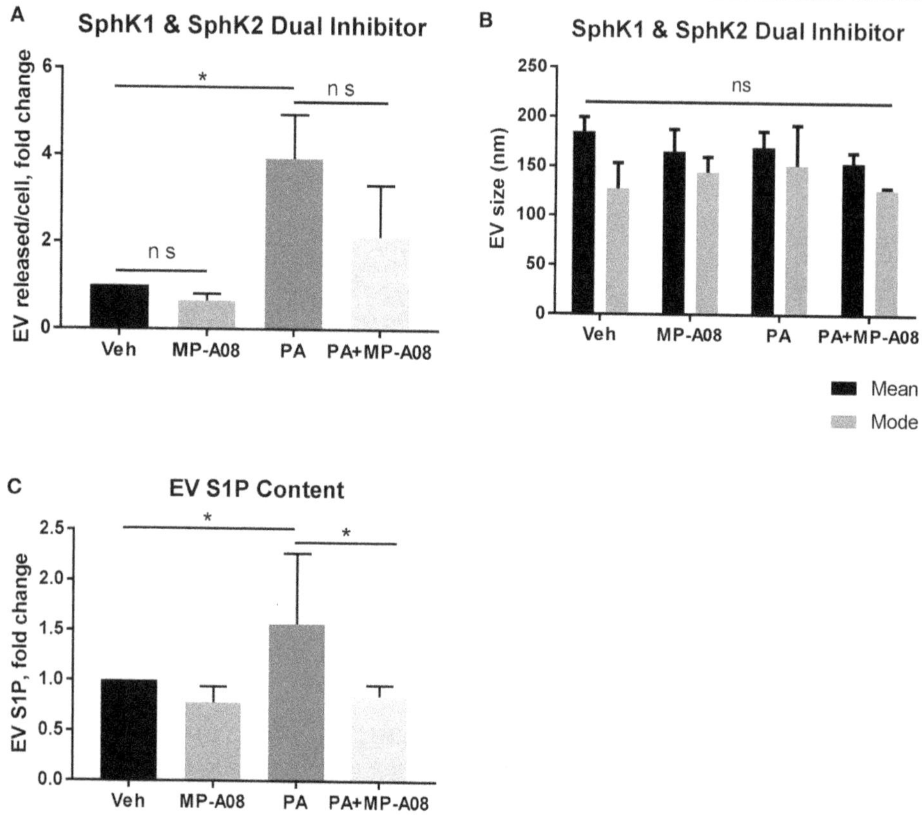

FIGURE 2 | EV S1P is not elevated under SphK1 and SphK2 inhibition. **(A)** IMH cells were treated with 400 μM PA, 400 μM PA + 2 μM MP-A08, vehicle, or vehicle + 2 μM MP-A08 for 20 h. EVs released were isolated by differential ultracentrifugation and characterized by NTA and normalized to cell numbers. Data are pooled from 4 experiments. **(B)** Size (nm, nanometers) of EVs released by IMH cells treated with vehicle, vehicle + 2 μM MP-A08, 400 μM PA, or 400 μM PA + 2 μM MP-A08 for 20 h. Data are pooled from 4 experiments. **(C)** EV S1P content was quantified by tandem mass spectrometry ($n = 2$). $^*p < 0.05$, ns, not significant. All error bars are SEM.

migratory persistence in Y [sum of the ratio of displacement along the gradient axis (Y axis) to total accumulated path length of all cell tracks, averaged] indicated that the direction of macrophage migration was toward the positive end of the PA-EV gradient (**Figure 1D**), and they did so over greater distances (**Figure 1E**). Together, these measured values show that macrophages migrate faster, longer, and in a more directionally persistent manner toward PA-EVs.

Inhibition of SphK1 and SphK2 Reduces S1P Levels in PA-Induced EVs

We next examined the EV S1P content and the significance of its formation in the release of PA-induced EVs. S1P is formed through the phosphorylation of sphingosine by SphK1 and SphK2 (24). We attempted to establish a double SphK1 and SphK2 knockout cell line using CRISPR/Cas9 gene editing technology. However, this was not successfully achieved likely due to lethality in the absence of both SphK isoenzymes, similar to observations in mice (37). It is also known that the downregulation of one SphK results in the compensatory upregulation of the other (38). Henceforth, we used a pharmacologic approach in the subsequent experiments. We asked whether SphK1 and SphK2 mediate the formation of S1P in PA-induced EVs by using the dual SphK pharmacologic inhibitor, MP-A08. We treated hepatocytes with vehicle, vehicle + MP-A08, PA, and PA + MP-A08 for 20 h, isolated the EVs released and normalized to cell number. We confirmed the absence of MP-A08-induced apoptosis by the biochemical and morphologic assessment of apoptosis (**Supplementary Figures 2A,B**). In hepatocytes treated with MP-A08, PA, or PA + MP-A08, both caspase 3/7 activity and percent apoptotic nuclei were comparable to vehicle treated cells. The inhibitory effect of MP-A08 was confirmed by measuring sphingosine kinase activity (**Supplementary Figure 2C**). We found almost a 3-fold increase in EV release in PA-treated cells compared to vehicle-treated cells, and no significant difference in EV release when SphK1 and SphK2 were inhibited by MP-A08 (**Figure 2A**). We did not find any difference in vesicle size (nm) between the groups (**Figure 2B**). We next quantified and analyzed the EV S1P content by tandem mass spectrometry. We found that PA-EVs were enriched in S1P cargo compared to those released by vehicle-treated, vehicle + MP-A08-treated and PA + MP-A08-treated cells (**Figure 2C**). Altogether, these data suggest that SphK1 and Sphk2 play a crucial role in the formation of S1P in PA-induced EVs, though the number of EV released is unaffected.

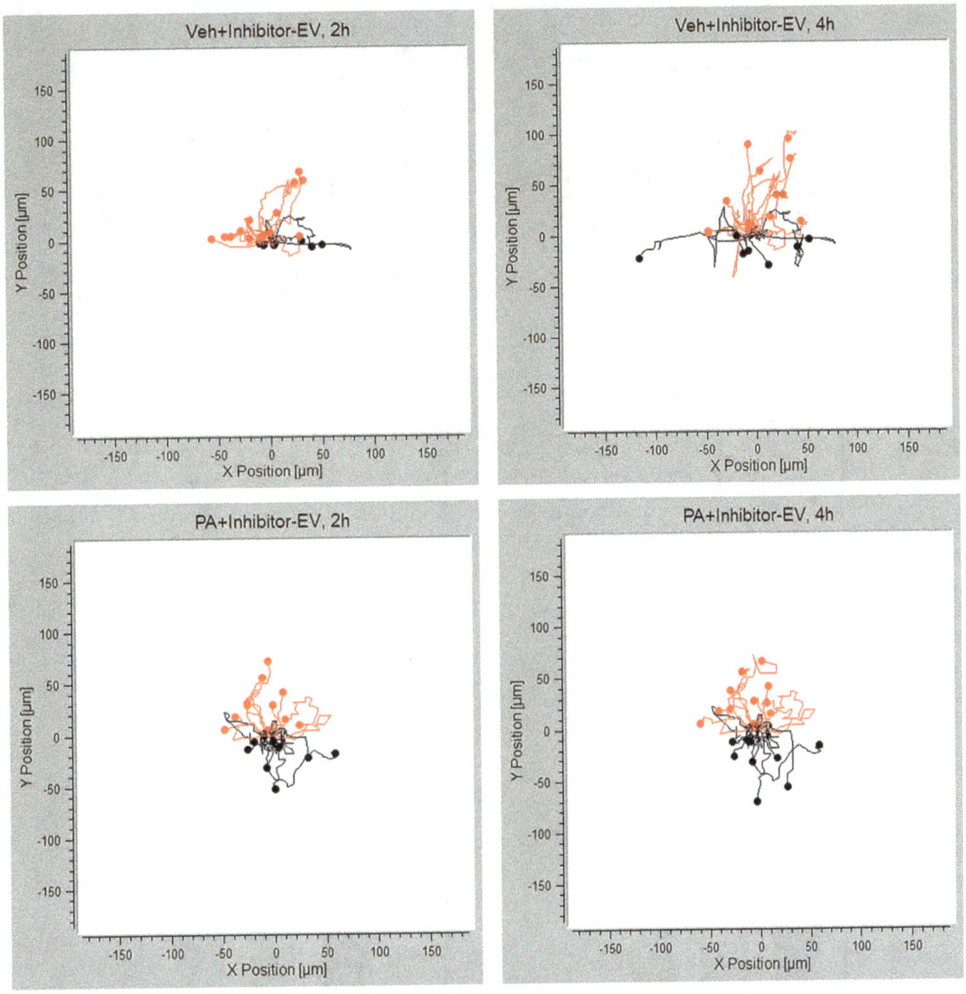

FIGURE 3 | PA-EV chemotactic response is attenuated through inhibition of SphK1 and SphK2. Migration plots of BMDMs migrating in a Veh + MP-A08-EV or PA + MP-A08-EV gradient for 4 h. Plots show migration trajectories of 20 randomly selected cells from each experiment ($n = 3$). The Rayleigh test for uniformity was used to test whether cell distribution was uniform. Cells highlighted in red are migrating up.

Macrophages Are Chemotactic Toward PA-Induced EVs Through the S1P Signaling Axis

Having demonstrated that PA-EVs attract macrophages, and that PA-EVs contain elevated levels of S1P through functional SphK1 and SphK2, we next asked whether SphK mediated formation of S1P plays a role in the chemoattractive effects of PA-EVs. If macrophages are stimulated by the SphK mediated formation of S1P cargo in PA-induced EVs, then the inhibition of both SphK1 & SphK2 should inhibit macrophage migration through impairment of the S1P signaling axis. BMDMs were exposed to 4 different gradients of EVs isolated from Veh-treated, Veh + MP-A08-treated, PA-treated, or PA + MP-A08-treated cells for 4 h. BMDMs did not migrate directionally (Rayleigh Test $P > 0.05$) in either the Veh + MP-A08-EV or PA + MP-A08-EV gradient (**Figure 3**). Migration velocity was significantly reduced toward PA + MP-A08-EVs compared to PA-EVs, similar to the response toward vehicle controls at both 2 and 4 h (**Figure 4A**). We speculate that this is due to the reduction in S1P content by the SphK inhibitor MP-A08. BMDMs in the PA + MP-A08-EV gradient migrated at less acute angles, or less in alignment with the gradient axis compared to those migrating toward PA-EVs (**Figure 4B**). Furthermore, the macrophages did not migrate persistently toward the positive end of the PA + MP-A08-EV gradient (**Figure 4C**), and migration distance was significantly reduced compared to that when exposed to PA-EVs (**Figure 4D**). Taken together, these data suggest that pharmacologic inhibition of SphK1 and SphK2 and the subsequent reduced levels of S1P in PA-EVs diminish their chemoattractive effects toward macrophages. We speculate that S1P mediated recruitment of macrophages is achieved through stimulating the $S1P_1$ receptor on macrophages.

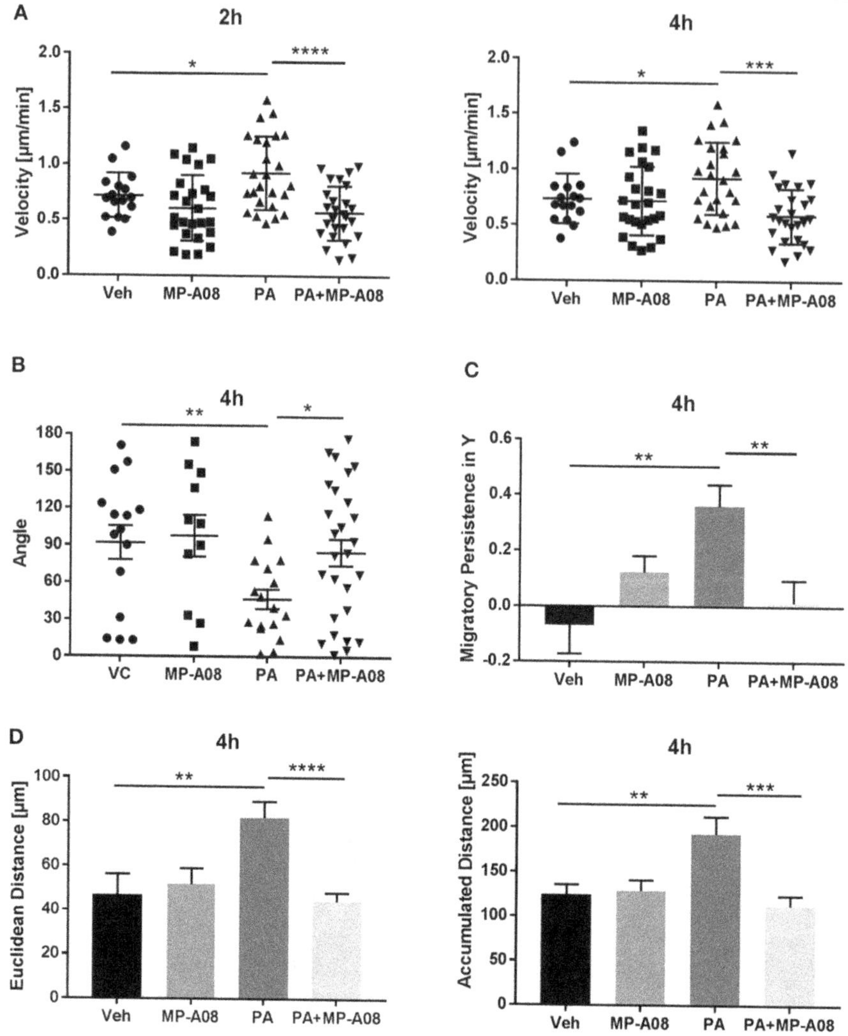

FIGURE 4 | Macrophages migrate persistently and directionally toward S1P-enriched EVs. **(A)** BMDM migration velocity when exposed to Veh-EV, Veh + MP-A08-EV, PA-EV, or PA + MP-A08-EV gradients at 2 and 4 h ($n = 3$). **(B)** The angle between the cell's leading edge and the gradient axis for BMDMs migrating in 4 types of EV gradients for 4 h ($n = 3$). **(C)** Migratory persistence in Y, comparing chemotaxis efficiency of BMDMs migrating in 4 types of EV gradients for 4 h ($n = 3$). **(D)** Comparison of the Euclidean distance and accumulated distance between BMDMs migrating in 4 types of EV gradients for 4 h ($n = 3$). $^{*}p < 0.05$, $^{**}p < 0.01$, $^{***}p < 0.001$, $^{****}p < 0.0001$. All error bars are SEM.

Intrahepatic Macrophages Express $S1P_1$ Receptor

As $S1P_1$ receptor is known to be expressed by macrophages (39), we characterized its expression on intrahepatic macrophages in normal mouse livers through FACS analysis. We defined intrahepatic leukocytes as the $CD45^{hi}$ population and further defined the macrophage population as $F4/80^{hi}$. We found that a significant percentage of the $CD45^{hi}$ population expressed both F4/80 and $S1P_1$ receptor (22.5 ± 2% of the $CD45^{hi}$ population, $n = 4$) (**Figures 5A,B**). Having demonstrated that this receptor is expressed by intrahepatic macrophages, we next asked whether it is upregulated in NASH, which would be in keeping with our proposed model. For this we utilized available archived mouse liver RNA and tissue samples from a previously published study (30). In this study mice were fed a diet known to induce obesity, insulin resistance and NASH, thus recapitulate cardinal features of human NASH, as previously reported by us and others (30, 40). Liver injury and macrophage accumulation in these mouse livers have been previously reported (30). In this dietary NASH model we found a significant increase in the hepatic expression of $S1P_1$ receptor by immunohistochemistry (**Figures 5C,D**), in regions of inflammatory cell infiltration. The mRNA abundance in this dietary NASH model was similar to the protein expression observed by immunohistochemistry (**Figure 5E**). Altogether, these data support an increase in $S1P_1$ receptor expression in the liver in NASH, and are consistent with our model that $S1P_1$ receptor expressing macrophages are recruited into the liver in NASH.

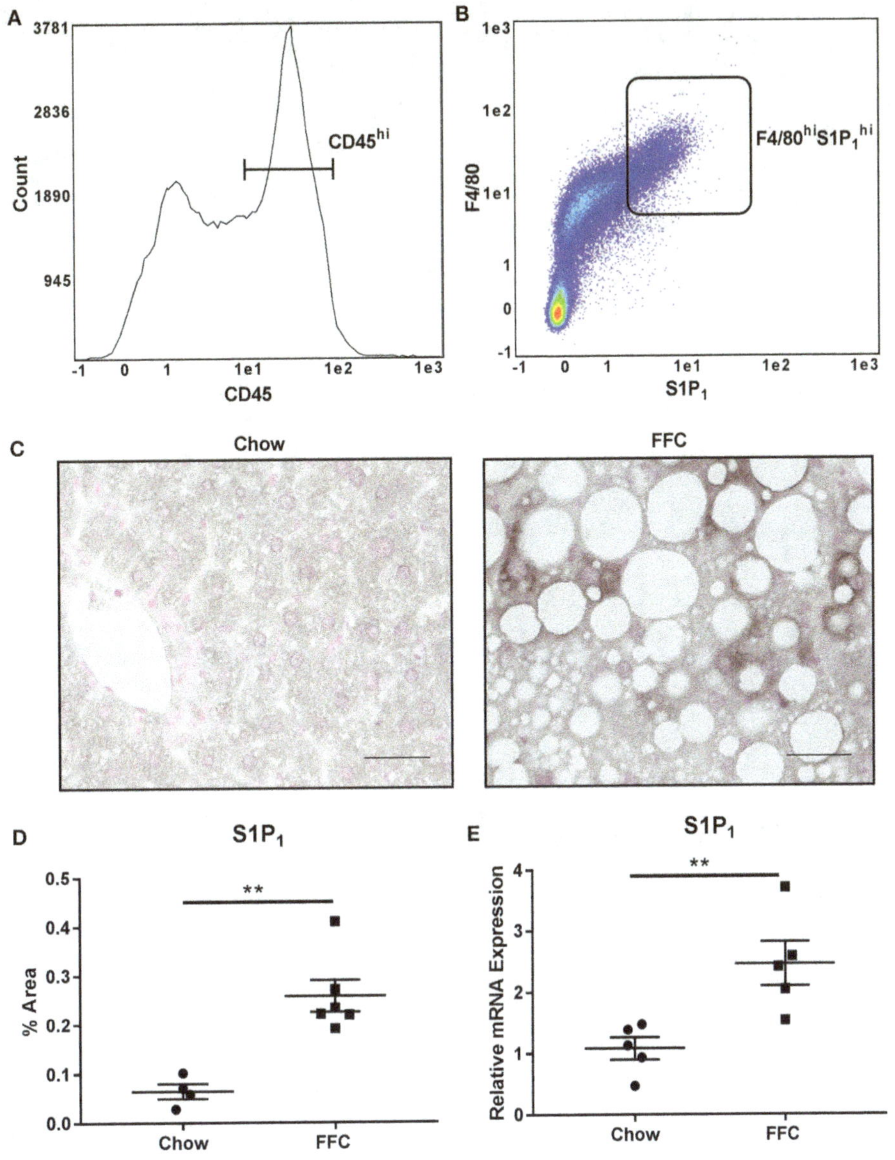

FIGURE 5 | Intrahepatic macrophages express the $S1P_1$ receptor. **(A)** CD45 expression and **(B)** F4/80 and $S1P_1$ receptor expression of $CD45^{hi}$ intrahepatic macrophages was determined in normal mouse livers by FACS analysis. **(C)** $S1P_1$ receptor immunohistochemistry was performed in livers from mice fed a diet high in fat, fructose and cholesterol (FFC) or chow for 20 weeks. Scale bar = 50 μM, $n = 4$ for chow and $n = 6$ for FFC. **(D)** Quantification of immunohistochemistry for $S1P_1$ receptor in chow fed ($n = 4$) and FFC fed ($n = 6$) mice. **(E)** mRNA expression for $S1P_1$ receptor in chow fed ($n = 5$) and FFC fed ($n = 5$) mice. $^{**}p < 0.01$.

Chemotactic Effect Toward PA-EVs Is Attenuated in the Absence of $S1P_1$ Receptor

Having demonstrated the presence of $S1P_1$ receptor on intrahepatic macrophages, we next wanted to confirm whether $S1P_1$ receptor plays a role in macrophage chemotaxis toward S1P in PA-EVs. BMDM $S1P_1$ receptor knockout was confirmed by RT-PCR (**Supplementary Figure 3**); the mRNA expression of S1P receptors 2–5 was unaffected by knockout of $S1P_1$ receptor. $S1P_1$ receptor KO BMDMs were exposed to Veh-EV or PA-EV gradients in the microfluidic gradient generator for 4 h. $S1P_1$ receptor KO BMDMs did not migrate directionally (Rayleigh Test $P > 0.05$) toward PA-EVs compared to WT BMDMs (Rayleigh Test $P<0.05$) when exposed to a PA-EV gradient for 4 h (**Figures 6A,B**). The migration of $S1P_1$ receptor KO BMDMs was similar toward Veh-EVs and PA-EVs and comparable to WT BMDMs migration toward Veh-EVs. This suggests that the $S1P_1$ receptor is crucial in mediating chemotactic effects in macrophages during S1P signaling. This was further confirmed by measuring migration velocity at 2 and 4 h, showing that $S1P_1$

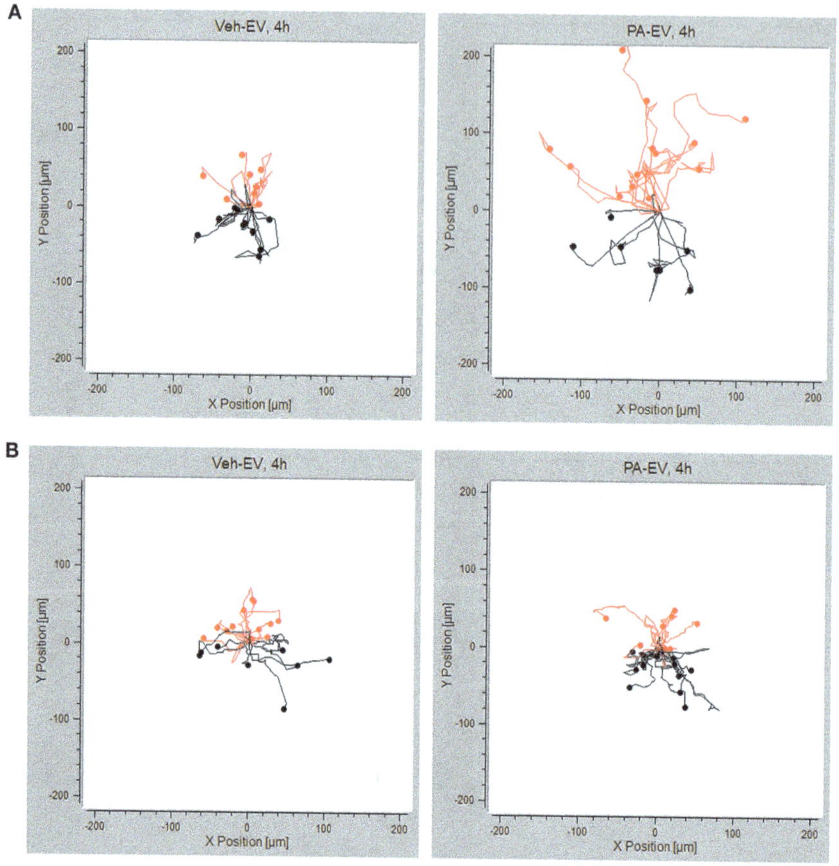

FIGURE 6 | Migration toward PA-EVs is reduced in the absence of the $S1P_1$ receptor. **(A)** Migration plots of WT BMDMs migrating in a Veh-EV and PA-EV gradient for 4 h (*n* = 3). **(B)** Migration plots of $S1P_1$ receptor KO BMDMs migrating in a Veh-EV and PA-EV gradient for 4 h (*n* = 2). Twenty randomly selected cells from each experiment are shown in each plot. The Rayleigh test of uniformity was used to test whether the cell distribution was uniform. Cells highlighted in red are migrating up toward the positive end of the gradient.

receptor KO BMDMs migrate significantly slower toward PA-EVs compared to WT BMDMs (**Figure 7A**). KO BMDMs also migrated at less acute angles, with significantly less persistence, and decreased Euclidean and accumulated distances toward PA-EVs (**Figures 7B–D**). Thus, in the absence of $S1P_1$ receptor, all measured parameters show attenuated migration toward PA-EVs, similar to the migration patterns toward MP-A08 treated EVs. This evidence further confirms the involvement of the $S1P_1$ receptor in S1P signaling in macrophage chemotaxis.

DISCUSSION

Macrophage-mediated sterile inflammation is a salient feature of NASH. The signals that lead to the recruitment of proinflammatory monocyte-derived macrophages such that they infiltrate the hepatic parenchyma are not well-understood. In this paper we report that: (i) lipotoxic hepatocyte-derived extracellular vesicles attract macrophages by chemotaxis; (ii) intrahepatic leukocytes express the sphingosine 1-phosphage 1 ($S1P_1$) receptor; and (iii) macrophage chemotaxis is mediated by the sphingosine 1-phosphate signaling axis. These *in vitro* findings advance our understanding of how lipotoxic hepatocyte-derived extracellular vesicles are proinflammatory and provide an explanation for the infiltration of macrophages into the hepatic cords by responding to EV gradients in the tissue microenvironment.

Lipotoxicity, summarized as accumulation of toxic lipid species with concomitant tissue or cellular injury, is a fundamental observation in obesity-associated disorders such as NASH (3). Several lipid classes have been implicated in lipotoxicity, including saturated free fatty acids, ceramides, lysophosphatidyl choline and free cholesterol (3, 41, 42). Among these lipids, the saturated free fatty acid palmitate, which is most abundant physiologically, and accumulates further in lipotoxic states is best characterized as being lipotoxic (18). Additionally, lipids, that can be synthesized directly from palmitate, such as ceramide via the *de novo* biosynthesis pathway (43), and indirectly such as lysophosphatidyl choline via phospholipase A2 (44), can induce hepatocyte cell death or stress responses. Though rarely observed in standard H&E stained liver biopsies, lipotoxic hepatocyte cell death correlates with features of progressive

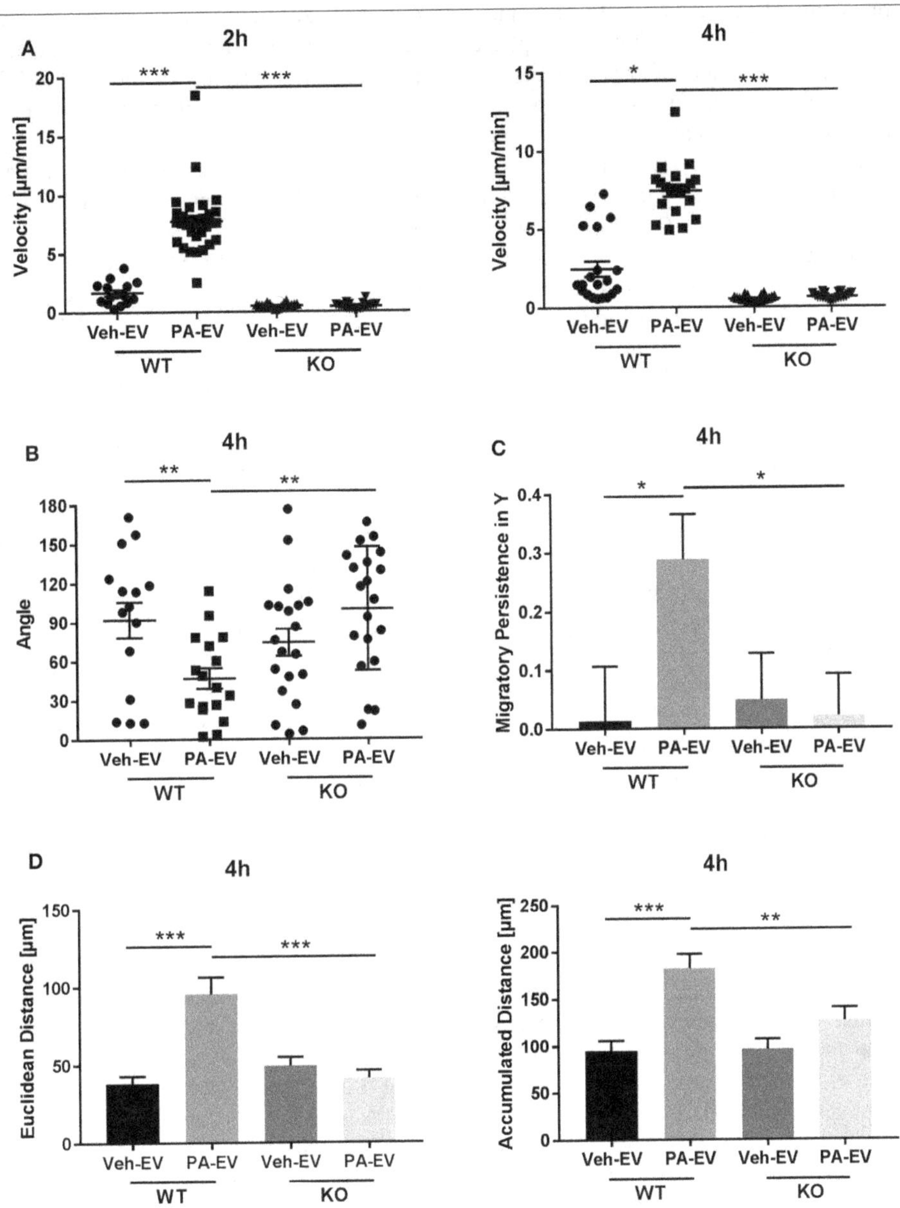

FIGURE 7 | S1P$_1$ receptor KO BMDMs migrate at reduced speeds, distances and persistence toward PA-EVs. **(A)** Migration velocity of WT vs. S1P$_1$ receptor KO BMDMs in Veh-EV and PA-EV gradients at 2 and 4 h ($n = 2$). **(B)** Angle between the cell's leading edge and gradient axis for WT and S1P$_1$ receptor KO BMDMs in Veh-EV and PA-EV gradients for 4 h ($n = 2$). **(C)** Migratory persistence in Y of WT and S1P$_1$ receptor KO BMDMs migrating in Veh-EV and PA-EV gradients for 4 h ($n = 2$). **(D)** Euclidean distance and accumulated distance for WT and S1P$_1$ receptor KO BMDMs migrating in Veh-EV and PA-EV gradients for 4 h ($n = 2$). $^{*}p < 0.05$, $^{**}p < 0.01$, $^{***}p < 0.001$. All error bars are SEM.

NASH (45, 46). However, death is a terminal outcome and there is emerging interest in events that occur in "at-risk" cells prior to the terminal outcome of cell death, which we and others have termed sublethal cellular stress (21). The "at-risk" cells may be defined in many ways including, but not limited to, cells that demonstrate activation of cell stress pathways such as endoplasmic reticulum stress (47), activation of death receptor signaling without cell death (48), secretion of soluble factors, and increasingly, as we demonstrate here, the release of extracellular vesicles (49). EVs are heterogeneous, membrane-enclosed, nanoparticles that most cells secrete into the extracellular space and into circulation (6). EV number and cargo, including lipids, proteins and nucleic acids, changes with disease states and there is immense interest in identifying disease-specific EV signatures, both for their utility as liquid biopsy and as a potentially targetable pathophysiologic mechanism (6, 50, 51). Here we advance the understanding of EV-mediated communication between donor cell, i.e., lipotoxic hepatocytes, and recipient cell, i.e., macrophages.

Proinflammatory activation of the innate immune system, manifest as macrophage infiltration of the hepatic parenchyma, is linked to key features of NASH including hepatocyte injury, hepatocyte cell death and fibrosis (45, 46). While macrophage activation by itself can lead to secretion of proinflammatory cytokines, death ligands and promote fibrosis, in lipotoxic disorders, where hepatocytes are a key cell that accumulates toxic lipids and lipid accumulation precedes the development of overt inflammation, hepatocyte-to-macrophage signals are important in understanding this key signaling axis. Our laboratory has focused on lipotoxic hepatocyte derived EVs as mediators of this cellular cross talk, and in particular signaling lipid mediators on EVs. We have previously demonstrated that palmitate-treated hepatocytes release ceramide-enriched extracellular vesicles, that these vesicles are also enriched in the ceramide-derived signaling sphingolipid S1P, and that their release is dependent on the endoplasmic reticulum stress sensor, inositol requiring protein 1 alpha (IRE1α) (5). Furthermore, we have recently demonstrated that the release of extracellular vesicles in PA-treated hepatocytes is preserved in the presence of caspase inhibitors, highlighting the potential importance of lipotoxic stress-induced EVs in cellular cross talk with the innate immune system (49). Here we extend our earlier observations by demonstrating persistent and directional migration of macrophages toward an EV S1P gradient. Not only are PA-induced EVs enriched in S1P, PA-stimulated cells release more EVs than vehicle-treated cells raising the possibility that macrophage chemotaxis toward S1P may be occurring toward a higher number of EVs. While this is possible, we show a lack of EV-S1P enrichment in cells treated with sphingosine kinase inhibitor MP-A08 and PA without a significant reduction in EV numbers, suggesting that EV cargo, S1P in this case, is mediating the observed macrophage chemotaxis. Others have reported proinflammatory, proangiogenic and profibrotic EVs in NASH models (52–54). Here, we focused on macrophage chemotaxis toward lipotoxic EVs in order to provide an explanation for macrophage infiltration, as chemotaxis to a site of injury and activation are both important components of macrophage effector responses. Though transwell macrophage migration has been reported by us and others in response to lipotoxic EVs, it does not differentiate between chemokinesis and chemotaxis. This is the first report of true directional chemotaxis of macrophages toward a lipotoxic EV gradient in response to EV S1P. We have previously demonstrated that EV S1P is increased in human and murine NASH (5). Thus, lipotoxic PA-EVs may play a role in macrophage recruitment *in vivo* in addition to the previously defined role of chemokines such as CCL2 and chemokine receptors CCR2 and CCR5 (10).

S1P is a potent bioactive sphingolipid, formed by phosphorylation of sphingosine by two isoenzymes of sphingosine kinase, SphK1 and SphK2. The cellular and subcellular distribution of SphK1 and 2 vary, accounting for distinct roles in the compartmental formation of S1P. Sphingosine, in turn, is formed by the deacylation of ceramide. Studies have shown that S1P is involved in the pathogenesis and progression of NASH, with concurrent upregulation of SphK1 and occasionally SphK2 (24). Both ceramide and S1P are implicated in the formation of intraluminal vesicles (ILVs) in multivesicular bodies and in cargo sorting into intraluminal vesicles (5, 22); however, when we inhibited SphK1 and 2 we did not observe a significant reduction in the number of EVs released by hepatocytes; predictably, EV S1P was significantly reduced to levels comparable to basal levels. S1P is the ligand of a family of 5 G-protein couple receptors, $S1P_1$-$S1P_5$, that regulate downstream signaling to mediate a variety of cellular responses including: immunity, cellular migration, angiogenesis, vascular and cardiac development (55, 56). Of these, $S1P_1$ receptor expression and S1P gradients in the microenvironment are known to influence T lymphocyte trafficking (57), NK cell trafficking (25), dendritic cell trafficking (58). Here, we confirmed the cell surface expression of $S1P_1$ on intrahepatic macrophages (59) and demonstrate that macrophage chemotaxis is attenuated in response to S1P deficient EVs. Our observations of macrophage chemotaxis toward EV-S1P are consistent with earlier reports of macrophage chemotaxis induced by S1P (60). Further, we have demonstrated that the chemotaxis responses of macrophages genetically deficient in $S1P_1$ receptor toward PA-EVs are attenuated, confirming that macrophage chemotaxis toward lipotoxic EVs is mediated by an intact S1P-$S1P_1$ signaling axis. Of the 5 known S1P receptors, $S1P_1$, $S1P_2$, $S1P_3$, and $S1P_4$ are expressed by human macrophages and $S1P_1$, $S1P_2$, and $S1P_4$ by monocytes (39). Our data suggest that the role of $S1P_1$ warrants investigation in human NASH.

Taken together these data provide an *in vitro* mechanism for lipotoxic hepatocyte-derived S1P-enriched EVs in macrophage chemotaxis responses. Recognizing that proinflammatory macrophages are derived from proinflammatory monocytes, we propose a model wherein multiple hepatocyte-derived signals act in concert to mediate macrophage attraction and activation in the microenvironment of NASH livers. Soluble signals such as CCL2 may lead to the egress of proinflammatory monocytes from the bone marrow and their recruitment in to the liver (10, 61); other soluble or EV-mediated signals might home proinflammatory monocytes to the sinusoidal endothelium; and promote adhesion of proinflammatory monocytes to give rise to macrophages which then infiltrate hepatic cords in response to an EV S1P gradient in the local microenvironment. Our data support a key role for S1P-$S1P_1$ in the last process, though we cannot exclude a role in adhesion or homing either. Here we demonstrate that $S1P_1$ receptor expression is increased in mouse livers in a NASH model, and in previous experiments we have demonstrated that pharmacologic inhibition of this signaling axis with FTY720 ameliorates murine NASH (23). However, the macrophage-specific role of S1P signaling has not been examined in this context. In ongoing experiments we are interrogating the *in vivo* role of myeloid cell $S1P_1$ in NASH models, as a corollary to our *in vitro* findings.

AUTHOR CONTRIBUTIONS

C-YL designed and conducted experiments, analyzed and graphed data and wrote the manuscript. MS, YG, and AM designed and conducted experiments. AR designed and supervised experiments. HM designed and supervised experiments, analyzed data, and wrote the manuscript. All authors reviewed and approved the manuscript.

ACKNOWLEDGMENTS

The authors are grateful to Dr. Anuradha Krishnan and Dr. Debanjali Dasgupta for their assistance with flow cytometry.

REFERENCES

1. Rinella ME. Nonalcoholic fatty liver disease: a systematic review. *JAMA* (2015) 313:2263–73. doi: 10.1001/jama.2015.5370
2. Argo CK, Iezzoni JC, Al-Osaimi AM, Caldwell SH. Thiazolidinediones for the treatment in NASH: sustained benefit after drug discontinuation? *J Clin Gastroenterol.* (2009) 43:565–8. doi: 10.1097/MCG.0b013e31818f4fc2
3. Musso G, Cassader M, Paschetta E, Gambino R. Bioactive lipid species and metabolic pathways in progression and resolution of nonalcoholic steatohepatitis. *Gastroenterology* (2018) 155:282–302.e8. doi: 10.1053/j.gastro.2018.06.031
4. Soltis AR, Kennedy NJ, Xin X, Zhou F, Ficarro SB, Yap YS, et al. Hepatic dysfunction caused by consumption of a high-fat diet. *Cell Rep.* (2017) 21:3317–28. doi: 10.1016/j.celrep.2017.11.059
5. Kakazu E, Mauer AS, Yin M, Malhi H. Hepatocytes release ceramide-enriched pro-inflammatory extracellular vesicles in an IRE1α-dependent manner. *J Lipid Res.* (2016) 57:233–45. doi: 10.1194/jlr.M063412
6. Hirsova P, Ibrahim SH, Verma VK, Morton LA, Shah VH, LaRusso NF, et al. Extracellular vesicles in liver pathobiology: small particles with big impact. *Hepatology* (2016) 64:2219–33. doi: 10.1002/hep.28814
7. Ganz M, Szabo G. Immune and inflammatory pathways in NASH. *Hepatol Int.* (2013) 7(Suppl. 2):771–81. doi: 10.1007/s12072-013-9468-6
8. Brunt EM. Histological assessment of nonalcoholic fatty liver disease in adults and children. *Clin Liver Dis.* (2012) 1:108–11. doi: 10.1002/cld.31
9. Gadd VL, Skoien R, Powell EE, Fagan KJ, Winterford C, Horsfall L, et al. The portal inflammatory infiltrate and ductular reaction in human nonalcoholic fatty liver disease. *Hepatology* (2014) 59:1393–405. doi: 10.1002/hep.26937
10. Tacke F. Cenicriviroc for the treatment of non-alcoholic steatohepatitis and liver fibrosis. *Expert Opin Investig Drugs* (2018) 27:301–11. doi: 10.1080/13543784.2018.1442436
11. Krenkel O, Puengel T, Govaere O, Abdallah AT, Mossanen JC, Kohlhepp M, et al. Therapeutic inhibition of inflammatory monocyte recruitment reduces steatohepatitis and liver fibrosis. *Hepatology* (2018) 67:1270–83. doi: 10.1002/hep.29544
12. Friedman SL, Ratziu V, Harrison SA, Abdelmalek MF, Aithal GP, Caballeria J, et al. A randomized, placebo-controlled trial of cenicriviroc for treatment of nonalcoholic steatohepatitis with fibrosis. *Hepatology* (2018) 67:1754–67. doi: 10.1002/hep.29477
13. Devhare PB, Ray RB. Extracellular vesicles: novel mediator for cell to cell communications in liver pathogenesis. *Mol Aspects Med.* (2018) 60:115–22. doi: 10.1016/j.mam.2017.11.001
14. Raposo G, Stoorvogel W. Extracellular vesicles: exosomes, microvesicles, and friends. *J Cell Biol.* (2013) 200:373–83. doi: 10.1083/jcb.201211138
15. Tauzin S, Starnes TW, Becker FB, Lam PY, Huttenlocher A. Redox and Src family kinase signaling control leukocyte wound attraction and neutrophil reverse migration. *J Cell Biol.* (2014) 207:589–98. doi: 10.1083/jcb.201408090
16. McLaughlin T, Ackerman SE, Shen L, Engleman E. Role of innate and adaptive immunity in obesity-associated metabolic disease. *J Clin Invest.* (2017) 127:5–13. doi: 10.1172/JCI88876
17. Wiesner C, Le-Cabec V, El Azzouzi K, Maridonneau-Parini I, Linder S. Podosomes in space: macrophage migration and matrix degradation in 2D and 3D settings. *Cell Adh Migr.* (2014) 8:179–91. doi: 10.4161/cam.28116
18. de Almeida IT, Cortez-Pinto H, Fidalgo G, Rodrigues D, Camilo ME. Plasma total and free fatty acids composition in human non-alcoholic steatohepatitis. *Clin Nutr.* (2002) 21:219–23. doi: 10.1054/clnu.2001.0529
19. Akazawa Y, Nakao K. To die or not to die: death signaling in nonalcoholic fatty liver disease. *J Gastroenterol.* (2018) 53:893–906. doi: 10.1007/s00535-018-1451-5
20. Hirsova P, Ibrahim SH, Gores GJ, Malhi H. Lipotoxic lethal and sublethal stress signaling in hepatocytes: relevance to NASH pathogenesis. *J Lipid Res.* (2016) 57:1758–70. doi: 10.1194/jlr.R066357
21. Ibrahim SH, Hirsova P, Gores GJ. Non-alcoholic steatohepatitis pathogenesis: sublethal hepatocyte injury as a driver of liver inflammation. *Gut* (2018) 67:963–72. doi: 10.1136/gutjnl-2017-315691
22. Kajimoto T, Okada T, Miya S, Zhang L, Nakamura S. Ongoing activation of sphingosine 1-phosphate receptors mediates maturation of exosomal multivesicular endosomes. *Nat Commun.* (2013) 4:2712. doi: 10.1038/ncomms3712
23. Mauer AS, Hirsova P, Maiers JL, Shah VH, Malhi H. Inhibition of sphingosine 1-phosphate signaling ameliorates murine nonalcoholic steatohepatitis. *Am J Physiol Gastrointest Liver Physiol.* (2017) 312:G300–13. doi: 10.1152/ajpgi.00222.2016
24. Kleuser B. Divergent role of sphingosine 1-phosphate in liver health and disease. *Int J Mol Sci.* (2018) 19:E722. doi: 10.3390/ijms19030722
25. Jenne CN, Enders A, Rivera R, Watson SR, Bankovich AJ, Pereira JP, et al. T-bet-dependent S1P5 expression in NK cells promotes egress from lymph nodes and bone marrow. *J Exp Med.* (2009) 206:2469–81. doi: 10.1084/jem.20090525
26. Hannun YA, Obeid LM. Principles of bioactive lipid signalling: lessons from sphingolipids. *Nat Rev Mol Cell Biol.* (2008) 9:139–50. doi: 10.1038/nrm2329
27. Rohrbach T, Maceyka M, Spiegel S. Sphingosine kinase and sphingosine-1-phosphate in liver pathobiology. *Crit Rev Biochem Mol Biol.* (2017) 52:543–53. doi: 10.1080/10409238.2017.1337706
28. Malhi H, Kropp EM, Clavo VF, Kobrossi CR, Han J, Mauer AS, et al. C/EBP homologous protein-induced macrophage apoptosis protects mice from steatohepatitis. *J Biol Chem.* (2013) 288:18624–42. doi: 10.1074/jbc.M112.442954
29. Idrissova L, Malhi H, Werneburg NW, LeBrasseur NK, Bronk SF, Fingas C, et al. TRAIL receptor deletion in mice suppresses the inflammation of nutrient excess. *J Hepatol.* (2015) 62:1156–63. doi: 10.1016/j.jhep.2014.11.033
30. Bandla H, Dasgupta D, Mauer AS, Nozickova B, Kumar S, Hirsova P, et al. Deletion of endoplasmic reticulum stress-responsive co-chaperone p58(IPK) protects mice from diet-induced steatohepatitis. *Hepatol Res.* (2018) 48:479–94. doi: 10.1111/hepr.13052
31. Allende ML, Yamashita T, Proia RL. G-protein-coupled receptor S1P1 acts within endothelial cells to regulate vascular maturation. *Blood* (2003) 102:3665–7. doi: 10.1182/blood-2003-02-0460
32. Malhi H, Bronk SF, Werneburg NW, Gores GJ. Free fatty acids induce JNK-dependent hepatocyte lipoapoptosis. *J Biol Chem.* (2006) 281:12093–101. doi: 10.1074/jbc.M510660200
33. van der Pol E, Coumans FA, Grootemaat AE, Gardiner C, Sargent IL, Harrison P, et al. Particle size distribution of exosomes and microvesicles determined by transmission electron microscopy, flow cytometry, nanoparticle tracking analysis, and resistive pulse sensing. *J Thromb Haemost.* (2014) 12:1182–92. doi: 10.1111/jth.12602
34. Gao Y, Sun J, Lin WH, Webb D, Li D. A compact microfluidic gradient generator using passive pumping. *Microfluid Nanofluidics* (2012) 12:887–95. doi: 10.1007/s10404-011-0908-0
35. Li Jeon N, Baskaran H, Dertinger SK, Whitesides GM, Van de Water L, Toner M. Neutrophil chemotaxis in linear and complex gradients of interleukin-8 formed in a microfabricated device. *Nat Biotechnol.* (2002) 20:826–30. doi: 10.1038/nbt712
36. Machado MV, Diehl AM. Pathogenesis of nonalcoholic steatohepatitis. *Gastroenterology* (2016) 150:1769–77. doi: 10.1053/j.gastro.2016.02.066
37. Mizugishi K, Yamashita T, Olivera A, Miller GF, Spiegel S, Proia RL. Essential role for sphingosine kinases in neural and vascular development. *Mol Cell Biol.* (2005) 25:11113–21. doi: 10.1128/MCB.25.24.11113-11121.2005
38. Haddadi N, Lin Y, Simpson AM, Nassif NT, McGowan EM. "Dicing and splicing" sphingosine kinase and relevance to cancer. *Int J Mol Sci.* (2017) 18:E1891. doi: 10.3390/ijms18091891
39. Duong CQ, Bared SM, Abu-Khader A, Buechler C, Schmitz A, Schmitz G. Expression of the lysophospholipid receptor family and investigation of lysophospholipid-mediated responses in human macrophages. *Biochim Biophys Acta* (2004) 1682:112–9. doi: 10.1016/j.bbalip.2004.03.002

40. Charlton M, Krishnan A, Viker K, Sanderson S, Cazanave S, McConico A, et al. Fast food diet mouse: novel small animal model of NASH with ballooning, progressive fibrosis, and high physiological fidelity to the human condition. *Am J Physiol Gastrointest Liver Physiol.* (2011) 301:G825–34. doi: 10.1152/ajpgi.00145.2011
41. Malhi H, Gores GJ. Molecular mechanisms of lipotoxicity in nonalcoholic fatty liver disease. *Semin Liver Dis.* (2008) 28:360–9. doi: 10.1055/s-0028-1091980
42. Musso G, Gambino R, Cassader M. Cholesterol metabolism and the pathogenesis of non-alcoholic steatohepatitis. *Prog Lipid Res.* (2013) 52:175–91. doi: 10.1016/j.plipres.2012.11.002
43. Gault CR, Obeid LM, Hannun YA. An overview of sphingolipid metabolism: from synthesis to breakdown. *Adv Exp Med Biol.* (2010) 688:1–23. doi: 10.1007/978-1-4419-6741-1_1
44. Kakisaka K, Cazanave SC, Fingas CD, Guicciardi ME, Bronk SF, Werneburg NW, et al. Mechanisms of lysophosphatidylcholine-induced hepatocyte lipoapoptosis. *Am J Physiol Gastrointest Liver Physiol.* (2012) 302:G77–84. doi: 10.1152/ajpgi.00301.2011
45. Feldstein AE, Canbay A, Angulo P, Taniai M, Burgart LJ, Lindor KD, et al. Hepatocyte apoptosis and fas expression are prominent features of human nonalcoholic steatohepatitis. *Gastroenterology* (2003) 125:437–43. doi: 10.1016/S0016-5085(03)00907-7
46. Ribeiro PS, Cortez-Pinto H, Sola S, Castro RE, Ramalho RM, Baptista A, et al. Hepatocyte apoptosis, expression of death receptors, and activation of NF-kappaB in the liver of nonalcoholic and alcoholic steatohepatitis patients. *Am J Gastroenterol.* (2004) 99:1708–17. doi: 10.1111/j.1572-0241.2004.40009.x
47. Malhi H, Kaufman RJ. Endoplasmic reticulum stress in liver disease. *J Hepatol.* (2011) 54:795–809. doi: 10.1016/j.jhep.2010.11.005
48. Guicciardi ME, Gores GJ. Life and death by death receptors. *FASEB J.* (2009) 23:1625–37. doi: 10.1096/fj.08-111005
49. Fukushima M, Dasgupta D, Mauer AS, Kakazu E, Nakao K, Malhi H. StAR-related lipid transfer domain 11 (STARD11)-mediated ceramide transport mediates extracellular vesicle biogenesis. *J Biol Chem.* (2018) 293:15277–89. doi: 10.1074/jbc.RA118.002587
50. Royo F, Moreno L, Mleczko J, Palomo L, Gonzalez E, Cabrera D, et al. Hepatocyte-secreted extracellular vesicles modify blood metabolome and endothelial function by an arginase-dependent mechanism. *Sci Rep.* (2017) 7:42798. doi: 10.1038/srep42798
51. Royo F, Schlangen K, Palomo L, Gonzalez E, Conde-Vancells J, Berisa A, et al. Transcriptome of extracellular vesicles released by hepatocytes. *PLoS ONE* (2013) 8:e68693. doi: 10.1371/journal.pone.0068693
52. Hirsova P, Ibrahim SH, Krishnan A, Verma VK, Bronk SF, Werneburg NW, et al. Lipid-induced signaling causes release of inflammatory extracellular vesicles from hepatocytes. *Gastroenterology* (2016) 150:956–67. doi: 10.1053/j.gastro.2015.12.037
53. Povero D, Eguchi A, Niesman IR, Andronikou N, de Mollerat du Jeu X, Mulya A, et al. Lipid-induced toxicity stimulates hepatocytes to release angiogenic microparticles that require Vanin-1 for uptake by endothelial cells. *Sci Signal.* (2013) 6:ra88. doi: 10.1126/scisignal.2004512
54. Povero D, Panera N, Eguchi A, Johnson CD, Papouchado BG, de Araujo Horcel L, et al. Lipid-induced hepatocyte-derived extracellular vesicles regulate hepatic stellate cell via microRNAs targeting PPAR-gamma. *Cell Mol Gastroenterol Hepatol.* (2015) 1:646–63e4. doi: 10.1016/j.jcmgh.2015.07.007
55. Spiegel S, Milstien S. Sphingosine-1-phosphate: an enigmatic signalling lipid. *Nat Rev Mol Cell Biol.* (2003) 4:397–407. doi: 10.1038/nrm1103
56. Kihara Y, Maceyka M, Spiegel S, Chun J. Lysophospholipid receptor nomenclature review: IUPHAR Review 8. *Br J Pharmacol.* (2014) 171:3575–94. doi: 10.1111/bph.12678
57. Zachariah MA, Cyster JG. Neural crest-derived pericytes promote egress of mature thymocytes at the corticomedullary junction. *Science* (2010) 328:1129–35. doi: 10.1126/science.1188222
58. Rathinasamy A, Czeloth N, Pabst O, Forster R, Bernhardt G. The origin and maturity of dendritic cells determine the pattern of sphingosine 1-phosphate receptors expressed and required for efficient migration. *J Immunol.* (2010) 185:4072–81. doi: 10.4049/jimmunol.1000568
59. Hughes JE, Srinivasan S, Lynch KR, Proia RL, Ferdek P, Hedrick CC. Sphingosine-1-phosphate induces an antiinflammatory phenotype in macrophages. *Circ Res.* (2008) 102:950–8. doi: 10.1161/CIRCRESAHA.107.170779
60. Gude DR, Alvarez SE, Paugh SW, Mitra P, Yu J, Griffiths R, et al. Apoptosis induces expression of sphingosine kinase 1 to release sphingosine-1-phosphate as a "come-and-get-me" signal. *FASEB J.* (2008) 22:2629–38. doi: 10.1096/fj.08-107169
61. Jung H, Mithal DS, Park JE, Miller RJ. Localized CCR2 activation in the bone marrow niche mobilizes monocytes by desensitizing CXCR4. *PLoS ONE* (2015) 10:e0128387. doi: 10.1371/journal.pone.0128387

3

Liver, Tumor and Viral Hepatitis: Key Players in the Complex Balance Between Tolerance and Immune Activation

Matti Sällberg and Anna Pasetto*

Division of Clinical Microbiology, Department of Laboratory Medicine, Karolinska Institutet, Stockholm, Sweden

***Correspondence:**
Matti Sällberg
matti.sallberg@ki.se

Liver cancer is the third most common cause of cancer related death in the World. From an epidemiological point of view the risk factors associated to primary liver cancer are mainly viral hepatitis infection and alcohol consumption. Even though there is a clear correlation between liver inflammation, cirrhosis and cancer, other emerging liver diseases (like fatty liver) could also lead to liver cancer. Moreover, the liver is the major site of metastasis from colon, breast, ovarian and other cancers. In this review we will address the peculiar status of the liver as organ that has to balance between tolerance and immune activation. We will focus on macrophages and other key cellular components of the liver microenvironment that play a central role during tumor progression. We will also discuss how current and future therapies may affect the balance toward immune activation.

Keywords: liver, macrophage, T cell, T cell therapy, cancer

INTRODUCTION

The liver is a multi-tasking organ responsible for many crucial functions in the body. It is mostly known for its metabolic and detox work, in fact, it participates in the metabolism of fats (making bile), it stores and releases glucose and it clears harmful substances from the blood. The liver receives about 1.5 L of blood every minute coming from the digestive tract and its job is also to prevent and fight infections coming from the bloodstream. With such massive amount of blood, it is easy to imagine the countless potential antigens that the liver encounters at any given time. To prevent unnecessary inflammation and autoimmune disease the liver harbors different cellular components that work together with complex loops of interactions to maintain the organism homeostasis (1). Immune tolerance is therefore needed in the liver as safe measure to prevent tissue damage that would compromise the metabolic functions of this organ (2). The down side of this protective effect is that some infections, like viruses targeting hepatocytes (3) and even cancer have the possibility to escape the immune-response and give rise to potentially lethal liver diseases (4–7). A general view is that tolerance can be induced by both an insufficient/tolerogenic priming of effector T cells (8, 9) and directly through a regulatory T-cell response (10, 11). Kupffer cells, the specific tissue-resident macrophages of the liver, have a key role in promoting tolerance (12). This review will examine the major cellular components of the liver and tumor microenvironment, their role in controlling the balance between tolerance and activation and the potential therapeutic interventions to tilt the balance against liver cancer progression.

ANTIGEN PRESENTATION IN THE LIVER

Role of Kupffer Cells

Kupffer cells (KCs) are liver-resident macrophages, they originate from fetal liver-derived erythromyeloid progenitors and their population is maintained by self-renewal and not by infiltrating monocytes (**Figure 1**; 13, 14). KCs are located in the hepatic sinusoid as represented in **Figure 2**, where pathogens enter the liver via portal or arterial circulation (15). The KC population represent a first line defense against infectious particles and potentially immune reactive particles entering the blood stream from the gut (16, 17). KCs express several scavenger receptors (18) such as Toll-like, complement, antibody receptors which allow them to activate danger-associated molecular patterns and internalize, and kill pathogens (15, 19). They also contribute to the initiation of an innate immune response by secretion of cytokines and chemokines (20). The KCs have a potent phagocytic activity not only for the above-mentioned blood-born pathogens but also for other particles/complexes/debris originating from dead erythrocytes and cells of the hepatic parenchyma. Other functions of KCs are related to the iron (21), bilirubin (22) and cholesterol metabolism (23).

The role of KCs in antigen presentation has been considered to be limited based on experiments where isolated mouse KCs only induced a low T-cell proliferation against soluble antigens *in vitro* (24). Other experimental *in vivo* set-ups (12) showed that KC were able not only to phagocytize particle-bound antigens but also subsequently induce a tolerogenic T-cell response against those antigens. This could be measured by induction of local T-cell proliferation, expansion of Foxp3 + IL-10 + OTII T regs *in vivo*. A high level expression of PDL-1 and secretion of IL-10 by KCs strongly suggests that this cell type can present antigens to CD4+ T cells but then with the goal of inducing tolerance (12, 25).

It is important in this regard to keep in mind that KCs are not a homogenous population. As with other macrophage-like cells, two distinct subsets have been identified, one "M1 immunogenic" type that has phagocytic properties and secretes high levels of IL-12 and low levels of IL-10 (26) and another "M2 alternatively activated" type that secretes high levels of IL-10, TGF-b and low levels of IL-12 (27). When TLRs are engaged the KCs usually act as M2 type (28). When it comes to antigen presentation, several evidences implicate KCs as capable antigen presenting cells (APCs) but due to their up-regulation of inhibitory molecules like PD-L1 (29) and also Fas ligand (30) their major role is likely to be suppression T cell activation and induction of Tregs (10). The classification in M1 and M2 types is not exhaustive and does not reflect the complexity and diversity of functions among this cell population. Further subgrouping of the M2 type in M2a, M2b, and M2c has indeed been proposed. These subgroups express different markers and respond to different stimuli (17, 31). It is important to note that tumor-associated macrophages, which will be discussed later, have a M2 phenotype but a distinct transcriptional profile that promotes tumor angiogenesis (17, 32).

Antigen Presentation by Other Cell Types

A schematic representation of antigen presentation to CD4+ and CD8+ T cells is depicted in **Figure 3**. Kupffer cells are not the only cell type in the liver that function as APC but inducing tolerance instead of immune activation. Human hepatic myeloid dendritic cells (DC) (phenotypically characterized as CD11b+, CD11c+, and CD1c+) secrete IL-10 and induce IL-10 secretion by T cells (33) upon release by hepatic stromal cells of macrophage colony stimulating factor (34). Plasmacytoid DC (phenotypically characterized by expression of BDCA-2 and CD123) are also present in the liver and up-regulate PD-L1 in response to TLR agonists, promoting Treg cell differentiation (35, 36). Even though the liver APCs are skewed toward inducing tolerance there is also a population of myeloid DC (CD141+) that is able to cross-present antigen to CD8+ cells and induce IFN-g secretion (37, 38).

Other liver parenchymal cells also express MHC and costimulatory molecules and are capable of antigen presentation, although most of them still induce tolerance against the antigens presented. Endothelial cells, located at the liver sinusoids and termed liver sinusoidal endothelial cells (LSECs), promote tolerance in CD8+ T cells (39, 40) and lead CD4+ T cells toward Tregs differentiation (11) by secreting IL-10, TGF-b, PGE2 (41) and upregulating PD-L1 (42).

Hepatic stellate cells (HSCs) reside along the sinusoids and regulate the blood flow through these veins. HSCs can present antigens to T cells but again to promote Treg differentiation (43–45).

Lastly hepatocytes seem to be able to present antigens to CD8+ and CD4+ T cells but fail to sustain their proliferation and induce apoptosis instead (46, 47).

Viral Hepatitis Infection: Chronic Inflammation and Liver Cancer

The three major viruses responsible for viral hepatitis are the hepatitis B virus (HBV), the hepatitis C virus (HCV), and the hepatitis D virus (HDV), each estimated to be chronically infect 257 milion, 140 milion, and 15 milion people worldwide, respectively (48). While the viruses are quite different as HBV is a double stranded-DNA virus belonging to the Hepadnaviridae family, HCV is a single-stranded + RNA virus belonging to the Flaviviridae family, and HDV a single stranded circular -RNA viroid, they share common pathological paths. All viruses infect hepatocytes but are not directly cytolytic, the cell damage in fact is due to the anti-viral immune response, such as direct killing by cytotoxic CD8+ T cells or NK cells (49) or the action of inflammatory cytokines (50). During immune activation, liver resident APCs can activate virus-specific T cells which are then responsible for recognition and killing of infected hepatocytes and secretion of inflammatory cytokines (50). Acute hepatitis is associated with viral clearance in 95% of HBV infections in adults but only 5% of vertical infections, and in about (49). 25% of HCV infections For HDV, a satellite virus to HBV, acute infections occur when HBV and HDV coinfect a host (clearance rate is 95%), whereas most become chronically infected by HDV when appearing as a superinfection of HBV carriers. When viral

Cell type	Functions
Kupffer cells 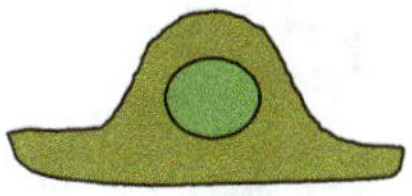	• High level of MHC and costimulatory molecules [7] • High level of PDL-1 and secretion of IL-10 [12, 25] • Not a homogenous population: "M1 immunogenic" type that has phagocytic properties and secretes high levels of IL-12 and low levels of IL-10 [26]; "M2 alternatively-activated" type secretes high levels of IL-10, TGF-b and low levels of IL-12 [27]. Further subgrouping ofthe M2 type in M2a, M2b and M2c has been proposed [17, 31]
Human hepatic myeloid dendritic cells (CD11b+, CD11c+ and CD1c+) 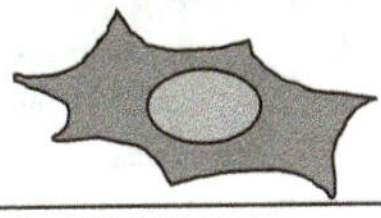	• Phenotype CD11b+, CD11c+ and CD1c+ • Secretion of IL-10 and induction of IL-10 secretion by T cells [33] upon release by hepatic stromal cells of macrophage colony stimulating factor [34]
Human hepatic myeloid dendritic cells (CD141+) 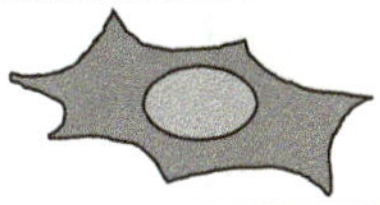	• Phenotype CD141+ • Antigen cross-presentation to CD8+ cells and induction of IFN-g secretion [37, 38]
Plasmacytoid dendritic cells (BDCA-2+ and CD123+) 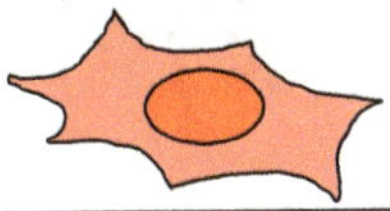	• Phenotype BDCA-2+ and CD123+ • Up-regulation of PD-L1 in response to TLR agonists, promoting Treg cell differentiation [35, 36]
Liver sinusoidal endothelial cells 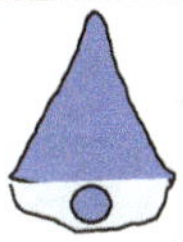	• Promote tolerance in CD8+ T cells [40, 41] • Lead CD4+ T cells toward Tregs differentiation [11] by secreting IL-10, TGF-b, PGE2 [42] and upregulating PD-L1 [43] • In the tumor have an accelerated cell cycle, greater migratory abilities and also secrete factors like IL-6, IL-8, MCP-1, GRO-a that can promote tumor progression and metastasis [51, 66, 67]
Hepatic stellate cells 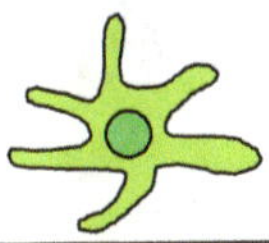	• Promote Treg differentiation [44-46] • Secretion of several soluble factors like cytokines (IL-6, IL-1B) [52], chemokines (CCL5, CCL21) [53] and growth factors (TGFa, TGFb, EGF, PDGF, bFGF) [54] • When activated HSCs can infiltrate in the HCC stroma [57] and promote tumor vascularization by secreting PDGF that attracts pericytes which also secrete VEGF [51, 58]
Hepatocytes 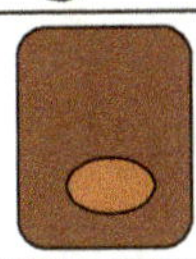	• Able to present antigens to CD8+ and CD4+ T cells butfail to sustain their proliferation and induce apoptosis instead [47, 48]
Cancer-associated fibroblasts 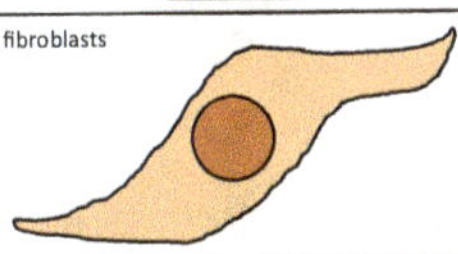	• Secretion of growth factors, cytokines and chemokines (e.g. EGF, FGF, HGF, TGFb, IL-6) that stimulate also tumor growth and proliferation [59], as well as a more malignant phenotype [60, 61] • Play an important role during HCC growth and metastasis [51, 62-64]
Tumor associated macrophages 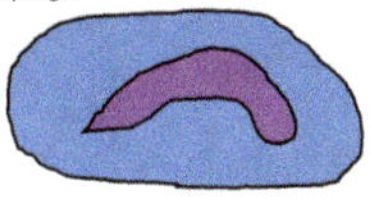	• Promote tumor initiation by secretion ofinflammatory molecules like IFN -g, TNF-a and IL-6 in response to chronic infection or irritation and this chronic inflammation [79] • Promote tumor progression and malignancy by switching to an immunosuppressive phenotype [78] • Supportthe metastatic process by promoting tumor cell migration and angiogenesis [78, 80-82]
Cytotoxic lymphocytes 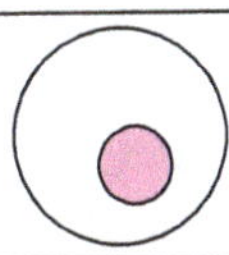	• Can kill tumor cells and recruite macrophages • An immune response against common tumor antigens has been identified from both TIL and blood of HCC patients [68]
Tregs 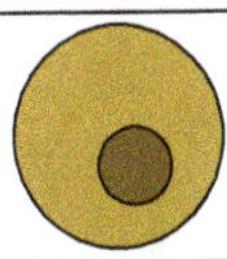	• Suppression ofimmune response by inhibiting CD8+ T cell effector functions like degranulation, and production of perforin and granzymes [70]
Mucosal-associated invariant T cells 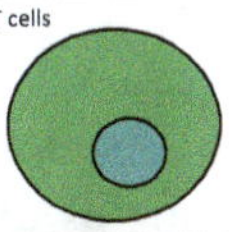	• Expression of cytokines [71] and other effector molecules [72] • Negatively affected by chronic viral hepatitis infection [73]
Natural Killer Cells 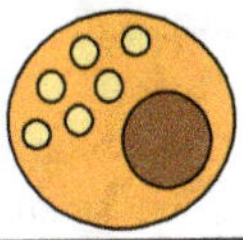	• Protective role in the liver especially during chronic viral hepatitis infection even though they are still functionally impaired by HBV and HCV [74]

FIGURE 1 | Key cellular components of liver tumor microenvironment. Schematic representation of cell types and summary of functions in tumor microenvironment.

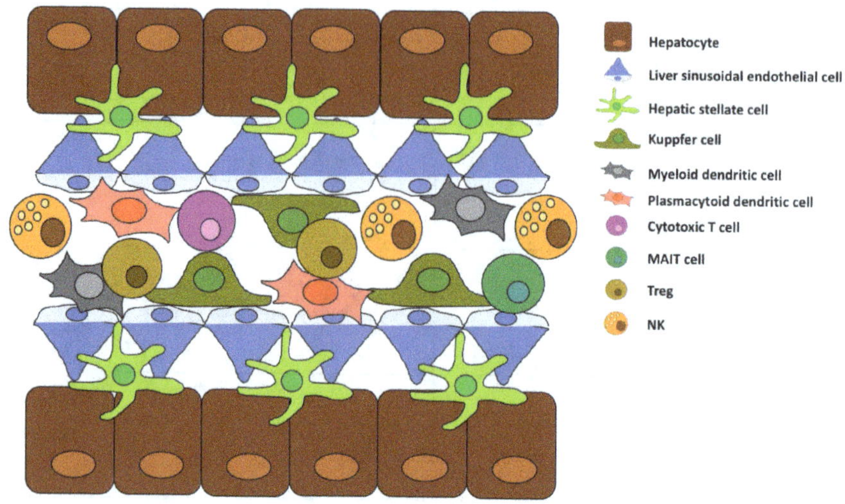

FIGURE 2 | Schematic structure of liver sinusoid. Key cell types and their spatial location are schematically represented.

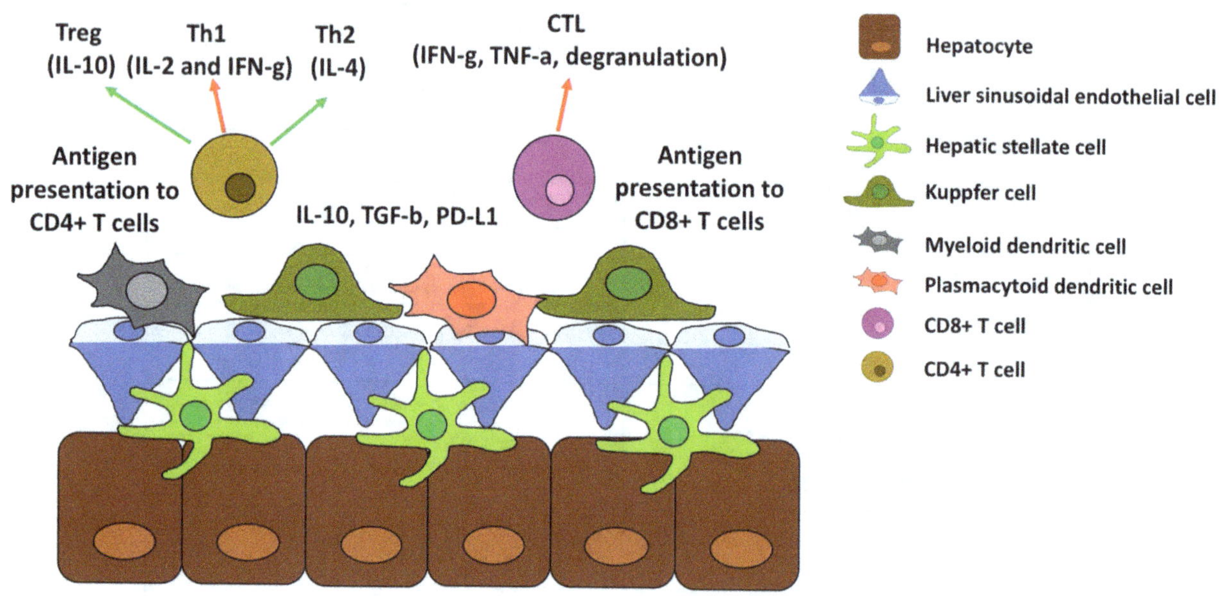

FIGURE 3 | Antigen presentation in the liver. Schematic representation of antigen presentation to CD4+ and CD8+ T cells and its effect toward tolerance (red arrows) or immune activation (green arrow).

clearance is not achieved and the virus is able to persist in the host, this is associated with a chronic inflammation of the liver that can lead to fibrosis, cirrhosis and also cancer. Thus, it is most likely that the persisting hepatic inflammation is the key driver for transformation of hepatocytes to cancer cells. The mechanisms of persistence differs for the different viruses, although a common strategy is to disturb and impair the host immune response. For HBV T cell tolerance, or dysfunction, is a key mechanism of persistence (51). In neonatal vertical infection, the high rate of chronicity is most likely explained by the immature immune response of the host in combination with overproduction of some HBV proteins. In particular one of these proteins is able to pass the placenta and thereby, when presented during schooling of the immunesystem, is perceived as self proteins (52, 53). Hence, these T cell clones are deleted. Other mechanisms of persistence used by HBV, are the constant presence of viral antigens causing immunactivation and then anergy or dysfunction. Finally, the over production and secretion of HBV surface antigen (HBsAg) particles mainly composed of small HBsAg, effectively blocks neutralizing anti-HBs antibodies. Thus, viral particles whose surface is mainly composed of PreS1 and PreS2 can escape these antibodies and infect new cells. Taken together, these factors most likely explain why HBV is able to persist, despite being a genetically stable virus. In contrast, several observations point to the fact that the higher rate of chronic infections due to HCV as compared to HBV is associated with the better ability of HCV to evade adaptive immunity (54–56), probably due to its extreme mutation rate (57). Thus, HCV persists as a virus constantly changing to evade both B and T cells. For HDV the mechanisms of persistence are less well known, except that HDV accelerates the tissue damage and disease during dual infection. Chronic hepatitis, regardless of the virus causing it, is characterized by a persistent presence of the viral antigens, which cause a continuous T cell stimulation. This chronic stimulation is regulated by immune checkpoint (i.e., expression of PD-1) that limit the effector functions of the virus-specific T cells resulting in a loop of low-grade inflammation and ineffective viral clearance (58, 59). Another important actor in the balance between immune activation and suppression are Tregs. Effective viral clearance is achieved through cytotoxicity that can be very dangerous if uncontrolled, or too massive. An excessive tissue damage needs to be prevented for the sake of host survival, and therefore the role of Tregs can be seen as a safe measure against fatal liver injury. Mouse studies modeling acute HBV infection observed an increased liver damage after Treg depletion (60), also HCV mouse models showed a transient peak of Tregs during acute infection, and a persistent increase in Tregs frequency in chronic infection (61). It is not yet clear wheather Tregs expansion is a cause or a consequence of chronic infection, but certainly this phenomenon is highlighting the complex interplay and immunological balance occurring in the liver during viral infection. The major long-term consequence of chronic infection is the occurrence of fibrosis and cirrhosis that impair liver functionality and also the insurgence of cancer. Treg expansion has been observed in samples of hepatocellular carcinomas (HCCs) and cirrhotic tissue (62). In this study (62), the expression of OX40 (a activation marker) correlates with intratumoral Treg frequency and other markers of proliferation like Ki67; OX40L on the other hand is expressed on myeloid liver infiltrating cells that co-localize with Tregs and directly correlates with HCV viral load. So this is an example of interplay between the host and the virus that is trying to escape the immune system by inducing Tregs via OX40L-OX40 interaction (63, 64).

PRIMARY TUMORS IN THE LIVER (HCC)

Hepatocellular carcinoma is one of the leading causes for cancer-related death in the world. HCC is mostly asymptomatic and the diagnosis is usually made at a late stage, whereby the prognosis generally is poor. Several risk factors have been identified for HCC, such as chronic viral hepatitis, excessive alcohol consumption, obesity, fatty liver, and diabetes (65). Although the presence of these risk factors aid in monitoring specific patient populations, the molecular mechanism(s) behind tumor initiation, progression, and metastasis are poorly understood and this poses a limitation to find efficient therapeutic approaches.

Hepatocellular carcinoma is associated with the dysregulated growth of hepatocytes that form dysplastic nodules resulting in chronic liver damage or cirrhosis. Mouse models have shown that the hepatocytes in this context have a higher expression of vimentin and type I collagen, suggesting that they are acquiring mesenchymal phenotype (66).

Although the specific mechanism has not been clarified, increasing evidence is pointing at the role of tumor microenvironment in HCC pathogenesis (67). In the following sections we will describe the main cellular components of the liver tumor microenvironment considering the primary tumor but also the metastatic deposits originated from other common tumor types like colon and breast cancer.

MAIN CELLULAR COMPONENTS OF THE TUMOR MICROENVIRONMENT

Hepatic Stellate Cells (HSCs)

A summary of cellular components of the tumor microenvironment is represented in **Figure 1**. These cells are part of the liver connective tissue and are located on the perisinusoidal space. HSCs have many homeostatic functions such as vitamin A accumulation, synthesis of collagen, expression of several soluble factors like cytokines (IL-6, IL-1B) (68), chemokines (CCL5, CCL21) (69), and growth factors (TGFa, TGFb, EGF, PDGF, and bFGF) (70). Liver damage can cause proliferation of HSCs and cytoskeleton remodeling (71, 72). When activated HSCs can infiltrate in the HCC stroma (73) and promote tumor vascularization by secreting PDGF that attracts pericytes which also secrete VEGF (67, 74).

Cancer-Associated Fibroblasts (CAFs)

This type of fibroblasts mediates several interactions between the tumor and the liver stroma. They secrete growth factors, cytokines and chemokines (e.g., EGF, FGF, HGF, TGFb, and IL-6) that stimulate also tumor growth and proliferation (75), as well as a more malignant phenotype (76, 77). Several evidences showed that CAFs play an important role during HCC growth and metastasis (67, 78–80).

Endothelial Cells

The main role of these cells is to promote tissue vascularization. The morphology of blood vessels is different in tumors compared to normal tissues, probably due to increased permeability, and this seems to be related to molecular and functional differences of epithelial cells (81). In particular, the endothelial cells present in the tumor have an accelerated cell cycle, greater migratory abilities and also secrete factors like IL-6, IL-8, MCP-1, and GRO-a that can promote tumor progression and metastasis (67, 82, 83).

Immune Cells

Tumor Infiltrating Lymphocytes (TILs)

Tumor Infiltrating Lymphocytes can play an important role for tumor progression, like Tregs, but can also be the source of powerful anti-tumor cells that can be used for therapy. An immune response against common tumor antigens has indeed been identified from both TIL and blood of HCC patients (84). The presence of Tregs in tumor is usually associated with a worse prognosis (85) since this cell type suppress the immune response by inhibiting CD8+ T cell effector functions like degranulation, and production of perforin and granzymes (86). Recent studies are also highlighting the importance of a mucosal-associated invariant T cell population (MAIT) that is able to activate and express cytokines (87) and other effector molecules (88), MAIT cells seem also to be negatively affected by chronic viral hepatitis infection (89).

Natural killer cells (NK) account for up to 50% of the total number of lymphocytes present in the liver. It has been shown that NK have a protective role in the liver especially during chronic viral hepatitis infection even though they are still functionally impaired by HBV and HCV (90). In HCC, it seems that the NK functionality is also impaired but the use of genetically modified NK cells in combination with kinase inhibitors has provided promising results by *in vivo* models (91, 92).

Tumor Associated Macrophages (TAMs)

Macrophages are frequently found in tumors and according to a high number of clinical and experimental data they seem to promote tumor initiation, progression and even metastasis (93, 94). The mechanism behind the contribution of macrophages to cancer initiation and progression seems to be caused at two major steps: initially macrophages secrete inflammatory molecules like IFN-g, TNF-a and IL-6 in response to chronic infection or irritation and this chronic inflammation seems to be causal to tumor initiation (95). Once the tumor is established, the macrophages switch to an immunosuppressive phenotype promoting progression and malignancy (94). Moreover, TAMs support the metastatic process by promoting tumor cell migration and angiogenesis (94, 96–98). In HCC a role of infiltrating monocytes and KCs seems to be to drive tumor progression and metastasis (99). The presence of TAMs is also associated with increase tumor burden an higher metastasis rate in both HCC patients and mouse models of liver cancer (100). In particular the ability of macrophages to secrete cytokines, chemokines and growth factors seems to be a crucial component of tumor initiation and proliferation (99, 101). KCs have a pro-inflammatory function that seems to be particularly important for HCC initiation (102). At later stages when the tumor is already established their ability to express PD-L1 and secrete immunosuppressive cytokines like IL-10 further contribute to promote tumor progression due to inhibition of effector lymphocytes like CD8+ T cells (14, 103, 104).

Microenvironment of Metastatic Deposits in the Liver

As already mentioned the liver receives a massive amount of blood which may help to explain the transport and hepatic entry of metastatic tumor cells coming from other organs of the body. The liver is indeed the main site of metastasis for several types of cancer, like colon, pancreas, melanoma, breast cancer, and sarcomas (105). The same cellular components that play an important role for tumor initiation and progression of primary liver cancer are also likely to be involved in facilitating the establishment of metastasis (106, 107). Another cell type that has been recently shown to be an important player for development of metastasis are marrow-derived immune cells recruited to the liver. A mouse model of metastatic pancreatic ductal adenocarcinoma revealed an interplay between the different cellular types in the liver that ultimately favored the metastatic deposit formation (108). In this model, tumor cells secrete exosomes that are taken up by KCs that then increase TGFb production affecting HSC that also increase fibronectin production with ultimate recruitment of bone marrow-derived macrophages. Another study found that exosomes from pancreatic cell lines able to metastasize in the liver, contain integrins that can fuse preferentially with KCs. These data also suggest that exosomes may have a role in disease progression and specific organ metastasis depending on the integrins that they contain (109). In general as a metastatic circulating cell survive the first line of defense offered by KCs and HSC (110), the liver milieu, rich of growth factors, proinflammatory molecule such as S100A8, and immune-suppressive cytokines, favors the formation of pre-metastatic niches (109, 111–114). In mouse models, NK cells are shown to play an important role in immune surveillance and prevention or delay of metastatic formation in the liver (115–117). Cancer cells are able to escape direct NK cytotoxicity by forming clusters with other cancer cells (118).

TARGETS FOR THERAPY: CAN WE TILT THE BALANCE?

As described above the level of complexity of the liver and liver-cancer microenvironment is very high. Due to the multiple cellular components, cytokines, chemokines, and physical disposition around the liver sinusoid, it is unlikely that one single approach could be able to break the vicious loop of inflammation, growth stimulation, and immune-tolerance that characterize the interplay between liver and cancer. Despite this, we believe that a combined approach of several therapies targeting different components of the tumor microenvironment may be effective. In the following sessions the available and potential future therapies for liver cancer are reviewed.

Target Microenvironment With Drugs

It is possible to specifically block the signaling pathways used by cancer cells to take advantage of the stroma cells and their growth stimulation (119). For HCC the two most studied pathways are the ones that promotes inflammation and angiogenesis (120). The only approved drug for advanced HCC is Sorafenib, a multi-kines inhibitor that target VEGFR, Raf-kinase and PDGFR, but unfortunately its efficacy is limited (121). Other drugs with similar mechanism of action are currently in experimental evaluation (122, 123).

Target Microenvironment With Physical Agents

One curative option for early stage HCC is ablative surgery. If the tumor is removed completely or the liver is transplanted there is a chance that the tumor will not come back. Most of patients are unfortunately diagnosed at a very late stage when surgical alternatives are not a possibility anymore (65). Common ablative procedures like radiation, cryoablation, and trans arterial chemoembolization (TACE) are also used at a late stage as palliative treatment. Physically destroying tumor cells may have the advantage to release tumor-antigens that can be taken-up by APCs and be cross-presented to T cells. Increased tumor-specific cytotoxicity has indeed been detected after this type of therapies (124–126). The potential side effect of this treatment is that the presence of PD-L1 on most of APCs in the liver could actually inhibit the tumor-specific T cell response (127) so one obvious measure would be to combine ablation therapy with PD-1 blockade treatment (128, 129). This is currently tested in various clinical trials.

Target Microenvironment With Immunotherapy

Immune suppression and tolerance are key factors in the induction, progression and metastasis of cancer in the liver. It is logical to assume that targeting the immune cells in the liver, reverting what cause their anergic state, may offer a solution for cancer treatment. Several immunotherapy trials have been conducted for HCC with cell therapy (LAK and TIL), cytokines and check-point inhibitors, dendritic cells vaccines and combinations of the above (129). The outcomes of these trials are promising but still not enough to offer a complete remission for HCC. Possibly, the particular microenvironment of the liver presents more challenges compared to other epithelial cancers that were successfully treated by adoptive cell therapy (130–134).

One current promising immunotherapeutic approach is the use of check-point inhibitors that target PD-1 and CTLA-4 promoting T cell activation (135). Recent clinical trials with the anti-PD-1 monoclonal antibodies Nivolumab showed promising anti-tumor activity in some patients with advanced HCC (136).

CONCLUSION

In this review we focused on the interplay within the liver between non-parechymal phagocytig and APCs, viruses, and liver cancer microenvironments. This highlights the complexity and intricate interplay of different factors. Due to the huge number of antigens going through the liver, the physiological need of having a "safe-guard" mechanism to prevent harmful immune-activation and liver damage is very understandable. The draw-back of this safe-guard mechanism is that pathogens like viruses or cancer, both primary and metastatic tumor cells, may establish and proliferate. We discussed some of the potential targets in the tumor microenvironment that can promote activation for the immune-system and potentially reverse the tolerance against cancer antigens. The milieu in the liver is highly complex and it is probably unrealistic to think that just a single "magic bullet" therapy could tilt the balance an mediate cure. It is most likely necessary to attack many or all the key players to effectively intervene with tumor progression. A combination of physical ablation, immunotherapy and other molecular drugs may indeed be needed.

One of the key components in the tumor microenvironments are TAMs. The biology of macrophages in general is very complex and to some extent still unknown. There are several evidences that suggest a different role of macrophage subgroups depending on their origin (e.g., fetal liver, bone marrow, etc.) and their location in the organism. What is clear is that they can have multiple, and sometimes opposite functions, that can influence clearance or disease progression. More research is needed to better understand the extent of their influence on tumor formation and progression.

AUTHOR CONTRIBUTIONS

All authors contributed to the conception and the writing of the review.

REFERENCES

1. Josefowicz SZ, Lu LF, Rudensky AY. Regulatory T cells: mechanisms of differentiation and function. *Annu Rev Immunol.* (2012) 30:531–64. doi: 10.1146/annurev.immunol.25.022106.141623
2. Medzhitov R, Schneider DS, Soares MP. Disease tolerance as a defense strategy. *Science.* (2012) 335:936–41. doi: 10.1126/science.1214935
3. Rehermann B. Pathogenesis of chronic viral hepatitis: differential roles of T cells and NK cells. *Nat Med.* (2013) 19:859–68. doi: 10.1038/nm.3251
4. Racanelli V, Rehermann B. The liver as an immunological organ. *Hepatology.* (2006) 43(2 Suppl. 1):S54–62.
5. Tiegs G, Lohse AW. Immune tolerance: what is unique about the liver. *J Autoimmun.* (2010) 34:1–6. doi: 10.1016/j.jaut.2009.08.008
6. Crispe IN. Immune tolerance in liver disease. *Hepatology.* (2014) 60:2109–17. doi: 10.1002/hep.27254
7. Doherty DG. Immunity, tolerance and autoimmunity in the liver: a comprehensive review. *J Autoimmun.* (2016) 66:60–75. doi: 10.1016/j.jaut.2015.08.020
8. Schurich A, Berg M, Stabenow D, Böttcher J, Kern M, Schild HJ, et al. Dynamic regulation of CD8 T cell tolerance induction by liver sinusoidal endothelial cells. *J Immunol.* (2010) 184:4107–14. doi: 10.4049/jimmunol.0902580
9. Tay SS, Lu B, Sierro F, Benseler V, McGuffog CM, Bishop GA, et al. Differential migration of passenger leukocytes and rapid deletion of naive alloreactive CD8 T cells after mouse liver transplantation. *Liver Transpl.* (2013) 19:1224–35. doi: 10.1002/lt.23720
10. Breous E, Somanathan S, Vandenberghe LH, Wilson JM. Hepatic regulatory T cells and Kupffer cells are crucial mediators of systemic T cell tolerance to antigens targeting murine liver. *Hepatology.* (2009) 50:612–21. doi: 10.1002/hep.23043
11. Kruse N, Neumann K, Schrage A, Derkow K, Schott E, Erben U, et al. Priming of CD4+ T cells by liver sinusoidal endothelial cells induces CD25low forkhead box protein 3- regulatory T cells suppressing autoimmune hepatitis. *Hepatology.* (2009) 50:1904–13. doi: 10.1002/hep.23191
12. Heymann F, Peusquens J, Ludwig-Portugall I, Kohlhepp M, Ergen C, Niemietz P, et al. Liver inflammation abrogates immunological tolerance induced by Kupffer cells. *Hepatology.* (2015) 62:279–91. doi: 10.1002/hep.27793
13. Gomez Perdiguero E, Klapproth K, Schulz C, Busch K, Azzoni E, Crozet L, et al. Tissue-resident macrophages originate from yolk-sac-derived erythro-myeloid progenitors. *Nature.* (2015) 518:547–51. doi: 10.1038/nature13989
14. Krenkel O, Tacke F. Liver macrophages in tissue homeostasis and disease. *Nat Rev Immunol.* (2017) 17:306–21.
15. Jenne CN, Kubes P. Immune surveillance by the liver. *Nat Immunol.* (2013) 14:996–1006. doi: 10.1038/ni.2691
16. Thomson AW, Knolle PA. Antigen-presenting cell function in the tolerogenic liver environment. *Nat Rev Immunol.* (2010) 10:753–66. doi: 10.1038/nri2858
17. Dixon LJ, Barnes M, Tang H, Pritchard MT, Nagy LE. Kupffer cells in the liver. *Compr Physiol.* (2013) 3:785–97.
18. Eckert C, Klein N, Kornek M, Lukacs-Kornek V. The complex myeloid network of the liver with diverse functional capacity at steady state and in

inflammation. *Front Immunol.* (2015) 6:179. doi: 10.3389/fimmu.2015.00179
19. Tu Z, Bozorgzadeh A, Pierce RH, Kurtis J, Crispe IN, Orloff MS. TLR-dependent cross talk between human Kupffer cells and NK cells. *J Exp Med.* (2008) 205:233–44. doi: 10.1084/jem.20072195
20. Tacke F, Zimmermann HW. Macrophage heterogeneity in liver injury and fibrosis. *J Hepatol.* (2014) 60:1090–6. doi: 10.1016/j.jhep.2013.12.025
21. Gammella E, Buratti P, Cairo G, Recalcati S. Macrophages: central regulators of iron balance. *Metallomics.* (2014) 6:1336–45. doi: 10.1039/c4mt00104d
22. Naito M, Hasegawa G, Ebe Y, Yamamoto T. Differentiation and function of Kupffer cells. *Med Electron Microsc.* (2004) 37:16–28. doi: 10.1007/s00795-003-0228-x
23. Wang Y, van der Tuin S, Tjeerdema N, van Dam AD, Rensen SS, Hendrikx T, et al. Plasma cholesteryl ester transfer protein is predominantly derived from Kupffer cells. *Hepatology.* (2015) 62:1710–22. doi: 10.1002/hep.27985
24. You Q, Cheng L, Kedl RM, Ju C. Mechanism of T cell tolerance induction by murine hepatic Kupffer cells. *Hepatology.* (2008) 48:978–90. doi: 10.1002/hep.22395
25. Erhardt A, Biburger M, Papadopoulos T, Tiegs G. IL-10, regulatory T cells, and Kupffer cells mediate tolerance in concanavalin a-induced liver injury in mice. *Hepatology.* (2007) 45:475–85.
26. Kinoshita M, Uchida T, Sato A, Nakashima M, Nakashima H, Shono S, et al. Characterization of two F4/80-positive Kupffer cell subsets by their function and phenotype in mice. *J Hepatol.* (2010) 53:903–10. doi: 10.1016/j.jhep.2010.04.037
27. Davies LC, Jenkins SJ, Allen JE, Taylor PR. Tissue-resident macrophages. *Nat Immunol.* (2013) 14:986–95. doi: 10.1038/ni.2705
28. Zhang M, Xu S, Han Y, Cao X. Apoptotic cells attenuate fulminant hepatitis by priming Kupffer cells to produce interleukin-10 through membrane-bound TGF-beta. *Hepatology.* (2011) 53:306–16. doi: 10.1002/hep.24029
29. Wu K, Kryczek I, Chen L, Zou W, Welling TH. Kupffer cell suppression of CD8+ T cells in human hepatocellular carcinoma is mediated by B7-H1/programmed death-1 interactions. *Cancer Res.* (2009) 69:8067–75. doi: 10.1158/0008-5472.CAN-09-0901
30. Sun Z, Wada T, Maemura K, Uchikura K, Hoshino S, Diehl AM, et al. Hepatic allograft-derived Kupffer cells regulate T cell response in rats. *Liver Transpl.* (2003) 9:489–97.
31. Mosser DM, Edwards JP. Exploring the full spectrum of macrophage activation. *Nat Rev Immunol.* (2008) 8:958–69. doi: 10.3389/fpls.2013.00334
32. Lawrence T, Natoli G. Transcriptional regulation of macrophage polarization: enabling diversity with identity. *Nat Rev Immunol.* (2011) 11:750–61. doi: 10.1038/nri3088
33. Bamboat ZM, Stableford JA, Plitas G, Burt BM, Nguyen HM, Welles AP, et al. Human liver dendritic cells promote T cell hyporesponsiveness. *J Immunol.* (2009) 182:1901–11. doi: 10.4049/jimmunol.0803404
34. Xia S, Guo Z, Xu X, Yi H, Wang Q, Cao X. Hepatic microenvironment programs hematopoietic progenitor differentiation into regulatory dendritic cells, maintaining liver tolerance. *Blood.* (2008) 112:3175–85. doi: 10.1182/blood-2008-05-159921
35. Moseman EA, Liang X, Dawson AJ, Panoskaltsis-Mortari A, Krieg AM, Liu YJ, et al. Human plasmacytoid dendritic cells activated by CpG oligodeoxynucleotides induce the generation of CD4+CD25+ regulatory T cells. *J Immunol.* (2004) 173:4433–42.
36. Castellaneta A, Sumpter TL, Chen L, Tokita D, Thomson AW. NOD2 ligation subverts IFN-alpha production by liver plasmacytoid dendritic cells and inhibits their T cell allostimulatory activity via B7-H1 up-regulation. *J Immunol.* (2009) 183:6922–32. doi: 10.4049/jimmunol.0900582
37. Haniffa M, Shin A, Bigley V, McGovern N, Teo P, See P, et al. Human tissues contain CD141hi cross-presenting dendritic cells with functional homology to mouse CD103+ nonlymphoid dendritic cells. *Immunity.* (2012) 37:60–73. doi: 10.1016/j.immuni.2012.04.012
38. Kelly A, Fahey R, Fletcher JM, Keogh C, Carroll AG, Siddachari R, et al. CD141(+) myeloid dendritic cells are enriched in healthy human liver. *J Hepatol.* (2014) 60:135–42. doi: 10.1016/j.jhep.2013.08.007
39. Limmer A, Ohl J, Kurts C, Ljunggren HG, Reiss Y, Groettrup M, et al. Efficient presentation of exogenous antigen by liver endothelial cells to CD8+ T cells results in antigen-specific T-cell tolerance. *Nat Med.* (2000) 6:1348–54.
40. von Oppen N, Schurich A, Hegenbarth S, Stabenow D, Tolba R, Weiskirchen R, et al. Systemic antigen cross-presented by liver sinusoidal endothelial cells induces liver-specific CD8 T-cell retention and tolerization. *Hepatology.* (2009) 49:1664–72. doi: 10.1002/hep.22795
41. Uhrig A, Banafsche R, Kremer M, Hegenbarth S, Hamann A, Neurath M, et al. Development and functional consequences of LPS tolerance in sinusoidal endothelial cells of the liver. *J Leukoc Biol.* (2005) 77:626–33.
42. Diehl L, Schurich A, Grochtmann R, Hegenbarth S, Chen L, Knolle PA. Tolerogenic maturation of liver sinusoidal endothelial cells promotes B7-homolog 1-dependent CD8+ T cell tolerance. *Hepatology.* (2008) 47:296–305. doi: 10.1002/hep.21965
43. Charles R, Chou HS, Wang L, Fung JJ, Lu L, Qian S. Human hepatic stellate cells inhibit T-cell response through B7-H1 pathway. *Transplantation.* (2013) 96:17–24. doi: 10.1097/TP.0b013e318294caae
44. Jiang G, Yang HR, Wang L, Wildey GM, Fung J, Qian S, et al. Hepatic stellate cells preferentially expand allogeneic CD4+ CD25+ FoxP3+ regulatory T cells in an IL-2-dependent manner. *Transplantation.* (2008) 86:1492–502. doi: 10.1097/TP.0b013e31818bfd13
45. Yang HR, Chou HS, Gu X, Wang L, Brown KE, Fung JJ, et al. Mechanistic insights into immunomodulation by hepatic stellate cells in mice: a critical role of interferon-gamma signaling. *Hepatology.* (2009) 50:1981–91. doi: 10.1002/hep.23202
46. Bertolino P, Trescol-Biemont MC, Rabourdin-Combe C. Hepatocytes induce functional activation of naive CD8+ T lymphocytes but fail to promote survival. *Eur J Immunol.* (1998) 28:221–36.
47. Qian S, Wang Z, Lee Y, Chiang Y, Bonham C, Fung J. Hepatocyte-induced apoptosis of activated T cells, a mechanism of liver transplant tolerance, is related to the expression of ICAM-1 and hepatic lectin. *Transplant Proc.* (2001) 33:226. doi: 10.1016/s0041-1345(00)01985-0
48. Lanini S, Pisapia R, Capobianchi MR, Ippolito G. Global epidemiology of viral hepatitis and national needs for complete control. *Expert Rev Anti Infect Ther.* (2018) 16:625–39. doi: 10.1080/14787210.2018.1505503
49. Shin EC, Sung PS, Park SH. Immune responses and immunopathology in acute and chronic viral hepatitis. *Nat Rev Immunol.* (2016) 16:509–23. doi: 10.1038/nri.2016.69
50. Guidotti LG, Inverso D, Sironi L, Di Lucia P, Fioravanti J, Ganzer L, et al. Immunosurveillance of the liver by intravascular effector CD8(+) T cells. *Cell.* (2015) 161:486–500. doi: 10.1016/j.cell.2015.03.005
51. Park JJ, Wong DK, Wahed AS, Lee WM, Feld JJ, Terrault N, et al. Hepatitis B virus–specific and global T-Cell dysfunction in chronic hepatitis B. Gastroenterology. (2016) 150:684–95.e5. doi: 10.1053/j.gastro.2015.11.050
52. Chen MT, Billaud JN, Sällberg M, Guidotti LG, Chisari FV, Jones J, et al. A function of the hepatitis B virus precore protein is to regulate the immune response to the core antigen. *Proc Natl Acad Sci USA.* (2004) 101:14913–8.
53. Chen M, Sällberg M, Hughes J, Jones J, Guidotti LG, Chisari FV, et al. Immune tolerance split between hepatitis B virus precore and core proteins. *J Virol.* (2005) 79:3016–27.
54. Mutz P, Metz P, Lempp FA, Bender S, Qu B, Schöneweis K, et al. HBV bypasses the innate immune response and does not protect HCV from antiviral activity of interferon. *Gastroenterology.* (2018) 154:1791–804.e22. doi: 10.1053/j.gastro.2018.01.044
55. Tan A, Koh S, Bertoletti A. Immune response in hepatitis B virus infection. *Cold Spring Harb Perspect Med.* (2015) 5:a021428. doi: 10.1101/cshperspect.a021428
56. Chen SL, Morgan TR. The natural history of hepatitis C virus (HCV) infection. *Int J Med Sci.* (2006) 3:47–52. doi: 10.7150/ijms.3.47
57. Lazarevic I. Clinical implications of hepatitis B virus mutations: recent advances. *World J Gastroenterol.* (2014) 20:7653–64. doi: 10.3748/wjg.v20.i24.7653
58. Barnaba V. Hepatitis C virus infection: a "liaison a trois" amongst the virus, the host, and chronic low-level inflammation for human survival. *J Hepatol.* (2010) 53:752–61. doi: 10.1016/j.jhep.2010.06.003
59. Guidotti LG, Isogawa M, Chisari FV. Host-virus interactions in hepatitis B virus infection. *Curr Opin Immunol.* (2015) 36:61–6. doi: 10.1016/j.coi.2015.06.016
60. Stross L, Günther J, Gasteiger G, Asen T, Graf S, Aichler M, et al. Foxp3+ regulatory T cells protect the liver from immune damage and compromise virus control during acute experimental hepatitis B virus infection in mice. *Hepatology.* (2012) 56:873–83. doi: 10.1002/hep.25765

61. Billerbeck E, Wolfisberg R, Fahnøe U, Xiao JW, Quirk C, Luna JM, et al. Mouse models of acute and chronic hepacivirus infection. *Science.* (2017) 357:204–8. doi: 10.1126/science.aal1962
62. Piconese S, Timperi E, Pacella I, Schinzari V, Tripodo C, Rossi M, et al. Human OX40 tunes the function of regulatory T cells in tumor and nontumor areas of hepatitis C virus-infected liver tissue. *Hepatology.* (2014) 60:1494–507. doi: 10.1002/hep.27188
63. Zhang JY, Wu XL, Yang B, Wang Y, Feng GH, Jiang TJ, et al. Upregulation of OX40 ligand on monocytes contributes to early virological control in patients with chronic hepatitis C. *Eur J Immunol.* (2013) 43:1953–62. doi: 10.1002/eji.201243097
64. Pollmann J, Götz JJ, Rupp D, Strauss O, Granzin M, Grünvogel O, et al. Hepatitis C virus-induced natural killer cell proliferation involves monocyte-derived cells and the OX40/OX40L axis. *J Hepatol.* (2018) 68:421–30. doi: 10.1016/j.jhep.2017.10.021
65. El-Serag HB. Hepatocellular carcinoma. *N Engl J Med.* (2011) 365:1118–27.
66. Nitta T, Kim JS, Mohuczy D, Behrns KE. Murine cirrhosis induces hepatocyte epithelial mesenchymal transition and alterations in survival signaling pathways. *Hepatology.* (2008) 48:909–19. doi: 10.1002/hep.22397
67. Novikova MV, Khromova NV, Kopnin PB. Components of the hepatocellular carcinoma microenvironment and their role in tumor progression. *Biochemistry (Mosc).* (2017) 82:861–73.
68. Marra F. Chemokines in liver inflammation and fibrosis. *Front Biosci.* (2002) 7:d1899–914. doi: 10.2741/marra
69. Schwabe RF, Bataller R, Brenner DA. Human hepatic stellate cells express CCR5 and RANTES to induce proliferation and migration. *Am J Physiol Gastrointest Liver Physiol.* (2003) 285:G949–58.
70. Pinzani M, Marra F, Carloni V. Signal transduction in hepatic stellate cells. *Liver.* (1998) 18:2–13. doi: 10.1111/j.1600-0676.1998.tb00120.x
71. Friedman SL. Hepatic stellate cells: protean, multifunctional, and enigmatic cells of the liver. *Physiol Rev.* (2008) 88:125–72. doi: 10.1152/physrev.00013.2007
72. Kluwe J, Pradere JP, Gwak GY, Mencin A, De Minicis S, Osterreicher CH, et al. Modulation of hepatic fibrosis by c-Jun-N-terminal kinase inhibition. *Gastroenterology.* (2010) 138:347–59. doi: 10.1053/j.gastro.2009.09.015
73. Wynn TA. Cellular and molecular mechanisms of fibrosis. *J Pathol.* (2008) 214:199–210.
74. Bergers G, Song S. The role of pericytes in blood-vessel formation and maintenance. *Neuro Oncol.* (2005) 7:452–64.
75. Pietras K, Ostman A. Hallmarks of cancer: interactions with the tumor stroma. *Exp Cell Res.* (2010) 316:1324–31. doi: 10.1016/j.yexcr.2010.02.045
76. Jia CC, Wang TT, Liu W, Fu BS, Hua X, Wang GY, et al. Cancer-associated fibroblasts from hepatocellular carcinoma promote malignant cell proliferation by HGF secretion. *PLoS One.* (2013) 8:e63243. doi: 10.1371/journal.pone.0063243
77. Liu F, Zhang W, Yang F, Feng T, Zhou M, Yu Y, et al. Interleukin-6-stimulated progranulin expression contributes to the malignancy of hepatocellular carcinoma cells by activating mTOR signaling. *Sci Rep.* (2016) 6:21260. doi: 10.1038/srep21260
78. Mazzocca A, Dituri F, Lupo L, Quaranta M, Antonaci S, Giannelli G. Tumor-secreted lysophostatidic acid accelerates hepatocellular carcinoma progression by promoting differentiation of peritumoral fibroblasts in myofibroblasts. *Hepatology.* (2011) 54:920–30. doi: 10.1002/hep.24485
79. Gaggioli C, Hooper S, Hidalgo-Carcedo C, Grosse R, Marshall JF, Harrington K, et al. Fibroblast-led collective invasion of carcinoma cells with differing roles for RhoGTPases in leading and following cells. *Nat Cell Biol.* (2007) 9:1392–400.
80. Fransvea E, Mazzocca A, Antonaci S, Giannelli G. Targeting transforming growth factor (TGF)-betaRI inhibits activation of beta1 integrin and blocks vascular invasion in hepatocellular carcinoma. *Hepatology.* (2009) 49:839–50. doi: 10.1002/hep.22731
81. Baluk P, Morikawa S, Haskell A, Mancuso M, McDonald DM. Abnormalities of basement membrane on blood vessels and endothelial sprouts in tumors. *Am J Pathol.* (2003) 163:1801–15.
82. Benetti A, Berenzi A, Gambarotti M, Garrafa E, Gelati M, Dessy E, et al. Transforming growth factor-beta1 and CD105 promote the migration of hepatocellular carcinoma-derived endothelium. *Cancer Res.* (2008) 68:8626–34. doi: 10.1158/0008-5472.CAN-08-1218
83. Knipe L, Meli A, Hewlett L, Bierings R, Dempster J, Skehel P, et al. A revised model for the secretion of tPA and cytokines from cultured endothelial cells. *Blood.* (2010) 116:2183–91. doi: 10.1182/blood-2010-03-276170
84. Flecken T, Schmidt N, Hild S, Gostick E, Drognitz O, Zeiser R, et al. Immunodominance and functional alterations of tumor-associated antigen-specific CD8+ T-cell responses in hepatocellular carcinoma. *Hepatology.* (2014) 59:1415–26. doi: 10.1002/hep.26731
85. Gao Q, Qiu SJ, Fan J, Zhou J, Wang XY, Xiao YS, et al. Intratumoral balance of regulatory and cytotoxic T cells is associated with prognosis of hepatocellular carcinoma after resection. *J Clin Oncol.* (2007) 25:2586–93.
86. Chen W, Jin W, Hardegen N, Lei KJ, Li L, Marinos N, et al. Conversion of peripheral CD4+CD25- naive T cells to CD4+CD25+ regulatory T cells by TGF-beta induction of transcription factor Foxp3. *J Exp Med.* (2003) 198:1875–86.
87. Sobkowiak MJ, Davanian H, Heymann R, Gibbs A, Emgård J, Dias J, et al. Tissue-resident MAIT cell populations in human oral mucosa exhibit an activated profile and produce IL-17. *Eur J Immunol.* (2019) 49:133–43. doi: 10.1002/eji.201847759
88. Sundström P, Szeponik L, Ahlmanner F, Sundquist M, Wong JSB, Lindskog EB, et al. Tumor-infiltrating mucosal-associated invariant T (MAIT) cells retain expression of cytotoxic effector molecules. *Oncotarget.* (2019) 10:2810–23. doi: 10.18632/oncotarget.26866
89. Dias J, Hengst J, Parrot T, Leeansyah E, Lunemann S, Malone DFG, et al. Chronic hepatitis delta virus infection leads to functional impairment and severe loss of MAIT cells. *J Hepatol.* (2019) 71:301–12. doi: 10.1016/j.jhep.2019.04.009
90. Sun C, Sun HY, Xiao WH, Zhang C, Tian ZG. Natural killer cell dysfunction in hepatocellular carcinoma and NK cell-based immunotherapy. *Acta Pharmacol Sin.* (2015) 36:1191–9. doi: 10.1038/aps.2015.41
91. Kamiya T, Chang YH, Campana D. Expanded and activated natural killer cells for immunotherapy of hepatocellular carcinoma. *Cancer Immunol Res.* (2016) 4:574–81. doi: 10.1158/2326-6066.CIR-15-0229
92. Hong ZF, Zhao WX, Yin ZY, Xie CR, Xu YP, Chi XQ, et al. Natural killer cells inhibit pulmonary metastasis of hepatocellular carcinoma in nude mice. *Oncol Lett.* (2016) 11:2019–26.
93. Sica A, Mantovani A. Macrophage plasticity and polarization: in vivo veritas. *J Clin Invest.* (2012) 122:787–95. doi: 10.1172/JCI59643
94. Qian BZ, Pollard JW. Macrophage diversity enhances tumor progression and metastasis. *Cell.* (2010) 141:39–51. doi: 10.1016/j.cell.2010.03.014
95. Balkwill FR, Mantovani A. Cancer-related inflammation: common themes and therapeutic opportunities. *Semin Cancer Biol.* (2012) 22:33–40. doi: 10.1016/j.semcancer.2011.12.005
96. DeNardo DG, Andreu P, Coussens LM. Interactions between lymphocytes and myeloid cells regulate pro- versus anti-tumor immunity. *Cancer Metastasis Rev.* (2010) 29:309–16. doi: 10.1007/s10555-010-9223-6
97. Hanahan D, Coussens LM. Accessories to the crime: functions of cells recruited to the tumor microenvironment. *Cancer Cell.* (2012) 21:309–22. doi: 10.1016/j.ccr.2012.02.022
98. Wynn TA, Chawla A, Pollard JW. Macrophage biology in development, homeostasis and disease. *Nature.* (2013) 496:445–55. doi: 10.1038/nature12034
99. Ju C, Tacke F. Hepatic macrophages in homeostasis and liver diseases: from pathogenesis to novel therapeutic strategies. *Cell Mol Immunol.* (2016) 13:316–27. doi: 10.1038/cmi.2015.104
100. Medina-Echeverz J, Eggert T, Han M, Greten TF. Hepatic myeloid-derived suppressor cells in cancer. *Cancer Immunol Immunother.* (2015) 64:931–40. doi: 10.1007/s00262-015-1736-y
101. Wan S, Kuo N, Kryczek I, Zou W, Welling TH. Myeloid cells in hepatocellular carcinoma. *Hepatology.* (2015) 62:1304–12. doi: 10.1002/hep.27867
102. Wu J, Li J, Salcedo R, Mivechi NF, Trinchieri G, Horuzsko A. The proinflammatory myeloid cell receptor TREM-1 controls Kupffer cell activation and development of hepatocellular carcinoma. *Cancer Res.* (2012) 72:3977–86. doi: 10.1158/0008-5472.CAN-12-0938
103. Eggert T, Wolter K, Ji J, Ma C, Yevsa T, Klotz S, et al. Distinct functions of senescence-associated immune responses in liver tumor surveillance and tumor progression. *Cancer Cell.* (2016) 30:533–47. doi: 10.1016/j.ccell.2016.09.003
104. Makarova-Rusher OV, Medina-Echeverz J, Duffy AG, Greten TF. The yin and yang of evasion and immune activation in HCC. *J Hepatol.* (2015) 62:1420–9. doi: 10.1016/j.jhep.2015.02.038
105. Hess KR, Varadhachary GR, Taylor SH, Wei W, Raber MN, Lenzi R, et al. Metastatic patterns in adenocarcinoma. *Cancer.* (2006) 106:1624–33.

106. Kmiec Z. Cooperation of liver cells in health and disease. *Adv Anat Embryol Cell Biol.* (2001) 161:1–151.
107. Smedsrød B, Le Couteur D, Ikejima K, Jaeschke H, Kawada N, Naito M, et al. Hepatic sinusoidal cells in health and disease: update from the 14th International Symposium. *Liver Int.* (2009) 29:490–501. doi: 10.1111/j.1478-3231.2009.01979.x
108. Costa-Silva B, Aiello NM, Ocean AJ, Singh S, Zhang H, Thakur BK, et al. Pancreatic cancer exosomes initiate pre-metastatic niche formation in the liver. *Nat Cell Biol.* (2015) 17:816–26.
109. Hoshino A, Costa-Silva B, Shen TL, Rodrigues G, Hashimoto A, Tesic Mark M, et al. Tumour exosome integrins determine organotropic metastasis. *Nature.* (2015) 527:329–35. doi: 10.1038/nature15756
110. Braet F, Nagatsuma K, Saito M, Soon L, Wisse E, Matsuura T. The hepatic sinusoidal endothelial lining and colorectal liver metastases. *World J Gastroenterol.* (2007) 13:821–5.
111. Kowanetz M, Wu X, Lee J, Tan M, Hagenbeek T, Qu X, et al. Granulocyte-colony stimulating factor promotes lung metastasis through mobilization of Ly6G+Ly6C+ granulocytes. *Proc Natl Acad Sci USA.* (2010) 107:21248–55. doi: 10.1073/pnas.1015855107
112. Seubert B, Grünwald B, Kobuch J, Cui H, Schelter F, Schaten S, et al. Tissue inhibitor of metalloproteinases (TIMP)-1 creates a premetastatic niche in the liver through SDF-1/CXCR4-dependent neutrophil recruitment in mice. *Hepatology.* (2015) 61:238–48. doi: 10.1002/hep.27378
113. Zhang Y, Davis C, Ryan J, Janney C, Peña MM. Development and characterization of a reliable mouse model of colorectal cancer metastasis to the liver. *Clin Exp Metastasis.* (2013) 30:903–18. doi: 10.1007/s10585-013-9591-8
114. Brodt P. Role of the microenvironment in liver metastasis: from pre- to prometastatic niches. *Clin Cancer Res.* (2016) 22:5971–82.
115. Bertin S, Neves S, Gavelli A, Baqué P, Brossette N, Simões S, et al. Cellular and molecular events associated with the antitumor response induced by the cytosine deaminase/5-fluorocytosine suicide gene therapy system in a rat liver metastasis model. *Cancer Gene Ther.* (2007) 14:858–66.
116. Takehara T, Uemura A, Tatsumi T, Suzuki T, Kimura R, Shiotani A, et al. Natural killer cell-mediated ablation of metastatic liver tumors by hydrodynamic injection of IFNalpha gene to mice. *Int J Cancer.* (2007) 120:1252–60.
117. Tatsumi T, Takehara T, Yamaguchi S, Sasakawa A, Miyagi T, Jinushi M, et al. Injection of IL-12 gene-transduced dendritic cells into mouse liver tumor lesions activates both innate and acquired immunity. *Gene Ther.* (2007) 14:863–71.
118. Paschos KA, Majeed AW, Bird NC. Natural history of hepatic metastases from colorectal cancer–pathobiological pathways with clinical significance. *World J Gastroenterol.* (2014) 20:3719–37. doi: 10.3748/wjg.v20.i14.3719
119. Coulouarn C, Clement B. Stellate cells and the development of liver cancer: therapeutic potential of targeting the stroma. *J Hepatol.* (2014) 60:1306–9. doi: 10.1016/j.jhep.2014.02.003
120. Taketomi A. Clinical trials of antiangiogenic therapy for hepatocellular carcinoma. *Int J Clin Oncol.* (2016) 21:213–8. doi: 10.1007/s10147-016-0966-0
121. Llovet JM, Ricci S, Mazzaferro V, Hilgard P, Gane E, Blanc JF, et al. Sorafenib in advanced hepatocellular carcinoma. *N Engl J Med.* (2008) 359:378–90. doi: 10.1056/NEJMoa0708857
122. Montella L, Palmieri G, Addeo R, Del Prete S. Hepatocellular carcinoma: will novel targeted drugs really impact the next future? *World J Gastroenterol.* (2016) 22:6114–26. doi: 10.3748/wjg.v22.i27.6114
123. Tahmasebi Birgani M, Carloni V. Tumor microenvironment, a paradigm in hepatocellular carcinoma progression and therapy. *Int J Mol Sci.* (2017) 18:405.
124. Zerbini A, Pilli M, Penna A, Pelosi G, Schianchi C, Molinari A, et al. Radiofrequency thermal ablation of hepatocellular carcinoma liver nodules can activate and enhance tumor-specific T-cell responses. *Cancer Res.* (2006) 66:1139–46.
125. Mizukoshi E, Yamashita T, Arai K, Sunagozaka H, Ueda T, Arihara F, et al. Enhancement of tumor-associated antigen-specific T cell responses by radiofrequency ablation of hepatocellular carcinoma. *Hepatology.* (2013) 57:1448–57. doi: 10.1002/hep.26153
126. Ayaru L, Pereira SP, Alisa A, Pathan AA, Williams R, Davidson B, et al. Unmasking of alpha-fetoprotein-specific CD4(+) T cell responses in hepatocellular carcinoma patients undergoing embolization. *J Immunol.* (2007) 178:1914–22.
127. Zeng Z, Shi F, Zhou L, Zhang MN, Chen Y, Chang XJ, et al. Upregulation of circulating PD-L1/PD-1 is associated with poor post-cryoablation prognosis in patients with HBV-related hepatocellular carcinoma. *PLoS One.* (2011) 6:e23621. doi: 10.1371/journal.pone.0023621
128. Shi L, Chen L, Wu C, Zhu Y, Xu B, Zheng X, et al. PD-1 blockade boosts radiofrequency ablation-elicited adaptive immune responses against tumor. *Clin Cancer Res.* (2016) 22:1173–84. doi: 10.1158/1078-0432.CCR-15-1352
129. Rai V, Abdo J, Alsuwaidan AN, Agrawal S, Sharma P, Agrawal DK. Cellular and molecular targets for the immunotherapy of hepatocellular carcinoma. *Mol Cell Biochem.* (2018) 437:13–36. doi: 10.1007/s11010-017-3092-z
130. Rosenberg SA, Yang JC, Sherry RM, Kammula US, Hughes MS, Phan GQ, et al. Durable complete responses in heavily pretreated patients with metastatic melanoma using T-cell transfer immunotherapy. *Clin Cancer Res.* (2011) 17:4550–7. doi: 10.1158/1078-0432.CCR-11-0116
131. Tran E, Turcotte S, Gros A, Robbins PF, Lu YC, Dudley ME, et al. Cancer immunotherapy based on mutation-specific CD4+ T cells in a patient with epithelial cancer. *Science.* (2014) 344:641–5. doi: 10.1126/science.1251102
132. Tran E, Robbins PF, Lu YC, Prickett TD, Gartner JJ, Jia L, et al. T-cell transfer therapy targeting mutant KRAS in cancer. *N Engl J Med.* (2016) 375: 2255–62.
133. Stevanoviæ S, Pasetto A, Helman SR, Gartner JJ, Prickett TD, Howie B, et al. Landscape of immunogenic tumor antigens in successful immunotherapy of virally induced epithelial cancer. *Science.* (2017) 356:200–5. doi: 10.1126/science.aak9510
134. Zacharakis N, Chinnasamy H, Black M, Xu H, Lu YC, Zheng Z, et al. Immune recognition of somatic mutations leading to complete durable regression in metastatic breast cancer. *Nat Med.* (2018) 24:724–30. doi: 10.1038/s41591-018-0040-8
135. Sangro B, Gomez-Martin C, de la Mata M, Iñarrairaegui M, Garralda E, Barrera P, et al. A clinical trial of CTLA-4 blockade with tremelimumab in patients with hepatocellular carcinoma and chronic hepatitis C. *J Hepatol.* (2013) 59:81–8. doi: 10.1016/j.jhep.2013.02.022
136. Kudo M. Immune checkpoint inhibition in hepatocellular carcinoma: basics and ongoing clinical trials. *Oncology.* (2017) 92(Suppl. 1):50–62. doi: 10.1159/000451016

4

Addressing Profiles of Systemic Inflammation Across the Different Clinical Phenotypes of Acutely Decompensated Cirrhosis

Jonel Trebicka [1,2,3,4,5], Alex Amoros [1], Carla Pitarch [1], Esther Titos [6], José Alcaraz-Quiles [6], Robert Schierwagen [2,5], Carmen Deulofeu [1], Javier Fernandez-Gomez [7], Salvatore Piano [8], Paolo Caraceni [9], Karl Oettl [10], Elsa Sola [7], Wim Laleman [11], Jane McNaughtan [12], Rajeshwar P. Mookerjee [12], Minneke J. Coenraad [13], Tania Welzel [5], Christian Steib [14], Rita Garcia [15], Thierry Gustot [16], Miguel A. Rodriguez Gandia [17], Rafael Bañares [15], Agustin Albillos [17], Stefan Zeuzem [5], Victor Vargas [18], Faouzi Saliba [19], Frederic Nevens [11], Carlo Alessandria [20], Andrea de Gottardi [21], Heinz Zoller [22], Pere Ginès [7], Tilman Sauerbruch [2], Alexander Gerbes [14], Rudolf E. Stauber [10], Mauro Bernardi [9], Paolo Angeli [8], Marco Pavesi [1], Richard Moreau [1,23,24,25,26], Joan Clària [1,6], Rajiv Jalan [12] and Vicente Arroyo [1] on behalf of the CANONIC Study Investigators of the EASL-CLIF Consortium the European Foundation for the Study of Chronic Liver Failure (EF-CLIF)*

[1] European Foundation for the Study of Chronic Liver Failure, Barcelona, Spain, [2] Department of Internal Medicine I, University of Bonn, Bonn, Germany, [3] Faculty of Health Sciences, University of Southern Denmark, Odense, Denmark, [4] Department of Mechanical Biology, Institute for Bioengineering of Catalonia, Barcelona, Spain, [5] J.W. Goethe University Hospital, Frankfurt, Germany, [6] Department of Biochemistry and Molecular Genetics, Hospital Clínic, IDIBAPS and CIBERehd, Barcelona, Spain, [7] Liver Unit, Hospital Clínic, IDIBAPS and CIBERehd, Barcelona, Spain, [8] Unit of Internal Medicine and Hepatology, Department of Medicine, DIMED, University of Padova, Padova, Italy, [9] Department of Medical and Surgical Sciences, University of Bologna, Bologna, Italy, [10] Department of Gastroenterology and Hepatology, Medical University of Graz, Graz, Austria, [11] University Hospital Gasthuisberg, KU Leuven, Leuven, Belgium, [12] Royal Free Hospital, London, United Kingdom, [13] Department of Gastroenterology and Hepatology, Leiden University Medical Center, Leiden, Netherlands, [14] Department of Medicine II, Liver Center Munich, University Hospital LMU Munich, Munich, Germany, [15] Department of Digestive Diseases and CIBERehd, Facultad de Medicina, Hospital General Universitario Gregorio Marañón, Instituto de Investigación Sanitaria Gregorio Marañón, Universidad Complutense, Madrid, Spain, [16] Erasme Hospital, Université Libre de Bruxelles, Brussels, Belgium, [17] Hospital Ramón y Cajal, Madrid, Spain, [18] Vall'd Hebron Hospital, Barcelona, Spain, [19] Hôpital Paul Brousse, Université Paris-Sud, Villejuif, France, [20] Division of Gastroenterology and Hepatology, San Giovanni Battista Hospital, Torino, Italy, [21] Department of Hepatology, Inselspital, Bern, Switzerland, [22] Department of Hepatology and Gastroenterology, University Clinic Innsbruck, Innsbruck, Austria, [23] Inserm, U1149, Centre de Recherche sur l'Inflammation (CRI), UMRS1149, Paris, France, [24] Université Paris Diderot-Paris 7, Département Hospitalo-Universitaire (DHU) UNITY, Paris, France, [25] Service d'Hépatologie, Hôpital Beaujon, Assistance Publique-Hôpitaux de Paris, Paris, France, [26] Laboratoire d'Excellence Inflamex, ComUE Sorbonne Paris Cité, Paris, France

***Correspondence:**
Jonel Trebicka
jonel.trebicka@efclif.com

Background: Patients with acutely decompensated cirrhosis (AD) may or may not develop acute-on-chronic liver failure (ACLF). ACLF is characterized by high-grade systemic inflammation, organ failures (OF) and high short-term mortality. Although patients with AD cirrhosis exhibit distinct clinical phenotypes at baseline, they have low short-term mortality, unless ACLF develops during follow-up. Because little is known about the association of profile of systemic inflammation with clinical phenotypes of patients with AD cirrhosis, we aimed to investigate a battery of markers of systemic inflammation in these patients.

Methods: Upon hospital admission baseline plasma levels of 15 markers (cytokines, chemokines, and oxidized albumin) were measured in 40 healthy controls, 39 compensated cirrhosis, 342 AD cirrhosis, and 161 ACLF. According to EASL-CLIF criteria, AD cirrhosis was divided into three distinct clinical phenotypes (AD-1: Creatinine<1.5, no HE, no OF; AD-2: creatinine 1.5–2, and or HE grade I/II, no OF; AD-3: Creatinine<1.5, no HE, non-renal OF).

Results: Most markers were slightly abnormal in compensated cirrhosis, but markedly increased in AD. Patients with ACLF exhibited the largest number of abnormal markers, indicating "full-blown" systemic inflammation (all markers). AD-patients exhibited distinct systemic inflammation profiles across three different clinical phenotypes. In each phenotype, activation of systemic inflammation was only partial (30% of the markers). Mortality related to each clinical AD-phenotype was significantly lower than mortality associated with ACLF ($p < 0.0001$ by gray test). Among AD-patients baseline systemic inflammation (especially IL-8, IL-6, IL-1ra, HNA2 independently associated) was more intense in those who had poor 28-day outcomes (ACLF, death) than those who did not experience these outcomes.

Conclusions: Although AD-patients exhibit distinct profiles of systemic inflammation depending on their clinical phenotypes, all these patients have only partial activation of systemic inflammation. However, those with the most extended baseline systemic inflammation had the highest the risk of ACLF development and death.

Keywords: acute decompensation, cirrhosis, signature, ACLF, organ failure, organ dysfunction

INTRODUCTION

Natural history of patients with acutely decompensated (AD) cirrhosis may be complicated by acute-on-chronic liver failure (ACLF) (1). ACLF, which has been intensively investigated during the recent years, is characterized by the presence of organ failure(s) (OFs) and high short-term mortality (1–4). The diagnosis of OFs is based on the CLIF-C OF scoring system which assesses the deterioration in the function of the six major organ systems, including liver, kidney, coagulation, brain, circulation, and respiration (1). ACLF is recognized when patients have either a single renal failure; moderate renal dysfunction (creatinine between 1.5 and 1.9 mg/dl) and/or cerebral dysfunction (grade I and II hepatic encephalopathy) in combination with any isolated non-renal OF; or two OFs or more (1). ACLF is also characterized by the presence of high-grade systemic inflammation. Many biomarkers of systemic inflammation are elevated in ACLF, and associated with outcome (5–12).

Unlike patients with ACLF, patients with AD have low short-term mortality (1). AD-patients without ACLF at hospital admission may present three distinct clinical phenotypes which do no overlap (1). The first phenotype (hereafter called AD-1) includes patients without any single OF, who have serum creatinine of <1.5 mg/dL and do not have hepatic encephalopathy (HE). The second phenotype (AD-2) includes patients with isolated renal dysfunction and/or HE I or II, but without any associated single non-renal OF. Finally, the third phenotype (AD-3) includes patients with a single non-renal OF without any kidney dysfunction. Although it is known that some AD-patients without ACLF at hospital admission can subsequently develop ACLF and die (1), the baseline profile of systemic inflammation in these patients developing or not ACLF during short-term follow-up is unknown. Also the profiles of systemic inflammation across the three distinct clinical phenotypes have not been investigated. Expanding our knowledge about the profile of systemic inflammation associated with each clinical phenotype should deliver not only insights into the pathogenesis of ACLF, and also provide clinical tools for stratification of patients and therapy (e.g., anti-TNF, G-CSF).

We hypothesized that each of the three distinct clinical phenotypes which compose the group of patients with AD cirrhosis who were free of ACLF may have a distinctive baseline inflammatory profile. In addition, we wondered whether, among the patients with AD cirrhosis without ACLF, the baseline inflammatory profile was able to distinguish those who will develop ACLF during follow-up from who will not, as well as differentiate those who will die from those who will remain alive. To address these hypotheses, we investigated a battery of markers of systemic inflammation in a large cohort of 582 individuals including healthy controls, patients with compensated cirrhosis

Abbreviations: ACLF, acute-on-chronic liver failure; AD, acute decompensation; ADH, antidiuretic hormone; ALT, alanine aminotransferase; BUN, blood urea nitrogen; BT, bacterial translocation; CHE, cholinesterase; G-CSF, granulocyte-colony stimulating factor; GM-CSF, granulocyte-macrophage colony-stimulating factor; HE, hepatic encephalopathy; HNA2, human non-mercaptalbumin-2; HRS, hepatorenal syndrome; HPLC, high performance liquid chromatography; IL, interleukin; IL-1ra, IL-1 receptor antagonist; INFγ, interferon gamma; INR, international normalized ratio; IP-10 (CXCL10), 10kDa interferon gamma-induced protein (C-X-C-motif chemokine 10); MCP-1 (CCL2), monocyte chemotactic protein 1 (C-C-motif chemokine 2); MELD, model for end-stage liver disease; MIP-1β, macrophage inflammatory protein 1-beta; NASH, non-alcoholic steatohepatitis; PBC, primary biliary cirrhosis; SD, standard deviation; SEM, standard error of the mean; SI, systemic inflammation; TNFα, tumor necrosis factor alpha.

without prior decompensation, patients with AD who were free of ACLF, and patients with ACLF.

PATIENTS AND METHODS

Patients

In all patients, presence of cirrhosis was diagnosed either by unequivocal signs in imaging, presence of complications of portal hypertension or development of AD and/or ACLF. This study analyzed a total of 582 individuals, of whom 542 were patients with cirrhosis. Three hundred and forty-two of these had been enrolled in the CANONIC study and were selected because they had AD cirrhosis but no ACLF at enrollment (1). These 342 patients were compared to 39 patients with compensated cirrhosis who had never presented an episode of decompensation, and 40 healthy volunteers as negative controls. Moreover, 161 patients with ACLF (95 ACLF grade 1, 66 patients with ACLF grade 2) enrolled in the CANONIC study were selected to serve as positive controls, since those patients have an extensive elevation of all systemic inflammation markers. The selection of the CANONIC study patients was based on the availability of blood samples within the first 2 days after enrollment from patients under intensive surveillance during hospitalization (5). All patients gave their written informed consent. Each center obtained the ethics approval from the local ethics committee for the CANONIC study (1, 5).

Definition of AD Cirrhosis, OF, and ACLF

AD of cirrhosis was defined according to criteria established by the CANONIC study (1). Briefly, it includes acute development of large ascites, hepatic encephalopathy, gastrointestinal hemorrhage, bacterial infection, or any combination of these (1).

Individual OFs were diagnosed according to the CLIF-C OF score (1). Liver failure was defined by serum bilirubin of 12 mg/dl or more, kidney failure by creatinine of 2 mg/dl or more (or renal replacement therapy), coagulation failure by INR of 2.5 or more. Circulatory failure was diagnosed when vasopressors were used, and respiratory failure when the patient received mechanical ventilation (not due to HE-induced coma) or PaO_2/FiO_2 was 200 or lower. Finally, cerebral failure was defined as HE grade III and IV (1).

As mentioned earlier, three distinct phenotypes characterized of patients with AD without ACLF at admission, and ACLF was defined according to criteria established by the CANONIC study (1).

Data Collection

Healthy controls were recruited among 45–65 year-old medical and non-medical staff from the Hospital Clinic, while patients with compensated cirrhosis were recruited from the University Hospital Bologna, University Hospital Padova and Royal Free Hospital London and the data at baseline were recorded. Data from the CANONIC study patients were obtained as previously described (1, 5). Briefly, data from previous medical history, physical examination, and laboratory parameters were recorded at baseline, including etiology, previous episodes of acute decompensation, potential precipitating events and reason for hospitalization. Moreover, close 28-day follow-up data were collected according to the CANONIC protocol (1). Finally, information on liver transplantation, mortality and causes of death were obtained on day 28, and at 3 and 6 months and 1 year after enrollment.

Sample Collection and Analysis of biomarkers

The baseline blood samples were obtained in Vacutainer EDTA tubes at the time of enrollment in the study and/or within the first 2 days after enrolment in the study (48 h of hospital admission). Samples at the last assessment could be obtained in 132 patients. In all cases, blood was rapidly centrifuged at 4°C and the plasma frozen at −80°C until analysis.

We measured TNF-α, IL-6, IL-8, MCP-1, IP-10, MIP-1β, G-CSF, GM-CSF, IL-10, IL-1ra, INFγ, IL-17A, IL-7, and eotaxin in 25 μl of plasma using a multiplexed bead-based immunoassay (Milliplex MAP Human Cytokine/Chemokine Magnetic Bead Panel (Merck Millipore, Darmstadt, Germany) on a Luminex 100 Bioanalyzer (Luminex Corp., Austin, TX). The readouts were analyzed with the standard version of the Milliplex Analyst software (Merck Millipore). A five-parameter logistic regression model was used to create standard curves (pg/mL) and to calculate the concentration of each sample. Finally, the levels of irreversibly oxidized albumin (HNA2) were assessed by high performance liquid chromatography (5) as marker of systemic oxidative stress. The levels of systemic inflammation markers in patients with ACLF have been published previously (5).

Statistical Analysis

Plasma levels were above detection limits in most patients. In healthy subjects and patients with values of cytokines or any other measurement below the detection limit, the threshold of detection was assigned as the determined value. Results are presented as frequencies and percentages for categorical variables, means and SDs for normally distributed continuous variables and medians with interquartile range for not normally distributed continuous variables. Hierarchical clustering analysis was performed using the GP plot package from R software. Intensity of inflammation was evaluated according to the relationship between the set of cytokines in different combinations stratifying for different groups of patients. In univariate statistical comparisons, Chi-square test was used for categorical variables, Student's t-test or ANOVA for normal continuous variables and Mann-Whitney U-test or Kruskal-Wallis test for non-normal continuous variables. Multiple-testing was corrected by the Bonferroni correction (corrected p-value for 15 markers $0.05/15 = 0.003$). To assess the strength of the association between each marker and ACLF, logistic regression models were performed. Factors showing a clinically and statistically significant association to the outcome in univariate analyses were selected for the initial model. The final models were fitted using a stepwise forward method based on likelihood ratios with the same significance level ($p < 0.05$) for entering and dropping variables. The proportional hazards model for competing risks proposed by Fine and Gray was used to identify independent predictors of mortality as previously described (1). This model was chosen to account for liver transplantation as an event "competing" with mortality. Variables with a skewed distribution were log-transformed for statistical analyses and graphical comparisons. A p- ≤ 0.05 was considered statistically significant. Analyses were done with SPSS V. 23.0, SAS V.9.4, and R V.3.4.2 statistical packages.

RESULTS

General Characteristics of the Patients

This study investigated 15 markers of systemic inflammation and oxidative stress in 342 AD-patients but without ACLF at admission. These were compared to the levels measured in 161 patients admitted to the hospital with ACLF grade 1 or 2, 39 patients with compensated cirrhosis and no prior decompensation episode, and 40 healthy controls (**Supplementary Tables 1,2**). The reason for selecting only patients with ACLF grade 1 or 2 was to exclude severely diseased patients who had three OFs or more, since the enormous elevation of inflammatory markers in these patients may make difficult the comparison of their profile of systemic inflammation with that of patients with AD and without ACLF.

Importantly, our patients with compensated cirrhosis had never experienced any decompensation, despite the fact that these patients were at risk of developing it. Briefly, these patients had a mean value of 37.8 kPa (21.4–49.7 kPa) measured by Fibroscan® (Echosense, France) and median platelet count of 108 x 10^9/L (72–159 × 10^9/L), surrogates suggesting the presence of clinical significant portal hypertension (13). Moreover, in 18 (46%) patients, esophageal varices were already diagnosed. Of note, levels of systemic inflammation markers were only moderately altered in patients with compensated cirrhosis compared to healthy controls (**Supplementary Table 1**), indicating the absence of significant systemic inflammation in most of these patients. Of note, patients with compensated cirrhosis were analyzed only in a cross-sectional manner, precluding any assessment of the development of AD disease in these patients (**Supplementary Table 1**).

While the demography was similar, there were important, but expected between-group differences, with the most abnormal values being observed in the ACLF group (**Supplementary Table 2**).

Markers of Systemic Inflammation According to the Three Clinical Phenotypes in AD Patients

The profile of systemic inflammation markers significantly differed across the three phenotypes of AD without ACLF (AD-1, AD-2, and AD-3; **Figure 1**, **Table 1** depicting median values). Interestingly, lower levels of TNF-α (OR, 0.52; 95%-CI, 0.34–0.79), eotaxin (OR, 0.57; 95% CI, 0.38–0.86) and HNA2 (OR,

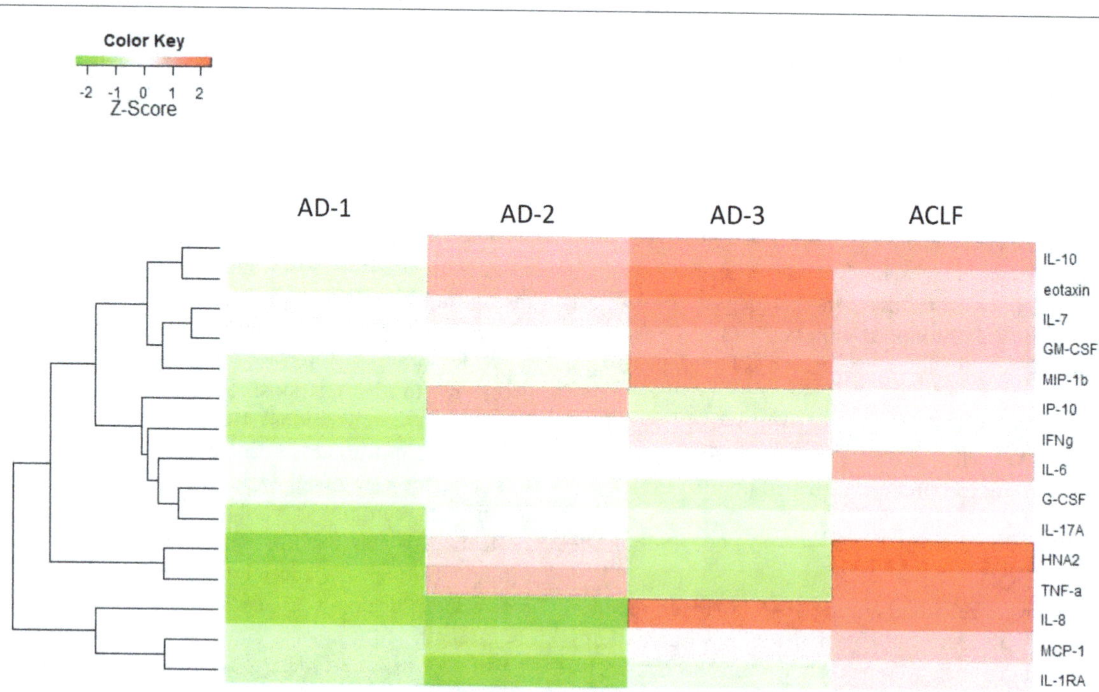

FIGURE 1 | Heat-map highlighting medians of the levels of the different biomarkers of systemic inflammation in patients with acutely decompensated (AD) cirrhosis (with and without ACLF). The patients with "ACLF-free" AD cirrhosis were stratified into three phenotypes. The first phenotype (AD-1) included patients without any single OF, who have serum creatinine of <1.5 mg/dL and do not have hepatic encephalopathy. The second phenotype (AD-2) included patients with isolated renal dysfunction and/or cerebral dysfunction, i.e., without any associated single non-renal, non-cerebral OF. The third phenotype (AD-3) included patients with a single non-renal OF, without any kidney dysfunction. The magnitude of the levels is color-coded and the clustering for each marker with the rest of the markers is shown to the left of the heat-map.

TABLE 1 | Clinical characteristics, routine laboratory tests, and inflammatory mediators, all at enrollment, across the three distinct phenotypes of patients with acutely decompensated (AD) cirrhosis who were free of ACLF (AD-1, AD-2, AD-3), and the group of patients with ACLF.

Variable	AD-1 (*N* = 155)	AD-2 (*N* = 121)	AD-3 (*N* = 66)	ACLF (*N* = 161)	*P*-value
CLINICAL CHARACTERISTICS					
Age—year	57.6 ± 11.90	59.2 ± 10.35	51.7 ± 11.25	57.3 ± 11.45	<0.001
Male gender—no./total no. (%)	99/155 (63.9)	83/121 (68.6)	45/66 (68.2)	108/161 (67.1)	0.843
Mean arterial pressure—mm Hg	84.1 ± 10.87	83.1 ± 13.02	84.9 ± 10.63	80.8 ± 13.40	0.050
PRECIPITATING EVENTS—NO./TOTAL NO. (%)					
Alcohol consumption	19/144 (13.2)	7/112 (6.3)	14/59 (23.7)	27/150 (18.0)	0.008
Mortality at 90 days	22/155 (14.2)	21/121 (17.4)	12/66 (18.2)	59/161 (36.6)	<0.001
ETIOLOGY OF CIRRHOSIS—NO./TOTAL NO. (%)					
Alcoholic	66/145 (45.5)	55/113 (48.7)	36/63 (57.1)	90/152 (59.)	0.080
HCV	40/145 (27.6)	28/113 (24.8)	10/63 (15.9)	27/152 (17.8)	0.109
Alcohol ± HCV	11/145 (7.6)	13/113 (11.5)	5/63 (7.9)	17/152 (11.2)	0.623
Others	28/145 (19.3)	17/113 (15.0)	12/63 (19.0)	18/152 (11.8)	0.300
MEDIAN VALUES FOR ROUTINE LABORATORY TESTS (IQR)					
Serum albumin—g/dl	2.9 (2.50–3.25)	2.9 (2.60–3.30)	2.8 (2.40–3.10)	3.0 (2.40–3.40)	0.157
Serum bilirubin—mg/d	2.5 (1.49–5.18)	2.8 (1.56–5.20)	13.7 (4.90–22.30)	6.1 (2.00–14.37)	< 0.001
Serum creatinine—mg/dl	0.8 (0.66–1.00)	1.5 (0.98–1.70)	0.8 (0.70–1.05)	2.2 (0.98–3.04)	< 0.001
C-reactive protein—mg/L	16.7 (6.80–41.40)	17.9 (6.50–43.00)	19.9 (6.50–34.00)	25.0 (9.70–50.40)	0.163
International Normalized Ratio	1.5 (1.27–1.73)	1.5 (1.27–1.66)	1.7 (1.39–2.20)	1.7 (1.37–2.30)	< 0.001
Platelets—× 10^9/L	95.0 (63.00–131.00)	84.5 (53.50–139.50)	81.0 (43.00–135.00)	76.0 (53.00–121.00)	0.094
White-cell count—×1 0^9/L	6.5 (4.38–9.88)	6.1 (4.60–7.90)	6.6 (4.08–10.72)	8.0 (5.30–12.20)	< 0.001
MEDIAN VALUES FOR INFLAMMATORY MEDIATORS (IQR)					
TNF-α—pg/ml	17.9 (13.43–26.64)	24.2 (17.88–34.23)	19.9 (13.05–29.26)	29.0 (17.38–42.83)	<0.001
IL-6—pg/ml	21.2 (11.71–44.47)	25.0 (12.75–54.20)	24.6 (14.49–47.12)	36.7 (13.79–106.83)	<0.001
IL-8—pg/ml)	35.9 (19.45–75.22)	37.3 (21.84–63.59)	78.4 (41.69–220.92)	84.5 (38.64–165.10)	<0.001
MCP-1—pg/ml	316.8 (235.9–395.7)	323.1 (209.49–455.92)	372.2 (254.60–494.73)	410.3 (293.88–690.00)	<0.001
IP-10—pg/ml	904.6 (530.4–1499.0)	1200.0 (627.0–2255.0)	950.3 (639.9–1718.0)	1147.0 (651.2–2123.0)	0.022
MIP-1ß—pg/ml	20.1 (13.55–37.43)	22.6 (12.93–34.30)	30.2 (16.88–45.41)	26.2 (17.89–42.55)	0.002
G-CSF—pg/ml	22.6 (12.32–54.85)	24.0 (11.19–52.24)	23.0 (12.80–46.65)	30.5 (13.85–81.63)	0.186
GM-CSF—pg/ml	5.0 (2.28–9.08)	4.5 (1.75–10.98)	7.5 (3.68–15.87)	6.8 (3.47–15.97)	0.003
IL-10—pg/ml	3.0 (0.90–9.36)	4.0 (1.37–13.07)	5.3 (1.88–13.39)	7.2 (1.90–25.78)	<0.001
IL1-ra—pg/ml	11.9 (5.40–25.90)	10.4 (4.52–23.03)	13.4 (6.14–40.97)	18.7 (8.56–50.48)	< 0.001
IFNγ—pg/ml	4.4 (1.65–19.38)	6.7 (2.38–24.29)	7.8 (2.82–18.85)	6.0 (2.32–23.12)	0.107
Eotaxin—pg/ml	103.7 (68.43–152.08)	120.4 (90.48–162.49)	137.0 (94.67–173.76)	123.5 (86.55–177.21)	0.008
IL-17A—pg/ml	3.1 (1.37–13.10)	4.2 (2.03–10.00)	3.8 (1.75–11.31)	4.8 (1.62–14.90)	0.376
IL-7—pg/ml	2.5 (0.85–7.46)	2.7 (1.13–11.74)	4.3 (1.38–8.80)	3.5 (1.62–11.07)	0.135
HNA2—%	4.2 (2.35–8.07)	6.9 (3.79–10.99)	5.6 (3.07–8.85)	11.0 (6.25–15.15)	<0.001

Patients with acutely decompensated cirrhosis were classified as having the AD-1, AD-2, or AD-3 phenotype or having ACLF according to the EASL-CLIF Consortium criteria (1, 2). Data are shown as means ± SD or median (range). P-values were calculated by unpaired Students' t-test or Kruskall-Wallis test where appropriate.

HCV denotes hepatitis C virus; IQR interquartile range; TNF, umor necrosis factor; IL, interleukin; MCP-1, monocyte chemotactic protein 1; IP-10, 10 kDa interferon gamma-induced protein; MIP-1ß, macrophage inflammatory protein 1-beta; G-CSF, granulocyte colony-stimulating factor; GM-CSF, granulocyte-macrophage colony-stimulating factor; IL-1ra, interleukin-1 receptor antagonist protein; IFN, interferon; HNA2, human non-mercaptalbumin 2.

0.64; 95% CI, 0.45–0.91) were independently associated with AD-1, while higher levels of TNF-α (OR, 3.25; 95% CI, 2.00–5.28) and HNA2 (OR, 1.75; 95% CI, 1.20–2.55) but lower levels of IL-8 (OR, 0.67; 95% CI, 0.53–0.85) were independently associated with AD-2 (renal and/or cerebral dysfunction, **Supplementary Table 3**).

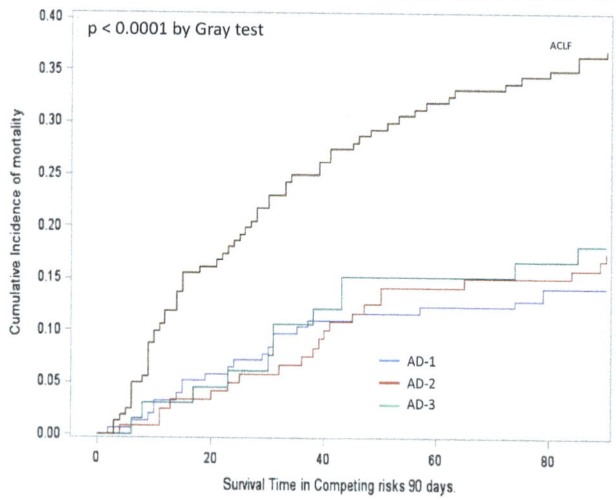

FIGURE 2 | Cumulative incidence function assessing survival in patients' groups analyzed in **Figure 1**. Mortality was significantly higher in patients with ACLF than in those without, irrespective of their phenotype, AD-1, AD-2, or AD-3 (Gray's test $p < 0.0001$). Mortality did not significantly differ between the three phenotypes AD-1, AD-2, and AD-3. For definitions of these phenotypes, see **Figure 1** legend.

By contrast, higher levels of IL-8 (OR, 2.30; 95% CI, 1.72–3.06) and lower levels of G-CSF (OR, 0.78; 95% CI, 0.64–0.94) were independently associated with isolated non-renal OF (AD-3, **Supplementary Table 3**). Importantly, all these results were independent of presence of infection, since we could not find any association of those markers with the presence of infection in the respective stratification of the patients, while IL-6 was independently associated with infection in the entire cohort (OR, 1.36; 95%-CI 1.13–1.65; $p = 0.01$).

Interestingly, the pattern of elevated markers for patients in AD-2 and AD-3 were opposite to each other, i.e., markers that were elevated in AD-2 were lower in AD-3 and vice-versa (**Figure 1**). The addition of elevated markers in AD-2 with the elevated markers in AD-3, recapitulated the profile of systemic inflammation seen in ACLF (**Figure 1**).

Importantly, not only the distribution of elevated biomarkers, but also the quantitative changes in their levels defined their affiliation to either AD-1, AD-2, or AD-3 (**Figure 1**, **Table 1**). Another interesting finding was that patients with ACLF did not show the highest levels of the single markers, but the highest number of elevated markers (**Figure 1**), suggesting a "full-blown" systemic inflammation in this group of patients and a rather attenuated systemic inflammation in the groups of patients without ACLF.

Another important observation was that despite the significant differences between the severity and profile of systemic inflammation markers across the three clinical phenotypes of "ACLF-free" AD cirrhosis, the cumulative incidence of death by 90 days, was similar irrespective

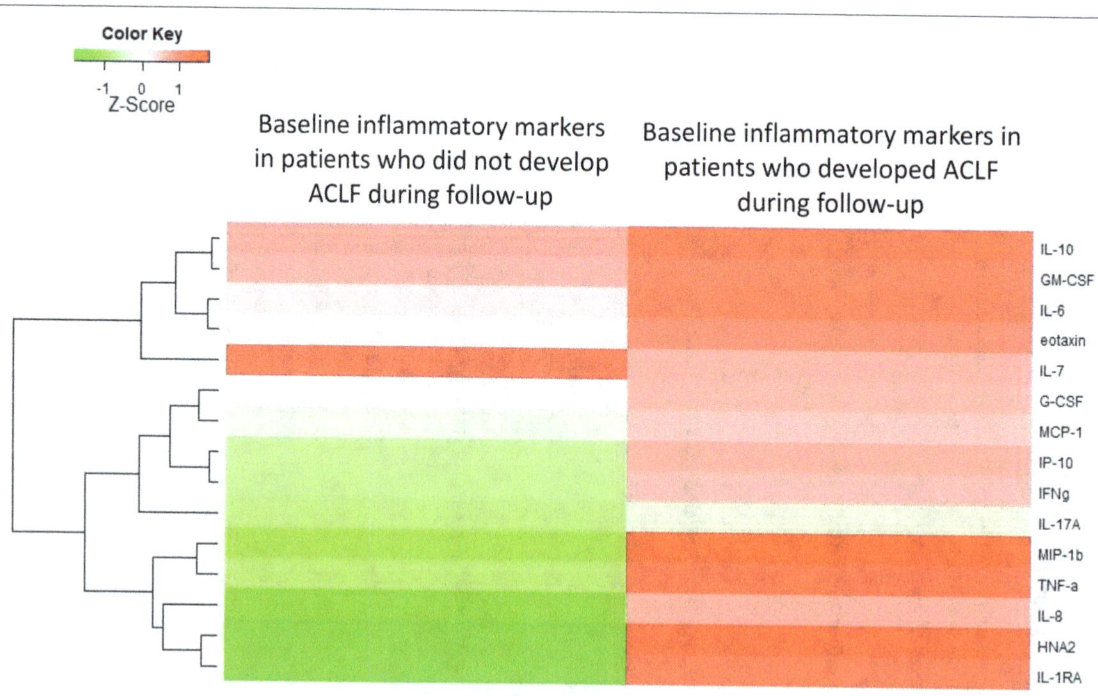

FIGURE 3 | Heat-map showing the median levels of systemic inflammation markers at enrollment of patients with acutely decompensated cirrhosis who were free of ACLF. For the comparison, patients were divided into two groups according to their outcome (i.e., development of ACLF or not, during 28 days of follow-up). The magnitude of the levels is color-coded and the clustering for each marker with the rest of the markers is shown to the left of the heat-map.

of the phenotype (**Figure 2**). In contrast, the "full-blown" systemic inflammation observed in patients with ACLF was associated with increased cumulative incidence of death by 90 days (**Figure 2**).

Predicting ACLF Development Using Baseline Systemic Inflammation Profiles

Next, we asked whether among AD-patients without ACLF at admission, the baseline systemic inflammation profile differed between those who will subsequently develop ACLF relative to those who will not develop this syndrome. Among the 342 patients with AD at admission, 57 developed ACLF within 28 days after admission. Importantly, baseline levels of systemic inflammation markers were significantly higher among patients who subsequently developed ACLF than among those who remained free of ACLF during the 28-day follow-up (**Figure 3**, **Table 2**). Therefore, in AD-patients without ACLF at admission, the development of ACLF can be predicted using the baseline profile of systemic inflammation-related markers.

When observing the magnitude of specific markers among patients with AD cirrhosis who were free of ACLF on admission, we saw that higher baseline levels of IL-6 (OR, 1.43; 95% CI, 1.04–1.96; $p = 0.03$), IL-1ra (OR, 1.46; 95%-CI 1.10–1.93; $p = 0.009$) and HNA2 (OR, 2.84; 95%-CI 1.52–5.34; $p = 0.001$) were independently associated with development of ACLF within 28 days.

Baseline Profiles Predicting Survival in Patients With "ACLF-free" AD cirrhosis

Among AD-patients without ACLF at hospital admission 55 died and 28 received a liver transplant. The baseline levels of several markers were significantly higher in patients who subsequently died than in those patients who survived (**Supplementary Table 4**; **Figure 4**). In particular, TNF-α, IL-6, IL-8, IL-10, eotaxin, IL-17A, IL-7, and HNA2 were higher in patients who died (**Supplementary Table 4**). Nevertheless, only IL-8 and HNA2 were independently associated with mortality in the patients with AD at baseline (**Table 3**).

DISCUSSION

This study offers a homogeneous classification way in the heterogeneous population of patients with acutely decompensated cirrhosis, which is related to ACLF development and death. Beyond the large sample size, our study provides novel information by showing that each of the three distinct clinical phenotypes, which compose the group of patients with AD cirrhosis who were free of ACLF had a distinctive baseline inflammatory profile. A second aspect of the novelty in our results is that, among the patients with AD cirrhosis without ACLF, the baseline inflammatory profile was able to distinguish those who will develop ACLF during follow-up from who will not. Finally, we showed that among the patients with AD cirrhosis without ACLF, the baseline inflammatory profile was different between those who will die at short-term and those who will survive.

This novel point of view is demonstrated in four major findings of the present study discussed in the following. The first was that inflammatory markers were only slightly altered in patients with compensated cirrhosis and no prior episode of decompensation. This finding is surprising and interesting considering that many of these patients had clinical significant portal hypertension, as assessed either by the presence of esophageal varices and/or high liver stiffness and low platelets (15). By contrast, most inflammatory mediators were markedly increased in patients admitted to hospital with AD (with or without ACLF). Indeed, this observation is of importance since it shows that severe systemic inflammation and acute decompensation of cirrhosis are concomitant processes, as proposed in the so-called "Systemic Inflammation Hypothesis" (16). This novel finding is probably a result of the careful review of the medical history of the patients included in the compensated control group, excluding any patients with compensated cirrhosis who had prior history of AD episodes. Although it remains unclear which of these processes (acute decompensation or severe systemic inflammation) occurs first, it is tempting to assume that systemic inflammation is a prerequisite for the development of AD cirrhosis. In any case, our findings suggest that systemic inflammation may serve to classify the stage of disease in patients with cirrhosis.

The second important observation was that patients with AD but without ACLF at admission had a very heterogeneous profile of circulating inflammatory mediators. There were three distinct clinical phenotypes (AD-1, AD-2, and AD-3) characterizing those AD patients; each phenotype being associated with distinct profile of systemic inflammation, irrespective of the fact that infection was present or not. The patients hospitalized with AD cirrhosis and neither OF, renal dysfunction nor cerebral dysfunction (AD-1 phenotype), had very mild systemic inflammation, while the patients with an isolated non-renal OF (AD-3 phenotype), and those with isolated renal and/or cerebral dysfunction (AD-2 phenotype) had a higher number of markedly increased markers of systemic inflammation. Moreover, our results obtained in patients with "ACLF-free" AD cirrhosis, suggest a potential explanation for the systemic inflammation signature of ACLF, which can be seen as a result of continuum of activation of systemic inflammation. Indeed, according to the EASL-CLIF consortium definition, the combination of any single non-renal, non-cerebral OF with renal and/or cerebral dysfunction defines ACLF grade 1. While some markers of inflammation were elevated in patients with AD-3 phenotype, other markers were elevated in patients with AD-2 phenotype. As suggested by **Figure 1**, the profile of systemic inflammation in ACLF could be seen as merging of the inflammatory profile of the AD-2 phenotype and that of the AD-3 phenotype. It could be argued that the division of ACLF-free AD cirrhosis into three phenotypes was arbitrary, one phenotype (AD-2) being more severe than the two others. However, several features do not support this contention. First, the rationale for dividing this group of patients into three distinct phenotypes was based on clinical evidence provided by the CANONIC study (1). Second, the results of the present study now provide a biological support to this distinction by showing that each clinical phenotype was

TABLE 2 | Baseline characteristics of 342 patients with acutely decompensated cirrhosis who were free of ACLF at enrollment, divided into two groups according to the development or the absence of development of ACLF during 28 days of follow-up.

Characteristic	Without ACLF development (*N* = 285)	With ACLF development (*N* = 57)	*P*–value
Age– year	56.7 ± 11.63	58.5 ± 11.00	0.2847
Male gender – no./total no. (%)	191/285 (67.0)	36/57 (63.2)	0.5734
Mean arterial pressure – mm Hg	83.8 ± 11.84	84.2 ± 10.46	0.8259
PRECIPITATING EVENTS – NO./TOTAL NO. (%)			
Alcohol consumption	33/265 (12.5)	7/50 (14.0)	0.7631
Mortality 90 days	29/285 (10.2)	26/57 (45.6)	< 0.0001
ETIOLOGY OF CIRRHOSIS – NO./TOTAL NO. (%)			
Alcoholic	128/269 (47.6)	29/52 (55.8)	0.2797
HCV	66/269 (24.5)	12/52 (23.1)	0.8224
Alcohol + HCV	26/269 (9.7)	3/52 (5.8)	0.5957
Others	49/269 (18.2)	8/52 (15.4)	0.6248
MEDIAN VALUES FOR LABORATORY VARIABLES (IQR)			
Serum albumin–g/dl	2.9 (2.60–3.30)	2.7 (2.19–3.01)	0.0049
Serum bilirubin–mg/d	3.0 (1.60–6.70)	4.4 (1.69–9.06)	0.0963
Serum creatinine–mg/dl	0.9 (0.70–1.32)	1.1 (0.80–1.40)	0.1285
C-reactive protein–mg/L	16.2 (6.00–39.60)	25.8 (10.00–45.60)	0.0887
International Normalized Ratio	1.5 (1.27–1.70)	1.7 (1.42–1.94)	0.0004
Platelets–x10^9/L	87.0 (57.00–139.00)	94.5 (57.50–119.50)	0.9581
White-cell count–x10^9/L	6.1 (4.08–9.03)	7.3 (5.04–10.53)	0.0146
MEDIAN VALUES FOR INFLAMMATORY MEDIATORS (IQR)			
TNF-α–pg/ml	19.5 (14.14–27.37)	26.7 (17.69–36.52)	<0.001
IL-6–pg/ml	21.2 (11.27–41.32)	34.3 (19.85–105.54)	<0.001
IL-8–(pg/ml)	37.3 (20.45–76.41)	58.7 (40.89–108.34)	<0.001
MCP-1–pg/ml	318.0 (228.03–436.02)	360.0 (276.53–586.47)	0.013
IP-10–pg/ml	965.2 (557.62–1676.00)	1272.0 (760.31–2150.00)	0.053
MIP-1ß–pg/ml	20.1 (13.14–33.55)	36.9 (23.88–56.10)	<0.001
G-CSF–pg/ml	22.6 (11.19–49.93)	31.0 (15.86–69.19)	0.048
GM-CSF–pg/ml	4.7 (1.96–9.48)	10.7 (3.76–20.05)	<0.001
IL-10–pg/ml	3.4 (1.12–9.15)	8.0 (2.45–26.42)	0.002
IL1-ra–pg/ml	9.9 (4.72–22.47)	24.0 (12.81–62.11)	<0.001
IFNγ–pg/ml	5.5 (2.00–18.11)	9.2 (3.20–31.34)	0.013
Eotaxin–pg/ml	110.4 (80.76–155.42)	135.8 (94.97–186.19)	0.008
IL-17A–pg/ml	3.7 (1.57–10.25)	3.4 (1.98–24.37)	0.214
IL-7–pg/ml	2.6 (0.99–8.50)	5.1 (1.88–14.52)	0.032
HNA2–%	4.5 (2.50–8.82)	8.1 (4.89–9.95)	<0.001

Patients with acutely decompensated cirrhosis were classified as being free of ACLF or having ACLF according to the EASL-CLIF Consortium criteria (1, 14). Data are shown as means ± SD or median (range). P-values were calculated by unpaired Students' t-test or Man-Whitney U-test where appropriate.

HCV, hepatitis C virus; IQR, interquartile range; TNF, umor necrosis factor; IL, interleukin; MCP-1, monocyte chemotactic protein 1; IP-10, 10 kDa interferon gamma-induced protein; MIP-1ß, macrophage inflammatory protein 1-beta; G-CSF, granulocyte colony-stimulating factor; GM-CSF, granulocyte-macrophage colony-stimulating factor; IL-1ra, interleukin-1 receptor antagonist protein; IFN, interferon; HNA2, human non-mercaptalbumin 2.

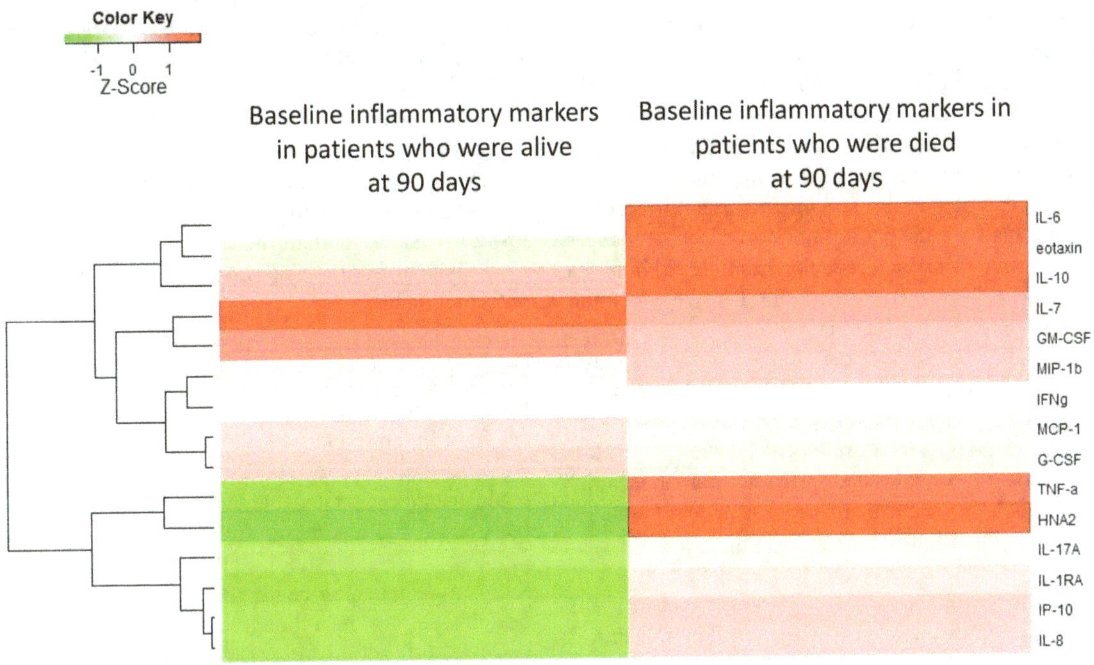

FIGURE 4 | Heat-map showing the median levels of systemic inflammation markers at enrollment of patients with acutely decompensated cirrhosis who were free of ACLF. For the comparison, patients were divided into two groups according to their outcome (i.e., occurrence of death or not during 90 days of follow-up). The magnitude of the levels is color-coded and the clustering for each marker with the rest of the markers is shown to the left of the heat-map.

TABLE 3 | Hazard ratios for death at 90 days in univariate and multivariable analyses of inflammatory mediators assessed at enrolment of 342 patients with acutely decompensated cirrhosis who were free of ACLF.

Inflammatory mediator	Univariate analysis			Multivariate analysis		
	Hazard ratio	95% IC	*P*-value	Hazard ratio	95% IC	*P*-value
Tumor necrosis factor-α	1.650	(1.056–2.578)	0.028	–	–	–
Interleukin-6	1.389	(1.094–1.764)	0.007	–	–	–
Interleukin-8	1.521	(1.256–1.842)	<0.001	1.608	(1.304–1.982)	<0.001
Eotaxin	2.765	(1.392–5.492)	0.004	–	–	–
Interleukin-17A	1.217	(1.033–1.434)	0.019	–	–	–
Interleukin-7	1.221	(1.047–1.422)	0.011	–	–	–
Human non-mercaptalbumin 2	2.116	(1.456–3.074)	<0.001	2.237	(1.506–3.323)	<0.001

The final models were fitted using a stepwise forward method based on likelihood ratios with the same significance level ($p < 0.05$) for entering and dropping variables. IC denotes confidence interval.

associated with a specific inflammatory profile. Third, none of these inflammatory profiles was as intense as the profile found in patients with ACLF. It was also interesting that, although marked differences in systemic inflammation profiles existed between the three clinical phenotypes of "ACLF-free" AD cirrhosis, there were no significant differences in survival between these three phenotypes. Together these findings indicate that the division into 3 phenotypes was not arbitrary, and more importantly did not underestimate the severity of one phenotype, in particular of the AD-2 phenotype. Our data are novel and very important, indicating that not a maximum level of a specific biomarker, but rather the extension (number of elevated markers) of systemic inflammation, such as that observed in ACLF, must be reached to determine increased mortality. Yet further studies are required to refine the risk assessment in these phenotypes.

There were, however, some differences in the pattern of systemic inflammation across the three clinical phenotypes of "ACLF-free" AD cirrhosis. For example, the presence of an isolated renal and/or cerebral dysfunction was independently associated with high TNF-α levels, while an isolated single non-renal OF was associated with low TNF-α levels. The reasons for these between-group differences in TNF-α expression are unclear but may explain some interesting observations of prior studies. Thus, large-scale trials in severe alcoholic hepatitis showed that anti-TNF approaches (e.g., pentoxifylline) might not work in patients with severe disease and liver failure, but had positive effects in the presence of renal failure (17, 18). Pentoxifylline has also been shown to improve outcomes in patients with alcoholic hepatitis and hepato-renal syndrome (19, 20).

In our study, some markers (i.e., TNF-alpha, HNA2, and IP-10) were elevated in AD-2 patients and lower in AD-3 patients, features, which could seem counterintuitive. We have no clear explanation for these differences, which contribute to the fact that each clinical phenotype has a specific inflammatory profile. We can only speculate on the pathophysiological consequences of differences in some marker levels. For example, TNF-alpha is known to protect the liver by stimulating liver regeneration (21). Therefore, increased TNF-alpha levels in AD-2 may be involved in the absence of liver failure in this group, and, conversely, low TNF-alpha levels could favor the development of liver failure in AD-3 patients. Obviously, future studies are needed. Surprisingly, TNF-alpha and MCP-1 levels were both lower in patients with compensated cirrhosis than in healthy subjects. We do not have clear explanations for these differences, only hypotheses. As mentioned earlier, TNF-alpha is known to stimulate liver regeneration. Therefore, low TNF-alpha levels in patients with compensated cirrhosis may reflect an insufficient TNF-alpha production in the liver, playing a role in subclinical liver failure in these patients. Regarding MCP-1, one should have in mind that this chemokine is produced by damaged tissues to attract monocytes whose function, once migrated, is to restore tissue homeostasis. Therefore, low MCP-1 levels in compensated cirrhosis may result in defective tissue homeostasis.

A third highly relevant finding was the observation that patients with AD cirrhosis who were free of ACLF at enrollment but subsequently developed ACLF within 28 days, had significantly higher baseline levels of inflammatory mediators. Moreover, these patients showed a distinct signature of systemic inflammation, relative to those who did not develop ACLF. These findings reveal that systemic inflammation precedes the development of ACLF, suggesting a cause-to-effect relationship. Importantly, in our study, higher IL-6 levels independently predict ACLF development, a finding which is consistent with previous results showing that elevated IL-6 levels were strongly associated with ACLF and its progression (5). Moreover, higher IL-1ra levels were independently associated with development of ACLF, which is fully in line with previous data demonstrating that polymorphisms of IL-1ra predispose to ACLF (22). Finally, HNA2, a marker for oxidative stress, was independently associated with ACLF development (5, 23). This latter finding calls for an important discussion not only on the pathogenesis of ACLF, but also on the prophylactic treatment since albumin is a potent immune modulator involved in reducing oxidative stress. In fact, there is strong evidence that albumin administration during an episode of spontaneous bacterial peritonitis prevents type I HRS—which represents a special form of ACLF—and improves survival (24). This has also recently been confirmed in the ANSWER trial, a randomized controlled trial in almost 400 patients, showing that long-term weekly albumin administration reduces the incidence of organ failure and thereby improves overall survival in decompensated cirrhotic patients (25). Further studies (e.g., PRECIOSA, NCT03451292) are underway.

Finally, in patients with "ACLF-free" AD cirrhosis, the extension of systemic inflammation at baseline was associated with 90-day mortality. The independent predictors of death were higher levels of IL-8 and HNA2 suggesting that decreasing the levels of these two inflammation-related markers may be an objective for future therapies aiming to increase survival in the group of patients with AD who are at high risk of death. Of note, among patients with AD at enrollment, those who will die had lower G-CSF levels than those who will survive. These patients might benefit from G-CSF therapy as recently shown in patients with ACLF (26).

Although the present study tested a large number of patients and a large number of systemic inflammation mediators, it has its limitations. The concept of this study is to observe systemic inflammation associated with AD cirrhosis (with and without ACLF) without taking into account specific events that could have precipitated the acute decompensation of cirrhosis (e.g., data about use of anti-inflammatory drugs, although unlikely since contraindicated in these patients). Moreover, there might be inter-center heterogeneity in the diagnosis of portal hypertension, although each liver unit participating in the CANONIC study had expertise in the diagnosis and treatment of complications of cirrhosis, therefore limiting the inter-center heterogeneity. Finally, this study did not aim to elaborate on a specific score, but rather to offer pathophysiologic insight into the role of systemic inflammation in patients with AD. Future studies are needed to further elaborate the specific events in AD cirrhosis.

In conclusion, baseline inflammatory markers exhibit no or slight abnormalities in compensated cirrhosis, while in "ACLF-free" AD cirrhosis their profile was heterogeneous, being markedly elevated in those who developed ACLF during follow up. Moreover, among patients with AD cirrhosis who were free of ACLF, this study showed a specific baseline profile of circulating inflammatory mediators in patients who died during follow-up.

AUTHOR CONTRIBUTIONS

JT, PG, RJ, AG, MB, PA, MP, RM, JC, and VA: study concept and design; JT, AlA, CP, ET, JA-Q, CD, JF-G, SP, PC, KO, JM, ES, WL, MC, TW, CS, RG, TG, MR, and AdG: acquisition of data; JT, AlA, CP, JF-G, KO, JM, RPM, WL, AdG, MP, RM, JC, and VA: analysis and interpretation of data; JT, AlA, CP, AG, RM, JC, and VA: drafting of the manuscript; JT, AlA, CP, JA-Q, CD, SP, PC, MP, and JC: statistical analysis; All authors: critical revision of the manuscript regarding important intellectual content; JT and VA: funding recipient; ET, RoS, SP, RPM, WL, TG, RB, AgA, SZ, VV, FS, FN, CA, AdG, PG, RJ, TS, AG, RuS, MB, PA, RM, JA-Q, and VA: administrative, technical and material support; JT, JF-G, PC, RPM, WL, TG, RB, AgA, SZ, VV, FS, FN, CA, AdG, PG, RJ, TS, AG, RuS, MB, PA, RM, JA, and VA: study supervision.

ACKNOWLEDGMENTS

We thank all CANONIC collaborators for support during the study.

REFERENCES

1. Moreau R, Jalan R, Gines P, Pavesi M, Angeli P, Cordoba J, et al. Acute-on-chronic liver failure is a distinct syndrome that develops in patients with acute decompensation of cirrhosis. *Gastroenterology.* (2013) 144:1426–37, 1437.e1–9. doi: 10.1053/j.gastro.2013.02.042
2. Arroyo V, Moreau R, Jalan R, Ginès P, EASL-CLIF Consortium CANONIC Study. Acute-on-chronic liver failure: a new syndrome that will re-classify cirrhosis. *J Hepatol.* (2015) 62:S131–43. doi: 10.1016/j.jhep.2014.11.045
3. Arroyo V, Moreau R, Kamath PS, Jalan R, Ginès P, Nevens F, et al. Acute-on-chronic liver failure in cirrhosis. *Nat Rev Dis Primers.* (2016) 2:16041. doi: 10.1038/nrdp.2016.41
4. Hernaez R, Solà E, Moreau R, Ginès P. Acute-on-chronic liver failure: an update. *Gut.* (2017) 66:541–53. doi: 10.1136/gutjnl-2016-312670
5. Clària J, Stauber RE, Coenraad MJ, Moreau R, Jalan R, Pavesi M, et al. Systemic inflammation in decompensated cirrhosis: characterization and role in acute-on-chronic liver failure. *Hepatology.* (2016) 64:1249–1264. doi: 10.1002/hep.28740
6. Solé C, Solà E, Morales-Ruiz M, Fernàndez G, Huelin P, Graupera I, et al. Characterization of inflammatory response in acute-on-chronic liver failure and relationship with prognosis. *Sci Rep.* (2016) 6:32341. doi: 10.1038/srep32341
7. Grønbæk H, Rødgaard-Hansen S, Aagaard NK, Arroyo V, Moestrup SK, Garcia E, et al. Macrophage activation markers predict mortality in patients with liver cirrhosis without or with acute-on-chronic liver failure (ACLF). *J Hepatol.* (2016) 64:813–22. doi: 10.1016/j.jhep.2015.11.021
8. Ariza X, Graupera I, Coll M, Solà E, Barreto R, García E, et al. Neutrophil gelatinase-associated lipocalin is a biomarker of acute-on-chronic liver failure and prognosis in cirrhosis. *J Hepatol.* (2016) 65:57–65. doi: 10.1016/j.jhep.2016.03.002
9. Jansen C, Möller P, Meyer C, Kolbe CC, Bogs C, Pohlmann A, et al. Increase in liver stiffness after transjugular intrahepatic portosystemic shunt is associated with inflammation and predicts mortality. *Hepatology.* (2017) 67:1472–84. doi: 10.1002/hep.29612
10. Lehmann JM, Claus K, Jansen C, Pohlmann A, Schierwagen R, Meyer C, et al. Circulating CXCL10 in cirrhotic portal hypertension might reflect systemic inflammation and predict ACLF and mortality. *Liver Int.* (2017) 38:875–884. doi: 10.1111/liv.13610
11. Tan W, Xia J, Dan Y, Li M, Lin S, Pan X, et al. Genome-wide association study identifies HLA-DR variants conferring risk of HBV-related acute-on-chronic liver failure. *Gut.* (2018) 67:757–66. doi: 10.1136/gutjnl-2016-313035
12. Bernsmeier C, Triantafyllou E, Brenig R, Lebosse FJ, Singanayagam A, Patel VC, et al. CD14+ CD15- HLA-DR- myeloid-derived suppressor cells impair antimicrobial responses in patients with acute-on-chronic liver failure. *Gut.* (2018) 67:1155–67. doi: 10.1136/gutjnl-2017-314184
13. Berzigotti A, Seijo S, Arena U, Abraldes JG, Vizzutti F, García-Pagán JC, et al. Elastography, spleen size, and platelet count identify portal hypertension in patients with compensated cirrhosis. *Gastroenterology.* (2013) 144:102–11.e1. doi: 10.1053/j.gastro.2012.10.001
14. Angeli P, Bernardi M, Villanueva C, Francoz C, Mookerjee RP, Trebicka J, et al. EASL Clinical practice guidelines for the management of patients with decompensated cirrhosis. *J Hepatol.* (2018) 69:406–60.doi: 10.1016/j.jhep.2018.03.024
15. de Franchis R, Baveno VI. Expanding consensus in portal hypertension: report of the Baveno VI consensus workshop: Stratifying risk and individualizing care for portal hypertension. *J Hepatol.* (2015) 63:743–52. doi: 10.1016/j.jhep.2015.05.022
16. Bernardi M, Moreau R, Angeli P, Schnabl B, Arroyo V. Mechanisms of decompensation and organ failure in cirrhosis: from peripheral arterial vasodilation to systemic inflammation hypothesis. *J Hepatol.* (2015) 63:1272–84. doi: 10.1016/j.jhep.2015.07.004
17. Thursz M, Forrest E, Roderick P, Day C, Austin A, O'Grady J, et al. The clinical effectiveness and cost-effectiveness of STeroids or pentoxifylline for alcoholic hepatitis (stopah): a 2×2 factorial randomised controlled trial. *Health Technol Assess.* (2015) 19:1–104. doi: 10.3310/hta191020
18. Hendy P. Pentoxifylline is ineffective in treating severe alcoholic hepatitis. *Frontline Gastroenterol.* (2016) 7:80–81. doi: 10.1136/flgastro-2015-100615
19. Akriviadis E, Botla R, Briggs W, Han S, Reynolds T, Shakil O. Pentoxifylline improves short-term survival in severe acute alcoholic hepatitis: a double-blind, placebo-controlled trial. *Gastroenterology.* (2000) 119: 1637–1648.
20. Lebrec D, Thabut D, Oberti F, Perarnau JM, Condat B, Barraud H, et al. Pentoxifylline does not decrease short-term mortality but does reduce complications in patients with advanced cirrhosis. *Gastroenterology.* (2010) 138:1755–62. doi: 10.1053/j.gastro.2010.01.040
21. Dubuquoy L, Louvet A, Lassailly G, Truant S, Boleslawski E, Artru F, et al. Progenitor cell expansion and impaired hepatocyte regeneration in explanted livers from alcoholic hepatitis *Gut.* (2015) 64:1949–60. doi: 10.1136/gutjnl-2014-308410
22. Alcaraz-Quiles J, Titos E, Casulleras M, Pavesi M, López-Vicario C, Rius B, et al. Polymorphisms in the IL-1 gene cluster influence systemic inflammation in patients at risk for acute-on-chronic liver failure. *Hepatology.* (2017) 65:202–16. doi: 10.1002/hep.28896
23. Domenicali M, Baldassarre M, Giannone FA, Naldi M, Mastroroberto M, Biselli M, et al. Posttranscriptional changes of serum albumin: clinical and prognostic significance in hospitalized patients with cirrhosis. *Hepatology.* (2014) 60:1851–60. doi: 10.1002/hep.27322
24. Sort P, Navasa M, Arroyo V, Aldeguer X, Planas R, Ruiz-del-Arbol L, et al. Effect of intravenous albumin on renal impairment and mortality in patients with cirrhosis and spontaneous bacterial peritonitis. *N Engl J Med.* (1999) 341:403–9. doi: 10.1056/NEJM199908053410603
25. Caraceni P, Riggio O, Angeli P, Alessandria C, Neri S, Foschi FG, et al. Long-term albumin administration in decompensated cirrhosis (ANSWER): an open-label randomised trial. *Lancet.* (2018) 391:2417–2429. doi: 10.1016/S0140-6736(18)30840-7
26. Garg V, Garg H, Khan A, Trehanpati N, Kumar A, Sharma BC, et al. Granulocyte colony-stimulating factor mobilizes CD34(+) cells and improves survival of patients with acute-on-chronic liver failure. *Gastroenterology.* (2012) 142:505–512.e1. doi: 10.1053/j.gastro.2011.11.027

5

Hepatic Macrophages in Liver Injury

Zhao Shan[1] *and Cynthia Ju*[2*]

[1] *Center for Life Sciences, School of Life Sciences, Yunnan University, Kunming, China,* [2] *Department of Anesthesiology, McGovern Medical School, University of Texas Health Science Center at Houston, Houston, TX, United States*

***Correspondence:**
Cynthia Ju
changqing.ju@uth.tmc.edu

Ample evidence suggests that hepatic macrophages play key roles in the injury and repair mechanisms during liver disease progression. There are two major populations of hepatic macrophages: the liver resident Kupffer cells and the monocyte-derived macrophages, which rapidly infiltrate the liver during injury. Under different disease conditions, the tissue microenvironmental cues of the liver critically influence the phenotypes and functions of hepatic macrophages. Furthermore, hepatic macrophages interact with multiple cells types in the liver, such as hepatocytes, neutrophils, endothelial cells, and platelets. These crosstalk interactions are of paramount importance in regulating the extents of liver injury, repair, and ultimately liver disease progression. In this review, we summarize the novel findings highlighting the impact of injury-induced microenvironmental signals that determine the phenotype and function of hepatic macrophages. Moreover, we discuss the role of hepatic macrophages in homeostasis and pathological conditions through crosstalk interactions with other cells of the liver.

Keywords: Kupffer cells, monocyte-derived macrophages, liver injury, microenvironmental cues, cellular crosstalk

INTRODUCTION

Hepatic macrophages, consisting of liver resident Kupffer cells (KCs) and monocyte-derived macrophages (MoMϕs), play a central role in maintaining homeostasis of the liver as well as contributing to the progression of acute or chronic liver injury (1). Kupffer cells are the most abundant tissue macrophages in mammalian bodies, accounting for 80–90% of total tissue macrophages (2). In the liver, KCs are distributed along the hepatic sinusoids, preferentially near the periportal areas (3). In the healthy liver, a small number of MoMϕs are located mainly in the portal triad areas (4, 5). In mouse, KCs and MoMϕs can be distinguished by their differential expression of certain cell surface markers. Kupffer cells are defined as $CD11b^{low}$, $F4/80^{hi}$, C-type lectin domain family 4 member F, $CD68^{+}$, and CX3C chemokine receptor 1 $(CX_3CR1)^{-}$ (6, 7). MoMϕs are $CD11b^{+}$, $F4/80^{+}$, $Ly6C^{+}$, macrophage colony-stimulating factor 1 receptor $(CSF1R)^{+}$. Human KCs are not as well-characterized and normally identified as $CD68^{+}$ cells (8). Human MoMϕs are normally identified as $CD14^{+}$, CC-chemokine receptor 2 $(CCR2)^{+}$ cells (**Table 1**) (8, 9).

A salient function of macrophages is to remove pathogens and dead cells (3). In a healthy liver, KCs constantly phagocytose aged erythrocytes, neutrophils, and effector $CD8^{+}$ T cells, thereby maintaining homeostasis within the liver (10–12). Monocyte-derived macrophages are also able to phagocytose dead endothelial cells and maintain integrity of vasculature under normal condition (13). The phagocytosis function of macrophages and its contribution to liver homeostasis and disease have been recently highlighted in an excellent review (14). Aside from phagocytosis, macrophages act as antigen-presenting cells and regulate adaptive immune responses. It is known that KCs play a central role in inducing immune tolerance to innocuous antigens that reached the liver from the intestine (15). In contrast, MoMϕs that are recruited into the liver lose the tolerogenic phenotype and instead contribute to antigen-specific proinflammatory immune

TABLE 1 | Difference between KCs and MoMϕs.

	KCs	MoMϕs
Origins	Fetal liver-derived erythromyeloid progenitors	Circulatory monocytes from bone marrow-derived haematopoietic stem cells
Location	Along the hepatic sinusoids, preferentially near the periportal area	Mainly in the portal triad of the healthy liver
Cell surface markers in mice	$CD11b^{low}$, $F4/80^{hi}$, $Clec4F^+$, $CD68^+$, $CX3CR1^-$	$CD11b^+$, $F4/80^+$, $Ly6C^+$, $CSF1R^+$
Cell surface markers in humans	$CD68^+$	$CD14^+$, $CCR2^+$
Functional differences	Induce immune tolerance to innocuous antigens; defend against pathogens; sense alterations in tissue integrity and maintain tissue homeostasis; orchestrate tissue repair after injury; facilitate leukocyte recruitment	Contribute to anti-bacterial responses; replenish KCs after injury; co-existence of subsets with opposing functions of pro-inflammatory and anti-inflammatory; pro-fibrogenic and anti-fibrogenetic

KCs, Kuppfer cells; MoMϕs, Monocytes-derived macrophages; CD11b, cluster of differentiation molecule 11B; Clec4f, C-type lectin domain family 4 member f; CX3CR1, CX3C chemokine receptor 1; CSF1R, Colony-stimulating factor 1 receptor; CCR2, Chemokine (C-C motif) receptor 2.

responses (**Table 1**) (16). During liver injury, a large number of circulating monocytes infiltrate into the liver and further differentiate into MoMϕs (17). Injury-induced modulations of the liver tissue microenvironment, such as soluble mediators released by activated/stress cells and accumulation of dead cells, influence the phenotypes of both KCs and MoMϕs and determine their involvement in aggravation of liver injury or restoration of liver functions (6, 16, 17). Under healthy and disease conditions, we call any signals received from local microenvironment and prompted functional differentiation of hepatic macrophages as microenvironmental signals. Understanding how microenvironmental signals affect the heterogeneity of hepatic macrophages and how hepatic macrophages interact with other cells during liver injury is instrumental not only in gaining basic knowledge but also in designing therapeutic strategies to treat liver diseases. In this review, we summarize the latest findings about specific environmental signals that impact the phenotype and function of hepatic macrophages and discuss the functions of hepatic macrophages in healthy and diseased liver through interacting with other cells.

ORIGIN OF HEPATIC MACROPHAGES

The recent development and improvement of research tools have allowed us to gain novel insights into the origin of hepatic macrophages. Contrary to the notion that KCs are originated solely from bone marrow–derived circulating monocytes (18), recent evidence suggests that KCs are mainly derived from yolk sac erythromyeloid progenitors (EMPs). Erythromyeloid progenitors colonize the fetal liver at E8.5 and give rise to macrophage precursors (pMacs) at E9.5 in a CX3CR1-dependent manner. A distinct transcriptional programming involving the upregulation of DNA binding 3 (Id3) is important in the further differentiation of pMacs into KCs (19). With regard to the maintenance of tissue-resident macrophages including KCs, an interesting "niche competition" model has been put forth. This model proposes that bone marrow–derived circulating monocytes and EMPs have an almost identical potential to develop into KCs and that they compete for a restricted number of niches. However, during liver development, the majority of liver niches are taken by EMPs and few by monocytes. At steady state, the niches in liver are self-maintained and tightly controlled by specific Maf transcription repressors and enhancers (20). However, when a significant number of KCs die or depleted experimentally, circulating monocytes have been shown to contribute to the KCs pool, suggesting that circulating monocytes have the potential as their embryonic counterparts to develop into KCs (21–23).

Monocyte-derived macrophages are derived from circulatory monocytes, which are developed from bone marrow–resident hematopoietic stem cells (23). Hematopoietic stem cells first differentiate into common lymphoid progenitors and then into granulocyte–monocyte progenitors (24, 25). Granulocyte–monocyte progenitors further give rise to common monocyte progenitors (cMoPs) under the regulation of macrophage CSF-1 (26). Eventually, cMoPs differentiate into circulatory monocytes. These distinct steps of hepatic stellate cell (HSC) differentiation into monocytes are tightly regulated by a number of transcription factors and epigenetic DNA methylation mechanisms (23). In mice, there are two subsets of monocytes in the liver: $Ly6C^{hi}$ and $Ly6C^{low}$ monocytes. The $Ly6C^{hi}$ monocytes can differentiate into $Ly6C^{low}$ monocytes, which can further differentiate into MoMϕs (27, 28). In humans, the $CD14^{hi}CD16^-$ and $CD14^-CD16^{hi}$ monocytes correlate with $Ly6C^{hi}$ and $Ly6C^{low}$ monocytes in mice, respectively (29).

IMPACT OF TISSUE MICROENVIRONMENTAL FACTORS ON HEPATIC MACROPHAGES

Irrespective of the cellular origins of hepatic macrophages, they differentiate into different phenotypes depending on the stimulatory signals in the tissue environment (30). In disease conditions, there are two major types of stimulatory signals (**Table 2**), including danger-associated molecular patterns (DAMPs) and pathogen-associated molecular patterns (PAMPs).

Danger-associated molecular patterns are a diverse group of molecules including nucleic acid in various conformations (e.g., single-/double-stranded RNA or DNA), nuclear proteins

TABLE 2 | Microenvironment in the liver.

	Examples	Reported in liver diseases	References
DAMPs	HMGB-1	AILI, I/R injury, NASH	(31–36)
	HSP-70	AILI	(37, 38)
	Bile acids	Cholestatic liver disease	(39–43)
	Histones	I/R injury	(44)
	FFAs	NASH	(45)
	mtDNA	NASH	(45)
PAMPs	Bacteria-derived products, e.g. LPS	ALD, NASH	(46–49)
	Hepatitis virus, e.g. HBV, HCV, HEV	Hepatitis virus infection	(50–52)
Phagocytosis of cellular debris	Apoptotic cells	LPS/D-gal-induced hepatitis, CCL4-induced liver fibrosis, ALD	(53–55)

DAMPs, danger-associated molecular patterns; PAMPs, pathogen-associated molecular patterns; HMGB-1, high mobility group box 1; HSP-70, heat shock protein 70; FFAs, free fatty acids; mtDNA, mitochondrial DNA; LPS, Lipopolysaccharides; HBV, hepatitis B virus; HCV, hepatitis C virus; HEV, hepatitis E virus; AILI, Acetaminophen-induced liver injury; I/R, Ischemia/Reperfusion; NASH, Non-alcoholic steatohepatitis; ALD, Alcoholic liver disease.

[e.g., high mobility group box 1 (HMGB1)], cytosolic proteins [e.g., heat shock protein 70 (HSP-70)], purine nucleotides [e.g., adenosine triphosphate (ATP)], or mitochondrial compounds (e.g., mtDNA, N-formyl peptides). Danger-associated molecular patterns are recognized by pathogen recognition receptors (PRRs), which are expressed on hepatic macrophages and can activate the cells (56, 57). These PRR receptors include Toll-like receptors (TLRs), nucleotide-binding oligomerization domain–like receptors (NLRs), and retinoic acid-inducible gene 1–like receptors (56). Danger-associated molecular patterns play a critical role in activating macrophages during sterile liver injury, which can be caused by a variety of stimuli, such as overdose of acetaminophen (APAP), cholestatic obstruction, excess accumulation of free fatty acids (FFAs), or hepatic ischemia, and reperfusion (I/R) (31, 58). The release of DAMPs is common in these situations, and it may be an active process from viable or dying cells, or a passive process leaking out from necrotic cells (56).

In APAP-induced liver injury (AILI), hepatocyte damage leads to the release of HMGB1, which activates KCs to produce proinflammatory cytokines and chemokines (31). High mobility group box 1 is a nuclear-binding protein that can function as a DNA chaperone in nucleus, sustaining autophagy in cytosol and DAMP molecule outside the cell (32). High mobility group box 1–deficient mice show less inflammation and neutrophil recruitment post-APAP treatment when compared to their wild-type counterparts (31, 33). Mice lacking the receptor for advanced glycation end products, a receptor for HMGB1, on bone marrow–derived cells display a similar phenotype as the HMGB1-deficient mice (31, 33). Together, these data indicate that HMGB1 activates KCs and contributes to AILI (31, 33). Aside from HMGB1, HSP-70 has also been reported to be released by necrotic hepatocytes during AILI (37). Heat shock protein 70 is an important component of cellular machinery, facilitating protein folding, but also an inducible stress-response protein that can undergo translocation to the cell surface or is released into the extracellular milieu during cellular stress or necrotic death (38). Heat shock protein 70 can stimulate macrophages to promote immune response and inflammation (37).

Similar to the necroinflammatory injury pattern in AILI, cholestatic liver disease is also characterized by hepatocytes necrosis (59). Lesions in bile duct canaliculi cause an increase of bile acids, which result in liver injury, but appear to drive KCs into anti-inflammatory state (39, 59). Bile acids can bind to G-protein–coupled bile acid receptor (TGR5), which is expressed on hepatic macrophages (40). Activation of TGR5 in macrophages reduces proinflammatory cytokines while maintaining anti-inflammatory cytokines (41). The anti-inflammatory effect of TGR5 on macrophages is mediated by inhibiting nuclear factor κB and JNK signaling pathways and NLRP3 inflammasome (41, 43).

Hepatic I/R injury is another example of sterile tissue injury in which DAMPs are released. It is reported that after I/R injury hepatocytes actively secrete HMGB1, which binds to TLR4 and activates KCs (34). In addition to HMGB1, other DAMPs, such as histones, DNA fragments, ATP, and mitochondrial reactive oxygen species (ROS), also activate KCs via different PRRs, such as TLR9 (recognizing histones) (44), TLR3 (recognizing RNA) (60, 61), TLR4 (recognizing HSP-70) (62), and nucleotide-binding domain leucine-rich repeat containing family pyrin domain containing 3 (NLRP3) (recognizing ATP) (63, 64). As a result, KCs secrete ample proinflammatory cytokines to exacerbate I/R injury (65).

Non-alcoholic steatohepatitis (NASH) is characterized by steatosis with tissue injury and inflammation (35). Increased accumulation of fat in hepatocytes leads to lipotoxicity, which induces apoptotic and necrotic death of hepatocytes with concomitant release of DAMPs, such as HMGB1 and FFAs (35). Released HMGB1 activates KCs via TLR4 as in other liver injury cases (35, 36). Free fatty acids decrease the mitochondrial membrane potential and subsequently induce mtDNA release from the mitochondria to the cytoplasm (45). Released mtDNA causes NLRP3 inflammasome activation in KCs, which further promotes the production of proinflammatory interleukin 1β (IL-1β) (45).

Pathogen-associated molecular patterns include pathogen-specific polysaccharides, lipoproteins, and nucleic acids. They bind to PPRs expressed on hepatic macrophages and trigger inflammatory activation of these cells (66). In alcoholic liver disease (ALD), excess chronic ingestion of alcohol increases gut permeability and causes translocation of bacteria-derived products, such as lipopolysaccharides (LPSs), from the gut to the liver (67). Lipopolysaccharide binds to CD14 in association with TLR4 on KCs to initiate proinflammatory signaling (46). Numerous studies have demonstrated that KCs play a central role in alcohol-induced inflammation and injury of the liver (27, 28). Kupffer cells produce cytokines such as tumor necrosis factor α (TNF-α) and free radicals to promote ALD (68, 69). In addition to KCs, MoMϕs can be differentiated from the circulating monocytes that are recruited into the liver as a result of the inflammatory response during liver injury (28). Two types of MoMϕs ($Ly6C^{low}$ MoMϕs and $Ly6C^{hi}$ MoMϕs) have been reported to coexist in the liver of mice after chronic alcohol feeding. The $Ly6C^{low}$ MoMϕs exhibit restorative phenotype, whereas $Ly6C^{hi}$ MoMϕs exhibit proinflammatory phenotype. A large dose of alcohol binge after chronic alcohol feeding enhances liver inflammation and injury with an increased ratio of $Ly6C^{hi}/Ly6C^{low}$ MoMϕ. Moreover, $Ly6C^{hi}$ MoMϕ switches to $Ly6C^{low}$ MoMϕ upon phagocytosis of apoptotic hepatocytes. Taken together, KCs and MoMϕ are involved in the pathogenesis of ALD (27, 28, 70).

Whereas, translocation of LPS from the gut lumen to portal circulation in ALD may result from direct alcohol toxicity to intestinal epithelium (67), increased exposure to intestinal LPS has also been considered in the pathogenesis of NASH (71). Increased levels of LPS in the portal circulation have been observed during NASH development (72). The role of LPS-TLR4 signaling in non-alcoholic fatty liver disease (NAFLD) has been demonstrated in a number of studies (47). Toll-like receptor 4 expression on KCs is elevated both in patients with NASH and mice fed with methionine–choline–deficient diet (47, 48). Depletion of KCs by clodronate liposomes significantly reduced TLR4 expression and steatohepatitis (47). Together, endotoxin appears to play an important role in NAFLD through TLRs on KCs, particularly TLR4. However, the function of MoMϕ in response to endotoxin during NAFLD remains unclear.

Hepatitis virus infection is a leading cause of chronic liver diseases (49). Hepatitis B virus (HBV) modulates liver macrophage functions to favor viral replication and survival. These modulations include reduced production of antiviral cytokine IL-1β and enhanced levels of immunosuppressive IL-10 (73). Hepatitis C virus (HCV) can enter KCs through phagocytic uptake. Subsequently, viral RNA triggers myeloid differentiation primary response gene 88 (MyD88)–mediated TLR7 signaling to induce IL-1β expression. Hepatitis C virus uptake concomitantly induces a potassium efflux that activates the NLRP3 inflammasome and promotes the secretion of activated IL-1β. Interleukin 1β produced by KCs contributes to HCV disease severity (74). It has also been reported that the function of monocytes/macrophages is impaired in pregnant patients with hepatitis E virus (HEV)–induced acute hepatitis (50). Toll-like receptor 3 and TLR7 expressions are reduced, and MyD88 downstream molecules, IRF3 and IRF7, are decreased in macrophages from these patients (50). The macrophage phagocytic activity and *Escherichia coli*–induced ROS production are significantly impaired in macrophages from HEV patients as well (50). These data suggest that the impact of viruses on hepatic macrophages could result in immune suppression and/or inflammation and tissue damage.

Phagocytosis of Dead Cells

A salient function of macrophages is to remove dead cells and cellular debris, which is a key initial step in resolving tissue inflammation and promoting tissue repair from injury. It has been widely reported that phagocytosis of dead cells triggers transcriptional reprogramming of macrophages to switch from a proinflammatory to an anti-inflammatory and tissue restorative phenotype. For example, it is shown that the membrane-bound transforming growth factor β (TGF-β) on apoptotic cells can trigger KCs to produce IL-10, which suppresses the proinflammatory immune response in a mouse model of LPS/D-galactosamine–induced hepatitis (51, 52). In a mouse model of ALD, it is reported that phagocytosis of cellular debris triggers hepatic macrophages to switch from proinflammatory to an anti-inflammatory phenotype (28). Similarly, in a mouse model of carbon tetrachloride–induced liver fibrosis, phagocytosis of cellular debris induces $Ly6C^{hi}$ proinflammatory, profibrotic MoMϕs to differentiate into antifibrotic macrophages (52). The restorative macrophages are the most abundant subset in the liver during maximal fibrosis resolution and represent the predominant source of matrix metalloproteinases. Moreover, it has been demonstrated that phagocytosis of necrotic hepatocytes by macrophages activates Wnt ligand secretion, thereby promoting liver regeneration (53).

In summary, the particular function of KCs and MoMϕ is tightly regulated by microenvironmental signals, such as DAMPs and PAMPs. The same signals may play a similar role in different liver diseases; for example, HMGB1 released by hepatocytes triggers KC activation in AILI, I/R, and NASH, indicating similar functions of macrophages in various liver diseases (32–34, 37, 54, 56, 58, 75, 76). In certain liver diseases, such as NAFLD and ALD, DAMPs and PAMPs coexist to regulate macrophage functions (35, 56, 77, 78) However, more studies are warranted to better understand the differential functions of KCs and MoMϕs in a given disease situation.

COMMUNICATION BETWEEN HEPATIC MACROPHAGES AND OTHER CELLS IN THE LIVER

There are five major cell types in the liver including hepatocytes, biliary epithelial cells (cholangiocytes), liver sinusoidal endothelial cells (LSECs), KCs, and HSCs (66, 79). Hepatocytes account for roughly 80% of the liver's mass (79), and they perform a number of vital functions, including protein synthesis, detoxification, and metabolism of lipids and carbohydrates (79). Cholangiocytes are another type of epithelial cells in the liver, lining the lumen of the

TABLE 3 | The crosstalk of hepatic macrophages with other cells in the liver.

	Interacted cell types	Roles of hepatic macrophages in interaction	Reported in liver diseases	References
KCs	Hepatocytes	KCs activate Notch signaling in hepatocytes	ICC	(81)
	Hepatocytes	KCs are essential for proliferation of liver progenitor cells	Choline-deficient, ethionine-supplemented diet-mediated liver injury	(82)
	Hepatocytes	KCs trigger hepatocytes senescence	ALD	(83)
	Hepatocytes	KC are activated by hepatocytes-derived extracellular vesicles	ALD	(84, 85)
	HSCs	KCs activate HSCs and modulate fibrogenic responses in HSCs	Liver fibrosis	(86, 87)
	HSCs	KCs secrete IFN-γ to induce apoptosis of HSCs	Liver fibrosis	(88)
	HSCs	HSCs induce KCs differentiation and decrease its cytokine secretion	Liver fibrosis	(89)
	LSECs	KCs are essential for LSECs' uptake of hyaluronic acid	*In vitro* culture	(90)
	MoMϕs	KCs produce CCL2 to recruit MoMϕs	Amodiaquine-induced liver injury	(91)
	Neutrophils	The production of TNF-α and TGF-β by KCs is promoted by neutrophil-secreted IL-17; Express adhesion molecules to recruit neutrophils	Cholestatic liver injury, LPS-induced liver injury	(92, 93)
	NKT cells	KCs produce IL-1β to recruit and activate NKT cells	Alcoholic steatosis	(94)
	$CD4^+$ T cells	KCs produce ROS, IL-6 and TNF-α to recruit $CD4^+$ T cells.	Hepatic I/R injury	(95)
	T cells	KCs produce IL-10, TGF-β, ROS, IDO, PGE2/J2 to induce and maintain T cell tolerance or apoptosis	Liver transplantation, HBV infection, *in vitro* culture	(96–101)
	$CD8^+$ T cells	KCs prime $CD8^+$ T cells to differentiate into effector cells to kill viruses	HBV infection	
	Platelets	KCs promote adhesion of platelets on the KCs to encase the bacteria and facilitate anti-bacterial responses	Bacteria infection in the liver	
MoMϕs	cholangiocytes	MoMϕs release IL-6 to promote the proliferation of cholangiocytes	Cholestatic liver disease	(102, 103)
	cholangiocytes	MoMϕs are recruited by cholangiocytes-derived osteopontin and MCP-1	Partial Hepatectomy	(104)
	LSECs	LSECs are activated by MoMϕs	Partial Hepatectomy	(105)
	NKT cells	MoMϕs promote NKT cells over-activation and cell death	NAFLD	(106)
	NKT cells	MoMϕs produce IL-12 to activate NKT cells, which inhibits liver regeneration	Partial hepatectomy	(107)

KCs, Kuppfer cells; MoMϕs, Monocytes-derived macrophages; LSECs, liver sinusoidal endothelial cells; HSCs, hepatic stellate cells; NKT cells, natural killer T cell; IFN-γ, Interferon-gamma; CCL2, chemokine (C-C motif) ligand 2; TNF-α, tumor necrosis factor alpha; TGF-β, transforming growth factor beta; IL-17, interleukin 17; IL-1β, interleukin 1 beta; IL-6, interleukin 6; IL-10, interleukin 10; ROS, reactive oxygen species; IDO, indoleamine 2,3-dioxygenase; PGE2/J2, prostaglandin E2/J2; MCP-1, monocyte chemoattractant protein-1; ICC, intrahepatic cholangiocarcinoma; LPS, lipopolysaccharides; HBV, hepatitis B virus; I/R, ischemia/reperfusion.

bile ducts (79). Liver sinusoidal endothelial cells form the lining of the smallest blood vessels in the liver, part of the reticuloendothelial system (79). Liver sinusoidal endothelial cells regulate the passage of molecules from the blood vessels into the liver (79). Hepatic stellate cells are found in the space of Disse, between hepatocytes and LSECs. Hepatic stellate cells can transdifferentiate from a quiescent state to an activated, highly proliferative, and wound-healing myofibroblast (80). In addition, there are a variety of other immune cells such as monocytes, neutrophils, and platelets that contribute to liver homeostasis as well as disease progression (66). In different types and stages of liver diseases, hepatic macrophages are critically involved in the progression and regression via close communication with other cells in the liver (**Table 3**) (108).

Crosstalk Between Hepatic Macrophages and Hepatocytes

The crosstalk between hepatic macrophages and hepatocytes has been indicated in a number of studies. In a mouse model of thioacetamide (TAA)–induced intrahepatic cholangiocarcinoma, KCs accumulate around the central vein area and express Notch ligand Jagged-1 rapidly after the initiation of the TAA treatment, coinciding with the activation of Notch signaling in pericentral hepatocytes. Depletion of KCs prevents the Notch-mediated hepatocytes transformation to cholangiocytes, suggesting that KCs contribute to the cell fate change in hepatocytes (109). Another study has also demonstrated that KCs are required for the proliferation of liver progenitor cells that can differentiate into hepatocytes in a model of choline-deficient, ethionine-supplemented diet–mediated liver injury and regeneration (110). In ALD, it is shown that KC-produced IL-6 triggers hepatocyte senescence, which becomes resistant to apoptosis (81). Interestingly, recent studies also support that hepatocytes communicate with macrophages through the release of extracellular vesicles (EVs) that contain proteins and microRNAs (82, 83). *In vitro* studies using HepG2 cells have demonstrated that alcohol treatment induces an elevated release of EVs, which activate THP-1 cells, a human leukemia monocytic cell line into a proinflammatory phenotype through CD40 ligand (83). Another study also showed that exosomes derived from alcohol-treated hepatocytes mediated the transfer of liver-specific miRNA-122 to monocytes and sensitized monocytes to LPS stimulation (82). These studies suggest that hepatocytes release EVs that contain altered proteins and miRNAs to regulate the activation of monocytes/macrophages.

Interactions of Hepatic Macrophages With Cholangiocytes, HSCs, and LSECs

Macrophages secrete IL-6 during infection, and IL-6 can induce cholangiocyte proliferation leading to ductular reaction (84, 85). On the other hand, cholangiocytes are the major source of osteopontin and macrophage chemoattractant protein 1, which acts as chemotaxis to recruit MoMϕs during partial hepatectomy (102). Hepatic stellate cells and KCs are located in close proximity to each other (86, 103). In a mouse model of CCl_4-induced liver fibrosis, it is shown that depletion of hypoxia-inducible factor 1α in HSCs inhibits KC activation and reduces the release of proinflammatory cytokines, suggesting a function of HSCs in regulating KCs during liver fibrosis (87). On the other hand, KCs have also been reported to modulate HSC functions. Chemokine (C-X-C motif) ligand 6 stimulates the phosphorylation of epidermal growth factor receptor and the expression of TGF-β in KCs, which further activates HSCs and results in liver fibrosis (103). It is reported that ROS and IL-6 activate KCs, which in turn modulate fibrogenic responses of HSCs (104). Activated KCs secrete interferon γ, which subsequently induces HSC apoptosis in a STAT1-dependent manner and reduces liver fibrosis (111). Liver sinusoidal endothelial cells are the major source of intercellular adhesion molecule 1 (ICAM-1). In partial hepatectomy, ICAM-1 expressed on KCs and LSECs recruits leukocytes, which leads to TNF-α and IL-6 production, thereby promoting hepatocyte proliferation (89). Moreover, MoMϕs also play an important role in activating LSECs and contributing to vascular growth and liver regeneration (88). Kupffer cell depletion inhibits hyaluronic acid uptake by LSECs and impairs sinusoidal integrity, suggesting there is a crosstalk between KCs and LSECs (37, 112).

Interactions of Macrophages With Other Hepatic Immune Cells

Kupffer cell activation by pathogens results in CCL2 secretion, which promotes the recruitment of monocytes into the injured liver (105). It has been reported that alcohol treatment of THP-1 cells or human primary monocytes triggers the secretion of EVs, which induce the differentiation of naive monocytes into anti-inflammatory macrophages by delivering cargos, such as miR-27a (90).

Neutrophils are the most abundant white blood cells in the circulation, and they are recruited to the liver in various injury conditions (91). During cholestatic liver injury, neutrophils secrete IL-17, which promotes the production of TNF-α and TGF-β by KCs. On the other hand, KCs express adhesion molecules that induce neutrophil attachment and facilitate bacterial clearance in the liver (113). Another study reported that KCs coordinate with LSECs for neutrophil adhesion, recruitment, and activation through TLR4 during LPS-induced liver injury (78).

Natural killer T (NKT) cells are a group of "unconventional" T cells that express both natural killer (NK) cell receptors and T cell receptors. In the NASH liver, lipid accumulation causes an increase of the number of MoMϕs and activates the cells to a proinflammatory phenotype. Activated MoMϕs promote NKT cell activation and induce NKT cell deficiency, contributing to the pathogenesis of NAFLD (93). The importance of KC/NKT interaction in liver regeneration has also been described. After partial hepatectomy, MoMϕs produce IL-12 to activate hepatic NKT cells, which prohibit liver regeneration (114). In ALD, NLRP3 inflammasome activation results in IL-1β release by KCs. Released IL-1β recruits and activates hepatic invariant NKT cells, which promote liver inflammation, neutrophil infiltration, and liver injury (106). Furthermore, ample evidence supports the importance of macrophages in interacting with conventional T cells. It has been shown that KCs trigger the recruitment of $CD4^+$ T cells by ROS, IL-6, and TNF-α (107). Kupffer cells express high levels of MHC class II and act as antigen-presenting cells. In fact, a number of studies have shown that KCs play an important role in inducing and maintaining T cell tolerance, through producing tolerogenic mediators such as IL-10, TGF-β, ROS, indoleamine 2,3-dioxygenase, prostaglandin E_2/J_2 (94, 97). Moreover, it is reported that during liver transplantation KCs induce T cell apoptosis and thus promote immune tolerance (98). After HBV infection, KCs produce IL-10 and support liver tolerance by inducing anti-HBV $CD8^+$ T cell exhaustion (99). A recent study demonstrated that the induction of endoplasmic reticulum stress in HCC cell lines induces the secretion of EVs. The HCC-derived EVs induce elevated expression of programmed death ligand 1 on macrophages *in vivo* and *in vitro*, which causes T cell dysfunction and impaired proliferation (100). Recent studies showed that priming $CD8^+$ T cells by KCs leads to the differentiation of $CD8^+$ T cells into effector cells that have powerful killing activities against hepatitis viruses, such as HBV (101).

Moreover, interesting interactions between macrophages and platelets have been unveiled (115). Under basal conditions, platelets form transient "touch-and-go" interactions with von Willebrand factor constitutively expressed on KCs (115). During bacterial infection, platelets switch from "tough-and-go" to sustained GPIIb-mediated adhesion on the KCs to encase the bacteria and facilitate anti-bacterial responses (115).

In summary, hepatic macrophages interact with almost all cell types of the liver. In naive state, KCs, through these interactions, play a critical role in maintaining tissue homeostasis. Under injury or disease conditions, the crosstalk of macrophages with hepatocytes, cholangiocytes, LSECs, HSCs, and other immune cells contributes to exacerbation of tissue damage or promotion of liver repair and regeneration, depending on the cell type and signaling pathways involved.

AUTHOR CONTRIBUTIONS

All authors listed have made a substantial, direct and intellectual contribution to the work, and approved it for publication. ZS wrote the draft. CJ revised the manuscript.

REFERENCES

1. Ju C, Tacke F. Hepatic macrophages in homeostasis and liver diseases: from pathogenesis to novel therapeutic strategies. *Cell Mol Immunol.* (2016) 13:316–27. doi: 10.1038/cmi.2015.104
2. Bilzer M, Roggel F, Gerbes AL. Role of Kupffer cells in host defense and liver disease. *Liver Int.* (2006) 26:1175–86. doi: 10.1111/j.1478-3231.2006.01342.x
3. Abdullah Z, Knolle PA. Liver macrophages in healthy and diseased liver. *Pflugers Arch.* (2017) 469:553–60. doi: 10.1007/s00424-017-1954-6
4. Theurl I, Hilgendorf I, Nairz M, Tymoszuk P, Haschka D, Asshoff M, et al. On-demand erythrocyte disposal and iron recycling requires transient macrophages in the liver. *Nat Med.* (2016) 22:945–51. doi: 10.1038/nm.4146
5. Gammella E, Buratti P, Cairo G, Recalcati S. Macrophages: central regulators of iron balance. *Metallomics.* (2014) 6:1336–45. doi: 10.1039/C4MT00104D
6. Scott CL, Zheng F, De Baetselier P, Martens L, Saeys Y, De Prijck S, et al. Bone marrow-derived monocytes give rise to self-renewing and fully differentiated Kupffer cells. *Nat Commun.* (2016) 7:10321. doi: 10.1038/ncomms10321
7. Lavin Y, Winter D, Blecher-Gonen R, David E, Keren-Shaul H, Merad M, et al. Tissue-resident macrophage enhancer landscapes are shaped by the local microenvironment. *Cell.* (2014) 159:1312–26. doi: 10.1016/j.cell.2014.11.018
8. Krenkel O, Tacke F. Liver macrophages in tissue homeostasis and disease. *Nat Rev Immunol.* (2017) 17:306–21. doi: 10.1038/nri.2017.11
9. Dal-Secco D, Wang J, Zeng Z, Kolaczkowska E, Wong CH, Petri B, et al. A dynamic spectrum of monocytes arising from the in situ reprogramming of CCR2+ monocytes at a site of sterile injury. *J Exp Med.* (2015) 212:447–56. doi: 10.1084/jem.20141539
10. Terpstra V, van Berkel TJ. Scavenger receptors on liver Kupffer cells mediate the *in vivo* uptake of oxidatively damaged red blood cells in mice. *Blood.* (2000) 95:2157–63. doi: 10.1182/blood.V95.6.2157
11. Shi JL, Fujieda H, Kokubo Y, Wake K. Apoptosis of neutrophils and their elimination by Kupffer cells in rat liver. *Hepatology.* (1996) 24:1256–63. doi: 10.1002/hep.510240545
12. Crispe IN, Dao T, Klugewitz K, Mehal WZ, Metz DP. The liver as a site of T-cell apoptosis: graveyard, or krilling field? *Immunol. Rev.* (2000) 174:47–62. doi: 10.1034/j.1600-0528.2002.017412.x
13. Carlin LM, Stamatiades EG, Auffray C, Hanna RN, Glover L, Vizcay-Barrena G, et al. Nr4a1-dependent Ly6C(low) monocytes monitor endothelial cells and orchestrate their disposal. *Cell.* (2013) 153:362–75. doi: 10.1016/j.cell.2013.03.010
14. Horst AK, Tiegs G, Diehl L. Contribution of macrophage efferocytosis to liver homeostasis and disease. *Front Immunol.* (2019) 10. doi: 10.3389/fimmu.2019.02670
15. Crispe IN. Immune tolerance in liver disease. *Hepatology.* (2014) 60:2109–17. doi: 10.1002/hep.27254
16. Heymann F, Peusquens J, Ludwig-Portugall I, Kohlhepp M, Ergen C, Niemietz P, et al. Liver inflammation abrogates immunological tolerance induced by Kupffer cells. *Hepatology.* (2015) 62:279–91. doi: 10.1002/hep.27793
17. Zigmond E, Samia-Grinberg S, Pasmanik-Chor M, Brazowski E, Shibolet O, Halpern Z, et al. Infiltrating monocyte-derived macrophages and resident kupffer cells display different ontogeny and functions in acute liver injury. *J Immunol.* (2014) 193:344–53. doi: 10.4049/jimmunol.1400574
18. van Furth R, Cohn ZA. The origin and kinetics of mononuclear phagocytes. *J Exp Med.* (1968) 128:415–35. doi: 10.1084/jem.128.3.415
19. Mass E, Ballesteros I, Farlik M, Halbritter F, Gunther P, Crozet L, et al. Contribution of macrophage efferocytosis to liver homeostasis and disease. *Science.* (2016) 353:aaf4238. doi: 10.1126/science.aaf4238
20. Soucie EL, Weng Z, Geirsdottir L, Molawi K, Maurizio J, Fenouil R, et al. Lineage-specific enhancers activate self-renewal genes in macrophages and embryonic stem cells. *Science.* (2016) 351:aad5510. doi: 10.1126/science.aad5510
21. Sawai CM, Babovic S, Upadhaya S, Knapp D, Lavin Y, Lau CM, et al. Hematopoietic stem cells are the major source of multilineage hematopoiesis in adult animals. *Immunity.* (2016) 45:597–609. doi: 10.1016/j.immuni.2016.08.007
22. Guilliams M, Scott CL. Does niche competition determine the origin of tissue-resident macrophages? *Nat Rev Immunol.* (2017) 17:451–60. doi: 10.1038/nri.2017.42
23. Eaves CJ. Hematopoietic stem cells: concepts, definitions, and the new reality. *Blood.* (2015) 125:2605–13. doi: 10.1182/blood-2014-12-570200
24. Auffray C, Fogg DK, Narni-Mancinelli E, Senechal B, Trouillet C, Saederup N, et al. CX3CR1+ CD115+ CD135+ common macrophage/DC precursors and the role of CX3CR1 in their response to inflammation. *J Exp Med.* (2009) 206:595–606. doi: 10.1084/jem.20081385
25. Liu K, Victora GD, Schwickert TA, Guermonprez P, Meredith MM, Yao K, et al. *In vivo* analysis of dendritic cell development and homeostasis. *Science.* (2009) 324:392–7. doi: 10.1126/science.1170540
26. Dai XM, Ryan GR, Hapel AJ, Dominguez MG, Russell RG, Kapp S, et al. Targeted disruption of the mouse colony-stimulating factor 1 receptor gene results in osteopetrosis, mononuclear phagocyte deficiency, increased primitive progenitor cell frequencies, and reproductive defects. *Blood.* (2002) 99:111–20. doi: 10.1182/blood.V99.1.111
27. Wang M, Frasch SC, Li G, Feng D, Gao B, Xu L, et al. Role of gp91(phox) in hepatic macrophage programming and alcoholic liver disease. *Hepatol Commun.* (2017) 1:765–779. doi: 10.1002/hep4.1078
28. Wang M, You Q, Lor K, Chen F, Gao B, Ju C. Chronic alcohol ingestion modulates hepatic macrophage populations and functions in mice. *J Leukoc Biol.* (2014) 96:657–65. doi: 10.1189/jlb.6A0114-004RR
29. Ingersoll MA, Spanbroek R, Lottaz C, Gautier EL, Frankenberger M, Hoffmann R, et al. Comparison of gene expression profiles between human and mouse monocyte subsets. *Blood.* (2010) 115:e10–9. doi: 10.1182/blood-2009-07-235028
30. Xue J, Schmidt SV, Sander J, Draffehn A, Krebs W, Quester I, et al. Transcriptome-based network analysis reveals a spectrum model of human macrophage activation. *Immunity.* (2014) 40:274–88. doi: 10.1016/j.immuni.2014.01.006
31. Huebener P, Hernandez C, Schwabe RF. HMGB1 and injury amplification. *Oncotarget.* (2015) 6:23048–9. doi: 10.18632/oncotarget.5243
32. Chen RC, Hou W, Zhang QH, Kang R, Fan XG, Tang DL. Emerging role of high-mobility group box 1 (HMGB1) in liver diseases. *Mol. Med.* (2013) 19:357–66. doi: 10.2119/molmed.2013.00099
33. Huebener P, Pradere JP, Hernandez C, Gwak GY, Caviglia JM, Mu X, et al. The HMGB1/RAGE axis triggers neutrophil-mediated injury amplification following necrosis. *J Clin Invest.* (2015) 125:539–50. doi: 10.1172/JCI76887
34. Tsung A, Sahai R, Tanaka H, Nakao A, Fink MP, Lotze MT, et al. The nuclear factor HMGB1 mediates hepatic injury after murine liver ischemia-reperfusion. *J Exp Med.* (2005) 201:1135–43. doi: 10.1084/jem.20042614
35. Arrese M, Cabrera D, Kalergis AM, Feldstein AE. Innate immunity and inflammation in NAFLD/NASH. *Dig Dis Sci.* (2016) 61:1294–303. doi: 10.1007/s10620-016-4049-x
36. Li L, Chen L, Hu L, Liu Y, Sun HY, Tang J, et al. Nuclear factor high-mobility group box1 mediating the activation of Toll-like receptor 4 signaling in hepatocytes in the early stage of nonalcoholic fatty liver disease in mice. *Hepatology.* (2011) 54:1620–30. doi: 10.1002/hep.24552
37. Martin-Murphy BV, Holt MP, Ju C. The role of damage associated molecular pattern molecules in acetaminophen-induced liver injury in mice. *Toxicol Lett.* (2010) 192:387–94. doi: 10.1016/j.toxlet.2009.11.016
38. Wallin RP, Lundqvist A, More SH, von Bonin A, Kiessling R, Ljunggren HG. Heat-shock proteins as activators of the innate immune system. *Trends Immunol.* (2002) 23:130–5. doi: 10.1016/S1471-4906(01)02168-8
39. Fiorucci S, Biagioli M, Zampella A, Distrutti E. Bile acids activated receptors regulate innate immunity. *Front Immunol.* (2018) 9:1853. doi: 10.3389/fimmu.2018.01853
40. Perino A, Schoonjans K. TGR5 and Immunometabolism: Insights from Physiology and Pharmacology. *Trends Pharmacol Sci.* (2015) 36:847–57. doi: 10.1016/j.tips.2015.08.002
41. Reich M, Klindt C, Deutschmann K, Spomer L, Haussinger D, Keitel V. Role of the G protein-coupled bile acid receptor TGR5 in liver damage. *Dig Dis.* (2017) 35:235–40. doi: 10.1159/000450917
42. Lou G, Ma X, Fu X, Meng Z, Zhang W, Wang YD, et al. GPBAR1/TGR5 mediates bile acid-induced cytokine expression in murine Kupffer cells. *PLoS ONE.* (2014) 9:e93567. doi: 10.1371/journal.pone.0093567

43. Wang YD, Chen WD, Yu D, Forman BM, Huang W. The G-protein-coupled bile acid receptor, Gpbar1 (TGR5), negatively regulates hepatic inflammatory response through antagonizing nuclear factor kappa light-chain enhancer of activated B cells (NF-κB) in mice. *Hepatology.* (2011) 54:1421–32. doi: 10.1002/hep.24525
44. Huang H, Evankovich J, Yan W, Nace G, Zhang L, Ross M, et al. Endogenous histones function as alarmins in sterile inflammatory liver injury through Toll-like receptor 9 in mice. *Hepatology.* (2011) 54:999–1008. doi: 10.1002/hep.24501
45. Pan J, Ou Z, Cai C, Li P, Gong J, Ruan XZ, et al. Fatty acid activates NLRP3 inflammasomes in mouse Kupffer cells through mitochondrial DNA release. *Cell Immunol.* (2018) 332:111–20. doi: 10.1016/j.cellimm.2018.08.006
46. Rao R. Endotoxemia and gut barrier dysfunction in alcoholic liver disease. *Hepatology.* (2009) 50:638–44. doi: 10.1002/hep.23009
47. Rivera CA, Adegboyega P, van Rooijen N, Tagalicud A, Allman M, Wallace M. Toll-like receptor-4 signaling and Kupffer cells play pivotal roles in the pathogenesis of non-alcoholic steatohepatitis. *J Hepatol.* (2007) 47:571–9. doi: 10.1016/j.jhep.2007.04.019
48. Emontzpohl C, Stoppe C, Theissen A, Beckers C, Neumann UP, Lurje G, et al. The role of macrophage migration inhibitory factor in remote ischemic conditioning induced hepatoprotection in a rodent model of liver transplantation. *Shock.* (2019) 52:e124–e34. doi: 10.1097/SHK.0000000000001307
49. Bernal W, Auzinger G, Dhawan A, Wendon J. Acute liver failure. *Lancet.* (2010) 376:190–201. doi: 10.1016/S0140-6736(10)60274-7
50. Sehgal R, Patra S, David P, Vyas A, Khanam A, Hissar S, et al. Impaired monocyte-macrophage functions and defective Toll-like receptor signaling in hepatitis E virus-infected pregnant women with acute liver failure. *Hepatology.* (2015) 62:1683–96. doi: 10.1002/hep.28143
51. Zhang M, Xu S, Han Y, Cao X. Apoptotic cells attenuate fulminant hepatitis by priming Kupffer cells to produce interleukin-10 through membrane-bound TGF-beta. *Hepatology.* (2011) 53:306–16. doi: 10.1002/hep.24029
52. Ramachandran P, Pellicoro A, Vernon MA, Boulter L, Aucott RL, Ali A, et al. Differential Ly-6C expression identifies the recruited macrophage phenotype, which orchestrates the regression of murine liver fibrosis. *Proc Natl Acad Sci USA.* (2012) 109:E3186–95. doi: 10.1073/pnas.1119964109
53. Boulter L, Govaere O, Bird TG, Radulescu S, Ramachandran P, Pellicoro A, et al. Macrophage-derived Wnt opposes notch signaling to specify hepatic progenitor cell fate in chronic liver disease. *Nat Med.* (2012) 18:572–9. doi: 10.1038/nm.2667
54. Alisi A, Carsetti R, Nobili V. Pathogen- or damage-associated molecular patterns during nonalcoholic fatty liver disease development. *Hepatology.* (2011) 54:1500–2. doi: 10.1002/hep.24611
55. Evankovich J, Cho SW, Zhang R, Cardinal J, Dhupar R, Zhang L, et al. High mobility group box 1 release from hepatocytes during ischemia and reperfusion injury is mediated by decreased histone deacetylase activity. *J Biol Chem.* (2010) 285:39888–97. doi: 10.1074/jbc.M110.128348
56. Mihm S. Danger-Associated Molecular Patterns (DAMPs): Molecular Triggers for Sterile Inflammation in the Liver. *Int J Mol Sci.* (2018) 19:E3104. doi: 10.3390/ijms19103104
57. Shi Y, Evans JE, Rock KL. Molecular identification of a danger signal that alerts the immune system to dying cells. *Nature.* (2003) 425:516–21. doi: 10.1038/nature01991
58. Antoine DJ, Williams DP, Kipar A, Jenkins RE, Regan SL, Sathish JG, et al. High-mobility group box-1 protein and keratin-18, circulating serum proteins informative of acetaminophen-induced necrosis and apoptosis *in vivo*. *Toxicol Sci.* (2009) 112:521–31. doi: 10.1093/toxsci/kfp235
59. Li M, Cai SY, Boyer JL. Mechanisms of bile acid mediated inflammation in the liver. *Mol Aspects Med.* (2017) 56l:45–53. doi: 10.1016/j.mam.2017.06.001
60. Kariko K, Ni H, Capodici J, Lamphier M, Weissman D. mRNA is an endogenous ligand for Toll-like receptor 3. *J Biol Chem.* (2004) 279:12542–50. doi: 10.1074/jbc.M310175200
61. Cavassani KA, Ishii M, Wen H, Schaller MA, Lincoln PM, Lukacs NW, et al. TLR3 is an endogenous sensor of tissue necrosis during acute inflammatory events. *J Exp Med.* (2008) 205:2609–21. doi: 10.1084/jem.20081370
62. Calderwood SK, Gong J, Murshid A. Extracellular HSPs: the complicated roles of extracellular HSPs in immunity. *Front Immunol.* (2016) 7:159. doi: 10.3389/fimmu.2016.00159
63. Nomura J, So A, Tamura M, Busso N. Intracellular ATP decrease mediates NLRP3 inflammasome activation upon nigericin and crystal stimulation. *J Immunol.* (2015) 195:5718–24. doi: 10.4049/jimmunol.1402512
64. Baron L, Gombault A, Fanny M, Villeret B, Savigny F, Guillou N, et al. The NLRP3 inflammasome is activated by nanoparticles through ATP, ADP and adenosine. *Cell Death Dis.* (2015) 6:e1629. doi: 10.1038/cddis.2014.576
65. Chang WJ, Toledo-Pereyra LH. Toll-like receptor signaling in liver ischemia and reperfusion. *J Invest Surg.* (2012) 25:271–7. doi: 10.3109/08941939.2012.687802
66. Gao B, Jeong WI, Tian Z. Liver: an organ with predominant innate immunity. *Hepatology.* (2008) 47:729–36. doi: 10.1002/hep.22034
67. Parlesak A, Schafer C, Schutz T, Bode JC, Bode C. Increased intestinal permeability to macromolecules and endotoxemia in patients with chronic alcohol abuse in different stages of alcohol-induced liver disease. *J Hepatol.* (2000) 32:742–7. doi: 10.1016/S0168-8278(00)80242-1
68. Iimuro Y, Gallucci RM, Luster MI, Kono H, Thurman RG. Antibodies to tumor necrosis factor alfa attenuate hepatic necrosis and inflammation caused by chronic exposure to ethanol in the rat. *Hepatology.* (1997) 26:1530–37. doi: 10.1002/hep.510260621
69. Zhong Z, Connor H, Stachlewitz RF, VonFrankenberg M, Mason RP, Lemasters JJ, et al. Role of free radicals in primary nonfunction of marginal fatty grafts from rats treated acutely with ethanol. *Mol Pharmacol.* (1997) 52:912–19. doi: 10.1124/mol.52.5.912
70. Ju C, Liangpunsakul S. Role of hepatic macrophages in alcoholic liver disease. *J Investig Med.* (2016) 64:1075–7. doi: 10.1136/jim-2016-000210
71. Thuy S, Ladurner R, Volynets V, Wagner S, Strahl S, Konigsrainer A, et al. Nonalcoholic fatty liver disease in humans is associated with increased plasma endotoxin and plasminogen activator inhibitor 1 concentrations and with fructose intake. *J Nutr.* (2008) 138:1452–5. doi: 10.1093/jn/138.8.1452
72. Baffy G. Kupffer cells in non-alcoholic fatty liver disease: the emerging view. *J Hepatol.* (2009) 51:212–23. doi: 10.1016/j.jhep.2009.03.008
73. Faure-Dupuy S, Delphin M, Aillot L, Dimier L, Lebosse F, Fresquet J, et al. Hepatitis B virus-induced modulation of liver macrophage function promotes hepatocyte infection. *J Hepatol.* (2019) 71:1086–98. doi: 10.1016/j.jhep.2019.06.032
74. Negash AA, Ramos HJ, Crochet N, Lau DT, Doehle B, Papic N, et al. IL-1beta production through the NLRP3 inflammasome by hepatic macrophages links hepatitis C virus infection with liver inflammation and disease. *PLoS Pathog.* (2013) 9:e1003330. doi: 10.1371/journal.ppat.1003330
75. Dragomir AC, Laskin JD, Laskin DL. Macrophage activation by factors released from acetaminophen-injured hepatocytes: potential role of HMGB1. *Toxicol Appl Pharmacol.* (2011) 253:170–7. doi: 10.1016/j.taap.2011.04.003
76. McDonald KA, Huang H, Tohme S, Loughran P, Ferrero K, Billiar T, et al. Toll-like receptor 4 (TLR4) antagonist eritoran tetrasodium attenuates liver ischemia and reperfusion injury through inhibition of high-mobility group box protein B1 (HMGB1) signaling. *Mol Med.* (2015) 20:639–48. doi: 10.2119/molmed.2014.00076
77. Ganz M, Szabo G. Immune and inflammatory pathways in NASH. *Hepatol Int.* (2013) 7(Suppl 2):771–81. doi: 10.1007/s12072-013-9468-6
78. McDonald B, Jenne CN, Zhuo L, Kimata K, Kubes P. Kupffer cells and activation of endothelial TLR4 coordinate neutrophil adhesion within liver sinusoids during endotoxemia. *Am J Physiol Gastrointest Liver Physiol.* (2013) 305:G797–806. doi: 10.1152/ajpgi.00058.2013
79. Trefts E, Gannon M, Wasserman DH. The liver. *Curr Biol.* (2017) 27:R1147–51. doi: 10.1016/j.cub.2017.09.019
80. Tsuchida T, Friedman SL. Mechanisms of hepatic stellate cell activation. *Nat Rev Gastro Hepat.* (2017) 14:397–411. doi: 10.1038/nrgastro.2017.38
81. Wan J, Benkdane M, Alons E, Lotersztajn S, Pavoine C. M2 kupffer cells promote hepatocyte senescence: an IL-6-dependent protective mechanism against alcoholic liver disease. *Am J Pathol.* (2014) 184:1763–72. doi: 10.1016/j.ajpath.2014.02.014
82. Momen-Heravi F, Bala S, Kodys K, Szabo G. Exosomes derived from alcohol-treated hepatocytes horizontally transfer liver specific miRNA-122 and sensitize monocytes to LPS. *Sci Rep.* (2015) 5:9991. doi: 10.1038/srep09991
83. Verma VK, Li H, Wang R, Hirsova P, Mushref M, Liu Y, et al. Alcohol stimulates macrophage activation through caspase-dependent hepatocyte

derived release of CD40L containing extracellular vesicles. *J Hepatol.* (2016) 64:651–60. doi: 10.1016/j.jhep.2015.11.020
84. Park J, Tadlock L, Gores GJ, Patel T. Inhibition of interleukin 6-mediated mitogen-activated protein kinase activation attenuates growth of a cholangiocarcinoma cell line. *Hepatology.* (1999) 30:1128–33. doi: 10.1002/hep.510300522
85. Xiao Y, Wang J, Yan W, Zhou Y, Chen Y, Zhou K, et al. Dysregulated miR-124 and miR-200 expression contribute to cholangiocyte proliferation in the cholestatic liver by targeting IL-6/STAT3 signalling. *J Hepatol.* (2015) 62:889–96. doi: 10.1016/j.jhep.2014.10.033
86. Weiskirchen R, Tacke F. Cellular and molecular functions of hepatic stellate cells in inflammatory responses and liver immunology. *Hepatobiliary Surg Nutr.* (2014) 3:344–63.
87. Mochizuki A, Pace A, Rockwell CE, Roth KJ, Chow A, O'Brien KM, et al. Hepatic stellate cells orchestrate clearance of necrotic cells in a hypoxia-inducible factor-1alpha-dependent manner by modulating macrophage phenotype in mice. *J Immunol.* (2014) 192:3847–57. doi: 10.4049/jimmunol.1303195
88. Melgar-Lesmes P, Edelman ER. Monocyte-endothelial cell interactions in the regulation of vascular sprouting and liver regeneration in mouse. *J Hepatol.* (2015) 63:917–25. doi: 10.1016/j.jhep.2015.05.011
89. Selzner N, Selzner M, Odermatt B, Tian Y, Van Rooijen N, Clavien PA. ICAM-1 triggers liver regeneration through leukocyte recruitment and Kupffer cell-dependent release of TNF-alpha/IL-6 in mice. *Gastroenterology.* (2003) 124:692–700. doi: 10.1053/gast.2003.50098
90. Saha B, Momen-Heravi F, Kodys K, Szabo G. MicroRNA cargo of extracellular vesicles from alcohol-exposed monocytes signals naive monocytes to differentiate into M2 macrophages. *J Biol Chem.* (2016) 291:149–59. doi: 10.1074/jbc.M115.694133
91. Prame Kumar K, Nicholls AJ, Wong CHY. Partners in crime: neutrophils and monocytes/macrophages in inflammation and disease. *Cell Tissue Res.* (2018) 371:551–65. doi: 10.1007/s00441-017-2753-2
92. Bendelac A, Savage PB, Teyton L. The biology of NKT cells. *Annu Rev Immunol.* (2007) 25:297–336. doi: 10.1146/annurev.immunol.25.022106.141711
93. Tang T, Sui Y, Lian M, Li Z, Hua J. Pro-inflammatory activated Kupffer cells by lipids induce hepatic NKT cells deficiency through activation-induced cell death. *PLoS ONE.* (2013) 8:e81949. doi: 10.1371/journal.pone.0081949
94. You Q, Cheng L, Kedl RM, Ju C. Mechanism of T cell tolerance induction by murine hepatic Kupffer cells. *Hepatology.* (2008) 48:978–90. doi: 10.1002/hep.22395
95. Grohmann U, Fallarino F, Bianchi R, Belladonna ML, Vacca C, Orabona C, et al. IL-6 inhibits the tolerogenic function of CD8 alpha+ dendritic cells expressing indoleamine 2,3-dioxygenase. *J Immunol.* (2001) 167:708–14. doi: 10.4049/jimmunol.167.2.708
96. Bissell DM, Wang SS, Jarnagin WR, Roll FJ. Cell-specific expression of transforming growth factor-beta in rat liver. Evidence for autocrine regulation of hepatocyte proliferation. *J Clin Invest.* (1995) 96:447–55. doi: 10.1172/JCI118055
97. Knolle PA, Uhrig A, Protzer U, Trippler M, Duchmann R, zum Buschenfelde KHM, et al. Interleukin-10 expression is autoregulated at the transcriptional level in human and murine Kupffer cells. *Hepatology.* (1998) 27:93–9. doi: 10.1002/hep.510270116
98. Chen GS, Qi HZ. Effect of Kupffer cells on immune tolerance in liver transplantation. *Asian Pac J Trop Med.* (2012) 5:970–972. doi: 10.1016/S1995-7645(12)60184-9
99. Li M, Sun R, Xu L, Yin WW, Chen YY, Zheng XD, et al. Kupffer cells support hepatitis B virus-mediated CD8(+) T cell exhaustion via hepatitis B core antigen-TLR2 interactions in mice. *J Immunol.* (2015) 195:3100–9. doi: 10.4049/jimmunol.1500839
100. Liu J, Fan L, Yu H, Zhang J, He Y, Feng D, et al. Endoplasmic reticulum stress causes liver cancer cells to release exosomal miR-23a-3p and up-regulate programmed death ligand 1 expression in macrophages. *Hepatology.* (2019) 70:241–58. doi: 10.1002/hep.30607
101. Benechet AP, De Simone G, Di Lucia P, Cilenti F, Barbiera G, Le Bert N, Fumagalli V, et al. Dynamics and genomic landscape of CD8(+) T cells undergoing hepatic priming. *Nature.* (2019) 574:200–5. doi: 10.1038/s41586-019-1620-6
102. Wen Y, Feng D, Wu H, Liu W, Li H, Wang F, et al. Defective initiation of liver regeneration in osteopontin-deficient mice after partial hepatectomy due to insufficient activation of IL-6/Stat3 pathway. *Int J Biol Sci.* (2015) 11:1236–47. doi: 10.7150/ijbs.12118
103. Cai X, Li Z, Zhang Q, Qu Y, Xu M, Wan X, et al. CXCL6-EGFR-induced Kupffer cells secrete TGF-beta1 promoting hepatic stellate cell activation via the SMAD2/BRD4/C-MYC/EZH2 pathway in liver fibrosis. *J Cell Mol Med.* (2018) 22:5050–61. doi: 10.1111/jcmm.13787
104. Nieto N. Oxidative-stress and IL-6 mediate the fibrogenic effects of [corrected] Kupffer cells on stellate cells. *Hepatology.* (2006) 44:1487–501. doi: 10.1002/hep.21427
105. Mak A, Uetrecht J. Involvement of CCL2/CCR2 macrophage recruitment in amodiaquine-induced liver injury. *J Immunotoxicol.* (2019) 16:28–33. doi: 10.1080/1547691X.2018.1516014
106. Cui KL, Yan GX, Xu CF, Chen YY, Wang J, Zhou RB, et al. Invariant NKT cells promote alcohol-induced steatohepatitis through interleukin-1 beta in mice. *J Hepatology.* (2015) 62:1311–8. doi: 10.1016/j.jhep.2014.12.027
107. Hanschen M, Zahler S, Krombach F, Khandoga A. Reciprocal activation between CD4(+) T cells and Kupffer cells during hepatic ischemia-reperfusion. *Transplantation.* (2008) 86:710–8. doi: 10.1097/TP.0b013e3181821aa7
108. Tacke F, Weiskirchen R. Liver immunology: new perspectives. *Hepatobiliary Surg Nutr.* (2014) 3:330. doi: 10.3978/j.issn.2304-3881.2014.11.07
109. Terada M, Horisawa K, Miura S, Takashima Y, Ohkawa Y, Sekiya S, et al. Kupffer cells induce Notch-mediated hepatocyte conversion in a common mouse model of intrahepatic cholangiocarcinoma. *Sci Rep.* (2016) 6:34691. doi: 10.1038/srep34691
110. Elsegood CL, Chan CW, Degli-Esposti MA, Wikstrom ME, Domenichini A, Lazarus K, et al. Kupffer cell-monocyte communication is essential for initiating murine liver progenitor cell-mediated liver regeneration. *Hepatology.* (2015) 62:1272–84. doi: 10.1002/hep.27977
111. Jeong WI, Park O, Radaeva S, Gao B. STAT1 inhibits liver fibrosis in mice by inhibiting stellate cell proliferation and stimulating NK cell cytotoxicity. *Hepatology.* (2006) 44:1441–51. doi: 10.1002/hep.21419
112. Deaciuc IV, Bagby GJ, Lang CH, Spitzer JJ. Hyaluronic acid uptake by the isolated, perfused rat liver: an index of hepatic sinusoidal endothelial cell function. *Hepatology.* (1993) 17:266–72. doi: 10.1002/hep.1840170217
113. Gregory SH, Cousens LP, van Rooijen N, Dopp EA, Carlos TM, Wing EJ. Complementary adhesion molecules promote neutrophil-Kupffer cell interaction and the elimination of bacteria taken up by the liver. *J Immunol.* (2002) 168:308–15. doi: 10.4049/jimmunol.168.1.308
114. Wu X, Sun R, Chen Y, Zheng X, Bai L, Lian Z, et al. Oral ampicillin inhibits liver regeneration by breaking hepatic innate immune tolerance normally maintained by gut commensal bacteria. *Hepatology.* (2015) 62:253–64. doi: 10.1002/hep.27791
115. Wong CH, Jenne CN, Petri B, Chrobok NL, Kubes P. Nucleation of platelets with blood-borne pathogens on Kupffer cells precedes other innate immunity and contributes to bacterial clearance. *Nat Immunol.* (2013) 14:785–92. doi: 10.1038/ni.2631

6

A Role for MK2 in Enhancing Neutrophil-Derived ROS Production and Aggravating Liver Ischemia/Reperfusion Injury

*Lei Sun[1], Qiong Wu[2], Yunjuan Nie[1], Ni Cheng[3], Rui Wang[2], Gang Wang[4], Dan Zhang[2], Huiqiong He[1], Richard D. Ye[1,5] and Feng Qian[1,2,4]**

[1] Engineering Research Center of Cell & Therapeutic Antibody, Ministry of Education, School of Pharmacy, Shanghai Jiao Tong University, Shanghai, China, [2] Anhui Province Key Laboratory of Translational Cancer Research, Bengbu Medical College, Bengbu, China, [3] Department of Pharmacology, University of Illinois College of Medicine, Chicago, IL, United States, [4] Jiangsu Center for the Collaboration and Innovation of Cancer Biotherapy, Cancer Institute, Xuzhou Medical University, Xuzhou, China, [5] Institute of Chinese Medical Sciences, University of Macau, Macau, China

***Correspondence:**
Feng Qian
fengqian@sjtu.edu.cn

Increased inflammatory responses and enhanced reactive oxygen species contribute to hepatic ischemia/reperfusion (I/R) injury, however the modulatory mechanisms haven't been completely unveiled. Here, we report that genetic deficiency of MAPK-activated protein kinase 2 (MK2) protected against hepatic I/R injury and decreased hepatic neutrophil accumulation in $MK2^{-/-}$ mice. Depletion of neutrophil attenuated hepatic I/R injury in wide type mice. In response to C5a stimulation, $MK2^{-/-}$ neutrophils generated less superoxide in which both NADPH oxidase activation and $p47^{phox}$ phosphorylation were decreased. Furthermore, Ser329 of $p47^{phox}$ was identified for enhancement of superoxide production. The Ser329 phosphorylation was reduced in $MK2^{-/-}$ neutrophils. To determine whether MK2 modulates hepatic I/R injury via activating neutrophils, we generated myeloid-specific MK2 deletion mice ($MK2^{Lyz2-KO}$) and liver I/R injury was reduced in $MK2^{Lyz2-KO}$ mice. Our results indicate that MK2 augments hepatic I/R injury and induces ROS production with increased $p47^{phox}$ phosphorylation and MK2 is a potential drug target for treating hepatic I/R injury.

Keywords: MK2, ROS, $p47^{phox}$, neutrophils, hepatic ischemia/reperfusion injury

INTRODUCTION

Hepatic ischemia/reperfusion (I/R) is a pathophysiologic process that can be triggered by liver transplantation, elective liver surgery, toxic liver injury, and hepatic sinusoidal obstruction syndrome (1). Hepatic I/R injury is induced by reperfusion of blood flow and hypoxia accentuation in ischemic tissues, which leading to traumatic hemorrhagic shock, live damage, and graft dysfunction (2). Despite the recent improvements in liver preservation and surgical techniques, hepatic I/R injury remains an important clinical problem during liver surgery. Therefore, it is of importance to comprehensively understand the mechanisms of hepatic I/R and develop novel therapeutic approaches.

Hepatic I/R injury is a complex pathophysiological process. Initial phase of hepatic I/R injury is associated with oxidative stress, anaerobic metabolism, and calcium overload. At late phase, an increase in the cellular damage and, immune response contribute to the progression of parenchymal injury (3). Overall, reactive oxygen species (ROS), pro-inflammatory cytokines and chemokines as well as Kupffer cells (KCs), neutrophils and lymphocytes are involved in the process and are closely interlocked (4–6).

Neutrophils have a pivotal role in the pathogenesis of hepatic I/R injury (7). During hepatic I/R injury, neutrophils are first activated by chemokines, and migrate across the endothelium to the hepatocytes (7, 8). Then neutrophils further damage endothelial cells and destroy the integrity of the microvasculature through release of ROS, proteinases (cathepsin G, granulocytes elastase) and cationic peptides. Inhibition of neutrophil infiltration can protect against hepatocellular injury following I/R (7). However, the molecular mechanisms and regulation of neutrophils-derived ROS production have not been defined.

MAPK-activating protein kinase 2 (MK2) is a major effector serine/threonine-protein kinase downstream of p38-alpha (p38α) MAPK (9, 10). Once activated, MK2 phosphorylates many substrates and is implicated in many cellular processes including stress and inflammatory responses, cytoskeleton modulation, nuclear export, gene expression and cell proliferation (10, 11). MK2 plays a vital role in several diseases, such as cancer (12, 13), neurodegenerative disease (14), and inflammatory diseases (10, 15). Recently, Ashraf et al. reported that p38 MAPK activity is increased upon reperfusion and p38 MAPK inhibition prevents severe functional impairment caused by I/R (16). However, It has not been demonstrated how p38 MAPK modulates hepatic I/R and whether MK2 is a critical gene in modulation of hepatic I/R injury.

Using a mouse model of hepatic I/R injury, we found that complete MK2 deficiency markedly alleviated liver damage, serum alanine aminotransferase levels, intrahepatic macrophage/neutrophil trafficking, and pro-infiammatory cytokine production. Depletion of neutrophils *in vivo* reduced hepatic I/R injury and MK2 was required for NADPH oxidase activation and superoxide production. We also identify $p47^{phox}$ as a substrate of MK2, in which MK2 phosphorylated serine 329 residue of $p47^{phox}$ and this modification was required for NADPH oxidase activation. Furthermore, we proved that conditional depletion of MK2 in neutrophils also protected against hepatic I/R injury. Collectively, our findings reveal a critical role of MK2 in promoting ROS production and accentuating hepatic I/R injury.

RESULTS

Genetic MK2 Deficiency Alleviates Liver Injury Caused by Hepatic I/R in Mice

MK2 plays a critical role in inflammation and cell proliferation (10), however its role in hepatic I/R injury remains unknown. To determine the effect of MK2 on hepatic I/R, we performed a hepatic I/R mouse model in genetic MK2 deficiency mice (referred to as $MK2^{-/-}$ mice) with 60 min of partial liver warm ischemia followed by reperfusion for 6 and 18 h. Compared to that in $MK2^{+/+}$ mice, the serum ALT levels in $MK2^{-/-}$ mice were significantly reduced at 6 and 18 h (**Figure 1A**). Based on H&E staining, the liver damage was concordant with the change of serum ALT so that liver necrosis area was attenuated in $MK2^{-/-}$ mice (**Figure 1B**). Image-Pro Plus software analysis revealed statistically significant decreased necrosis area in livers from $MK2^{-/-}$ mice, compared to that from $MK2^{+/+}$ mice (**Figure 1C**). Collectively, these results indicated that MK2 deficiency dramatically ameliorates liver damage during hepatic I/R injury.

MK2 Deficiency Reduces Inflammatory Cytokine Production

Given that inflammatory cytokines contribute to the occurrence and development of hepatic I/R injury (6), we further determined whether MK2 modulates cytokine production in hepatic I/R injury. Six hours after hepatic I/R injury, significant increases of IL-6, TNF-α and KC mRNA of liver were observed in $MK2^{+/+}$ mice (**Figures 1D,E**). However, deletion of MK2 resulted in dramatic decrease of these cytokine at 6 h after I/R injury (**Figure 1D**). Similarly, compared with that in $MK2^{+/+}$ mice, the levels of IL-6, TNF-α and KC in serum were remarkably attenuated in $MK2^{-/-}$ mice at 6 h after hepatic I/R (**Figure 1E**). These results indicate that MK2 contributes to the hepatic I/R-induced increase of inflammatory cytokines in mice.

MK2 Is Required for Neutrophil Infiltration During Hepatic I/R Injury

Because neutrophil infiltration is associated with hepatic I/R injury, we firstly determined whether neutrophils contribute to hepatic I/R injury by depleting neutrophils with anti-Gr-1 antibody (1A8). As showed in **Figure 2A**, administration of anti-Gr-1 intraperitoneally (i.p.) effectively reduced neutrophil count in peripheral blood to 0.3%, compared to control mice receiving isotype-IgG which showed 39.8% of neutrophils in peripheral blood (**Figure 2A**). Then, mice received anti-Gr-1 antibody or an IgG control were subjected to hepatic I/R. As shown in **Figure 2B**, mice receiving anti-Gr-1 antibody displayed significantly reduced ALT in the serum. In the I/R groups, less necrotic areas were observed after neutrophil depletion based on histologic analysis and statistical analysis (**Figures 2C,D**). Additionally, to evaluate the infiltration and activation of neutrophils, we assessed the myeloperoxidase (MPO) activity. As shown in **Figure 2E**, mice receiving anti-Gr-1 antibody displayed a lower MPO activity. Furthermore, we investigated the role for MK2 in the accumulation of neutrophils during hepatic I/R injury. As showed in **Figure 2F**, increased MPO activity was significantly decreased after MK2 deletion during hepatic I/R injury (**Figure 2F**). Taken together, these results indicate that neutrophils are required for hepatic I/R injury and MK2 contributes to local accumulation of neutrophils during hepatic I/R injury.

Abbreviations: I/R injury, Hepatic ischemia/reperfusion injury; ROS, reactive oxygen species; MK2, MAPK-activating protein kinase 2; ALT, alanine amino transferase; AST, aspartate amino transferase; PMA, phorbol ester phorbol 12-myristate 13-acetate; fMLF, N-formyl-Met-Leu-Phe; MPO, Myeloperoxidase; NADPH oxidase, nicotinamide adenine dinucleotide phosphate oxidase; PMN, polymorphonuclear neutrophils; KCs, Kupffer cells.

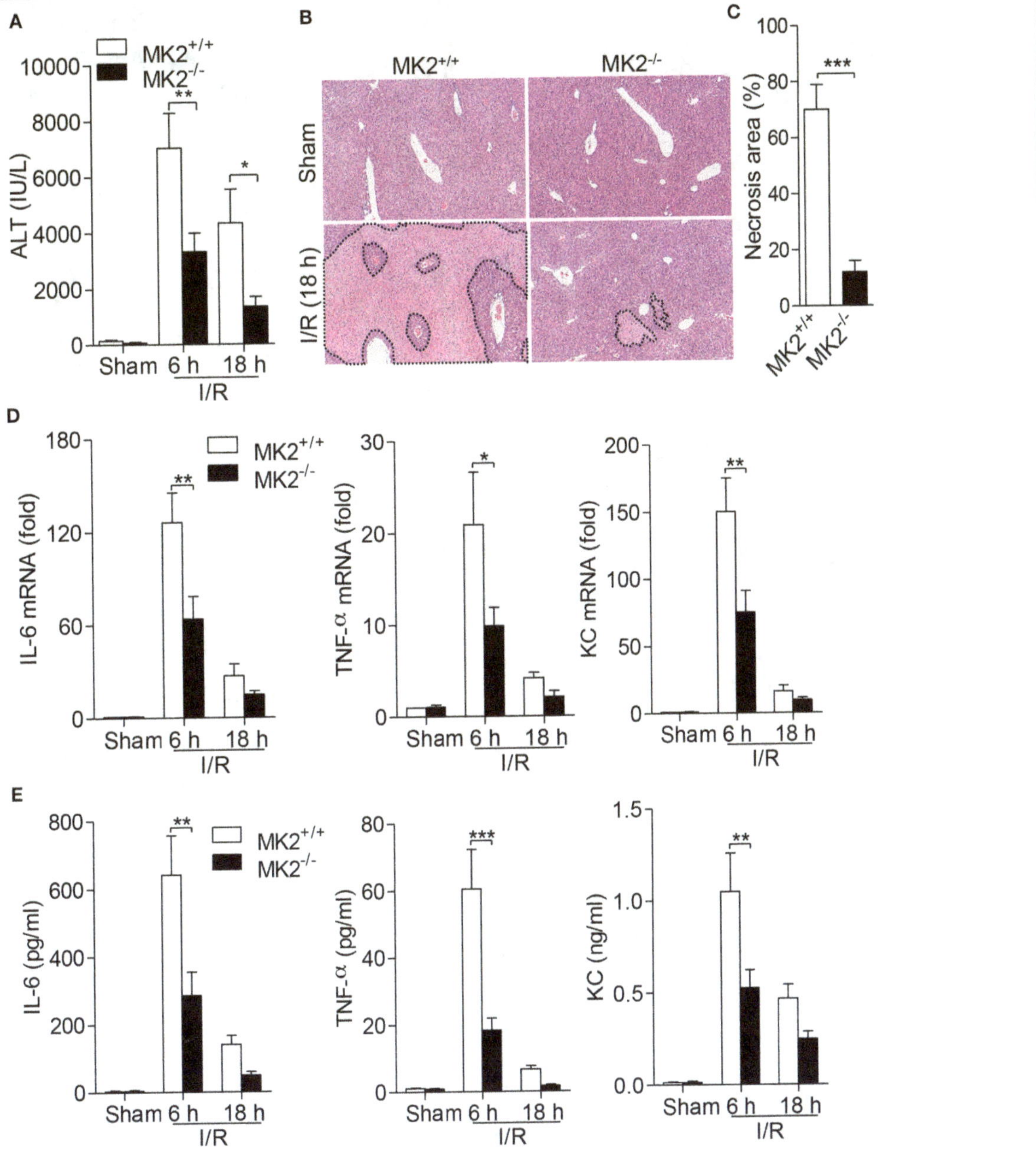

FIGURE 1 | Genetic MK2 deficiency alleviated hepatic I/R injury and inflammatory cytokine production. $MK2^{+/+}$ and $MK2^{-/-}$ mice were subjected to 60 min of partial liver warm ischemia, followed by reperfusion for 6 and 18 h. **(A)** Mouse blood was collected and serum ALT was detected. **(B)** Hepatic I/R injury was evaluated by hematoxylin-and-eosin (H&E) staining of injury liver tissues. Original magnification ×100. **(C)** The necrosis area was quantified by using ImageJ software. **(D)** The mRNA levels of IL-6, TNF-α, and KC in injury livers were detected by qPCR. **(E)** The protein levels of IL-6, TNF-α, and KC in serum were detected by ELISA. The results are shown as means ± SEM. $^{*}P < 0.05$; $^{**}P < 0.01$, $^{***}P < 0.001$, based on 5 mice in each group.

MK2 Is Required for Neutrophil Superoxide Production

It has been demonstrated that oxidant stress, especially the excessive reactive oxygen species (ROS), acts as one of the main modulators of hepatic I/R. Neutrophils are one of main sources of oxygen radicals in the post-ischemic liver, in which nicotinamide adenine dinucleotide phosphate (NADPH) oxidase is activated upon adhesion or by pro-inflammatory cytokines and the complement system (17). To determine the role of MK2 in oxygen radical production by neutrophils, we isolated polymorphonuclear neutrophils (PMN) from bone marrow of $MK2^{-/-}$ and $MK2^{+/+}$ mice. As shown in **Figures 3A,C,E**, the baseline of superoxide generation in neutrophils from $MK2^{-/-}$ were not changed compared with $MK2^{+/+}$ mice. Upon

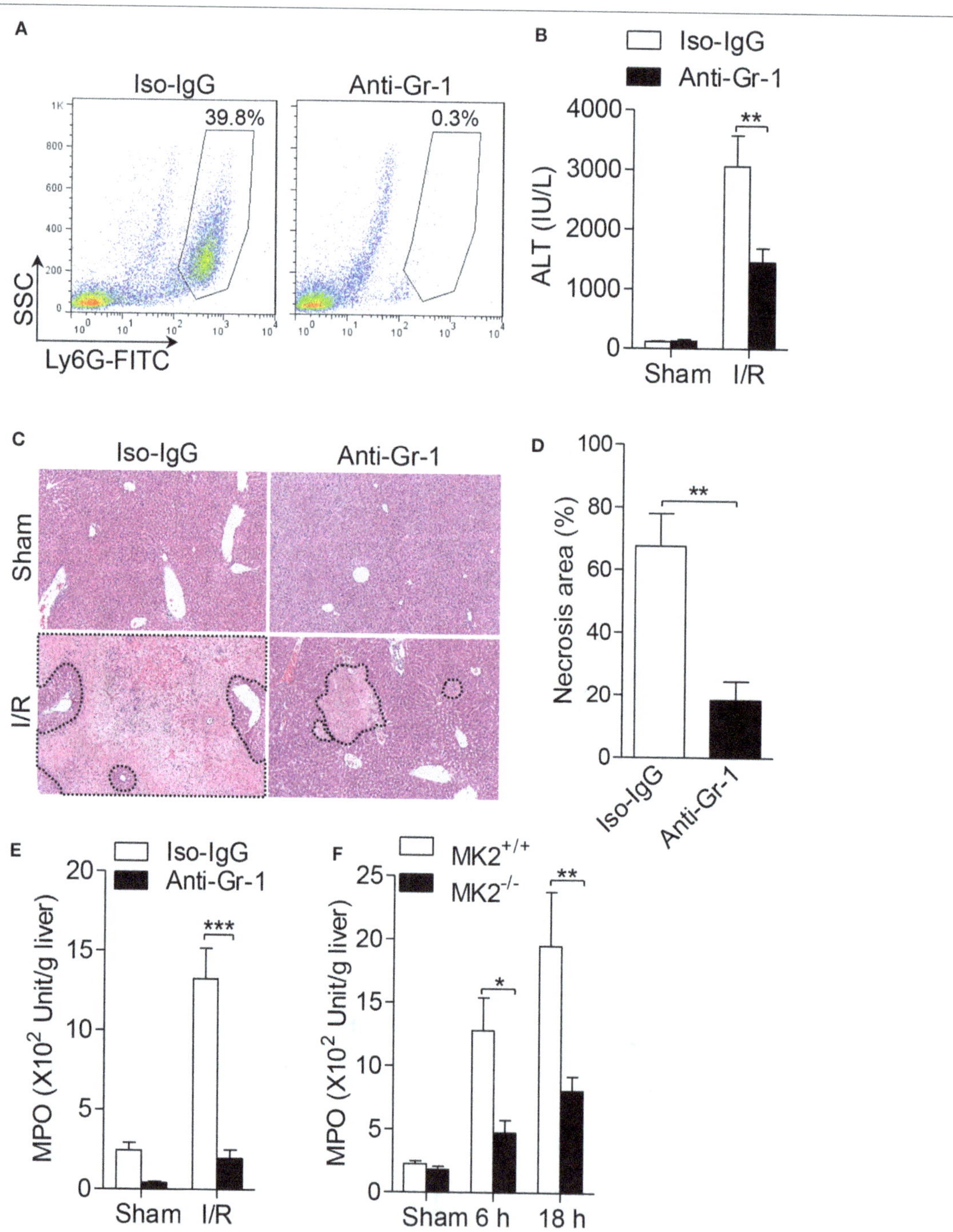

FIGURE 2 | Genetic MK2 deficiency reduced neutrophil trafficking in hepatic I/R injury. **(A)** The wild type mice ($MK2^{+/+}$) were intraperitoneally injected with anti-Gr-1 antibody (1A8), or isotype-matched IgG as control for 24 h, and then the percentage of neutrophils in peripheral blood were shown, as determined by anti-Ly6G-FITC FACS staining. **(B)** After injected with anti-Gr-1 antibody as in **(A)**, mice were subjected to hepatic ischemia for 60 min and reperfusion for 18 h. Serum ALT was detected for evaluation of liver injury. **(C)** Representative histological staining (H&E) of ischemic liver tissue was displayed. Original magnification ×100. **(D)** The necrosis area was quantified by ImageJ software. **(E)** The activities of MPO activity of injury liver tissues were detected. **(F)** $MK2^{+/+}$ and $MK2^{-/-}$ mice were subjected to hepatic I/R injury as in **Figure 1**, the activities of MPO in liver tissue extract were evaluated. The results are shown as means ± SEM. *$P < 0.05$; **$P < 0.01$, ***$P < 0.001$, based on 5 mice in each group.

treatment with C5a, neutrophils from $MK2^{-/-}$ mice generated significantly less superoxide compared to that from $MK2^{+/+}$ mice (**Figures 3A,B**). Besides activated complement component, bacterial derived formylated peptide formyl-methionyl-leucyl-phenylalanine (fMLF) also tightly regulates the activation of the NAPDH oxidase in a receptor specific manner (18). Here,

MK2$^{-/-}$ neutrophils treated with fMLF showed significantly impaired superoxide production compared to that from MK2$^{+/+}$ mice (**Figures 3C,D**). PMA is another NADPH oxidase agonist, which bypasses receptors and directly activates PKC. It is interesting that PMA-stimulated superoxide production showed no significant difference between neutrophils from MK2$^{+/+}$ and MK2$^{-/-}$ mice (**Figures 3E,F**). Collectively, these findings indicated that MK2 is involved in the regulation of chemoattractant receptor-dependent neutrophil NADPH oxidase activation and superoxide production.

MK2 Regulates AKT and P38 MAPK Phosphorylation in Neutrophils

Since several signaling pathways contribute to the activity of NADPH oxidase, we therefore reasoned whether MK2 has crosstalk with these signals. As shown in **Figure 4A**, neutrophils purified from the MK2$^{+/+}$ and MK2$^{-/-}$ mice were stimulated with 100 nM C5a for 5 min. Phosphorylation of AKT and p38 MAPK was determined by western blotting using respective antibodies. In response to C5a stimulation, the MK2$^{-/-}$ neutrophils exhibited attenuated phosphorylation of AKT (Ser473) and p38 MAPK with unaltered kinetics, compared to MK2$^{+/+}$ neutrophils (**Figures 4A–C**). In addition, the total level of p38 MAPK was also greatly decreased in MK2$^{-/-}$ neutrophils (**Figures 4A,D**). Altogether, these findings suggest that MK2 is required for C5a-induced activation of AKT and p38 MAPK, two critical kinases for modulation of NADPH oxidase activation.

MK2 Directly Phosphorylates P47 ^{phox} and Regulates Its Membrane Translocation

Phosphorylation of p47^{phox} leads to its membrane translocation that is critical for the formation of the active NADPH oxidase (19). Therefore, we further determined whether MK2 regulated p47^{phox} activation and membrane translocation. As shown in **Figures 5A,B**, C5a significantly induced p47^{phox} phosphorylation which was abolished after the neutrophils were pre-treated with the p38 inhibitor SB203580 for 15 min. In response to C5a stimulation, phospho-p47^{phox} was evaluated in neutrophils in 1 min, whereas the phospho-p47^{phox} was greatly decreased in neutrophils from MK2$^{-/-}$ mice, compared to that from MK2$^{+/+}$ mice (**Figures 5C,D**). Furthermore, to test whether MK2 directly phosphorylated p47^{phox}, we generated and purified human GST-p47^{phox} (hp47^{phox}) and mouse GST-p47^{phox} (mp47^{phox}) protein (20), which were then subjected MK2. Phosphorylation of p47^{phox} was evaluated by *in vitro* kinase assays. As showed in **Figure 6A**, both human p47^{phox} and mouse p47^{phox} protein were phosphorylated by MK2. The results suggested that MK2 could directly phosphorylate p47^{phox}.

Because p47^{phox} is responsible for transporting the whole cytosolic complex (p47^{phox}-p67^{phox}-p40^{phox}) to the docking site during NADPH oxidase activation (21), it is possible that MK2 modulates p47^{phox} membrane translocation via phosphorylation of p47^{phox}. In naïve neutrophils, the majority of p47^{phox} proteins were located in the cytoplasmic compartment (green) in image a (**Figure 6B**). Upon treatment with C5a for 2 min, p47^{phox} was translocated to the plasma membrane as shown in image b, which was greatly impaired in MK2$^{-/-}$ neutrophils in image d (**Figure 6B**). Thus, these data indicated that MK2 directly phosphorylates p47^{phox} and induces membrane translocation of p47^{phox}.

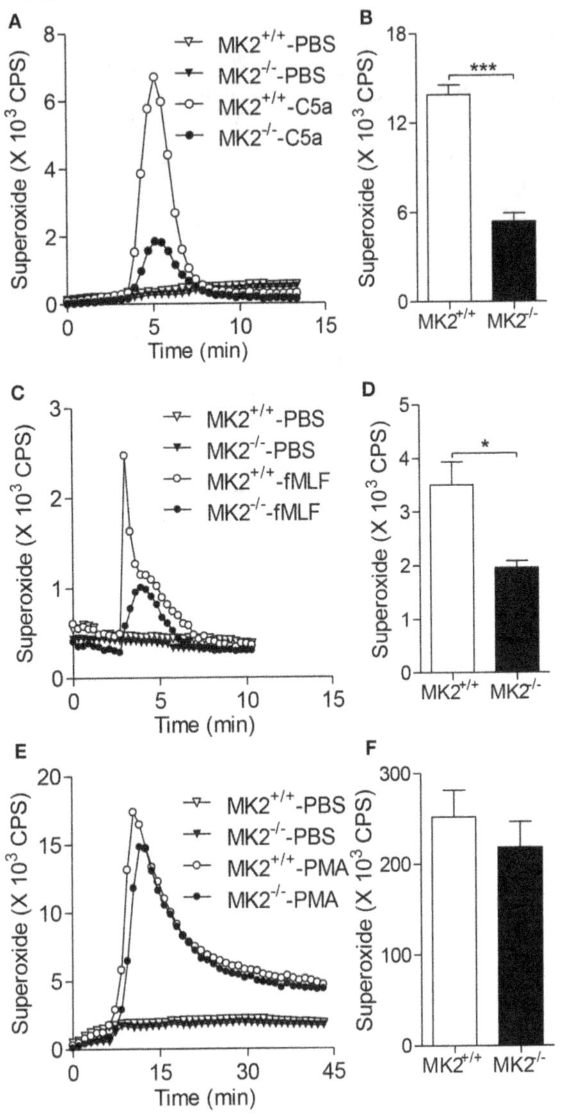

FIGURE 3 | MK2 modulated neutrophil superoxide production. Neutrophils were isolated from mice and isoluminol-ECL was used to measure superoxide production. Representative tracing showing the production of superoxide (left) and cumulative superoxide production was quantified based the area under tracing line (right). The MK2$^{+/+}$ and MK2$^{-/-}$ neutrophils were stimulated with 100 nM of C5a or PBS **(A,B)**, 10 μM of fMLF or PBS **(C,D)**, and 200 ng/ml of PMA or PBS **(E,F)**. The results were presented as means ± SEM, $^{*}P < 0.05$; $^{***}P < 0.001$, compared with similarly treated cells from MK2$^{+/+}$ mice. The experiments were repeated at least 3 times.

MK2 Phosphorylates P47^{Phox} on Ser329

The C terminus (between Ser303 and Ser379) of p47^{phox} is a regulatory domain for p47^{phox} activation and membrane translocation (19, 22, 23). To determine the specific phosphorylated site of $p47^{phox}$ by MK2, we compared mouse $p47^{phox}$ with human $p47^{phox}$ and found that Ser329 on mouse $p47^{phox}$ was conservative to human $p47^{phox}$ serine 328 (**Figure 7A**). To further identify whether Ser329 of p47phox is required for NAPDH oxidase activation, we generated lentivirus with full-length $p47^{phox}$ ($p47^{phox}$-WT) or Ala substitution Ser329 of $p47^{phox}$ ($p47^{phox}$-S329A) mutant and infected them into $p47^{phox}$ deficient neutrophils that were defective for superoxide generation. In response to C5a stimulation, $p47^{phox}$ deficient neutrophils with wide type $p47^{phox}$ ($p47^{phox}$-WT) produced more superoxide than that with $p47^{phox}$-S329A, although neutrophils with $p47^{phox}$-S329A still had capability to generate superoxide (**Figures 7B,C**). To evaluate whether MK2 modulated $p47^{phox}$ Ser329 phosphorylation, we used antibody specific to phosphorylated $p47^{phox}$ Ser329. Upon treatment with C5a, the phosphorylation of $p47^{phox}$ Ser329 were induced within 0.5 min and reached peak at 1 min (**Figures 7D,E**). $MK2^{-/-}$ neutrophils displayed an attenuated phosphorylation at Ser329 of $p47^{phox}$ compared to $MK2^{+/+}$ neutrophils. Thus, these data indicate that Ser329 in $p47^{phox}$ sequence is an important regulatory site for NADPH oxidase activation and can be modulated by MK2.

Myeloid-Specific Deletion of MK2 Alleviated Hepatic I/R Injury

To further prove that the loss of MK2 in neutrophils regulates hepatic I/R injury, we generated myeloid-specific deficiency of MK2 mice (referred to as $MK2^{Lyz2-KO}$) by mating $MK2^{loxP/loxP}$ mice with lysozyme 2-Cre mice (**Figure 8A**). The expression of MK2 was abolished in neutrophils from $MK2^{Lyz2-KO}$ mice compared with that from $MK2^{Lyz2-WT}$ mice (**Figure 8B**), which was no significant difference between the liver tissues from $MK2^{Lyz2-KO}$ or $MK2^{Lyz2-WT}$ mice (**Figure 8C**), suggesting MK2 was deficient in neutrophils. Then, the $MK2^{Lyz2-KO}$ and $MK2^{Lyz2-WT}$ mice were subjected to hepatic I/R. Compared to $MK2^{Lyz2-WT}$ mice, $MK2^{Lyz2-KO}$ mice displayed reduced ALT activities (**Figure 8D**) and decreased liver necrosis injury (**Figures 8E,F**) 6 h after hepatic I/R injury. Taken together, these data confirm that MK2 contributes to hepatic I/R injury and modulates neutrophil activation and ROS production.

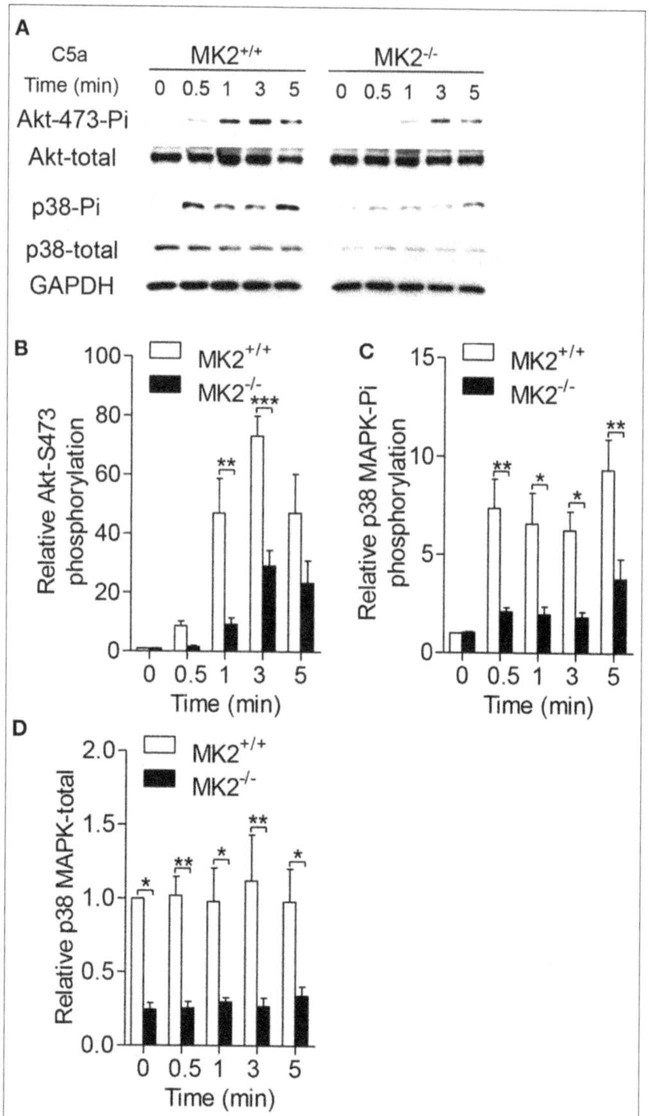

FIGURE 4 | MK2 was required for AKT and p38 MAPK phosphorylation in neutrophils. **(A)** Neutrophils from $MK2^{+/+}$ and $MK2^{-/-}$ mice were challenged with C5a (100 nM) for indicated time. Phosphorylation of AKT (Ser473) and p38 MAPK was determined by western blotting using anti-phospho-antibodies against the phospho-AKT (Ser473), total AKT, phospho-p38 MAPK, and total p38 MAPK. **(B–D)** Densitometry analysis was conducted to determine the relative level of induced AKT phosphorylation, p38 MAPK phosphorylation, and total p38 MAPK. Data shown are means ± SEM from three independent experiments. $^{*}P < 0.05$; $^{**}P < 0.01$; $^{***}P < 0.001$.

DISCUSSION

Hepatic ischemia/reperfusion (I/R) injury is a common pathological process in liver surgery and transplantation, influencing the patient's outcome post-surgery (8). Although p38 MAPK has been implicated in the pathogenesis of hepatic I/R injury (16), the modulatory mechanisms remain elusive. Here, we found that MK2, one of the downstream kinases of p38 MAPK, contributed to hepatic I/R. Genetic MK2 deficiency dramatically limited pathological damage, reduced serum ALT activities, decreased inflammatory cytokine production, and impaired neutrophil infiltration in mice. In *in vitro* study, MK2 deficiency abrogated superoxide production and activation of AKT and p38 MAPK in neutrophils. Furthermore, we identified that NADPH oxidase activation was regulated by MK2 that directly phosphorylated Ser329 of $p47^{phox}$. The myeloid-specific deletion of MK2 mice ($MK2^{Lyz2-KO}$) also displayed a reduced liver injury after I/R injury. Therefore, our findings demonstrated for the first time that down-regulation of MK2 protects against hepatic I/R injury, which could be a novel therapeutic target for I/R injury.

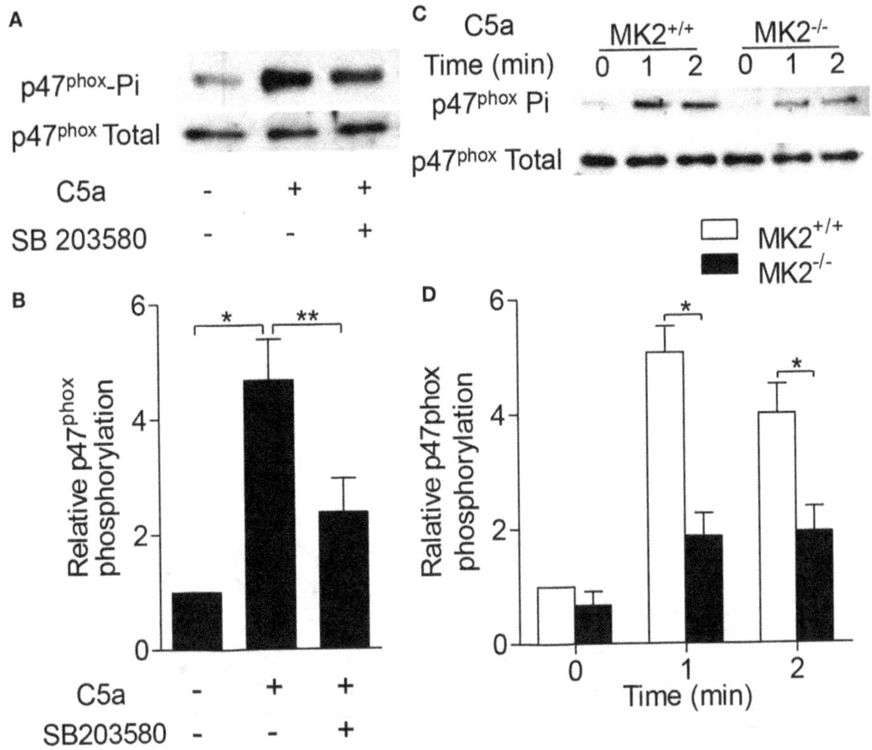

FIGURE 5 | MK2 was essential for p47^{phox} phosphorylation in response to C5a stimulation. **(A)** Neutrophils from WT mice were pre-treated with SB203580 (3 μM) for 15 min, and then stimulated with C5a (100 nM) for 1 min. The phosphorylation of p47^{phox} was determined. **(B)** Densitometry analysis was conducted to determine the 47^{phox} phosphorylation. **(C)** Neutrophils from MK2$^{+/+}$ and MK2$^{-/-}$ mice were stimulated with C5a (100 nM) for 1 and 2 min. The phosphorylation (Phospho) of p47^{phox} was determined. **(D)** Densitometry analysis was conducted to determine 47^{phox} phosphorylation in MK2$^{+/+}$ and MK2$^{-/-}$ neutrophils. The results are shown as means ± SEM. $^{*}P < 0.05$; $^{**}P < 0.01$, based on three independent experiments.

Hepatic I/R injury is closely related to innate immune cell activation and inflammatory processes. Although dendritic cells, natural killer T (NKT) cells, Kupffer cells are all involved in modulation of hepatic I/R injury (4), neutrophils play an nonredundant role in hepatic I/R injury because depletion of neutrophils or neutrophil specific deficiency of MK2 alleviating I/R injury (**Figures 2, 8**). Coincidentally, recent studies also reveal that neutrophils participate in the hepatic I/R injury. Honda M et al found that formyl-peptide receptor 1 (FPR1)-mediated neutrophil recruitment modulate hepatic I/R injury (24). Infiltrated neutrophils induce hepatocyte death and enhance Kupffer cells to produce inflammatory cytokines by releasing neutrophil extracellular trap (NET) (25). In addition to generation of NET, neutrophils can exacerbate tissue injury though releasing ROS, proteinases and cationic peptides (20). Although we couldn't exclude that MK2 may regulate hepatic I/R injury via modulating Kupffer cells or dendritic cells, our results suggest that MK2-mediated neutrophil activation is involved in hepatic I/R injury.

MK2 is one of the downstream kinases of p38 MAPK that is activated during hepatic I/R injury and regulates liver injury (16). Coxon et al. proved that MK2 regulates human neutrophil activation in p38-dependent and ERK-dependent signal pathways (26). Furthermore, MK2 is involved in neutrophils polarization and chemotaxis and regulates infectious diseases (27, 28). However, a particular role of MK2 in sterile inflammatory responses was not well investigated. In this study, we uncovered the alleviation of liver damage and reduction of liver neutrophil accumulation in genetic MK2 deficiency mice (MK2$^{-/-}$) and myeloid-specific deletion of MK2 mice (MK2$^{Lyz2-KO}$) during haptic I/R injury. These results indicate that MK2 regulates hepatic I/R injury through modulating neutrophil functions. However, it should be noted that, in our *in vivo* data, we only examined that several inflammatory cytokines and chemokines such as IL-6, TNF-α and KC within the liver tissue were decreased in MK2$^{-/-}$ mice. More adhesion molecules such as intercellular adhesion molecule 1 (ICAM-1), integrin need to be further studied to explore the molecular mechanism for the regulatory effect of MK2 in neutrophils chemotaxis, recruitment and transendothelial migration.

Oxidative stress has been considered to be a major part of liver damage induced by I/R injury, and oxygen free radicals are the principal components that lead to hepatocellular necrosis and apoptosis in I/R injury (8). Therefore, antioxidants including superoxide dismutase, catalase, glutathione, vitamin E, and beta-carotene protect against hepatic I/R injury (29). During reperfusion after liver ischemia, neutrophils are a potential source of oxygen free radicals by activation of

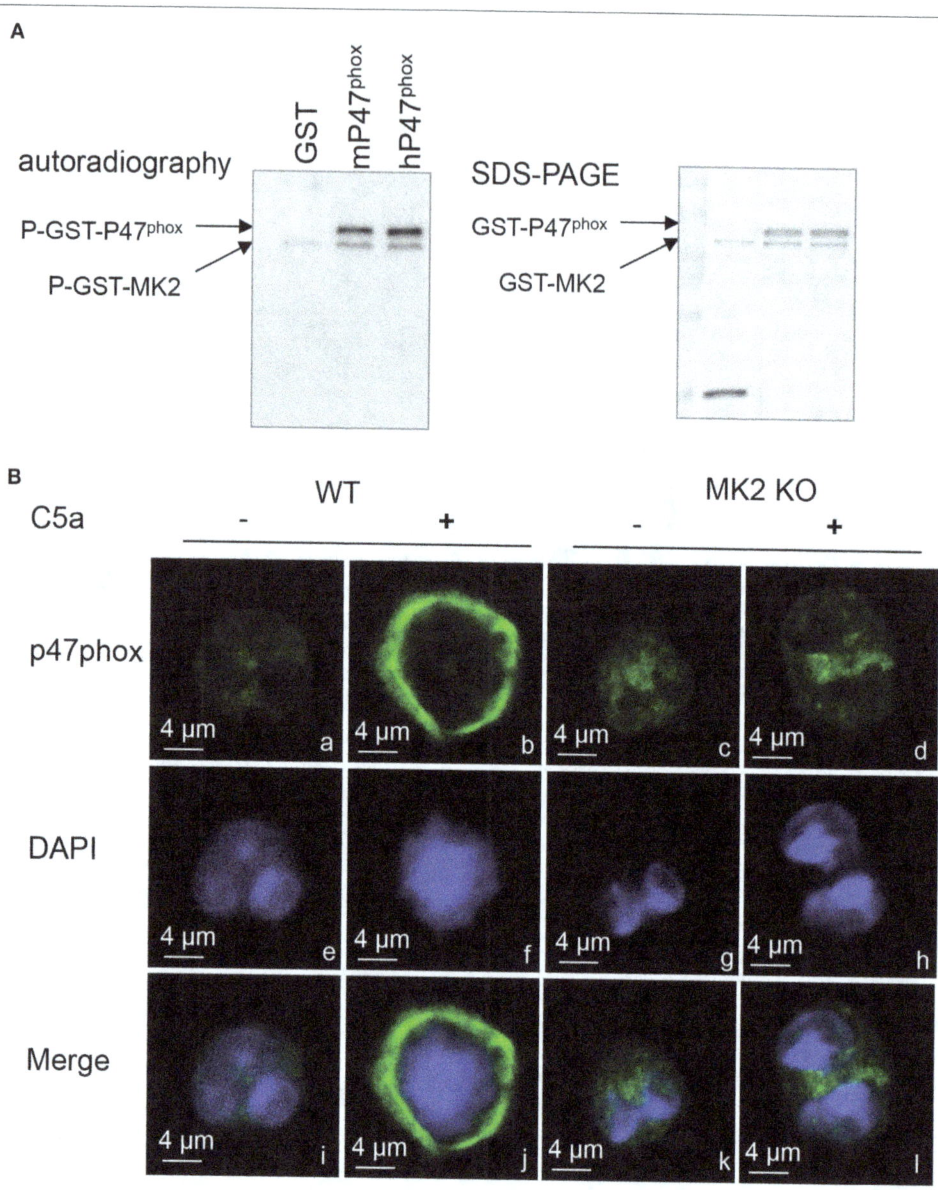

FIGURE 6 | MK2 directly regulated $p47^{phox}$ phosphorylation and membrane translocation. **(A)** Autoradiograph of *in vitro* kinase assay using full-length human $p47^{phox}$ ($hp47^{phox}$) or mouse $p47^{phox}$ ($mp47^{phox}$) fused to GST as substrates for GST-MK2. GST without $mp47^{phox}$ was used as a negative control. Two phosphorylated bands were identified in the autoradiograph: a phosphorylated GST–$p47^{phox}$, and an autophosphorylated GST-MK2. The loading levels of each protein were indicated in coomassie blue staining (right). **(B)** Neutrophils from $MK2^{+/+}$ and $MK2^{-/-}$ mice were treated with C5a (100 nM) for 2 min and immunofluorescence imaging was performed to detect the localization of $p47^{phox}$ (green). Nuclei were stained with DAPI (blue). The results are representatives of three independent experiments, scale bar is 4 μm.

NADPH oxidase. Here, our data showed that MK2 deficient neutrophils produced less superoxide production in response to C5a or fMLF stimulation but not to PMA. Given that PMA bypasses receptors and directly activates protein kinase C (PKC), MK2 mediates NADPH oxidase activation through specific cell-surface receptors and related molecules, such as phosphoinositide 3-kinase (PI3K), G protein-coupled receptor kinases (GRKs), small GTP-binding proteins, and mitogen-activated protein kinases (MAPK). Consistently, we also found that phosphorylation of AKT and p38 MAPK is reduced in MK2-deficient neutrophils in response to C5a stimulation (**Figure 4**). Thus, our data suggests that MK2 accentuate superoxide generation and hepatic I/R injury via modulating AKT and p38 MAPK signals.

MK2 is a stress-activated serine/threonine-protein kinase involved in different cellular functions through its kinase activity (9). NADPH oxidase is an inducible electron transport system assembled by several subunits ($gp91^{phox}$, $gp22^{phox}$,

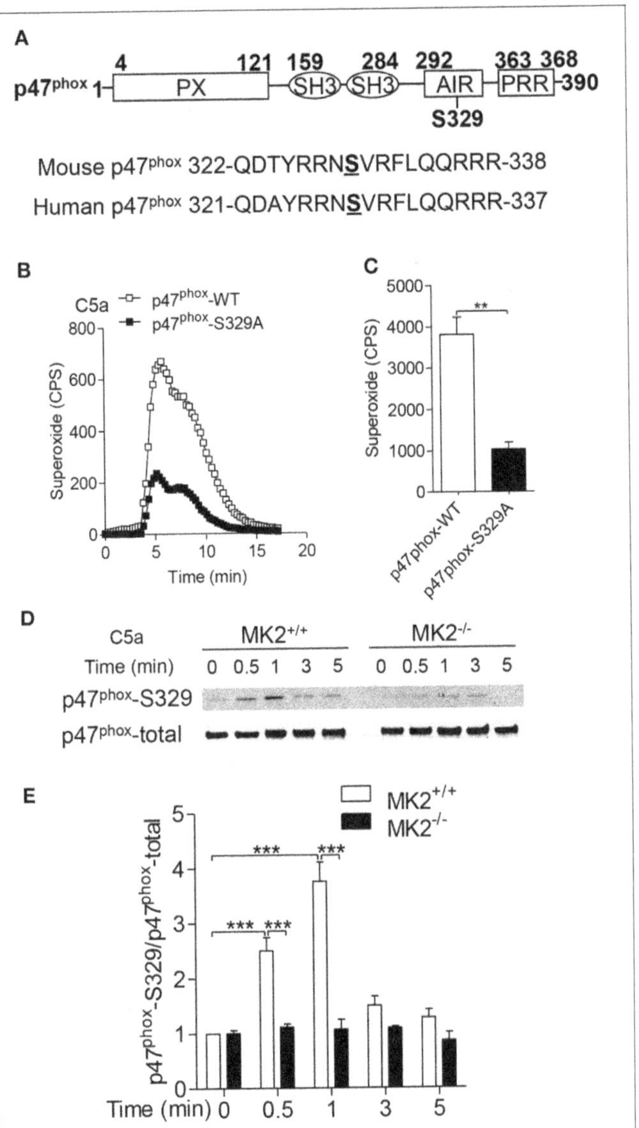

FIGURE 7 | MK2 regulated mouse p47^{phox} at Ser329 residue. **(A)** Alignment of sequence of human and mouse p47^{phox} proteins surrounding the potential MK2 phosphorylation site. **(B)** Neutrophils from *p47$^{phox--/-}$* mice were transiently transfected with full-length p47phox or its S329 mutant for 6 h, and followed challenge with 100 nM of C5a. The production of superoxide production was measured as described. **(C)** The quantitative analysis was performed based on results of B superoxide. **(D)** Neutrophils from MK2$^{+/+}$ and MK2$^{--/-}$ mice were challenged with 100 nM of C5a for 0.5, 1, 3, and 5 min, the phosphorylation of p47^{phox} (Ser329) was determined by western blotting with anti- p47phox-S329 antibody and p47^{phox}-total antibody. **(E)** Densitometry analysis was conducted to determine the relative level of p47^{phox}-S329. Data shown are means ± SEM from three independent experiments. $^{**}P < 0.01$, $^{***}P < 0.001$.

p47^{phox}, p67^{phox}, small GTPase Rac, and p40^{phox}) (17). The phosphorylation and membrane translocation of the subunit p47^{phox} is necessary for NADPH oxidase activation and regulation (21, 22). Although several kinases are implicated in regulating the phosphorylation of p47^{phox}, the mechanisms and dynamics of p47^{phox}-orchestrated NADPH activation haven't been completely revealed. In human neutrophils, phorbol myristate acetate (PMA), and fMLF induce MK2 phosphorylation at Ser334 and further increase NADPH oxidase activation (30). TNF-α, granulocyte-macrophage colony-stimulating factor (GM-CSF), and C5a can induce p47^{phox} phosphorylation through p38 MAPK (31). Thus, p38 MAPK and MK2 are involved in the modulation of NADPH oxidase activation. However, the regulatory mechanisms have not yet been defined. Our *in vitro* kinase assay showed that MK2 can directly regulated the phosphorylation of p47^{phox}, thereby reducing neutrophil superoxide production. Moreover, membrane translocation of p47^{phox} was impaired in MK2$^{-/-}$ neutrophils. Our data first demonstrate that MK2 regulates the ROS production in neutrophils through the direct regulatory effect on the phosphorylation of p47^{phox}.

Several phosphorylated sites of p47^{phox} are involved in NADPH oxidase activation. The p47^{phox} phosphorylation at Ser345 serves as a point of convergence for different MAPKs to induce priming of ROS production (23). We previously proved that Thr356 of p47^{phox} is a phosphorylation site for p38 MAPK (20). Here, we identified that Ser329 was a new phosphorylation site and could be modulated by MK2. The phosphorylation level of p47^{phox} on Ser329 was abrogated in MK2$^{-/-}$ neutrophils. The p47^{phox} has multiple serine residues ranging from Ser303 to Ser379 (23). Phosphorylation of some serine sites, such as Ser359 or Ser370, is an important initial step to activate p47^{phox} (32, 33). Other residue such as Ser379 can cause inhibition of NADPH oxidase activation (34). Although we identified Ser329 as a new residue that can be regulated by MK2, the synergistic and dynamic effects of these residues on p47^{phox} activation and ROS production should be further explored.

In conclusion, we demonstrated substantial and significant protection against the hepatic I/R injury in genetic MK2 knockout mice and MK2 myeloid-specific deletion mice. In addition, we found MK2 played a vital role in NADPH oxidase activation and ROS production through AKT and p38 signal pathways. Moreover, MK2 regulated NADPH oxidase activation by phosphorylation of p47^{phox} on Ser329 under complement component stimulation. Our findings not only reveal a novel regulatory mechanism for hepatic I/R injury, but also identify a novel therapeutic target for ameliorating hepatic I/R injury in liver transplantation.

METHODS

Mice

MK2 deficient mice, MK2$^{loxP/loxP}$ mice and lysozyme 2-Cre mice were purchased from The Jackson Laboratory. *MK2*$^{Lyz2-KO}$ Mice were generated by mating MK2$^{loxP/loxP}$ mice with lysozyme 2-Cre mice (35). The p47$^{phox-/-}$ mice was provided by Dr. Steven M Holland (NIH, Bethesda, MD, USA). All mice used in the study were on C57BL/6 background and 8–12 weeks of age. Mice were housed in a climate-controlled room (25°C, 55% humidity and 12 h light/darkness cycles) and all procedures were conducted with the use of protocols approved by the Institutional Animal Care and Use Committee at Shanghai Jiao Tong University.

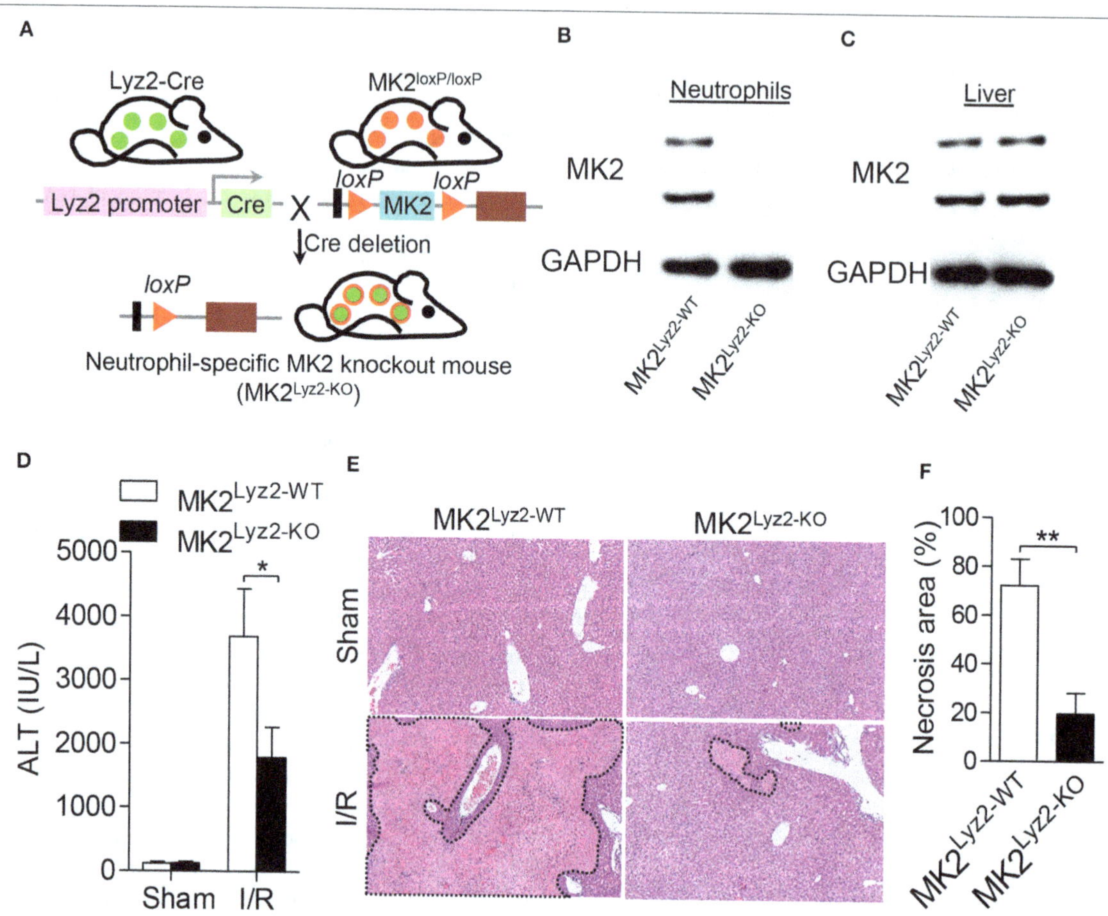

FIGURE 8 | Myeloid-specific deletion of MK2 decreased hepatocellular damage in hepatic I/R injury. **(A)** Schematic representation of the generation of $MK2^{Lyz2-KO}$ and $MK2^{Lyz2-WT}$ mice that $MK2^{loxP/loxP}$ mice were bred with Lysozyme (Lyz2)-Cre transgenic mice. The protein level of MK2 in neutrophils **(B)** and livers **(C)** from $MK2^{Lyz2-KO}$ and $MK2^{Lyz2-WT}$ mice was detected by western blot. $MK2^{Lyz2-KO}$ and $MK2^{Lyz2-WT}$ mice were subjected to hepatic I/R injury with 60 min of ischemia and 16 h of reperfusion. Serum and injury livers were collected for analysis. **(D)** Serum ALT levels were measured. **(E)** Representative H&E stained sections of injury livers were shown. Original magnification ×100. **(F)** The necrosis area was measured by ImageJ software. The results are shown as means ± SEM. $^*P < 0.05$; $^{**}P < 0.01$, based on 5 mice in each group.

Reagents

Phorbol ester phorbol 12-myristate 13-acetate (PMA), *N*-formyl-Met-Leu-Phe (fMLF), C5a and isoluminol were purchased from Sigma-Aldrich (St. Louis, MO, USA). The p38 MAPK inhibitor SB203580 was ordered from Selleck (Houston, TX, USA). Antibodies including Phosphor-Akt, Akt, Phosphor-p38 MAPK, p38 MAPK, MK2, and GAPDH were ordered from Cell Signaling Technology (Danvers, MA, USA). Anti-$p47^{phox}$ antibody was purchased from Santa Cruz Biotechnology and anti-phospho-$p47^{phox}$ (Ser329) antibody was generated by N.J. Compass Biotechnology (Nanjing, China). Other reagents were ordered from Sigma-Aldrich (St. Louis, MO, USA).

Partial Liver Ischemia/Reperfusion Injury (IRI) Mouse Model

All mice were anesthetized with pentobarbital (5 mg/kg) by intraperitoneal injection. The mouse abdominal cavities were opened with operating scissors. All structures in the portal triad (hepatic artery, portal vein, bile duct) to the left and median liver lobes were occluded with a microvascular clamp (Fine Science Tools) for 60 min; reperfusion was initiated by removal of the clamp. After 6 or 18 h of reperfusion, anesthetized animals were sacrificed, and liver tissue and serum were collected for analysis. Sham-operated groups underwent the same surgical procedure, except that the blood supply to the liver lobes was not interrupted.

Histopathological Analysis

Following euthanasia, representative pieces of ischemic lobes were quickly removed and fixed in ice cold 10% phosphate-buffered formalin for 24 h at 4°C, and then embedded in paraffin. Tissue blocks were sectioned at 4 μm thickness and slices were baked at 60°C for 4 h. After removal of the paraffin by using xylene and a graded ethanol series, the sections were cut to 4-μm-thick sections, stained with hematoxylin and eosin (Beyotime Institute of Biotechnology, China). Following staining, the observer was blinded to treatment group. The slides were viewed under a microscope (Olympus Optical Co. Ltd., Tokyo, Japan).

Activity Assay of ALT

Blood samples were centrifuged for 10 min at 3,000 rpm and serum were collected. The activities of serum alanine aminotransferase (ALT) were measured using the ALT Assay Reagent kit (NJJCBIO, Nanjing, China) according to the manufacturer's instructions with colorimetric evaluation on the microplate reader (FlexStation 3, Molecular Devices, CA, USA).

Myeloperoxidase Activity Assay

Frozen mouse liver was homogenized with a Teflon homogenizer in 50 mM phosphate buffer. After centrifugation at 13,000 *g* for 30 min, the cell pellet was resuspended in 1 ml 0.5% hexadecyl trimethylammonium bromide (Sigma-Aldrich, St. Louis, MO, USA), and treated with three cycles of freeze, thaw, and sonication. After centrifugation at 13,000 *g* for 20 min at 4°C, the supernatant was incubated with 16 mM 3,3′,5,5′-tetramethylbenzidine (Sigma-Aldrich, St. Louis, MO, USA) and 15 mM H_2O_2, and absorbance at 655 nm was determined. One unit of MPO activity was defined as the change of absorbance of 1.0 per min.

Superoxide Production Assays

Mouse polymorphonuclear neutrophils (PMN) were purified from bone marrow cell suspensions as described previously (20). Isolated neutrophils were incubated with 10 μM isoluminol at 37°C for 30 min, and then challenged with PMA (200 ng/mL) for 45 min, fMLF (10 μM) or C5a (100 nM) for 15–60 min. The generation of superoxide was detected by using a Wallac 1420 Multilabel Counter (PerkinElmer, Houston, TX, USA).

Neutrophil Depletion

To deplete neutrophils, mice were intraperitoneally injected with 5 mg/kg (100 μg/mouse) anti-Gr-1 antibody (1A8) that specifically recognized neutrophil surface mark Ly6G (Bio X Cell, West Lebanon, NH, USA) 24 h before ischemia/reperfusion challenge. Isotype-matched IgG of the same amount was used as a negative control.

Flow Cytometric Analysis

After treating with anti-Gr-1 antibody for neutrophils deletion, the mice were performed liver ischemia/reperfusion injury (IRI), the percentages of neutrophils were measured using Ly6G-FITC (BD Biosciences, West Lebanon, NH, USA) for flow cytometry. Data was analyzed using FlowJo 7.5 (Tree Star Software).

Immunofluorescence Microscopy

Neutrophils on glass coverslips coated with fibrinogen were stimulated with or without C5a, washed once with ice-cold phosphate-buffered saline (PBS), and then fixed with 3% paraformaldehyde in PBS. The anti-$p47^{phox}$ antibody were used at 1:250 dilution overnight, cells were incubated with a rhodamine green-X-conjugated goat anti-mouse IgG (secondary antibody) at room temperature for 1 h. After washing, the coverslips were mounted on glass slides with the use of ProLong Gold anti-fade reagent with DAPI. Fluorescence images were captured with a confocal microscope with custom software (Leica Micro-systems, CMS GMBH, and LAS AF).

Quantitative Real-Time Reverse Transcription Polymerase Chain Reaction

Total RNA was isolated from liver tissues, and first-strand cDNA was synthesized with Moloney murine leukaemia virus reverse transcriptase (Qiagen, USA). Quantitative real-time polymerase chain reaction (qRT-PCR) was performed with SYBR Green (Invitrogen) in a Bio-Rad real-time PCR detection system with primer sets for IL-6, forward 5′-TAGTCCTTCCTACCC CAATTTCC-3′, reverse 5′- TTGGTCCTTAGCCACTCCTTC-3′; TNF-α, forward 5′-CCCTCACACTCAGATC ATCTTCT-3′, reverse 5′-GCTACGACGTGGGCTACAG-3′; KC, forward 5′-TCCA GAGCTTGAAGGTGTTGCC-3′, reverse 5′-AACCAA GGGAGCTTCAGGGTCA-3′. The expression of each gene was normalized to GAPDH mRNA, and calculated with respect to the baseline control using $\Delta\Delta Ct$ method *via* StepOne 2.0.

Cytokine Production Detection

The concentration of TNF-α, IL-6, and KC in supernatants from liver tissues of liver ischemia/reperfusion injury (IRI) mice were evaluated by ELISA, according to manufacturer's instruction (R&D Systems, Minneapolis, MN, USA).

Kinase Assay

In vitro kinase assays were performed as previously described by using activate and a recombinant GST-mouse $p47^{phox}$ or GST-human $p47^{phox}$ fusion protein as substrates (20). The samples were analyzed by SDS-PAG autoradiography.

Western Blot Analysis

The neutrophils after treatment were washed with DPBS and lysed with RIPA lysis buffer (Thermo Fisher Scientific Inc., Rockford, IL, USA) containing protease inhibitor cocktail (Sigma-Aldrich, St Louis, MO, United States) and phosphatase inhibitor cocktail (Roche Applied Science, Indianapolis, IN, United States). The samples were resolved on SDS-PAGE, and underwent immunoblotting analysis using the indicated antibodies. The protein band intensities were normalized to those of GAPDH. The intensity was quantified by Image J software.

Lentiviral Production and Transduction

Full-length $p47^{phox}$ ($p47^{phox}$-WT) and Ala substitution Ser329 of $p47^{phox}$ ($p47^{phox}$-S329A) mutant were cloned into the pLVX-IRES-mCherry vector (Takara CA, USA). HEK293T cells were planted into 90 mm dish at 80% confluence and co-transfected with 10 μg of $p47^{phox}$ plasmid, 7.5 μg of the psPAX2 plasmid and 2.5 μg of pMD2.G plasmid (Addgene, Cambridge, MA) by using polyethyleneimine (Polyscience,USA). Culture supernatants of the HEK293T cells were collected after 72 h and concentrated to 300 μl with a concentration tube. For infection„ $p47^{phox}$ deficient neutrophils were incubated with lentiviral supernatants of different concentrations and Polybrene (Sigma, St. Louis, MO), followed by centrifugation at 2,000 x g for 90 min at 30°C and incubation at 37°C for 4 h. The supernatant was exchanged with fresh complete medium. The cells were stimulated with C5a (100 nM) and harvested for experiment after 6 h.

Statistical Analysis

Each experiment was performed independently for at least 3 times. The results are presented as the mean ± SEM. Statistical significance of differences between groups was analyzed with unpaired Student's t-test or one-way ANOVA when more than two groups were compared. Statistical significance was defined as $^{*}P < 0.05$, $^{**}P < 0.01$, and $^{***}P < 0.001$. Analysis and graphing were performed using the Prism software (ver. 5.0; GraphPad, San Diego, CA).

AUTHOR CONTRIBUTIONS

LS, QW, YN, NC, RW, GW, DZ, and HH performed the experiments. LS, NC, YN, and FQ analyzed the data. LS, RY, and FQ prepared the manuscript.

ACKNOWLEDGEMENTS

This work was supported by grants from the Nathonal Key Research and Development Program of China (2017YFC0908500), National Natural Science Foundation of China 81773741, 81573438, 81770633, and 31741038. RY was supported by Grant CPG2015-00018-ICMS, MYRG2016-00246-ICMS-QRCM from the University of Macau and Grant 026/2016/A1 from the Science and Technology Development Fund of Macau.

REFERENCES

1. Papadopoulos D, Siempis T, Theodorakou E, Tsoulfas G. Hepatic ischemia and reperfusion injury and trauma: current concepts. *Arch Trauma Res.* (2013) 2:63–70. doi: 10.5812/atr.12501
2. Peralta C, Jimenez-Castro MB, Gracia-Sancho J. Hepatic ischemia and reperfusion injury: effects on the liver sinusoidal milieu. *J Hepatol.* (2013) 59:1094–106. doi: 10.1016/j.jhep.2013.06.017
3. Jaeschke H. Molecular mechanisms of hepatic ischemia-reperfusion injury and preconditioning. *Am J Physiol Gastrointest Liver Physiol.* (2003) 284:G15–26. doi: 10.1152/ajpgi.00342.2002
4. Lutz J, Thurmel K, Heemann U. Anti-inflammatory treatment strategies for ischemia/reperfusion injury in transplantation. *J Inflamm.* (2010) 7:27. doi: 10.1186/1476-9255-7-27
5. Guan LY, Fu PY, Li PD, Li ZN, Liu HY, Xin MG, et al. Mechanisms of hepatic ischemia-reperfusion injury and protective effects of nitric oxide. *World J Gastrointest Surg.* (2014) 6:122–8. doi: 10.4240/wjgs.v6.i7.122
6. van Golen RF, van Gulik TM, Heger M. The sterile immune response during hepatic ischemia/reperfusion. *Cytokine Growth Factor Rev.* (2012) 23:69–84. doi: 10.1016/j.cytogfr.2012.04.006
7. Oliveira THC, Marques PE, Proost P, Teixeira MMM. Neutrophils: a cornerstone of liver ischemia and reperfusion injury. *Lab Invest.* (2018) 98:51–62. doi: 10.1038/labinvest.2017.90
8. Datta G, Fuller BJ, Davidson BR. Molecular mechanisms of liver ischemia reperfusion injury: insights from transgenic knockout models. *World J Gastroenterol.* (2013) 19:1683–98. doi: 10.3748/wjg.v19.i11.1683
9. ter Haar E, Prabhakar P, Liu X, Lepre C. Crystal structure of the p38 alpha-MAPKAP kinase 2 heterodimer. *J Biol Chem.* (2007) 282:9733–9. doi: 10.1074/jbc.M611165200
10. Roux PP, Blenis J. ERK and p38 MAPK-activated protein kinases: a family of protein kinases with diverse biological functions. *Microbiol Mol Biol Rev.* (2004) 68:320–44. doi: 10.1128/MMBR.68.2.320-344.2004
11. Li YY, Ochs S, Gao ZR, Malo A, Chen CJ, Lv S, et al. Regulation of HSP60 and the role of MK2 in a new model of severe experimental pancreatitis. *Am J Physiol Gastrointest Liver Physiol.* (2009) 297:G981–9. doi: 10.1152/ajpgi.00225.2009
12. Samulin Erdem J, Skaug V, Haugen A, Zienolddiny S. Loss of MKK3 and MK2 copy numbers in non-small cell lung cancer. *J Cancer* (2016) 7:512–5. doi: 10.7150/jca.13651
13. Franks HA, Wang Q, Lax SJ, Collins MK, Escors D, Patel PM, et al. Novel function for the p38-MK2 signaling pathway in circulating CD1c+ (BDCA-1+) myeloid dendritic cells from healthy donors and advanced cancer patients; inhibition of p38 enhances IL-12 whilst suppressing IL-10. *Int J Cancer* (2014) 134:575–86. doi: 10.1002/ijc.28398
14. Tietz SM, Hofmann R, Thomas T, Tackenberg B, Gaestel M, Berghoff M. MK2 and Fas receptor contribute to the severity of CNS demyelination. *PLoS ONE* (2014) 9:e100363. doi: 10.1371/journal.pone.0100363
15. Hegen M, Gaestel M, Nickerson-Nutter CL, Lin LL, Telliez JB. MAPKAP kinase 2-deficient mice are resistant to collagen-induced arthritis. *J Immunol.* (2006) 177:1913–7. doi: 10.4049/jimmunol.177.3.1913
16. Ashraf MI, Ebner M, Wallner C, Haller M, Khalid S, Schwelberger H, et al. A p38MAPK/MK2 signaling pathway leading to redox stress, cell death and ischemia/reperfusion injury. *Cell Commun Signal.* (2014) 12:6. doi: 10.1186/1478-811X-12-6
17. El-Benna J, Dang PM, Gougerot-Pocidalo MA. Priming of the neutrophil NADPH oxidase activation: role of p47phox phosphorylation and NOX2 mobilization to the plasma membrane. *Semin Immunopathol.* (2008) 30:279–89. doi: 10.1007/s00281-008-0118-3
18. Fu H, Bylund J, Karlsson A, Pellme S, Dahlgren C. The mechanism for activation of the neutrophil NADPH-oxidase by the peptides formyl-Met-Leu-Phe and Trp-Lys-Tyr-Met-Val-Met differs from that for interleukin-8. *Immunology* (2004) 112:201–10. doi: 10.1111/j.1365-2567.2004.01884.x
19. El-Benna J, Dang PM, Gougerot-Pocidalo MA, Marie JC, F. Braut-Boucher: p47phox, the phagocyte NADPH oxidase/NOX2 organizer: structure, phosphorylation and implication in diseases. *Exp Mol Med.* (2009) 41:217–25. doi: 10.3858/emm.2009.41.4.058
20. Qian F, Deng J, Cheng N, Welch EJ, Zhang Y, Malik AB, et al. A non-redundant role for MKP5 in limiting ROS production and preventing LPS-induced vascular injury. *EMBO J.* (2009) 28:2896–907. doi: 10.1038/emboj.2009.234
21. Faust LR, el Benna J, Babior BM, Chanock SJ. The phosphorylation targets of p47phox, a subunit of the respiratory burst oxidase. Functions of the individual target serines as evaluated by site-directed mutagenesis. *J Clin Invest.* (1995) 96:1499–505. doi: 10.1172/JCI118187
22. Dusi S, Della Bianca V, Grzeskowiak M, Rossi F. Relationship between phosphorylation and translocation to the plasma membrane of p47phox and p67phox and activation of the NADPH oxidase in normal and Ca(2+)-depleted human neutrophils. *Biochem J.* (1993) 290(Pt 1):173–8.
23. el Benna J, Faust LP, Babior BM. The phosphorylation of the respiratory burst oxidase component p47phox during neutrophil activation. Phosphorylation of sites recognized by protein kinase C and by proline-directed kinases. *J Biol Chem.* (1994) 269:23431–6.
24. Honda M, Takeichi T, Hashimoto S, Yoshii D, Isono K, Hayashida S, et al. Intravital imaging of neutrophil recruitment reveals the efficacy of FPR1 blockade in hepatic ischemia-reperfusion injury. *J Immunol.* (2017) 198:1718–28. doi: 10.4049/jimmunol.1601773
25. Huang H, Tohme S, Al-Khafaji AB, Tai S, Loughran P, Chen L, et al. Damage-associated molecular pattern-activated neutrophil extracellular trap exacerbates sterile inflammatory liver injury. *Hepatology* (2015) 62:600–14. doi: 10.1002/hep.27841

26. Coxon PY, Rane MJ, Uriarte S, Powell DW, Singh S, Butt W, et al. MAPK-activated protein kinase-2 participates in p38 MAPK-dependent and ERK-dependent functions in human neutrophils. *Cell Signal.* (2003) 15:993–1001. doi: 10.1016/S0898-6568(03)00074-3
27. Wu Y, Zhan L, Ai Y, Hannigan M, Gaestel M, Huang CK, et al. MAPKAPK2-mediated LSP1 phosphorylation and FMLP-induced neutrophil polarization. *Biochem Biophys Res Commun.* (2007) 358:170–5. doi: 10.1016/j.bbrc.2007.04.104
28. Wu Y, Hannigan MO, Kotlyarov A, Gaestel M, Wu D, Huang CK. A requirement of MAPKAPK2 in the uropod localization of PTEN during FMLP-induced neutrophil chemotaxis. *Biochem Biophys Res Commun.* (2004) 316:666–72. doi: 10.1016/j.bbrc.2004.02.107
29. Lee D, Park S, Bae S, Jeong D, Park M, Kang C, et al. Hydrogen peroxide-activatable antioxidant prodrug as a targeted therapeutic agent for ischemia-reperfusion injury. *Sci Rep.* (2015) 5:16592. doi: 10.1038a/srep 16592
30. Makni-Maalej K, Chiandotto M, Hurtado-Nedelec M, Bedouhene S, Gougerot-Pocidalo MA, Dang PM, et al. Zymosan induces NADPH oxidase activation in human neutrophils by inducing the phosphorylation of p47phox and the activation of Rac2: involvement of protein tyrosine kinases, PI3Kinase, PKC, ERK1/2 and p38MAPkinase. *Biochem Pharmacol.* (2013) 85:92–100. doi: 10.1016/j.bcp.2012.10.010
31. Mollapour E, Linch DC, Roberts PJ. Activation and priming of neutrophil nicotinamide adenine dinucleotide phosphate oxidase and phospholipase A(2) are dissociated by inhibitors of the kinases p42(ERK2) and p38(SAPK) and by methyl arachidonyl fluorophosphonate, the dual inhibitor of cytosolic and calcium-independent phospholipase A(2). *Blood* (2001) 97:2469–77. doi: 10.1182/blood.V97.8.2469
32. Giamas G, Hirner H, Shoshiashvili L, Grothey A, Gessert S, Kuhl M, et al. Phosphorylation of CK1delta: identification of Ser370 as the major phosphorylation site targeted by PKA *in vitro* and *in vivo*. *Biochem J.* (2007) 406:389–98. doi: 10.1042/BJ20070091
33. Gong J, Yao Y, Zhang P, Udayasuryan B, Komissarova EV, Chen J, et al. The C2 domain and altered ATP-binding loop phosphorylation at Ser(3)(5)(9) mediate the redox-dependent increase in protein kinase C-delta activity. *Mol Cell Biol.* (2015) 35:1727–40. doi: 10.1128/MCB.01436-14
34. Mizuki K, Takeya R, Kuribayashi F, Nobuhisa I, Kohda D, Nunoi H, et al. A region C-terminal to the proline-rich core of p47phox regulates activation of the phagocyte NADPH oxidase by interacting with the C-terminal SH3 domain of p67phox. *Arch Biochem Biophys.* (2005) 444:185–94. doi: 10.1016/j.abb.2005.10.012
35. Wu Y, He H, Ding Y, Liu S, Zhang D, Wang J, et al. MK2 mediates macrophage activation and acute lung injury by regulating let-7e miRNA. *Am J Physiol Lung Cell Mol Physiol.* (2018) 315:L371–81. doi: 10.1152/ajplung.00019.2018

7

Therapeutic Targeting of Hepatic Macrophages for the Treatment of Liver Diseases

Daphne van der Heide[1], *Ralf Weiskirchen*[2] *and Ruchi Bansal*[1*]

[1] Department of Biomaterials Science and Technology, Faculty of Science and Technology, Technical Medical Center, University of Twente, Enschede, Netherlands, [2] Institute of Molecular Pathobiochemistry, Experimental Gene Therapy and Clinical Chemistry (IFMPEGKC), RWTH University Hospital Aachen, Aachen, Germany

***Correspondence:**
Ruchi Bansal
r.bansal@utwente.nl

Hepatic macrophages play a central role in maintaining homeostasis in the liver, as well as in the initiation and progression of liver diseases. Hepatic macrophages are mainly derived from resident hepatic macrophages called Kupffer cells or circulating bone marrow-derived monocytes. Kupffer cells are self-renewing and typically non-migrating macrophages in the liver and are stationed in the liver sinusoids in contrast to macrophages originating from circulating monocytes. Kupffer cells regulate liver homeostasis by mediating immunity against non-pathogenic blood-borne molecules, while participating in coordinated immune responses leading to pathogen clearance, leukocyte recruitment and antigen presentation to lymphocytes present in the vasculature. Monocyte-derived macrophages infiltrate into the liver tissue when metabolic or toxic damage instigates and are likely dispensable for replenishing the macrophage population in homeostasis. In recent years, different populations of hepatic macrophages have been identified with distinct phenotypes with discrete functions, far beyond the central dogma of M1 and M2 macrophages. Hepatic macrophages play a central role in the pathogenesis of acute and chronic liver failure, liver fibrosis, non-alcoholic fatty liver disease, alcoholic liver disease, viral hepatitis, and hepatocellular carcinoma, as well as in disease resolution. The understanding of the role of hepatic macrophages in liver diseases provides opportunities for the development of targeted therapeutics for respective malignancies. This review will summarize the current knowledge of the hepatic macrophages, their origin, functions, their critical role in maintaining homeostasis and in the progression or resolution of liver diseases. Furthermore, we will provide a comprehensive overview of the therapeutic targeting strategies against hepatic macrophages developed for the treatment of liver diseases.

Keywords: hepatic macrophages, targeted therapeutics, liver diseases, monocytes, Kupffer cells

INTRODUCTION

The liver is the largest gland in the human body, weighing about 1.5 kg in an adult. It plays an important role in metabolism and mediate several functions including glycogen storage, plasma protein synthesis, and drug detoxification. Liver tissue is highly vascularized with a continuous blood flow and contain extremely permeable fenestrated endothelia facilitating the interaction between the bloodstream and liver cells. The liver is also a central immunological organ in the human body that is exposed to large amounts of circulating antigens and endotoxins from gut microbiota. To maintain liver homeostasis, the liver employs multiple mechanisms to suppress immune responses and create tolerance (1). Liver sinusoidal endothelial cells (LSECs), Kupffer cells (KCs) and dendritic cells are essential players in initiating and shaping liver immune responses, through antigen presentation, and cytokine and chemokine excretion along with neutrophils, B and T lymphocytes, and natural killer (NK) cells that circulate in the hepatic sinusoids (2).

In this review, we present the insights on hepatic macrophages [collectively referred to as resident KCs and monocyte-derived macrophages (MoMFs)], a heterogeneous population of immune cells that originate from different sources (3). Traditionally, macrophages are classified into a classical M1 pro-inflammatory phenotype, and a dichotomic M2 pro-resolving phenotype (3). However, in past years, tremendous heterogeneity in hepatic macrophages, with distinct functions and gene signatures, have been revealed highlighting their cruciality in liver diseases. While KCs represent the main hepatic macrophages during steady state involved in homeostasis, hepatic metabolic or toxic damage results in massive infiltration of MoMFs into the injured liver. Mice with injured livers showed that the infiltration of MoMFs resulted in antigen redistribution between myeloid cell populations and loss of specific markers for tolerogenic phenotype by KCs, due to amplification of the hepatic phagocytic compartment (4, 5). Hepatic macrophages generally maintain homeostasis, but when imbalance ensues this can result in liver inflammation and fibrosis. The imbalance in hepatic macrophage functioning can result in different liver diseases consequently liver inflammation that has been shown to be associated with the poor disease prognosis in patients.

During liver damage, hepatic macrophages interacts and communicates with hepatic stellate cells that are also known as the liver pericytes located in the space of Disse between parenchymal cells and LSECs of the hepatic lobule. Hepatic stellate cells have numerous functions like vitamin A storage, hemodynamic functions, immuno-regulation and extracellular matrix (ECM) remodeling (6). Upon liver injury, these cells transdifferentiate into activated proliferative, migratory and contractile myofibroblasts, and secrete multiple pro-inflammatory and pro-fibrotic factors (7, 8). In addition, these hepatic myofibroblasts promote the differentiation of liver macrophages with pro-inflammatory and pro-fibrotic functions (9), hence play a central role in the development of liver fibrosis and hepatocellular carcinoma (HCC) in combination with liver macrophages.

In the past decades, it has become apparent that macrophages play a central role in initiation, perpetuation and restoration of liver inflammation and damage. Tremendous progress has been made in the understanding of their origin, heterogeneity and functions that has provided with new therapeutics that have been—or currently being—explored in preclinical models and clinical trials. These increasing developments in understanding hepatic macrophage biology will provide new perspectives toward the effective treatment of liver diseases.

ORIGIN OF HEPATIC MACROPHAGES

Ninety percent of all macrophages in the human body reside in the liver. These macrophages can be derived from different cells. The diverse origins of the macrophages result in cellular heterogeneity in the liver, which is reflected in a high diversity in released cytokines, cell surface markers and transcriptional profiles (3, 10). Hepatic macrophages can be derived from either resident hepatic macrophages, called KCs and from distinct populations of infiltrating macrophages i.e., circulating bone marrow (BM)-derived macrophages, avascular peritoneal macrophages (PMs) that reside in subcapsular regions of the liver or splenic monocytes (3, 11–13) (**Figure 1**). In response to microenvironmental signals, macrophages can migrate and polarize toward different phenotypes with pro-inflammatory and/or anti-inflammatory responses (14).

Kupffer Cells

KCs are the resident, self-renewing and non-migrating macrophages, localized at the luminal side of the liver sinusoids (3, 10). KCs are the largest tissue-resident macrophage population that maintain liver integrity, restore tissue after injury and infection, and initiate the innate and adaptive immune responses (15). KCs form a highly dynamic and complex network in this defense and mediate tolerance, mostly via the interaction with hepatic regulatory T cells (Tregs) (2). KCs provide an anti-inflammatory microenvironment, during homeostasis, by secreting an anti-inflammatory cytokine interleukin (IL)-10 (4, 12). Antigen presentation to KCs induces CD4 T-cell arrest and secretion of immunosuppressive cytokine IL-10 producing antigen-specific Tregs, which results in promoting the immune tolerance. To maintain liver homeostasis, KCs do not only interact with T cells, but also with another macrophage population, circulating MoMFs and hepatic stellate cells (liver fibroblasts) (**Figure 1**).

The resident macrophages are developed asynchronously in three waves at multiple anatomical locations (**Figure 1**). The first wave, primitive hematopoiesis, starts at embryonic day 7.5. In the first wave, primitive erythroid progenitors are detected in the yolk sac (YS) and give rise to primitive erythroblasts (16, 17). In the second wave, transient hematopoiesis, fate-mapping studies in mice showed that resident macrophages descend from a Tie2^{+}, also called Tek receptor tyrosine kinase through a cellular pathway generating colony-stimulating factor 1 receptor (CSF1R) positive erythro-myeloid progenitors (EMPs). The EMPs are developed in the YS at embryonic day 8.5, they migrate *via* the bloodstream and colonize to the nascent fetal liver in a chemokine-receptor-dependent manner before embryonic day 10.5 and give rise to the pre-macrophages until embryonic day 16.5. KCs are marginally replaced by hematopoietic stem cells derived macrophages in 1-year-old mice, hereby generating macrophage diversity observed in postnatal tissues (18–20). Finally, the third wave, definitive hematopoiesis, hematopoietic stem cells can be distinguished from other hematopoietic progenitors by their self-renewal capacity, presence in adults and repopulation potential after

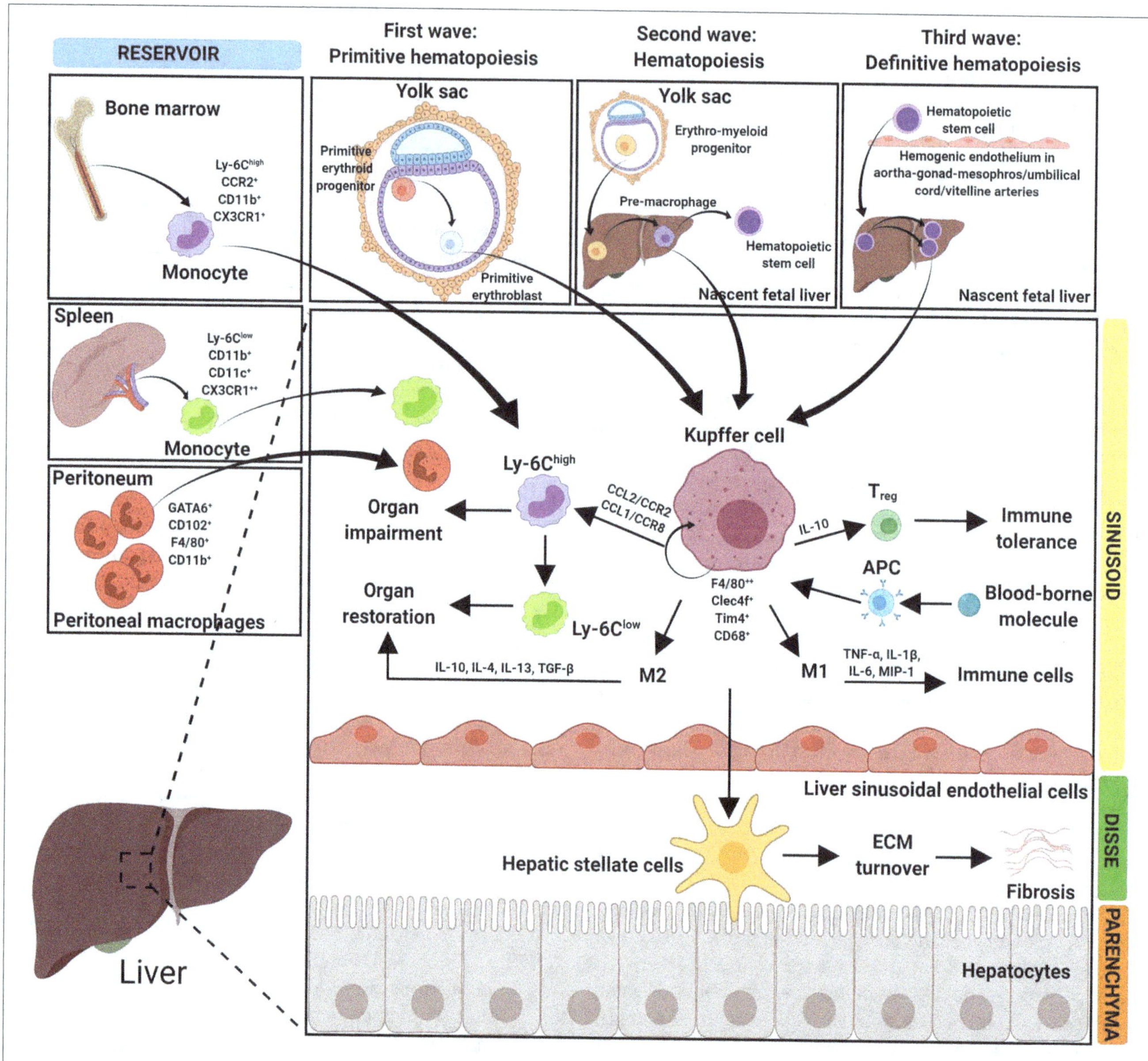

FIGURE 1 | Origin of hepatic macrophages. The figure depicts the diverse origin of hepatic macrophages. Hepatic macrophages can arise from bone marrow derived monocytes, spleen derived monocytes and peritoneum-derived macrophages. Resident hepatic macrophages (Kupffer cells, KCs) develop in three waves at multiple anatomical locations. In the first wave (primitive hematopoiesis), primitive erythroid progenitors originate and differentiate into primitive erythroblasts in the yolk sac. In the second wave (transient hematopoiesis), erythro-myeloid progenitors develop in the yolk sac and migrate into the nascent fetal liver. In the third wave (definitive hematopoiesis), hematopoietic stem cells arise intra-embryonically from hemogenic endothelium in the aorta-gonad-mesonephros region and in the umbilical and vitelline arteries. Hematopoietic stem cells migrate into the fetal liver and expand/differentiate into resident KCs. Hepatic macrophages mediate different functions in organ homeostasis, impairment, restoration, and in fibrosis. APC, antigen presenting cells; CCL, chemokine (C-C) motif ligand; CCR, chemokine (C-C) motif receptor; CD, cluster of differentiation; Clec4f, C-type lectin domain family 4 member F; CX3CR1, C-X3-C motif chemokine receptor 1; ECM, extracellular matrix; F4/80, EGF-like module-containing mucin-like hormone receptor-like 1; GATA6, GATA-binding factor 6; IL, interleukin; MIP-1, macrophage inflammatory protein 1; Tim4, T-cell membrane protein 4; TGFβ, transforming growth factor beta; TNF-α, tumor necrosis factor-α; Treg, regulatory T cells; Ly-6C, lymphocyte antigen 6 complex locus C1.

transplantation (21). Hematopoietic stem cells arise intra-embryonically from hemogenic endothelium in the aorta-gonad-mesonephros region and in the umbilical and vitelline arteries at embryonic days 10.5. The hematopoietic stem cells migrate to the fetal liver, expand and differentiate into resident macrophages (17, 22).

KCs are primarily identified as $CD45^{+}$ $F4/80^{+}$ $CD11b^{intermediate/int}$ cells expressing C-type lectin 4F (*Clec4f*) as a specific KC marker. Based on intravital microscopy, morphometric analysis and gene expression profiling, two distinct intrahepatic KCs subsets i.e., BM-derived KCs and YS-derived KCs, highlighting KCs heterogeneity (23).

YS-derived KCs express Macrophage Receptor with Collagenous Structure (MARCO) and T-cell immunoglobulin and mucin domain containing 4 (Tim4) and possess pro-inflammatory functions. On the other hand, BM-derived KCs display an immunoregulatory gene signature possessing protective functions in the maintenance of liver homeostasis (23). Interestingly, recent studies have highlighted a rapid KCs loss upon infection (24, 25), and in HCC (26), thereby questioning why and how KCs loss is established. Several hypotheses have been proposed e.g., KCs loss as a self-inflicted brake of immune system to prevent excessive inflammation, as supported by studies whereby KCs depletion attenuated chronic inflammatory diseases such as non-alcoholic steatohepatitis (NASH) (27, 28). However, in contrast, studies have revealed that tissue-resident macrophages inhibit inflammation after injury and maintain homeostasis (29, 30). With these contradicting findings, it is highly critical to understand if KCs loss is an essential to control liver inflammation or is a consequence of the inflammation. Considering the distinct KC populations (BM-derived and YS-derived) with different functions might explain these contradictions, however further studies are required to deeply understand the underlying mechanisms. These insights will improve our current understanding about liver diseases and will help in developing novel therapeutic strategies targeting specific KC phenotype for the efficient treatment of liver diseases.

Monocyte-Derived Macrophages

Circulating MoMFs mainly infiltrate into the liver when hepatic metabolic or toxic damage occurs and are likely dispensable for replenishing the macrophage population in homeostasis (**Figure 1**). MoMFs are mainly derived from a chemokine C-X3-C motif receptor 1 (CX3CR1)$^+$ CD117$^+$ Lin$^-$ (lineage-negative) BM progenitors and express CX3CR1, lymphocyte antigen 6 complex locus C1 (Ly-6C), CD11b and chemokine (C-C motif) receptor 2 (CCR2) (31). MoMFs recruitment is primarily initiated by activated toll-like receptor (TLR) signaling in KCs or hepatic stellate cells that results in increased secretion of chemokine (C-C motif) ligand 2 (CCL2) or monocyte chemoattractant protein 1 (MCP-1) (32–34).

Upon recruitment, MoMFs differentiate into a plethora of phenotypes with discrete functions depending on the microenvironmental cues. Studies in mice have shown that inflammatory lymphocyte antigen 6 complex, locus C1 (Ly-6C)^{high} expressing monocytes (analogous to CD14^{hi} CD16^{lo} human monocytes) are attracted and accumulated in the injured liver tissue depending on chemokine ligand/receptor interactions of CCL2/CCR2 or CCL1/CCR8 (3, 34–37). In acute liver injury mouse model, Ly-6C^{high} monocytes have been shown to express the increasing levels of T cell Ig Mucin 3 (*Havcr2*), toll-like receptors (*Tlr2*), C-type lectins (*Clec4d*, *Clec4e*, and *Clec5a*), CD209a and CD93 (38). Ly-6C^{high} monocytes provoke organ impairment, but can locally undergo a functional switch into restorative Ly-6C^{low} monocytes (analogous to CD14^{low} CD16^{high} human monocytes) that can restore liver damage. Therefore, this study showed a Ly-6C^{high}/Ly-6C^{low} phenotype beyond the traditional M1/M2 classification (39).

Ly-6C^{high} monocytes express high levels of CCR2 and activated hepatic stellate cells have been to secrete increasing levels of CCR2 ligand CCL2. It has been further suggested using CCR2 deficient mouse model, that CCR2 critically controls intrahepatic Ly-6C^{high} monocytes recruitment during liver injury via CCR2-dependent BM egress and promote the progression of liver fibrosis (39, 40). The CCL2/CCR2 signaling therefore critically mediates hepatic macrophage recruitment upon liver injury, leading to shaping of the inflammatory response in the injured liver. Furthermore, other CCRs such as CCR1 and CCR5, via CCL3/MIP1α, CCL4/MIP1β and CCL5/RANTES interaction have been implicated in liver fibrosis attributed to Ly-6C^{high} monocytes recruitment or stellate cells activation, respectively (39–41). CCR8 that interacts with CCL1 was also shown to be involved in the directed infiltration of infiltrating monocytes into injured liver (37). In the respective study, CCR8-deficient mice having reduced intrahepatic monocytes/macrophages showed significantly attenuated hepatic fibrosis that could be restored by adoptive transfer of CCR8-expressing Ly-6C^{high} BM-derived monocytes (37). These studies highlight the importance of MoMFs recruitment in disease progression and therefore the therapeutic potential of CCRs e.g., CCR2, CCR5, and CCR8 antagonists to inhibit MoMFs infiltration thereby limiting liver inflammation and fibrosis.

Peritoneal and Splenic Macrophages

Wang and Kubes have identified a distinct avascular population of macrophages, PMs, that are recruited through the visceral endothelium upon liver injury and contribute to liver regeneration (13). PMs, that reside in the peritoneal cavity with self-renewal abilities (42), exists as two distinct PM subsets i.e., large peritoneal macrophages (LPMs) and small peritoneal macrophages (SPMs). LPMs originate from embryonic precursors and represent the most abundant subset under steady conditions that display F4/80^{high} CD11b^{high} MHCII^{low} phenotype (**Figure 1**). While SPMs are the minor subset with F4/80^{low} CD11b^{low} MHCII^{high} phenotype and originate from BM-derived myeloid precursors and predominantly appear during infection (42). Flow cytometry studies confirmed the recruitment of subpopulation of mature PMs expressing CD102 and GATA-binding protein 6 (GATA6) transcription factor within 1 h at the site of thermal injury at the liver surface (13, 43). Furthermore, depletion of PMs prevented the early F4/80$^+$ macrophage influx and finally, macrophage recruitment and tissue regeneration was reported to be impaired in GATA6-deficient mice, suggesting an important role of PMs during resolution of liver diseases (13, 43).

Besides KCs, MoMFs and PMs, splenic derived monocytes may also contribute to hepatic macrophages during liver injury (11, 44) (**Figure 1**). Studies have unraveled spleen as a site for storage and deployment of monocytes, and have identified the contribution of splenic monocytes in regulating immune response during injury (44). Furthermore, splenic macrophages have been shown to promote monocytes infiltration and supports M1 dominant phenotype *via* secretion of CCL2, and regulate KCs activation and hepatic inflammation by releasing of factors such as lipocalin-2 in the portal vein (45, 46). However, more studies are vital to gain insights into distinct phenotypes and functions of splenic macrophages during liver diseases.

MACROPHAGE HETEROGENEITY: BEYOND M1 AND M2 POLARIZATION DOGMA

Within hepatic macrophage populations, there is a substantial heterogeneity characterized by a broad spectrum of released cytokines, cell surface markers and transcriptional profiles. Within the simplistic M1/M2 terminology, classically activated M1 macrophages—activated by interferon gamma (IFN-γ) and lipopolysaccharides (LPS)—are pro-inflammatory, microbicidal, tumoricidal, and release numerous inflammatory cytokines e.g., tumor necrosis factor (TNF)-α, IL-1, IL-6, IL-12, IL-15, and IL-18. While alternatively activated M2 macrophages downregulate inflammatory responses and facilitate tissue repair by secreting IL-10, IL-4/IL-13, transforming growth factor (TGF)-β and vascular endothelial growth factor (VEGF)-α. Due to the complex biological characteristics, M2 macrophages can be further sub-categorized into distinct phenotypes based on the stimuli: M2a (induced by IL-4 and IL-13), M2b (elicited by immune complexes), M2c (stimulated by IL-10, TGF-β and glucocorticoids) and M2d (activated by IL-6, TLR ligands and adenosine) (47, 48). M2a macrophages are wound healing macrophages that express high levels of mannose receptor (MR, also called CD206), secrete pro-fibrotic factors such as TGF-β, insulin-like growth factor (IGF), and fibronectin, and contribute to tissue repair. M2b macrophages possess both protective and pathogenic roles, and secrete both pro- and anti-inflammatory cytokines. M2c phenotype display regulatory phenotype, can repress inflammation and fibrosis, and promote tissue repair. In addition, M2c macrophages have the ability to induce regulatory T cells and are involved in the phagocytosis of apoptotic cells. M2d macrophages have phenotypic and functional attributes similar to tumor-associated macrophages (TAMs), and are distinct from M2a-c. M2d constitute the major inflammatory component in tumor, contributing to angiogenesis and metastasis (47, 48).

Strikingly, recent studies have unraveled a complex and spectrum of macrophage polarization states beyond the ancient dogma of M1 and M2 macrophages (11, 49). A recent study, using single-cell RNA sequencing, has provided a comprehensive map of the human liver at a single-cell resolution and revealed distinct intrahepatic monocyte/macrophage populations with unique functional pathways. Furthermore, this study highlighted the disparity between different macrophage populations and biological differences between livers from mice and humans. This recent study describing a transcriptional map of the human liver microenvironment provides a framework for understanding the human liver and the role of different cellular phenotypes that will provide a benchmark for the development of novel immunomodulatory therapies (49).

FUNCTION OF HEPATIC MACROPHAGES IN LIVER DISEASES

Homeostasis of the liver is important for tolerating and regulating immune responses. Hepatic immune tolerance is mostly dependent on the interaction between KCs and Tregs to create a local suppressive microenvironment, while the recruitment of MoMFs and crosstalk between hepatic stellate cells and macrophages are important determinant for the disease progression/pathogenesis, and tissue regeneration following liver injury. For the development of targeting therapies for liver diseases, especially targeting liver inflammation, it is highly crucial to gain insights into the origin, phenotypic heterogeneity and functions of hepatic macrophages. Here, the role of hepatic macrophages in different liver diseases has been described, including acute liver failure (ALF), liver fibrosis, non-alcoholic fatty liver disease (NAFLD), alcoholic liver disease (ALD), viral hepatitis and HCC.

As mentioned earlier, hepatic macrophages (KCs and MoMFs) are the key players in various types of liver disease. The understanding of their roles in different liver diseases defines them as promising targets to develop new therapies for different liver diseases. Several commendable reviews have detailed the divergent roles and mechanisms of hepatic macrophages in liver diseases (3, 10). The function of hepatic macrophages in these different liver diseases is briefly summarized below and depicted in **Figure 2**.

Acute Liver Failure

ALF is a syndrome that is characterized by peripheral vasodilation, encephalopathy and coagulopathy resulting in multiple organ dysfunction and death (50). Patients with ALF, without previously recognized liver disease, sustain a liver injury that results in a rapid loss of hepatic function. Hepatic insult activates KCs and MoMFs to release large amounts of pro-inflammatory cytokines and chemokines, such as TNF-α, IFN-γ, MCP-1/CCL2, and IL-8 (**Figure 2**). They also express death ligands resulting in hepatocyte apoptosis (50). KCs release wide range of cytokines that are critical in determining the subsequent reactions of other immune cells, hepatocytes and the degree of organ damage (51). MoMFs have been shown to be actively recruited and secrete large amounts of pro-inflammatory cytokines, present antigens *via* their surface HLA class II molecules and trigger the adaptive immune response. In ALF, a counter-regulatory process ensues that is intended to offset the damaging effects of unhindered pro-inflammatory KCs and MoMFs activation. This counter-regulatory process consists of KCs secreting cytokines, such as IL-6, IL-10, and IL-18, to compensate for the deleterious effects of the pro-inflammatory response (50, 52).

Liver Fibrosis

Liver fibrosis is the final common pathway of chronic liver diseases caused by toxic damage, viral infections, autoimmune conditions, and metabolic and genetic diseases (53). The advanced stage of liver fibrosis is called cirrhosis, which is characterized by a loss of architecture, function of the liver

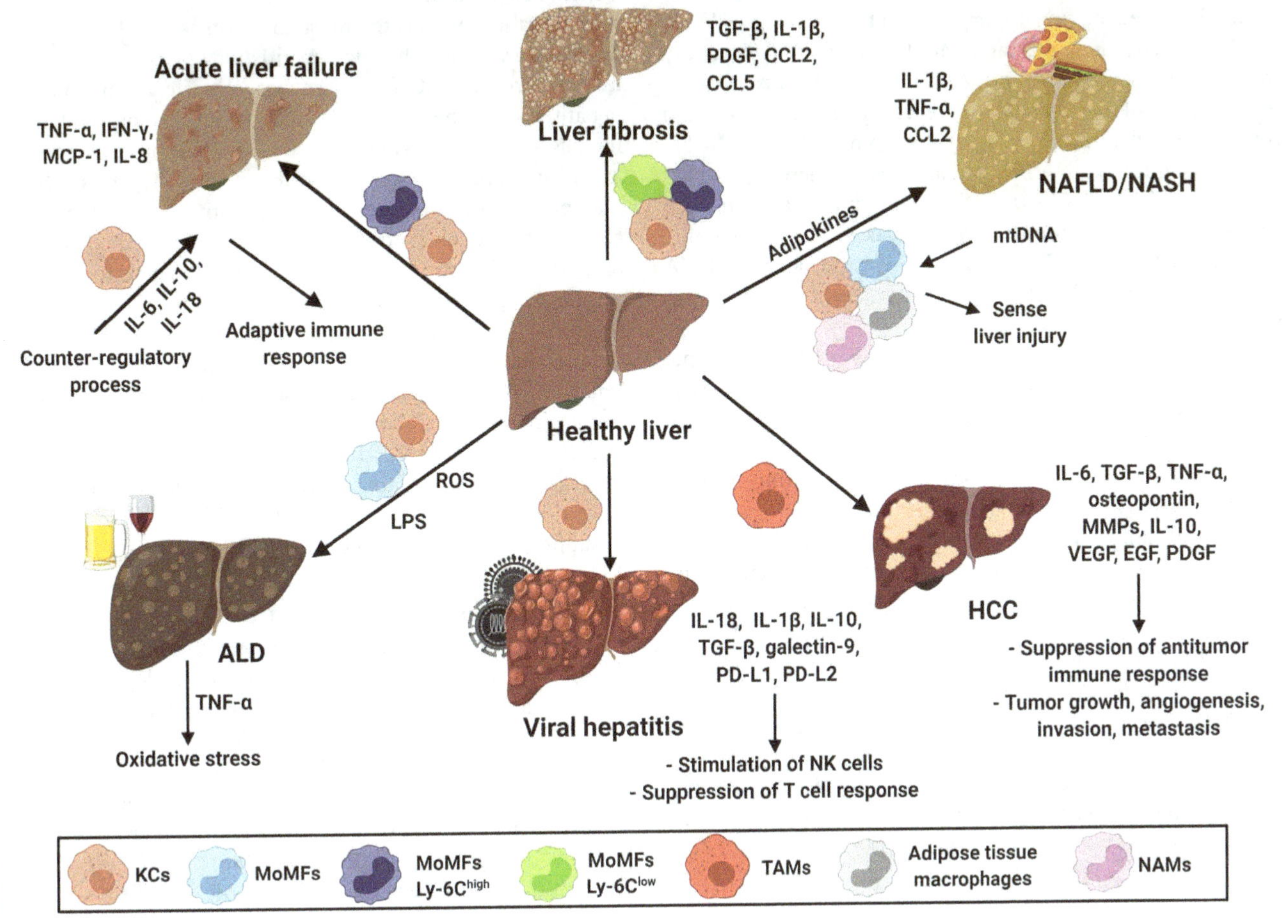

FIGURE 2 | Macrophages in hepatic disease. Hepatic macrophages, KCs and MoMFs, are the key players in various types of liver disease including acute liver failure (ALF), liver fibrosis, non-alcoholic fatty liver disease (NAFLD), alcoholic liver disease (ALD), viral hepatitis and hepatocellular carcinoma (HCC). They modulate adaptive immune responses, fibrosis progression/resolution, sense disease severity, contribute to the establishment of a tumorigenic environment, promote tumor growth, angiogenesis, invasion, and metastasis. CCL, chemokine (C-C) motif ligand; EGF, epidermal growth factor; HCC, hepatocellular carcinoma; IL, interleukin; IFN-γ, interferon-γ; KCs, Kupffer cells; LPS, lipopolysaccharides; Ly-6C, lymphocyte antigen 6 complex locus C1; MCP-1, monocyte chemoattractant protein 1; MMPs, matrix metalloproteinases; MoMFs, monocyte derived macrophages; mtDNA, mitochondrial DNA; NAFLD, non-alcoholic fatty liver disease; NASH, non-alcoholic steatohepatitis; NAMs, NASH-associated macrophages; PD-L, programmed death-ligand; PDGF, platelet-derived growth factor; ROS, reactive oxygen species; TAMs, tumor-associated macrophages; TGFβ, transforming growth factor beta; TNF-α, tumor necrosis factor-α; VEGF, vascular endothelial growth factor.

and development of life-threatening complications. Hepatocytes, cholangiocytes, hepatic stellate cells, LSECs, immune cells and especially macrophages have been identified in the pathogenesis of liver fibrosis (54). KCs are important in the initial response to injury, produce cytokines and chemokines, and recruit monocytes *via* secretion of CCL2 and CCL5 chemokines (39, 55). Studies have shown that that infiltration of Ly-6C^{high} MoMFs contributing to the expansion of hepatic macrophages to 3–5-fold. MoMFs could promote fibrosis by releasing factors like TGF-β, IL-1β, platelet-derived growth factor (PDGF) and CCL2, which activates hematopoietic stem cells (HSCs) and progresses the inflammation. Ly-6C^{high} MoMFs are pro-fibrogenic and pro-inflammatory (34) and can be switched to Ly-6C^{low} macrophages that are pro-restorative, anti-fibrotic and anti-inflammatory based on microenvironmental cues (39) (**Figure 2**). Importantly, when the injury in the liver is removed, macrophages are also responsible for the reversal of the liver fibrosis (55).

Non-alcoholic Fatty Liver Disease

NAFLD refers to a wide range of liver damage, from simple steatosis to NASH, advanced fibrosis, cirrhosis and liver failure (56). Pathological NAFLD resembles alcohol-induced liver disease but occurs in patients who do not abuse alcohol (57). NAFLD is a metabolic syndrome associated with unhealthy lifestyle and several risk factors, obesity, dyslipidemia and insulin resistance (58). Besides liver macrophages, adipose tissue macrophages are also shown to contribute to NAFLD and secretes adipokines and cytokines (59). Hepatic macrophages play the central role in NAFLD, the activation and polarization of macrophages affect the NAFLD progression. Dysregulation in macrophage polarization assist in progression to steatosis, the early stage of NAFLD (60). During chronic liver injury, KCs become activated and release inflammatory cytokines and chemokines. Endotoxins and bacterial components released due to increased intestinal permeability, (lipo)apoptotic hepatocytes, gut microbiota, free fatty acids, cholesterol etc. are the factors that mediate macrophage activation during NAFLD (61). Upon activation, KCs and MoMFs secrete inflammatory cytokines IL-1β, TNF-α and CCL2, that are involved in the development of steatosis, serve as lipogenic factors and promote the inflammatory progression from NAFLD to NASH (62–65) (**Figure 2**). NASH patients have increased levels of mitochondrial DNA (mtDNA) in serum, as damaged hepatocytes release exosomes/extracellular vesicles containing mitochondrial DNA. KCs recognizes this mitochondrial DNA *via* TLR9 and can therefore sense the severity of the liver injury (66, 67).

More recently, Krenkel et al., has reported the distinct fate of myeloid cells in liver and BM during obesity-related NASH. The study showed a unique, however common and functionally relevant, inflammatory signature in liver myeloid compartment and the BM precursors during NAFLD progression (68). This study suggests that myeloid cells, especially macrophages, adapt their phenotype in response to metabolic microenvironment, indicating the metabolic reprogramming of macrophages in NASH. Interestingly, using single-cell secretome gene analysis, Xiong et al., has identified NASH-associated macrophages (NAMs). NAMs markedly express high levels of triggering receptors expressed on myeloid cells 2 (Trem2) as a feature of mouse and human NASH correlating with disease severity, and responsive to pharmacological and dietary interventions. This study further provide insights into reprogramming of macrophages (and other non-parenchymal cells) in NASH (69).

Alcoholic Liver Disease

ALD includes different disease stages from simple steatosis to cirrhosis and HCC. Liver injury in ALD can be caused by the following factors: dose, duration and type of alcohol consumption, drinking patterns, sex, ethnicity, obesity, iron overload, viral hepatitis and genetic factors (70). Alcohol ingestion can cause alcohol-induced liver injury through activation of the innate and adaptive immune responses by cytotoxic and reactive oxygen species (ROS)-mediated effects of alcohol and its metabolite, acetaldehyde, on hepatocytes (71). Hepatic macrophages (both M1 and M2 phenotype) increases significantly during disease progression with increased intrahepatic inflammation e.g., increased expression of inflammatory genes, M1 and M2 markers, cytokines and chemokines (70–75).

KCs play a key role in ALD and alcohol consumption can lead to an increase in gut permeability resulting in endotoxemia. KCs can bind to endotoxin *via* CD14 receptor in combination with TLR4, leading to oxidative stress and release of pro-inflammatory cytokines such as TNF-α, causing alcohol-induced liver injury (72–75) (**Figure 2**). LPS levels are increased in ALD patients, which activates TLR4 signaling in KCs, HSCs and LSECs, and contributes to the regulation of angiogenesis and fibrogenesis, leading to fibrosis. Complement activation, TLR pathways and LPS-mediated pathways, including inflammasome activation could be potential therapeutic targets to develop new therapies for the treatment of ALD (74, 76).

Viral Hepatitis

Acute viral hepatitis is the most common cause of chronic liver disease worldwide. Chronic hepatitis may progress to cirrhosis, liver failure or HCC (77). A major obstacle in studying viral hepatitis is that there only exist a few immunocompetent animal models for chronic viral hepatitis (10). Hepatic macrophages are recognized as important cells in viral hepatitis. Hepatic macrophages can provide an efficient antiviral response but can also contribute to adverse effects as liver fibrosis or suppression of antiviral immunity (78). KCs play a pivotal role in both the hepatitis B virus (HBV) and the hepatitis C virus (HCV) infection. HBV can infect KCs, leading to the release of inflammatory cytokines, such as IL-18, and stimulation of NK cells (79, 80). The HCV can activate KCs through TLR2, which results in secretion of inflammatory molecules such as IL-1β and IL-18 (81, 82). KCs secrete IL-10, TGF-β, galectin-9 and induces expression of programmed death-ligands 1 and 2 (PD-L1 and PD-L2) during both HBV and HCV infection, resulting in suppression of T cell response (12) (**Figure 2**).

Hepatocellular Carcinoma

HCC is one of the most aggressive form of human cancer and a growing cause of cancer-related deaths worldwide (83, 84). Chronic inflammation seems to be essential in the initiation and development of HCC but idem for fibrosis and cirrhosis, which finally result in HCC. HBV and HCV as well as chronic alcohol abuse, biliary disease, metabolic disorders, drugs, toxins and genetic alterations are the major risk factors for the development of HCC (85, 86). TAMs are the key players in cancer-related inflammation (86, 87). TAMs originate from circulating monocytes that are recruited to the tumor microenvironment by CCL2, macrophage colony-stimulating factor (M-CSF), VEGF, and TGF-β, where they differentiate to mature hepatic macrophages (88). In the HCC tumor microenvironment, TAMs are mostly polarized into the M2 phenotype (87, 89) and promote HCC growth, angiogenesis, invasion and metastasis. They are also shown to suppress an antitumor immune response through the interaction with stromal and cancer cells in the tumor microenvironment. In the tumor microenvironment, TAMs release many cytokines, chemokines and growth factors. While IL-6 and TGF-β favor tumor growth, TNF-α, osteopontin, matrix metalloproteases (MMPs), and IL-6 supports invasion and metastasis. TGF-β in combination with IL-10 favors suppression of an antitumor immune response, and VEGF, epidermal growth factor (EGF), PDGF and TGF-β induces angiogenesis (86) (**Figure 2**).

As described above, hepatic macrophages play an highly essential role in liver diseases like ALF, liver fibrosis, NAFLD, ALD, viral hepatitis, and HCC. Therefore, hepatic macrophages represent the potential targets for therapeutic targeting for the treatment of liver diseases.

THERAPEUTIC TARGETING OF HEPATIC MACROPHAGES

Based on our increasing understanding about macrophages, several pathways have been identified that regulate their recruitment, differentiation/polarization and activation, based on which, a number of drugs have been designed and investigated in different preclinical murine models. Furthermore, it has been increasingly recognized that macrophages possess high scavenging ability thereby allowing their preferential targeting using nanoparticles (NPs).

However, there are several challenges that are hampering the drug development: (1) disparity in macrophage phenotypes in humans and in animal models resulting in poor translation of therapeutics studied in animal models to human patients; (2) greater macrophage heterogeneity in humans as compared to inbred mouse strains due to several intrinsic (genetics, ethnicity, sex, and age) and extrinsic factors (microbiota, infections, medications); (3) limited in-depth knowledge about human macrophage subsets as compared to mouse models. Importantly, macrophages display incredible heterogeneity with distinct functions in disease initiation and progression as well as protective role and maintain homeostasis. Therefore, it is crucial to target the pathogenic phenotypes of macrophages therapeutically without hindering the functions of so-called restorative or homeostatic macrophages.

Here, we summarize different approaches that have been explored for targeting of hepatic macrophages and are sub-categorized into three major categories: (a) modulation of macrophage polarization/reprogramming, (b) inhibition of KCs activation and (c) dampening of monocyte recruitment. These strategies have been investigated in experimental animal models, while some have been translated in the clinical settings (**Table 1** and **Figure 3**).

Modulation of Macrophage Polarization/Reprogramming

Macrophages phenotypes exert contrasting functions, therefore a therapeutic approach that promotes a switch from pathogenic phenotype to restorative phenotype is an interesting approach to accelerate disease resolution and promote liver regeneration. This can be achieved by using therapeutics that promote macrophage polarization and/or using nanoparticles that can selectively reprogram macrophages to restorative phenotype. Steroids (e.g., Dexamethasone), IL-4, IL-10, secretory leukocyte protease inhibitor (SLPI), prostaglandin E2 (PGE2) and colony-stimulating factor 1 receptor (CSF-1R) agonists are the promising therapeutics targeting different immuno-modulatory pathways that have been explored for macrophage reprogramming in liver diseases (90).

NPs are materials with dimensions between 10^{-9} and 10^{-7} m. Such particles can be used as nanocarriers for diagnosis and targeted delivery of therapeutic agents for liver diseases (109). There are several nanocarriers that can be used for diagnosis and therapy referred to as nano-theranostics. The NPs for drug and gene delivery systems include polymeric NPs, lipid NPs, organic and inorganic NPs (110). NPs provide multiple new properties, which can be exploited to improve the ability to detect, treat, monitor and prevent diseases. Moreover, the interactions between these nanomaterials and comparably sized physiological structures in the human body e.g., DNA, proteins and organelles, can be used in combination with existing medical diagnostic and treatment strategies to develop more efficacious approaches (111). These NPs could be loaded with small drug molecules, proteins, DNA or RNA. The drug release can be favorably tuned in different NPs, and in some cases, the release of the therapeutic agents could also be initiated by internal stimuli such as pH (112), or external stimuli such as light (113). Various surface modifications can be applied to NPs including small drug molecules, antibodies, fluorescent dyes, peptides, proteins, polyethylene glycol (PEG), DNA or RNA.

The NPs can be delivered at the targeted site *via* active or passive targeting. With active targeting, the NP surface can be modified with targeting ligands, e.g., targeting peptides, antibodies, which leads to specific binding to the targeted cells. Unlike active targeting, passive targeting does not use any targeting ligands, but uses the physiological properties e.g., enhanced permeability and retention (EPR) in tumors, due to leaky vasculature, to deliver the NPs to the target cells (114). To prolong the circulation time of the NPs in the circulatory system, with both active and passive targeting, the NPs can be surface modified with PEG.

NPs can be made out of different nanomaterials and are generally non-toxic. Gold NPs (AuNPs), which are similar to other inorganic NPs, are mostly non-toxic, but when used in small sizes of 1.4 nm they showed an increased toxicity. Silica NPs induces toxicity due to activation of macrophages. However, at higher doses, many nanotherapeutics have been shown to be toxic. To reduce non-specific uptake by macrophages and alter the response of immune cells, NPs can be modified with PEG or with peptides (115). Liver inflammation and fibrosis can be targeted by nanomedicine. This could be done by the therapeutic targeting of macrophages and especially KCs, because these macrophages have an inherent ability of efficient and non-specific uptake of most nanomaterials and these macrophages play a critical function during inflammation and fibrogenesis. KCs can be targeted by the mannose receptor in liver disease or become activated by specific nanomaterials like peptide-modified gold nanorods (AuNRs) to polarize them into the pro-inflammatory phenotype (115).

Different strategies have been proposed for hepatic macrophage targeting with nanomedicine in the preclinical setting (**Table 1** and **Figure 3**). A system studied by He et al., was to inhibit TNF-α using small interfering RNA (siRNA) delivered *via* mannose-modified trimethyl chitosan-cysteine (MTC) conjugated NPs that are mostly internalized by macrophages, due to macrophages-specific delivery route using the mannose receptor. With this strategy, inflammation-driven liver damage and lethality induced by acute lipopolysaccharide/D-galactosamine administration *in vivo* in mice was prevented. This system offers possibility for oral delivery, which is advantageous for clinical application (94).

Bartneck and colleagues showed that dexamethasone-loaded liposomes were efficient *in vivo* by ameliorating inflammatory liver diseases in a model of acute hepatitis and in chronic carbon tetrachloride (CCl_4)-based chronic toxic liver injury. This approach resulted in a M2 activation profile of macrophages and with a significant reduction in the number of T cells in the liver

TABLE 1 | Therapeutic targeting strategies of hepatic macrophages.

Strategy	(nano) Therapeutics	Mechanism/outcome	References
Modulation of macrophage polarization/macrophage reprogramming	Steroids e.g., glucocorticoids	Anti-inflammatory, anti-fibrotic	(90, 91)
	CSF-1R agonists CSF1-Fc	Proliferation of resident macrophages and recruitment of monocytes	(92)
	SLPI	Anti-inflammatory responses through modulation of monocyte/macrophage function	(93)
	MTC-TNF-α siRNA NPs	Inhibition of TNF-α production, reduction in liver inflammation	(94)
	Dexamethasone liposomes	Induction of T cells apoptosis	(95)
	COOH-micelles	Improvement, restoration of tolerance autoimmune disease and chronic inflammation	(96)
	Galectin-3	Inhibits inflammatory macrophage functions	(97)
	SYK pathway inhibitor R406	Anti-inflammatory, anti-fibrotic	(76)
	R406-PLGA NPs	Anti-inflammatory, anti-fibrotic	(98)
Inhibition of KCs activation	ASK1 inhibitor selonsertib	Anti-inflammatory, anti-fibrotic	(99)
	DAMPs (e.g., HMGB1) antagonists	Defected TLR9 signaling, decreased tumor cell proliferation Inhibits acute liver injury and bacterial translocation	(90, 100)
	PRR antagonists	Attenuates DAMPs/PAMPs mediated liver injury	(101)
	Curcumin and calcitriol liposomes	Immuno-modulatory	(102)
Dampening of monocyte recruitment	CCR2 antagonists Cenicriviroc, propagermanium	Anti-inflammatory, anti-fibrotic	(103–106)
	CCL2 antagonist mNOX-E36	Anti-inflammatory, anti-fibrotic	(33, 107)
	CCR5 antagonist Miraviroc	Anti-inflammatory, anti-fibrotic	(108)

ASK-1, apoptosis signal-regulating kinase 1; CCL, chemokine (C-C motif) ligand; CCR, chemokine (C-C) motif receptor; COOH-micelles, carboxy-modified micelles; CSF-1R, colony stimulating factor 1 receptor; CVC, cenicriviroc; KCs, Kupffer cells; DAMPs,/PAMPs damage-associated/pathogen-associated molecular patterns; HMGB1, High mobility group box 1 protein; SLPI, secretory leukocyte protease inhibitor; SYK, spleen tyrosine kinase; mNOX-E36, emapticap pegol; MTC, mannose-modified trimethyl chitosan-cysteine; NPs, nanoparticles; PLGA, poly(lactic-co-glycolic acid); siRNA, small interfering RNA.

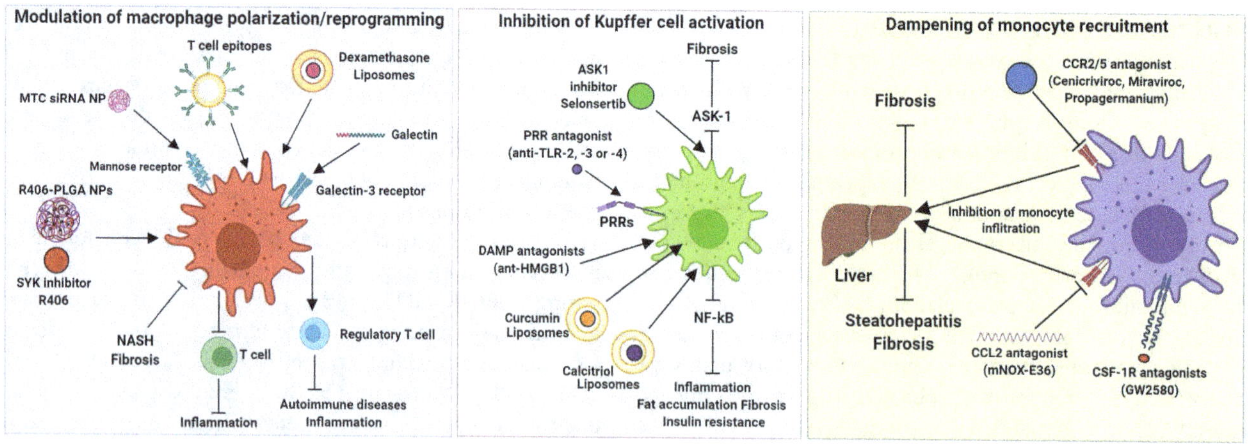

FIGURE 3 | Therapeutic targeting of hepatic macrophages. Modulation of macrophage polarization and function, inhibition of Kupffer cell activation, and dampening of monocyte recruitment into the inflamed liver are the three strategies that have been investigated for the resolution of hepatic inflammation and fibrogenesis. ASK1, Apoptosis signal-regulating kinase 1; CCL, chemokine (C-C) motif ligand; CCR, chemokine (C-C) motif receptor; CSF-1R, colony stimulating factor 1 receptor; DAMP, damage-associated molecular patterns; HMGB1, High mobility group box 1 protein; mNOX-E36, emapticap pegol; MTC, Mannose-modified trimethyl chitosan-cysteine; NASH, non-alcoholic steatohepatitis; NP, nanoparticle; PLGA, poly(lactic-co-glycolic acid); PRR, pattern recognition receptors; TLR, Toll like receptors.

(95). Herkel and co-workers published a patent based on a study of the induction of tolerance in liver by influencing Tregs by LSEC- and KC-directed carboxy-modified micelles. The micelles have been modified with T cell epitopes on their surface and were targeted to LSECs and KCs. These micelles can deliver antigens and induce the generation of Tregs to suppress autoimmunity.

These NPs are intended to induce tolerance against autoantigens and therefore ameliorating autoimmune diseases and chronic inflammation (96). Traber and Zomer used galactin-3 inhibitors to target inflammatory macrophage functions in liver diseases in mice. The treatment with galectin-3 resulted in regression of NASH and fibrosis. Therefore, they suggested that this galectin-targeting drugs have potential in treatment in human for NASH and fibrosis (97).

Furthermore, Bukong et al., demonstrated the central role of spleen tyrosine kinase (SYK) in multiple proinflammatory pathways involved in the ALD pathogenesis. Furthermore, SYK inhibitor R406 abrogated immune cell infiltration, macrophage and inflammasome activation, thereby ameliorated liver injury, liver inflammation, and reduced hepatic steatosis induced by alcohol (76). In another recent study, Kurniawan and colleagues reported an efficient delivery of small molecule SYK kinase inhibitor R406 using Poly(lactic-co-glycolic acid) (PLGA) NPs for the treatment of NASH in Methionine-Choline-deficient (MCD)-diet induced NASH mouse model (98).

Inhibition of Kupffer Cell Activation

When liver injury ensues, KCs initiate inflammatory cascades in the liver *via* different mechanisms. For instance, the early communication of cellular distress or hepatocyte damage is mediated by KCs through damage-associated molecular patterns (DAMPs)/pathogen-associated molecular patterns (PAMPs) via pattern recognition receptors (PRRs) and NF-κB signaling and inflammasome activation etc. Therefore, inhibition of PRRs using TLR2, TLR3, and TLR4 antagonists have been shown to ameliorate liver inflammation in murine models (101). Another interesting strategy that has been explored is targeting of released DAMPs such as high mobility group box 1 (HMGB1) proteins and histones. Intriguingly, HMGB1 neutralizing antibodies are shown to attenuate liver injury and reduce bacterial translocation *in vivo* in murine models (90). A possible targeting strategy to treat liver diseases is to influence KCs activation. There are several approaches for influencing KCs activation, such as reducing bacterial translocation and inhibition of TLR4-dependent macrophage activation using a broad spectrum of antibiotics. This could improve steatohepatitis, liver fibrosis and HCC (10).

Modifying KCs activation has been explored (**Table 1** and **Figure 3**). Hepatic macrophages and hepatocytes share some of the intracellular inflammatory signaling pathways like NF-κB, ASK1, JNK, or p38 (116). Loomba et al., developed selonsertib, an inhibitor of the inflammatory signaling pathway ASK1 (apoptosis signal-regulating kinase 1). Selonsertib treatment has been shown to have an effect on hepatocyte metabolism as well as macrophage activation. In a randomized phase 2 trial, selonsertib showed an improvement in fibrosis, lobular inflammation and serum biomarkers of apoptosis and necrosis in patients with NASH and fibrosis (99). However, in phase 3 randomized double-blind placebo-controlled STELLAR-3 and STELLAR-4 studies in patients with F3 fibrosis and compensated F4 cirrhosis respectively, due to NASH, selonsertib did not show a histologic improvement in fibrosis however well-tolerated safety results. In the study of Maradana et al., liposome-encapsulated lipophilic curcumin or 1,25-dihydroxy-vitamin D3, also called calcitriol, was investigated in mice with diet-induced NASH. Curcumin and calcitriol are both NF-κB inhibitors and were shown to be taken up by hepatic macrophages and dendritic cells, leading to the suppression of hepatic inflammation, fat accumulation, fibrosis and insulin resistance (102).

Dampening of Monocyte Recruitment

MoMFs are recruited by KCs to the liver, where they amplify and maintain liver inflammation. The recruitment of monocytes by KCs is driven by chemokine receptor interactions of CCL2/CCR2 or CCL1/CCR8 (16–19). A strategy to reduce the number of monocytes recruited into the liver include an interference with chemokine signaling. Interference with chemokine signaling can be achieved with monoclonal antibodies against chemokines or receptors, receptor antagonists, inhibition of chemokines by aptamer molecules or small molecule inhibitors blocking chemokine-induced intracellular signaling (10).

Chemokine interference as a targeting therapy for treating liver diseases has been intensively studied (**Table 1** and **Figure 3**). Lefebvre and co-workers as well as Krenkel and colleagues showed that the dual CCR2/CCR5 inhibitor, called cenicriviroc (CVC) that efficiently blocks CCL2-mediated monocyte recruitment to the liver and has an anti-fibrotic effect in mouse models of liver and kidney fibrosis (103, 104). In a randomized controlled trial, Friedman et al., showed $\geq$2-point improvement in NAS with no worsening of fibrosis after 1 year of CVC treatment in patients with NASH (NAS $\geq$ 4) and stage 1–3 liver fibrosis (105). Baeck et al., investigated CCL2 inhibitor, RNA-aptamer molecule mNOX-E36 in CCl_4 fibrosis model and MCD-diet induced NASH model. mNOX-E36 inhibited early influx of $Ly6C^+$ monocytes thereby shifting macrophage equilibrium to $Ly6C^-$-restorative monocytes hence favoring fibrosis resolution (33, 107). Furthermore, Mulder et al., showed that CCR2 has a crucial role in the recruitment of immune cells to white adipose tissue and the liver, and a CCR2 inhibitor, propagermanium, attenuated liver inflammation and NASH development (106). Interestingly, chemokine CCL5/RANTES has been documented to play an important role in the progression of hepatic inflammation and fibrosis. Maraviroc, a CCL5/RANTES inhibitor, ameliorated hepatic steatosis in a high-fat diet (HFD)-induced model of NAFLD (108). These studies suggest that significant involvement of CCL/CCR pathways in macrophage recruitment and that the inhibition of these pathways showed potential therapeutic effects. However, monocyte recruitment to the liver when injury ensues does not only have negative consequences, but can also have positive implications, as shown in a study in which CSF1-Fc fragment promoted KC proliferation and monocyte infiltration and differentiation, restored innate immunity (92). However, as described previously, monocytes can differentiate into a plethora of phenotypes with discrete functions depending on the microenvironmental cues. They can also differentiate into a phenotype that is involved in the restoration of organ damage depending on the liver disease and stage of the disease.

CONCLUSION AND FUTURE PROSPECTIVE

Research about the insights in the initiation and progression of liver diseases has given the opportunity to develop novel therapeutic targeting strategies for the treatment of different liver diseases. The liver consists of a heterogenic population of hepatic macrophages, called KCs and MoMFs. Multiple studies have shown that hepatic macrophages play a pivotal role in liver homeostasis and liver diseases. Hepatic macrophages have central functions in the progression and regression of liver inflammation, ALF, liver fibrosis, NAFLD, ALD, viral hepatitis, and HCC. Different approaches have been developed to target hepatic macrophages to treat these different liver diseases. Due to the rapid advancement in nanomedicine attributable to its versatile application from drug delivery to diagnosis and imaging, few nanotechnology-enabled therapeutic modalities such as liposomes and polymeric micelles have been successfully approved for cancer treatment while others are under clinical investigation. Liposome and micelles based nanomedicines cause low toxicity and have a cost-efficient production. These are recent advantages that could help in the clinical translation of these nanomedicines. However, most of them have not been extensively tested yet in context to liver (and macrophage) targeting. Another promising nanocarrier could be solid lipid nanoparticles (SLN), which are based on solid components and are stable at room- and body temperature, resulting in a prolonged drug release. SLN consist of a lipid core that can be functionalized and stabilized with polymers to reduce non-specific cellular uptake (115).

Targeting therapies based on reducing the activation of KCs have been investigated. These therapies are mostly based on inhibiting intracellular inflammatory signaling pathways. KCs activation could also be dampened by restoring the normal gut microbiome, with probiotics, antibiotics, fecal microbiota transfer and sequestration of bile acids (12). In another study, cadherin-11 (CDH11) was increased during liver fibrosis suggesting this protein as an important regulator during liver fibrosis (117). The expression of CDH11 in injured cells, such as HSCs and macrophages, has been shown to regulate myofibroblasts activation and ECM production during the development of fibrosis. Therefore, CDH11 could be a potential therapeutic target of macrophages for the treatment of liver fibrosis. Furthermore, therapies have been focused on reducing monocyte recruitment to the liver. These therapies are mostly based on interfering with the chemokine signaling for monocytes. But as mentioned earlier, MoMFs can be categorized as Ly-6C^{high} monocytes, that cause organ impairment, and Ly-6C^{low} monocytes, which are organ restorative (39). Another potential strategy is to restore normal liver function by switching Ly6C^{high} monocytes into Ly6C^{low} monocytes. With this switch the function of the MoMFs could be changed into restorative instead of destructive.

Furthermore, therapies have been focused on reducing monocyte recruitment to the liver. These therapies are mostly based on interfering with the chemokine signaling for monocytes. But as mentioned earlier, MoMFs can be categorized as Ly-6C^{high} monocytes, that cause organ impairment, and Ly-6C^{low} monocytes, which are organ restorative (39). Another potential strategy is to restore normal liver function by switching Ly-6C^{high} monocytes into Ly-6C^{low} monocytes. With this switch the function of the MoMFs could be changed into restorative instead of destructive.

The recent studies have unraveled the large spectrum of macrophage phenotypes suggesting the heterogeneity and immunomodulatory functions of macrophages in liver diseases. Inspired by the recent developments, the questions that remain unanswered are: what is the significance and function of different macrophage phenotypes, can we reprogram the selective phenotypic macrophages for disease resolution and, finally how can we induce disease regression without affecting functions of other macrophage phenotypes and other cell types thereby reducing adverse effects? Taken together, the understanding of macrophage heterogeneity and their role in liver diseases gives the opportunity to translate this knowledge into developing targeted therapies to treat these diseases in the clinic.

AUTHOR CONTRIBUTIONS

DH and RB drafted the manuscript and designed the figures. RB and RW made the final corrections. All authors corrected and approved the manuscript.

ACKNOWLEDGMENTS

The authors are grateful to Sabine Weiskirchen (Institute of Molecular Pathobiochemistry, Experimental Gene Therapy and Clinical Chemistry, RWTH University Hospital Aachen) for preparing **Figure 2**.

REFERENCES

1. Jenne CN, Kubes P. Immune surveillance by the liver. *Nat Immunol.* (2013) 14:996–1006. doi: 10.1038/ni.2691
2. Heymann F, Tacke F. Immunology in the liver-from homeostasis to disease. *Nat Rev Gastroenterol Hepatol.* (2016) 13:88–110. doi: 10.1038/nrgastro.2015.200
3. Tacke F, Zimmermann HW. Macrophage heterogeneity in liver injury and fibrosis. *J Hepatol.* (2014) 60:1090–6. doi: 10.1016/j.jhep.2013.12.025
4. Heymann F, Peusquens J, Ludwig-Portugall I, Kohlhepp M, Ergen C, Niemietz P, et al. Liver inflammation abrogates immunological tolerance induced by Kupffer cells. *Hepatology.* (2015) 62:279–91. doi: 10.1002/hep.27793
5. Breous E, Somanathan S, Vandenberghe LH, Wilson JM. Hepatic regulatory T cells and Kupffer cells are crucial mediators of systemic T cell tolerance to antigens targeting murine liver. *Hepatology.* (2009) 50:612–21. doi: 10.1002/hep.23043

6. Geerts A. History, heterogeneity, developmental biology, and functions of quiescent hepatic stellate cells. *Semin Liver Dis.* (2001) 21:311–35. doi: 10.1055/s-2001-17550
7. Hellerbrand C. Hepatic stellate cells–the pericytes in the liver. *Pflugers Arch.* (2013) 465:775–8. doi: 10.1007/s00424-012-1209-5
8. Weiskirchen R, Weiskirchen S, Tacke F. Recent advances in understanding liver fibrosis: bridging basic science and individualized treatment concepts. *F1000Res.* (2018) 7:F1000. doi: 10.12688/f1000research.14841.1
9. Chang J, Hisamatsu T, Shimamura K, Yoneno K, Adachi M, Naruse H, et al. Activated hepatic stellate cells mediate the differentiation of macrophages. *Hepatol Res.* (2007) 43:658–69. doi: 10.1111/j.1872-034X.2012.01111.x
10. Tacke F. Targeting hepatic macrophages to treat liver diseases. *J Hepatol.* (2017) 66:1300–12. doi: 10.1016/j.jhep.2017.02.026
11. Guillot A, Tacke F. Liver macrophages: old dogmas and new insights. *Hepatol Commun.* (2019) 3:730–43. doi: 10.1002/hep4.1356
12. Ju C, Tacke F. Hepatic macrophages in homeostasis and liver diseases: from pathogenesis to novel therapeutic strategies. *Cell Mol Immunol.* (2016) 13:316–27. doi: 10.1038/cmi.2015.104
13. Wang J, Kubes P. A reservoir of mature cavity macrophages that can rapidly invade visceral organs to affect tissue repair. *Cell.* (2016) 165:668–78. doi: 10.1016/j.cell.2016.03.009
14. Sica A, Invernizzi P, Mantovani A. Macrophage plasticity and polarization in liver homeostasis and pathology. *Hepatology.* (2014) 59:2034–42. doi: 10.1002/hep.26754
15. Abdullah Z, Knolle PA. Liver macrophages in healthy and diseased liver. *Pflugers Arch.* (2017) 469:553–60. doi: 10.1007/s00424-017-1954-6
16. Palis J, Robertson S, Kennedy M, Wall C, Keller G. Development of erythroid and myeloid progenitors in the yolk sac and embryo proper of the mouse. *Development.* (1999) 126:5073–84.
17. Mass E. Delineating the origins, developmental programs and homeostatic functions of tissue-resident macrophages. *Int Immunol.* (2018) 30:493–501. doi: 10.1093/intimm/dxy044
18. Gomez Perdiguero E, Klapproth K, Schulz C, Busch K, Azzoni E, Crozet L, et al. Tissue-resident macrophages originate from yolk-sac-derived erythro-myeloid progenitors. *Nature.* (2015) 518:547–51. doi: 10.1038/nature13989
19. Mass E, Ballesteros I, Farlik M, Halbritter F, Günther P, Crozet L, et al. Specification of tissue-resident macrophages during organogenesis. *Science.* (2016) 353:eaaf4238. doi: 10.1126/science.aaf4238
20. Hoeffel G, Chen J, Lavin Y, Low D, Almeida FF, See P, et al. C-Myb(+) erythro-myeloid progenitor-derived fetal monocytes give rise to adult tissue-resident macrophages. *Immunity.* (2015) 42:665–78. doi: 10.1016/j.immuni.2015.03.011
21. Cumano A, Godin I. Ontogeny of the hematopoietic system. *Annu Rev Immunol.* (2007) 25:745–85. doi: 10.1146/annurev.immunol.25.022106.141538
22. Bertrand JY, Jalil A, Klaine M, Jung S, Cumano A, Godin I. Three pathways to mature macrophages in the early mouse yolk sac. *Blood.* (2005) 106:3004–11. doi: 10.1182/blood-2005-02-0461
23. Beattie L, Sawtell A, Mann J, Frame TCM, Teal B, de Labastida Rivera F, et al. Bone marrow-derived and resident liver macrophages display unique transcriptomic signatures but similar biological functions. *J Hepatol.* (2016) 65:758–68. doi: 10.1016/j.jhep.2016.05.037
24. Borst K, Frenz T, Spanier J, Tegtmeyer PK, Chhatbar C, Skerra J, et al. Type I interferon receptor signaling delays Kupffer cell replenishment during acute fulminant viral hepatitis. *J Hepatol.* (2018) 68:682–90. doi: 10.1016/j.jhep.2017.11.029
25. Blériot C, Dupuis T, Jouvion G, Eberl G, Disson O, Lecuit M. Liver-resident macrophage necroptosis orchestrates type 1 microbicidal inflammation and type-2-mediated tissue repair during bacterial infection. *Immunity.* (2015) 42:145–58. doi: 10.1016/j.immuni.2014.12.020
26. Lefere S, Degroote H, Van Vlierberghe H, Devisscher L. Unveiling the depletion of Kupffer cells in experimental hepatocarcinogenesis through liver macrophage subtype-specific markers. *J Hepatol.* (2019) 71:631–3. doi: 10.1016/j.jhep.2019.03.016
27. Huang W, Metlakunta A, Dedousis N, Zhang P, Sipula I, Dube JJ, et al. Depletion of liver Kupffer cells prevents the development of diet-induced hepatic steatosis and insulin resistance. *Diabetes.* (2010) 59:347–57. doi: 10.2337/db09-0016
28. Reid DT, Reyes JL, McDonald BA, Vo T, Reimer RA, Eksteen B. Kupffer cells undergo fundamental changes during the development of experimental NASH and are critical in initiating liver damage and inflammation. *PLoS ONE.* (2016) 11:e0159524. doi: 10.1371/journal.pone.0159524
29. Roberts AW, Lee BL, Deguine J, John S, Shlomchik MJ, Barton GM. Tissue-resident macrophages are locally programmed for silent clearance of apoptotic cells. *Immunity.* (2017) 47:913–927.e6. doi: 10.1016/j.immuni.2017.10.006
30. Uderhardt S, Martins AJ, Tsang JS, Lämmermann T, Germain RN. Resident macrophages cloak tissue microlesions to prevent neutrophil-driven inflammatory damage. *Cell.* (2019) 177:541–55.e17. doi: 10.1016/j.cell.2019.02.028
31. Fogg DK., Sibon C, Miled C, Jung S, Aucouturier P, Littman DR., et al. A clonogenic bone marrow progenitor specific for macrophages and dendritic cells. *Science.* (2006) 311:83–7. doi: 10.1126/science.1117729
32. Miura K, Namba N, Fujiwara M, Ohata Y, Ishida H, Kitaoka T, et al. An overgrowth disorder associated with excessive production of cGMP due to a gain-of-function mutation of the natriuretic peptide receptor 2 gene. *PLoS ONE.* (2012) 7:e42180. doi: 10.1371/journal.pone.0042180
33. Baeck C, Wehr A, Karlmark KR, Heymann F, Vucur M, Gassler N, et al. Pharmacological inhibition of the chemokine CCL2 (MCP-1) diminishes liver macrophage infiltration and steatohepatitis in chronic hepatic injury. *Gut.* (2012) 61:416–26. doi: 10.1136/gutjnl-2011-300304
34. Karlmark KR, Weiskirchen R, Zimmermann HW, Gassler N, Ginhoux F, Weber C, et al. Hepatic recruitment of the inflammatory Gr1$^+$ monocyte subset upon liver injury promotes hepatic fibrosis. *Hepatology.* (2009) 50:261–74. doi: 10.1002/hep.22950
35. Miura K, Yang L, van Rooijen N, Ohnishi H, Seki E. Hepatic recruitment of macrophages promotes non-alcoholic steatohepatitis through CCR2. *Am J Physiol Gastrointest Liver Physiol.* (2012) 302:G1310–21. doi: 10.1152/ajpgi.00365.2011
36. Galastri S, Zamara E, Milani S, Novo E, Provenzano A, Delogu W, et al. Lack of CC chemokine ligand 2 differentially affects inflammation and fibrosis according to the genetic background in a murine model of steatohepatitis. *Clin Sci.* (2012) 123:459–71. doi: 10.1042/CS20110515
37. Heymann F, Hammerich L, Storch D, Bartneck M, Huss S, Rüsseler V, et al. Hepatic macrophage migration and differentiation critical for liver fibrosis is mediated by the chemokine receptor C-C motif chemokine receptor 8 in mice. *Hepatology.* (2012) 55:898–909. doi: 10.1002/hep.24764
38. Zigmond E, Samia-Grinberg S, Pasmanik-Chor M, Brazowski E, Shibolet O, Halpern Z, et al. Infiltrating monocyte-derived macrophages and resident Kupffer cells display different ontogeny and functions in acute liver injury. *J Immunol.* (2014) 193:344–53. doi: 10.4049/jimmunol.1400574
39. Ramachandran P, Pellicoro A, Vernon MA, Boulter L, Aucott RL, Ali A, et al. Differential Ly-6C expression identifies the recruited macrophage phenotype, which orchestrates the regression of murine liver fibrosis. *Proc Natl Acad Sci USA.* (2012) 109:E3186–95. doi: 10.1073/pnas.1119964109
40. Tacke F. Functional role of intrahepatic monocyte subsets for the progression of liver inflammation and liver fibrosis *in vivo*. *Fibrogenesis Tissue Repair.* (2012) 5(Suppl. 1):S27. doi: 10.1186/1755-1536-5-S1-S27
41. Seki E, De Minicis S, Gwak GY, Kluwe J, Inokuchi S, Bursill CA, et al. CCR1 and CCR5 promote hepatic fibrosis in mice. *J Clin Invest.* (2009) 119:1858–70. doi: 10.1172/jci37444
42. Cassado Ados A, D'Império Lima MR, Bortoluci KR. Revisiting mouse peritoneal macrophages: heterogeneity, development, and function. *Front Immunol.* (2015) 6:225. doi: 10.3389/fimmu.2015.00225
43. Rehermann B Mature peritoneal macrophages take an avascular route into the injured liver and promote tissue repair. *Hepatology.* (2017) 65:376–9. doi: 10.1002/hep.28883
44. Swirski FK, Nahrendorf M, Etzrodt M, Wildgruber M, Cortez-Retamozo V, Panizzi P, et al. Identification of splenic reservoir monocytes and their deployment to inflammatory sites. *Science.* (2009) 325:612–6. doi: 10.1126/science.1175202
45. Li L, Wei W, Li Z, Chen H, Li Y, Jiang W, et al. The spleen promotes the secretion of CCL2 and supports an M1 dominant phenotype in hepatic macrophages during liver fibrosis. *Cell Physiol Biochem.* (2018) 51:557–74. doi: 10.1159/000495276

46. Aoyama T, Kuwahara-Arai K, Uchiyama A, Kon K, Okubo H, Yamashina S, et al. Spleen-derived lipocalin-2 in the portal vein regulates Kupffer cells activation and attenuates the development of liver fibrosis in mice. *Lab Invest.* (2017) 97:890–902. doi: 10.1038/labinvest.2017.44
47. Roszer T. Understanding the mysterious M2 macrophage through activation markers and effector mechanisms. *Mediators Inflamm.* (2015) 2015:816460. doi: 10.1155/2015/816460
48. Wang LX, Zhang SX, Wu HJ, Rong XL, Guo J. M2b macrophage polarization and its roles in diseases. *J Leukoc Biol.* (2019) 106:345–58. doi: 10.1002/JLB.3RU1018-378RR
49. MacParland SA, Liu JC, Ma XZ, Innes BT, Bartczak AM, Gage BK, et al. Single cell RNA sequencing of human liver reveals distinct intrahepatic macrophage populations. *Nat Commun.* (2018) 9:4383. doi: 10.1038/s41467-018-06318-7
50. Antoniades CG, Berry PA, Wendon JA, Vergani D. The importance of immune dysfunction in determining outcome in acute liver failure. *J Hepatol.* (2008) 49:845–61. doi: 10.1016/j.jhep.2008.08.009
51. Wu Z, Han M, Chen T, Yan W, Ning Q. Acute liver failure: mechanisms of immune-mediated liver injury. *Liver Int.* (2010) 30:782–94. doi: 10.1111/j.1478-3231.2010.02262.x
52. Ju C, Reilly TP, Bourdi M, Radonovich MF, Brady JN, George JW, et al. Protective role of Kupffer cells in acetaminophen-induced hepatic injury in mice. *Chem Res Toxicol.* (2002) 15:1504–13. doi: 10.1021/tx0255976
53. Pellicoro A, Ramachandran P, Iredale JP, Fallowfield JA. Liver fibrosis and repair: immune regulation of wound healing in a solid organ. *Nat Rev Immunol.* (2014) 14:181–94. doi: 10.1038/nri3623
54. Weiskirchen R, Weiskirchen S, Tacke F. Organ and tissue fibrosis: Molecular signals, cellular mechanisms and translational implications. *Mol Aspects Med.* (2019) 65:2–15. doi: 10.1016/j.mam.2018.06.003
55. Campana L, Iredale JP. Regression of Liver Fibrosis. *Semin Liver Dis.* (2017) 37:1–10. doi: 10.1055/s-0036-1597816
56. Drescher HK, Weiskirchen S, Weiskirchen R. Current status in testing for non-alcoholic fatty liver disease (NAFLD) and non-alcoholic steatohepatitis (NASH). *Cells.* (2019) 8:845. doi: 10.3390/cells8080845
57. Angulo P. Nonalcoholic fatty liver disease. *N Engl J Med.* (2002) 346:1221–31. doi: 10.1056/NEJMra011775
58. Adams LA, Anstee QM, Tilg H, Targher G. Non-alcoholic fatty liver disease and its relationship with cardiovascular disease and other extrahepatic diseases. *Gut.* (2017) 66:1138–53. doi: 10.1136/gutjnl-2017-313884
59. Boutens L, Stienstra R. Adipose tissue macrophages: going off track during obesity. *Diabetologia.* (2016) 59:879–94. doi: 10.1007/s00125-016-3904-9
60. Krenkel O, Tacke F. Macrophages in non-alcoholic fatty liver disease: a role model of pathogenic immunometabolism. *Semin Liver Dis.* (2017) 37:189–97. doi: 10.1055/s-0037-1604480
61. Kazankov K, Jørgensen SMD, Thomsen KL, Møller HJ, Vilstrup H, George J, et al. The role of macrophages in non-alcoholic fatty liver disease and non-alcoholic steatohepatitis. *Nat Rev Gastroenterol Hepatol.* (2019) 16:145–59. doi: 10.1038/s41575-018-0082-x
62. Stienstra R, Saudale F, Duval C, Keshtkar S, Groener JE, van Rooijen N, et al. Kupffer cells promote hepatic steatosis via interleukin-1β-dependent suppression of peroxisome proliferator-activated receptor α activity. *Hepatology.* (2010) 51:511–22. doi: 10.1002/hep.23337
63. Miura K, Yang L, van Rooijen N, Brenner DA, Ohnishi H, Seki E. Toll-like receptor 2 and palmitic acid cooperatively contribute to the development of non-alcoholic steatohepatitis through inflammasome activation in mice. *Hepatology.* (2013) 57:577–89. doi: 10.1002/hep.26081
64. Negrin KA, Roth Flach RJ, DiStefano MT, Matevossian A, Friedline RH, Jung D, et al. IL-1 signaling in obesity-induced hepatic lipogenesis and steatosis. *PLoS ONE.* (2014) 9:e107265. doi: 10.1371/journal.pone.0107265
65. Clément S, Juge-Aubry C, Sgroi A, Conzelmann S, Pazienza V, Pittet-Cuenod B, et al. Monocyte chemoattractant protein-1 secreted by adipose tissue induces direct lipid accumulation in hepatocytes. *Hepatology.* (2008) 48:799–807. doi: 10.1002/hep.22404
66. Garcia-Martinez I, Santoro N, Chen Y, Hoque R, Ouyang X, Caprio S, et al. Hepatocyte mitochondrial DNA drives non-alcoholic steatohepatitis by activation of TLR9. *J Clin Invest.* (2016) 126:859–64. doi: 10.1172/JCI83885
67. Miura K, Ohnishi H. Role of gut microbiota and Toll-like receptors in non-alcoholic fatty liver disease. *World J Gastroenterol.* (2014) 20:7381–91. doi: 10.3748/wjg.v20.i23.7381
68. Krenkel O, Hundertmark J, Abdallah AT, Kohlhepp M, Puengel T, Roth T, et al. Myeloid cells in liver and bone marrow acquire a functionally distinct inflammatory phenotype during obesity-related steatohepatitis. *Gut.* (2019). doi: 10.1136/gutjnl-2019-318382. [Epub ahead of print].
69. Xiong X, Kuang H, Ansari S, Liu T, Gong J, Wang S, et al. Landscape of intercellular crosstalk in healthy and NASH liver revealed by single-cell secretome gene analysis. *Mol Cell.* (2019) 75:644–60.e5. doi: 10.1016/j.molcel.2019.07.028
70. O'Shea RS, Dasarathy S, McCullough AJ, Practice Guideline Committee of the American Association for the Study of Liver Diseases, Practice Parameters Committee of the American College of Gastroenterology. Alcoholic liver disease. *Hepatology.* (2010) 51:307–28. doi: 10.1002/hep.23258
71. Ju C, Liangpunsakul S. Role of hepatic macrophages in alcoholic liver disease. *J Investig Med.* (2016) 64:1075–7. doi: 10.1136/jim-2016-000210
72. Bala S, Marcos M, Gattu A, Catalano D, Szabo G. Acute binge drinking increases serum endotoxin and bacterial DNA levels in healthy individuals. *PLoS ONE.* (2014) 9:e96864. doi: 10.1371/journal.pone.0096864
73. Chen P, Stärkel P, Turner JR, Ho SB, Schnabl B. Dysbiosis-induced intestinal inflammation activates tumor necrosis factor receptor I and mediates alcoholic liver disease in mice. *Hepatology.* (2015) 61:883–94. doi: 10.1002/hep.27489
74. Gao B, Bataller R. Alcoholic liver disease: pathogenesis and new therapeutic targets. *Gastroenterology.* (2011) 141:1572–85. doi: 10.1053/j.gastro.2011.09.002
75. Gao B, Seki E, Brenner DA, Friedman S, Cohen JI, Nagy L, et al. Innate immunity in alcoholic liver disease. *Am J Physiol Gastrointest Liver Physiol.* (2011) 300:G516–25. doi: 10.1152/ajpgi.00537.2010
76. Bukong TN, Iracheta-Vellve A, Saha B, Ambade A, Satishchandran A, Gyongyosi B, et al. Inhibition of spleen tyrosine kinase activation ameliorates inflammation, cell death, and steatosis in alcoholic liver disease. *Hepatology.* (2016) 64:1057–71. doi: 10.1002/hep.28680
77. Reiss G, Keeffe EB. Review article: hepatitis vaccination in patients with chronic liver disease. *Aliment Pharmacol Ther.* (2004) 19:715–27. doi: 10.1111/j.1365-2036.2004.01906.x
78. Boltjes A, Movita D, Boonstra A, Woltman AM. The role of Kupffer cells in hepatitis B and hepatitis C virus infections. *J Hepatol.* (2014) 61:660–71. doi: 10.1016/j.jhep.2014.04.026
79. Tu Z, Bozorgzadeh A, Pierce RH, Kurtis J, Crispe IN, Orloff MS. TLR-dependent cross talk between human Kupffer cells and NK cells. *J Exp Med.* (2008) 205:233–44. doi: 10.1084/jem.20072195
80. Boltjes A, van Montfoort N, Biesta PJ, Op den Brouw ML, Kwekkeboom J, van der Laan LJ, et al. Kupffer cells interact with hepatitis B surface antigen *in vivo* and *in vitro*, leading to proinflammatory cytokine production and natural killer cell function. *J Infect Dis.* (2015) 211:1268–78. doi: 10.1093/infdis/jiu599
81. Shrivastava S, Mukherjee A, Ray R, Ray RB. Hepatitis C virus induces interleukin-1β (IL-1β)/IL-18 in circulatory and resident liver macrophages. *J Virol.* (2013). 87:12284–90. doi: 10.1128/JVI.01962-13
82. Chang S, Dolganiuc A, Szabo G. Toll-like receptors 1 and 6 are involved in TLR2-mediated macrophage activation by hepatitis C virus core and NS3 proteins. *J Leukoc Biol.* (2007) 82:479–87. doi: 10.1189/jlb.0207128
83. Yang JD, Nakamura I, Roberts LR. The tumor microenvironment in hepatocellular carcinoma: current status and therapeutic targets. *Semin Cancer Biol.* (2011) 21:35–43. doi: 10.1016/j.semcancer.2010.10.007
84. Bruix J, Boix L, Sala M, Llovet JM. Focus on hepatocellular carcinoma. *Cancer Cell.* (2004) 5:215–9. doi: 10.1016/S1535-6108(04)00058-3
85. Berasain C, Castillo J, Perugorria MJ, Latasa MU, Prieto J, Avila MA. Inflammation and liver cancer: new molecular links. *Ann N Y Acad Sci.* (2009) 1155:206–21. doi: 10.1111/j.1749-6632.2009.03704.x
86. Capece D, Fischietti M, Verzella D, Gaggiano A, Cicciarelli G, Tessitore A, et al. The inflammatory microenvironment in hepatocellular carcinoma: a pivotal role for tumor-associated macrophages. *Biomed Res Int.* (2013) 2013:187204. doi: 10.1155/2013/187204
87. Solinas G, Germano G, Mantovani A, Allavena P. Tumor-associated macrophages (TAM) as major players of the cancer-related inflammation. *J Leukoc Biol.* (2009) 86:1065–73. doi: 10.1189/jlb.0609385

88. Porta C, Larghi P, Rimoldi M, Totaro MG, Allavena P, Mantovani A, et al. Cellular and molecular pathways linking inflammation and cancer. *Immunobiology.* (2009) 214:761–77. doi: 10.1016/j.imbio.2009.06.014
89. Qian BZ, Pollard J W. Macrophage diversity enhances tumor progression and metastasis. *Cell.* (2010) 141:39–51. doi: 10.1016/j.cell.2010.03.014
90. Triantafyllou E, Woollard KJ, McPhail MJW, Antoniades CG, Possamai LA. The role of monocytes and macrophages in acute and acute-on-chronic liver failure. *Front Immunol.* (2018) 9:2948. doi: 10.3389/fimmu.2018.02948
91. LiverTox: *Clinical and Research Information on Drug-Induced Liver Injury.* Bethesda, MD: National Institute of Diabetes and Digestive and Kidney Diseases (2012). Available online at: http://www.ncbi.nlm.nih.gov/books/NBK548400/
92. Stutchfield BM, Antoine DJ, Mackinnon AC, Gow DJ, Bain CC, Hawley CA, et al. CSF1 restores innate immunity after liver injury in mice and serum levels indicate outcomes of patients with acute liver failure. *Gastroenterology.* (2015) 149:1896–909.e14. doi: 10.1053/j.gastro.2015.08.053
93. Antoniades CG, Khamri W, Abeles RD, Taams LS, Triantafyllou E, Possamai LA, et al. Secretory leukocyte protease inhibitor: a pivotal mediator of anti-inflammatory responses in acetaminophen-induced acute liver failure. *Hepatology.* (2014) 59:1564–76. doi: 10.1002/hep.26933
94. He C, Yin L, Tang C, Yin C. Multifunctional polymeric nanoparticles for oral delivery of TNF-α siRNA to macrophages. *Biomaterials.* (2013) 34:2843–54. doi: 10.1016/j.biomaterials.2013.01.033
95. Bartneck M, Scheyda KM, Warzecha KT, Rizzo LY, Hittatiya K, Luedde T, et al. Fluorescent cell-traceable dexamethasone-loaded liposomes for the treatment of inflammatory liver diseases. *Biomaterials.* (2015) 37:367–82. doi: 10.1016/j.biomaterials.2014.10.030
96. Freund B, Heeren J, Nielsen P, Carambia A, Herkel J, Bruns O, et al. *Nanoparticle Compositions for Generation of Regulatory T Cells and Treatment of Autoimmune Diseases and Other Chronic Inflammatory Conditions. United States Patent Application 20180325821.* Available online at: http://www.freepatentsonline.com/y2018/0325821.html (accessed August 22, 2019). (2018).
97. Traber PG, Zomer E. Therapy of experimental NASH and fibrosis with galectin inhibitors. *PLoS ONE.* (2013) 8:e83481. doi: 10.1371/journal.pone.0083481
98. Kurniawan DW, Jajoriya AK, Dhawan G, Mishra D, Argemi J, Bataller R, et al. Therapeutic inhibition of spleen tyrosine kinase in inflammatory macrophages using PLGA nanoparticles for the treatment of non-alcoholic steatohepatitis. *J Control Release.* (2018) 288:227–38. doi: 10.1016/j.jconrel.2018.09.004
99. Loomba R, Lawitz E, Mantry PS, Jayakumar S, Caldwell SH, Arnold H, et al. The ASK1 inhibitor selonsertib in patients with non-alcoholic steatohepatitis: a randomized, phase 2 trial. *Hepatology.* (2018) 67:549–59. doi: 10.1002/hep.29514
100. Liu Y, Yan W, Tohme S, Chen M, Fu Y, Tian D, et al. Hypoxia induced HMGB1 and mitochondrial DNA interactions mediate tumor growth in hepatocellular carcinoma through Toll-like receptor 9. *J Hepatol.* (2015) 63:1114–21. doi: 10.1016/j.jhep.2015.02.009
101. Brenner C, Galluzzi L, Kepp O, Kroemer G. Decoding cell death signals in liver inflammation. *J Hepatol.* (2013) 59:583–94. doi: 10.1016/j.jhep.2013.03.033
102. Maradana MR, Yekollu SK, Zeng B, Ellis J, Clouston A, Miller G, et al. Immunomodulatory liposomes targeting liver macrophages arrest progression of non-alcoholic steatohepatitis. *Metab Clin Exp.* (2018) 78:80–94. doi: 10.1016/j.metabol.2017.09.002
103. Lefebvre E, Moyle G, Reshef R, Richman LP, Thompson M, Hong F, et al. Antifibrotic effects of the dual CCR2/CCR5 antagonist cenicriviroc in animal models of liver and kidney fibrosis. *PLoS ONE.* (2016) 11:e0158156. doi: 10.1371/journal.pone.0158156
104. Krenkel O, Puengel T, Govaere O, Abdallah AT, Mossanen JC, Kohlhepp M, et al. Therapeutic inhibition of inflammatory monocyte recruitment reduces steatohepatitis and liver fibrosis. *Hepatology.* (2018) 67:1270–83. doi: 10.1002/hep.29544
105. Friedman SL, Ratziu V, Harrison SA, Abdelmalek MF, Aithal GP, Caballeria J, et al. A randomized, placebo-controlled trial of cenicriviroc for treatment of non-alcoholic steatohepatitis with fibrosis. *Hepatology.* (2018) 67:1754–67. doi: 10.1002/hep.29477
106. Mulder P, van den Hoek AM, Kleemann R. The CCR2 inhibitor propagermanium attenuates diet-induced insulin resistance, adipose tissue inflammation and non-alcoholic steatohepatitis. *PLoS ONE.* (2017) 12:e0169740. doi: 10.1371/journal.pone.0169740
107. Baeck C, Wie X, Bartneck M, Fech V, Heymann F, Gassler N, et al. Pharmacological inhibition of the chemokine C-C motif chemokine ligand 2 (monocyte chemoattractant protein 1) accelerates liver fibrosis regression by suppressing Ly-6C$^+$ macrophage infiltration in mice. *Hepatology.* (2014) 59:1060–72. doi: 10.1002/hep.26783
108. Pérez-Martínez L, Pérez-Matute P, Aguilera-Lizarraga J, Rubio-Mediavilla S, Narro J, Recio E, et al. Maraviroc, a CCR5 antagonist, ameliorates the development of hepatic steatosis in a mouse model of non-alcoholic fatty liver disease (NAFLD). *J Antimicrob Chemother.* (2014) 69:1903–10. doi: 10.1093/jac/dku071
109. Ferrari M. Cancer nanotechnology: opportunities and challenges. *Nat Rev Cancer.* (2005) 5:161–71. doi: 10.1038/nrc1566
110. Ranghar S, Sirohi P, Verma P, Agarwal V. Nanoparticle-based drug delivery systems: promising approaches against infections. *Brazilian Arch Biol Technol.* (2013) 57:209–22. doi: 10.1590/S1516-89132013005000011
111. Dreaden EC, Austin LA, Mackey MA, El-Sayed MA. Size matters: gold nanoparticles in targeted cancer drug delivery. *Ther Deliv.* (2012) 3:457–78. doi: 10.4155/tde.12.21
112. Polizzi MA, Stasko NA, Schoenfisch MH. Water-soluble nitric oxide-releasing gold nanoparticles. *Langmuir.* (2007) 23:4938–43. doi: 10.1021/la0633841
113. Han G, You CC, Kim BJ, Turingan RS, Forbes NS, Martin CT, et al. Light-regulated release of DNA and its delivery to nuclei by means of photolabile gold nanoparticles. *Angew Chem Int Ed Engl.* (2006) 45:3165–9. doi: 10.1002/anie.200600214
114. Maeda H. Tumor-selective delivery of macromolecular drugs via the EPR effect: background and future prospects. *Bioconjug Chem.* (2010) 21:797–802. doi: 10.1021/bc100070g
115. Bartneck M, Warzecha KT, Tacke F. Therapeutic targeting of liver inflammation and fibrosis by nanomedicine. *Hepatobiliary Surg Nutr.* (2014) 3:364–76. doi: 10.3978/j.issn.2304-3881.2014.11.02
116. Weiskirchen R, Tacke F. Liver fibrosis: from pathogenesis to novel therapies. *Dig Dis.* (2016) 34:410–22. doi: 10.1159/000444556
117. Pedroza M, To S, Smith J, Agarwal SK. Cadherin-11 contributes to liver fibrosis induced by carbon tetrachloride. *PLoS ONE.* (2019) 14:e0218971. doi: 10.1371/journal.pone.0218971

8

The Role of Myeloid-Derived Cells in the Progression of Liver Disease

Chris John Weston [1,2*†], *Henning Wolfgang Zimmermann* [3†] *and David H. Adams* [1,2]

[1] *Centre for Liver and Gastrointestinal Research, Institute of Immunology and Immunotherapy, Medical School, University of Birmingham, Birmingham, United Kingdom,* [2] *NIHR Birmingham Biomedical Research Centre, University Hospitals Birmingham NHS Foundation Trust and University of Birmingham, Birmingham, United Kingdom,* [3] *Medical Department III, University Hospital of Aachen, Aachen, Germany*

***Correspondence:**
Chris John Weston
c.j.weston@bham.ac.uk

† *These authors have contributed equally to this work*

Control of homeostasis and rapid response to tissue damage in the liver is orchestrated by crosstalk between resident and infiltrating inflammatory cells. A crucial role for myeloid cells during hepatic injury and repair has emerged where resident Kupffer cells, circulating monocytes, macrophages, dendritic cells and neutrophils control local tissue inflammation and regenerative function to maintain tissue architecture. Studies in humans and rodents have revealed a heterogeneous population of myeloid cells that respond to the local environment by either promoting regeneration or driving the inflammatory processes that can lead to hepatitis, fibrogenesis, and the development of cirrhosis and malignancy. Such plasticity of myeloid cell responses presents unique challenges for therapeutic intervention strategies and a greater understanding of the underlying mechanisms is needed. Here we review the role of myeloid cells in the establishment and progression of liver disease and highlight key pathways that have become the focus for current and future therapeutic strategies.

Keywords: hepatitis (general), hepatocellular carcinoma, cirrhosis, fibrosis, myeloid derived suppressor cell (MDSC), neutrophil (PMN), macrophage, circulating monocytes

INTRODUCTION

Myeloid cells arise from the common myeloid precursor and give rise to monocytes, dendritic cells and macrophages, and granulocytes. Myeloid cell functions include the recognition, ingestion and degradation of cellular debris, foreign material or pathogens, subsequent control of inflammatory responses, and maintenance of tissue architecture. There is increasing evidence implicating granulocytes in liver homeostasis and disease but this review will focus mainly on monocytes and macrophages. Macrophages are a diverse, heterogeneous population derived from short-lived, but plastic, precursor monocyte populations. Monocytes are rapidly recruited to sites of injury and their functions are imprinted in the bone marrow, whereas macrophages tend to be long-lived and tissue-resident, where their functions are dictated by environmental cues (1). A highly coordinated pathway of monocyte recruitment and subsequent imprinting of macrophage "identities," the mechanisms of which are only now beginning to be understood, controls local tissue inflammatory and regenerative functions and is critical in maintaining tissue architecture (2–4). Extensive rodent and human studies have demonstrated key roles for monocytes and macrophages in the establishment, progression and regression of liver disease including a critical role in directing tissue regeneration (5–7). This fine balance of pro- and anti-inflammatory mediators is crucial to determining the path of disease progression, and understanding how myeloid cells contribute to injury and repair will enable the rational design of novel therapies. In this review we summarize the identities and roles of myeloid cell populations in the liver, and describe approaches that are being developed to reduce inflammation through targeting this innate immune cell population.

HEPATIC MONOCYTE AND MACROPHAGE POPULATIONS

Kupffer Cells

The liver contains a population of self-renewing resident macrophages, termed Kupffer cells (KC), derived from yolk sac-derived progenitor cells (8, 9) or hematopoietic stem cells (10). In mice KC phenotype is thought to be controlled by a specific set of transcription factors including ID3 and ZEB2 through progenitor cell development and maintenance of the expression of LXRα permitting replenishment of the KC niche by progenitors from the circulation (2, 11–13) (**Figure 1**, **Table 1**). They are non-migratory, being retained in the sinusoids where they maintain a tolerogenic environment despite the presence of low levels of food particles and bacterial antigens delivered from the gut via the portal vein (4, 14, 15). This is achieved through highly effective phagocytic and scavenging mechanisms triggered by toll-like receptor (TLR) signaling and scavenger receptors such as CD36, scavenger receptor-A and galectin-3 (16, 17). Their expression of high levels of pattern recognition receptors (PRRs) allows macrophages to respond to a wide range of danger-associated molecular patterns (DAMPs) released during tissue injury, such as high mobility group protein B1 (HMGB1), ATP, uric acid, DNA fragments and cholesterol crystals (5) and pathogen-associated molecular patterns (PAMPs, such as lipopolysaccharide and flagellin) released from microbes. Activation of PRRs leads to the formation of the inflammasome (18) via multi-protein complexes including the NOD-, LRR- and pyrin domain-containing 3 (NLRP3) (19). Formation of the inflammasome promotes the release of potent signaling molecules including IL-1β, PGE_2, HMGB1, TNF-α, and IL-17, driving inflammation and fibrosis (20–24). KC from both mouse and human liver also secrete the anti-inflammatory cytokine IL-10 (25–27), express low levels of MHC class II and co-stimulatory molecules combined with high levels of the T-cell inhibitory molecule PDL-1 (27). This makes them unable to fully activate T cell effector function but rather to promote the development of regulatory T-cells (Treg). This is further enhanced through their secretion of PGE_2 (28) and upregulation of the indolamine 2,3-dioxygenase pathway which promotes immune cell tolerance (29).

Murine KC have been well characterized under homeostatic conditions and in experimental models of hepatic injury, where they express $CD11b^+F4/80^{++}CD68^+CD11c^{+/-}CLEC4F^+TIM4^+$ in addition to TLR4, TLR9, and CRIg, but are negative for the chemokine receptor CX_3CR1. Recent advances in proteomic analysis has revealed circadian regulation of not only KC numbers in uninjured mouse liver, but also components of the immune response pathway which peak during the daytime, including Tlr4, Myd88, Irak4, and Takl (30). Human KC are less well described but can be identified through expression of $CD68^+CD14^+TLR4^+$ and lack of CX_3CR1.

Infiltrating Monocytes

Circulating monocytes are actively recruited to the liver, guided by adhesion molecules and chemokine gradients generated at the sinusoidal endothelial interface (see below). In mice bone marrow derived myeloid cells expressing high levels of Ly6C and CCR2 rapidly infiltrate tissue and are associated with the expression of pattern recognition receptors (PRR) and inflammatory cytokines ($CD11b^+CCR2^+CX_3CR1^+CD43^-$). In contrast $Ly6C^{low}$ monocytes from the spleen express a broad range of scavenger receptors and exhibit a patrolling behavior that may enable the engulfment of apoptotic cells ($CD11b^+CCR2^-CX_3CR1^{++}CD43^+$) (27, 31–36). In humans there is no discriminatory expression of Ly6C and monocytes are classified according to the expression of CD14 and CD16 giving rise to classical ($CD14^{++}CD16^-$), intermediate ($CD14^+CD16^+$), and non-classical ($CD14^-CD16^+$) populations. Gene expression profiling of these subsets has determined that $CD14^{++}CD16^-$ monocytes resemble murine $Ly6C^{high}$ infiltrative cells and $CD14^-CD16^+$ monocytes more closely align with the patrolling $Ly6C^{low}$ population (31). Potent immunomodulatory myeloid derived suppressor cells (MDSC) are also present in both murine and human liver tissue. MDSCs are a heterogeneous population of cells which express markers shared with other immune cell populations ($CD11b^+Ly6C^+$ in mice, $CD14^+HLA\text{-}DR^{+/-}CD33^+$ in humans), therefore identification is usually confirmed by means of a T-cell suppression assay (37). MDSC suppress immune responses through production of arginase 1 (Arg1), inducible nitric oxide synthase (iNOS) and generation of reactive oxygen species (ROS), or secretion of IL-10 (38).

RECRUITMENT FROM THE CIRCULATION AND DIFFERENTIATION IN TISSUE

Damage to tissue results in an upregulation of adhesion molecules on liver sinusoidal endothelium (LSEC) and the secretion of chemokines, cytokines and other bioactive molecules that promote immune cell recruitment [reviewed in (39)]. Circulating $CCR2^+$ monocytes are recruited in response to local CCL2, released primarily by hepatic stellate cells (HSC) (40, 41), or through the CCR8/CCL1 and CXCR3/CXCL10 axes (42–44). In humans the migration of $CD14^-CD16^+$ monocytes is promoted through activation of CX_3CR1 by endothelial CX_3CL1, a transmembrane chemokine that is expressed at high levels during inflammation (45). Intermediate $CD14^+CD16^+$ monocyte populations are enriched in the diseased liver (46), partly due to their increased propensity when compared with other monocytes to migrate across LSEC. These cells exhibit high phagocytic activity and secrete pro-inflammatory and fibrogenic mediators (47). Bidirectional migration of monocytes affects the local balance of inflammatory and anti-inflammatory cells. Pro-inflammatory $CD14^-CD16^+$ subsets undergo reverse migration from tissue back into the circulation via across LSEC from

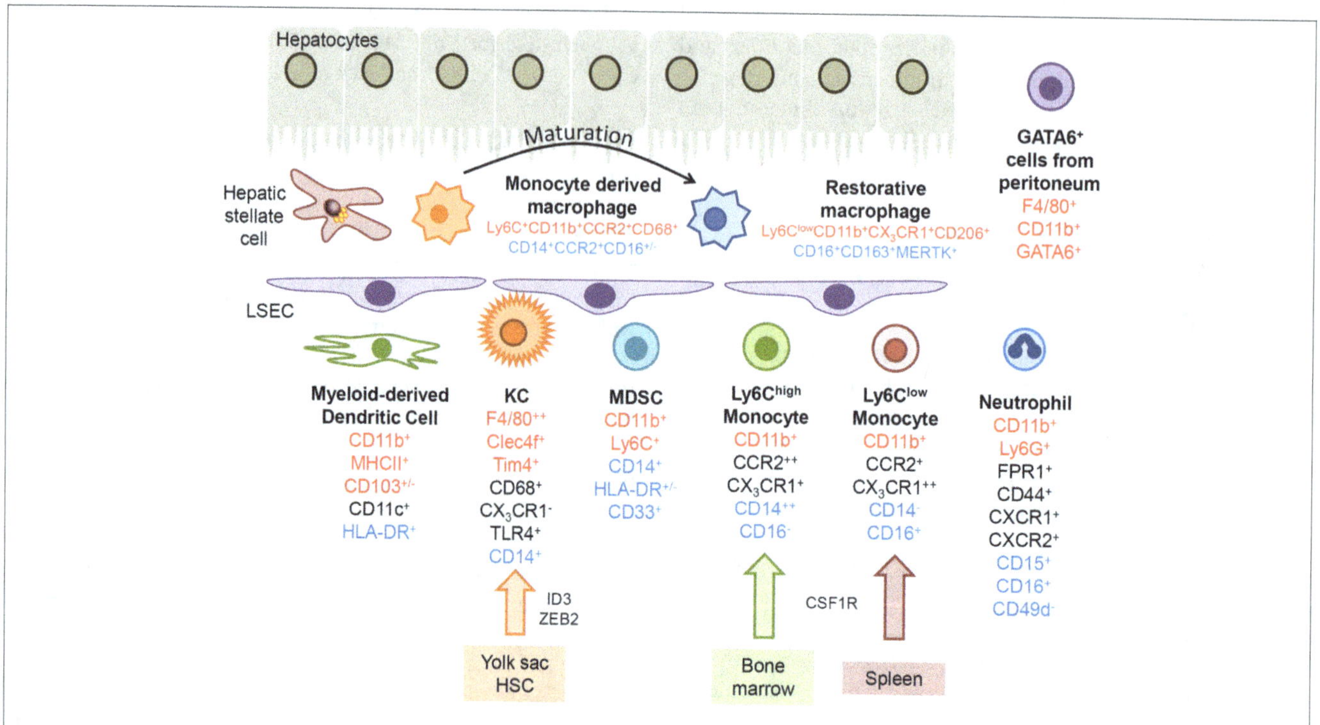

FIGURE 1 | Myeloid populations present within the liver. Kupffer cells are derived from the yolk sac or hematopoietic stem cells, under the control of transcription factors such as ID3 and ZEB2. Infiltrating monocytes originating in the bone marrow or spleen express the chemokine receptors CCR2 and CX_3CR1, and can differentiate into monocyte-derived dendritic cells. Following injury monocytes undergo transendothelial migration across LSEC and differentiate into monocyte derived macrophages, which can mature into a more restorative phenotype or replenish the KC pool. A $GATA6^+$ macrophage population that migrates from the peritoneum during hepatic injury has been identified in mice. Markers that identify hepatic macrophages in mice, humans or are common to both are highlighted in red, blue and black text, respectively.

where they may contribute to systemic inflammatory responses, whereas anti-inflammatory cells remain in the tissue where they suppress T-cells and promote endotoxin tolerance (48). A phenotypic switch in macrophage phenotype is observed during acute liver injury in humans where MAC387 (S100A9) can be used to identify circulation-derived macrophages in contrast to $CD68^+$ resident populations (49). Infiltrating monocytes also undergo local intrahepatic differentiation into anti-inflammatory MDSC following injury via contact-dependent mechanisms such as communication with hepatic stellate cells (HSC), or interaction with soluble mediators such as catalase (50, 51).

In mouse models of sterile injury $CCR2^+Ly6C^{high}$ monocytes form rings to demarcate the extent of injury (14), and subsequently mature into $Ly6C^{low}$ monocytes that promote the resolution of injury and fibrosis (52). These "pro-restorative" macrophages exhibited a phenotype distinct from the classical M1 (pro-inflammatory) or M2 (pro-resolution) dichotomy with increased expression of genes that promote tissue restoration including matrix metalloproteinases (MMPs), growth factors, and phagocytosis-related genes. Murine monocytes can also take unconventional routes into liver tissue. In a model of sterile liver injury GATA6-positive macrophages ($CD11b^+F4/80^+Gata6^+$) originating in the peritoneal compartment were observed within the hepatic compartment at a very early stage of tissue damage (53). These cells migrate directly across the mesothelium, dependent on adenosine triphosphate and the adhesion molecule CD44. The contribution of these cells to disease pathogenesis is currently unknown.

Thus, local polarization of myeloid cell populations, and recruitment of macrophages from other sites, has important implications in disease pathogenesis where the balance of pro-/anti- inflammatory mediators and fibrogenic responses dictates the course of the disease.

RESPONSE TO ACUTE AND CHRONIC LIVER DISEASE

Acute Liver Disease (Such as Acetaminophen Overdose, Acute Viral, or Alcoholic Hepatitis)

Acute liver failure (ALF) is associated with high mortality and toxic liver injury in response to overdose of drugs such as acetaminophen is a more common cause of ALF than immune-mediated injury arising from acute viral hepatitis (54, 55). Much of what we know of macrophage function during early disease is derived from experimental models of acute liver injury in rodents such as carbon tetrachloride toxicity (hepatocyte necrosis) (56), bacterial infection (57),

TABLE 1 | Myeloid cell populations in humans and mice.

Myeloid population	Murine markers	Human markers	Role
Myeloid-derived dendritic cell	$CD11b^+$ $MHCII^+$ $CD11c^+$ $CD103^{+/-}$	$CD11c^+$ $HLA\text{-}DR^+$	Tolerogenic in nature; Upon injury may adopt an inflammatory phenotype; Functional role in liver disease ill-defined
Kupffer cells	$CD11b^+$ $CD68^+$ $F4/80^{++}$ $CLEC4f^+$ $TIM4^+$ CX_3CR1^- $TLR4^+$ $TLR9^+$ $CRIg^+$	$CD68^+$ $CD14^+$ $TLR4^+$ CX_3CR1^-	Promote tolerance under steady-state conditions to restrict immune response against food-borne antigens; Activated during tissue damage; main source of cytokines / chemokines governing local inflammation
Myeloid derived suppressor cells	$CD11b^+$ $Ly6C^+$	$CD14^+$ $HLA\text{-}DR^{+/-}$ $CD33^+$	Immunosuppressive; Facilitate HCC growth by dampening T-cell activity
Monocyte derived macrophage	$CD11b^+$ $Ly6C^{+/-}$ $F4/80^{+/-}$ $CCR2^+$ CX_3CR1^+ $CD64^+$	$CD14^+$ $CCR2^+$ $CD16^{+/-}$	*See subsets below*
Inflammatory macrophage	$Ly6C^{high}$ $CD11b^+$ $CCR2^{++}$ CX_3CR1^+ $iNOS^+$ TNF^+	$CD14^{++}$ $CD16^-$ $CLEC5A^+$ $S100A9^+$	Pro-inflammatory, massively recruited during liver injury; elicits tissue damage; drive fibrogenesis by maintaining inflammation and activating fibrosis effector cells; can undergo phenotypic switch to restorative macrophages
Pro-resolution macrophage	$Ly6C^{low}$ $CD11b^+$ $CCR2^+$ CX_3CR1^{++} $CD206^+$ $MMP9^+$ $MMP12^+$	$CD14^-$ $CD16^+$ $CD163^+$ $CCR2^+$ CX_3CR1^{++} $Stabilin\text{-}1^+$ $(MERTK^+)$	Anti-inflammatory; restorative function in liver fibrosis; promote tissue repair after acute damage; in humans $CD16^+$ rather linked to fibrosis progression
Neutrophils	CD11b+ Ly6G+ Fpr1+ $CD44^+$ $CXCR1^+$ $CXCR2^+$	$CD15^+$ $CD16^+$ $CD49d^-$ $FPR1^+$ $CD44^+$ $CXCR1^+$ $CXCR2^+$	Ambiguous role in liver injury; functional role likely context-dependent; putatively profibrogenic in steatohepatitis
Peritoneal infiltrating cells	$CD11b^+$ $F4/80^+$ $GATA6^+$	Unknown	Currently not known

concanavalin A (T cell mediated hepatocyte destruction) (58), ischemia-reperfusion (I-R) injury (59), sterile injury (14), and viral infection (60). These models show that extensive hepatocyte damage mediated by heat/toxin/immune-mediated killing releases DAMPs such as HMGB1 and nuclear DNA which are sensed by KC leading to the release of cytokines and chemokines, creating an environment that drives the recruitment of inflammatory macrophage subsets (5). In the absence of persistent injury, tissue repair is initiated by the maturation of pro-inflammatory populations to a more restorative phenotype, associated with anti-inflammatory and pro-angiogenic responses (52) (**Figure 2**).

In acetaminophen (APAP) induced liver injury, perhaps the best described rodent model of ALF, KC respond to tissue damage through the rapid release of cytokines and chemokines including IL-1β, TNF-α, CCL2, and CCL5 (61). Initially the numbers of KC are reduced (<24 h) and early injury is associated with high numbers of infiltrating $Ly6C^{high}$ monocytes which produce proinflammatory cytokines such as TNF-α and IL-1β and chemokines such as CCL2 and CCL5 (62–65). Evidence that these early entrants drive tissue injury comes from data showing that (i) infiltration of these cells during acetaminophen-induced injury can be reduced through blockade of CCR2-mediated recruitment (mNOX-E36, a CCL2 inhibitor, or cenicriviroc, a CCR2/CCR5 dual inhibitor) and (ii) that adoptive transfer of bone marrow monocytes exacerbated tissue damage (66). Initiation of repair and control of inflammation is mediated following a phenotypic switch in hepatic macrophages toward a pro-resolution, hepatoprotective subset expressing IL-10, IL-4 and IL-13 (67–69). This maturation event is dependent on colony stimulating factor 1 (CSF1) and secretory leukocyte protease inhibitor (SLPI) in areas of hepatic necrosis (70–72). The emergence of $CCR2^{low}CX_3CR1^{high}$ cells is also associated with the expression of vascular endothelial growth factor A (VEGF-A) which promotes repair of the vascular architecture, and increased phagocytic capacity to remove dead and dying cells (72–74). In murine models this reparative pathway can be disrupted via modulation of CCR2 signaling or depletion of macrophages through treatment with liposomal clodronate, indicating that both tissue resident and infiltrating myeloid cell populations orchestrate repair (62, 63, 75).

Similar findings have been described in patients with ALF. Clusters of $CCR2^+$ macrophages are seen in patients with APAP-induced liver failure (66) and increased serum CCL2 levels are associated with an unfavorable prognosis (49). A pro-resolution population of $MerTK^+HLA\text{-}DR^{high}$ cells has been identified in circulatory and tissue compartments of patients with ALF (72, 76). Analysis of these macrophages determined that they secreted anti-inflammatory mediators and exhibited reduced responses to bacterial challenge, consistent with an anti-inflammatory immune tolerant function. This is supported by the fact that APAP-treated *Mer* knockout animals exhibited persistent liver injury and inflammation associated with a defect in efferocytosis (72).

The pathways involved in other acute injury settings also result in activation of KC following hepatocyte damage mediated by T-cells (concanavalin A), oxidative stress (I-R), heat (sterile injury), or virus induced apoptosis (hepatitis viruses). During viral infection of humans KC increase in number and drive the infiltration of other immune cell populations through the production of inflammatory cytokines such as IL-1β, IL-18, and TNF-α (77–80). KC expression of IL-6, IFN-γ, reactive oxygen species, FAS ligand, granzyme B and TRAIL has been shown to inhibit hepatitis C (HCV) replication, and induces apoptosis of infected hepatocytes (81, 82). Triggering of KC responses arises as a result of engulfment of hepatitis B viral particles (leading to production of IL-18 and NK cell stimulation) (83)

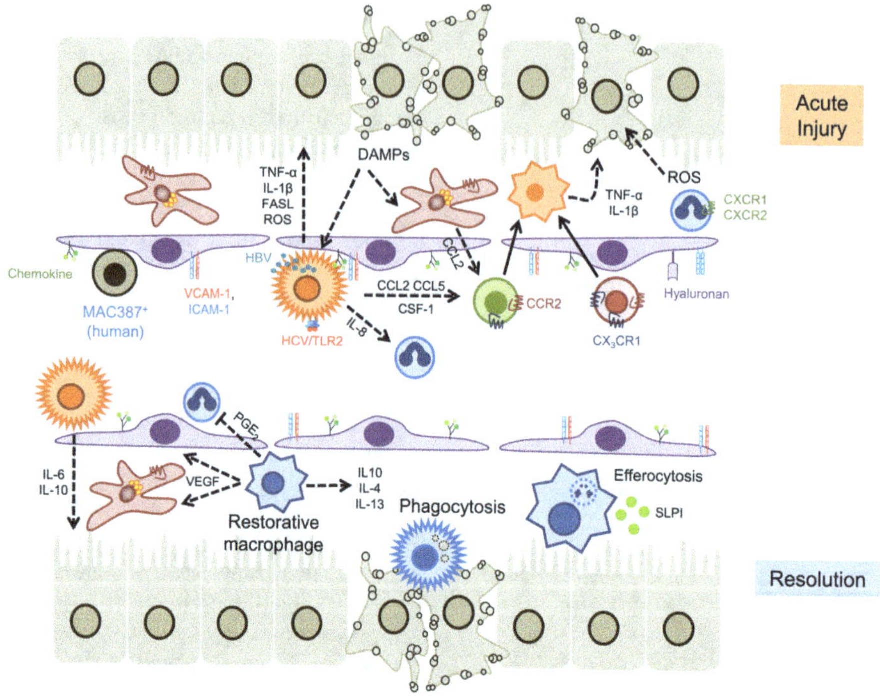

FIGURE 2 | The role of myeloid cells in acute liver injury. Hepatocyte cell death releases DAMPs that activate KC and hepatic stellate cells, leading to the release of chemokines such as CCL2 and IL-8 (CXCL8) that drives the recruitment of myeloid cells into local areas of inflammation (top). Neutrophils are recruited via CD44 and hyaluronan and generate ROS that promotes hepatocyte death, whereas infiltrating monocytes (and KCs) secrete proinflammatory cytokines such as TNFα and IL-1β. Hepatic viruses can also stimulate KC through internalization (HBV) or binding to TLR2 (HCV). Homeostasis is restored through the action of restorative macrophages (matured by phagocytosis) that secrete anti-inflammatory cytokines and promote angiogenesis, and secretion of IL-6 and IL-10 by KC (lower panel). Infiltrating neutrophils are removed through efferocytosis mediated by $MERTK^+$ macrophages and SLPI. Solid lines indicate cell migration, dashed lines represent the secretion of soluble mediators.

or via TLR2 signaling and formation of the inflammasome, with concomitant secretion of IL-18 and IL-1β, in the case of HCV (84, 85). Conversely in the setting of chronic hepatitis B viral infection the immune response is impaired through release of IL-10 (86), reduced IL-12 expression (87) or T-cell exhaustion (88) mediated by TLR2 signaling on KCs, via upregulation of galectin-9 expression driving further immune cell exhaustion following engagement with Tim-3 (89), or through increased expression of the inhibitory ligand PDL1 (90). An excess of hepatitis B virus antigen can also dampen TLR responses which contribute to viral evasion of innate and adaptive immune responses (91). This is thought to occur through suppression of proinflammatory cytokines and expression of tolerogenic mediators (IL-10 in particular) reminiscent of the tolerogenic effects of LPS, although the signaling pathways mediating this effect may be distinct.

Chronic Liver Disease and Contribution to Fibrosis

A prolonged cycle of iterative bursts of tissue damage and inflammation underlies chronic liver disease leading to fibrogenesis and ultimately in some cases cirrhosis. A proportion of patients will develop hepatocellular carcinoma on the background of continuing inflammation and fibrogenesis (92). The incidence of non-alcoholic fatty liver disease (NAFLD) and alcohol related liver disease (ARLD) has increased rapidly in recent years and following advances in the treatment of chronic viral hepatitis, attention is now switching to treating these increasingly common chronic conditions (93) (**Figure 3**).

NAFLD is a spectrum of disease ranging from simple steatosis (fatty liver) to non-alcoholic steatohepatitis (NASH), fibrosis and cirrhosis (with or without malignancy). The underlying pathology is driven by dysregulation of lipid metabolism and accumulation of lipid in hepatocytes. It is a systemic disease where dysregulated inflammation in adipose, and liver tissue and changes in the gut microbiome all drive the production of inflammatory mediators such as cytokines and chemokines (94). In patients with NAFLD enlarged and aggregated KC populations are seen in the liver and their presence correlates with the severity of the disease (95).

This is consistent with observations in diet-induced murine models of NAFLD where KC activation leads to triglyceride accumulation and production of proinflammatory cytokines such as TNF-α (96, 97). Murine hepatic macrophages can also receive activation signals from lipid-stimulated hepatocyte-derived extracellular vesicles via tumor necrosis factor-related apoptosis-inducing ligand receptor 2 (TRAIL-R2, also known as DR5) and receptor-interacting protein kinase 1 (98), and

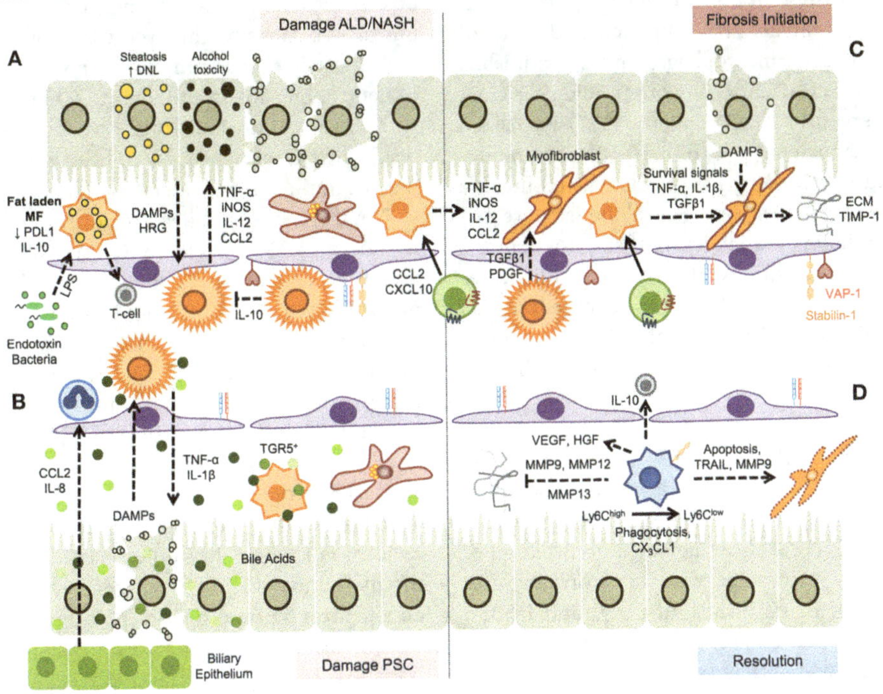

FIGURE 3 | A dual role for myeloid cells in the establishment and resolution of chronic liver disease. **(A)** Hepatocyte damage driven by steatosis or alcohol toxicity activates KC which secrete proinflammatory cytokines that drive disease progression and promotes infiltration of myeloid cells. In steatotic livers fat laden macrophages exhibit impaired endotoxin responses but may prime T-cell mediated immunity. **(B)** Cholangiocyte-derived chemokines promote recruitment of hepatic neutrophils and subsequent damage to hepatocytes promotes further inflammation. Bile acids promote KC inflammasome formation; however this can be suppressed through binding of bile salts to TGR5 expressed by monocyte-derived macrophages. **(C)** Secretion of soluble factors by KC and monocyte-derived macrophages promotes fibrosis through the activation and differentiation of hepatic stellate cells, promoting survival of myofibroblasts and the generation of extracellular matrix proteins. **(D)** Resolution of fibrosis is mediated by Ly6C^{low} macrophages, generated from Ly6C^{high} precursors, by degradation of ECM by matrix metalloproteinases, induced apoptosis of hepatic stellate cells and myofibroblasts, and secretion of anti-inflammatory cytokines.

obese mice also show reduced expression of the glucocorticoid-induced leucine zipper (GILZ) in macrophages associated with a proinflammatory phenotype (99). In this context the development of steatohepatitis arises from chronic inflammation associated with an influx of Ly6C$^+$ monocytes that enhances the proinflammatory environment through activation of liver resident cell populations (100, 101). These infiltrating monocyte subsets are recruited via chemokine receptor pairs such as CCR2-CCL2 (40, 102) and CXCR3-CXCL10 (44), or atypical adhesion molecules including vascular adhesion protein-1 and scavenger receptors (103).

Intestinal dysbiosis and hepatocyte apoptosis contribute to the inflammatory response via DAMP- and PAMP-mediated pathways respectively (104, 105) associated with increased expression and activation of receptors such as *TLR4* and *TLR9* in both humans and murine models of NASH (106). Changes in the microbiome can have complex effects on the liver altering metabolic response through the production of metabolites that enter the liver via the portal vein as well as through bacterial products such as LPS, and in the presence of a leaky gut intact bacteria are taken up by KC (107). KC also regulate anti-inflammatory responses through secretion of IL-10. In addition to its more general anti-inflammatory properties KC derived IL-10 also induces the apoptosis of proinflammatory KC allowing KC to self-regulate toward a more tolerogenic environment (108). The induction of a pro-resolution M2 KC phenotype is dependent on activation of RORα and KLF4, and provision of an activator of RORα (JC1-40) improved the symptoms of NASH in a high fat diet murine model suggesting that KC polarization is a viable therapeutic strategy (109). Immune checkpoint proteins such as Tim-3 have been detected on a range of macrophage subsets in murine models of NASH. The presence of TIM-3 limits steatohepatitis by controlling ROS induced activation of NOX2 and the NLRP3 inflammasome and secretion of IL-1β and IL-18 (110). Thus, therapeutic strategies could look at promoting the recruitment or differentiation of TIM-3 macrophages to shift the local environment toward resolution and suppression of inflammation.

Similar mechanisms of disease progression have been described for ARLD, where metabolism of alcohol in the liver drives hepatocyte cell death. In rodent models of ARLD such as the Lieber-DeCarli diet hepatic macrophages become activated to produce TNF-α, IL-6, CCL2 and ROS (111, 112) and depletion of macrophage populations with either $GdCl_3$ or liposomal clodronate attenuated alcohol-induced liver inflammation (111, 113). Expression of myeloid NADPH oxidase, specifically the catalytic subunit gp91^{phox}, contributes to the pathogenesis of murine ARLD by driving a switch between pro-inflammatory and pro-resolution macrophage populations. Thus, gp91^{phox}-deficient animals show an increased ratio of Ly6C^{high}/Ly6C^{low} intrahepatic macrophages and a diminished capacity for efferocytosis (114). Clustering of myeloid cells close to portal tracts is observed in ARLD patients (115) associated with increased levels of cytokines (IL-6, IL-8, IL-18), chemokines and macrophage activation markers that correlate with outcome and severity of disease (116–119). Gut permeability is increased in patients with ARLD leading to high levels of endotoxin in the liver resulting in a greater sensitivity of circulating monocytes from these patients to LPS (120, 121); a phenomenon also reported for resident KC isolated from alcohol-fed mice where increased sensitivity to endotoxin promoted expression of TNF-α and CCL2 (122, 123).

The role of macrophages in cholestatic diseases such as primary biliary cholangitis (PBC) and primary sclerosing cholangitis (PSC) is not well described. Accumulation of perisinusoidal hepatic macrophages in human tissue is reported in PSC but not in PBC (124) and increased infiltration of CD68$^+$/CCR2$^+$ cells was observed at later stages of disease in PSC including both CD206$^+$ (anti-inflammatory) and iNOS$^+$ (pro-inflammatory) macrophages (125). In diseases associated with cholestasis dysregulated bile acid production and excretion by cholangiocytes directly affects macrophage function and differentiation although the effects are complex. Although in mice hydrophobic bile acids have been reported to promote the formation of macrophage inflammasomes and IL-1β secretion (126, 127) other studies report activation of anti-inflammatory pathways in human macrophages by taurolithocholic acid through a PKA-mediated increase in IL-10 (128). Mice lacking the bile acid transporter *Mdr2* (*Abcb4*) develop hepatobiliary inflammation and fibrosis with some, but not all, features of PSC including an accumulation of peribiliary, proinflammatory macrophages recruited in response to cholangiocyte secretion of IL-8 and CCL2. Pharmacological treatment of mice with the CCR2/CCR5 antagonist cenicriviroc attenuated macrophage infiltration and liver injury consistent with an effector role for macrophages (125) and other rodent models have shown that the G-protein-coupled bile acid receptor, *Gpbar1* (TGR5) is expressed by macrophages to sense and respond to bile acids (129, 130). Activation of murine TGR5 leads to PKA-induced ubiquitination of NLRP3, acting as a brake on inflammasome activation (131) and dampening cytokine responses (129). In a murine model of colitis treatment with the TGR5 agonist BAR501 reduced the trafficking of Ly6C^{high} monocytes into the intestinal mucosa, reduced the expression of inflammatory genes (*Tnfa*, *Ifng*, *Il1b*, *Il6*, and *Ccl2*), and induced a regulatory T-cell environment through the production of IL-10 and TGF-β (132). The therapeutic potential of other TGR5 agonists such as 6α-ethyl-23(S)-methyl-cholic acid (6-EMCA, INT-777) are currently being explored in cholestatic liver disease (126, 133).

NEUTROPHIL MEDIATED LIVER INJURY

Neutrophils are derived from bone marrow and are released into the peripheral circulation where they play an important role in host defense and tissue healing (134), characterized by a high phagocytic capacity, the production of antimicrobial molecules and ability to shape immune responses (134, 135). The identities of neutrophil subsets and their functions are not clearly defined, with much of our knowledge arising from murine models. As a result their important roles in liver homeostasis and disease are only beginning to be understood (136, 137).

Neutrophil recruitment from the circulation into the liver is independent of selectins (138) and in many conditions is also independent of α2 integrin and ICAM-1 (139). Instead, neutrophils use CD44 to bind hyaluronan (HA) on LSEC and respond to chemokine ligands of CXCR2. A signaling network of TLR2, S100A9 and CXCL2 was shown to be necessary for neutrophil recruitment in a chronic model of liver injury in the mouse (140), while activation of TLR4 on LSEC was sufficient to induce the deposition of serum-associated hyaluronan-associated protein within the hepatic sinusoids which promoted CD44-dependent neutrophil migration in a murine model of endotoxemia (141). In sterile rodent injury models such as local thermal injury, HA-CD44 driven recruitment is less important and neutrophils use αMβ2 (Mac-1) binding to ICAM-1 (21). This pathway plays little role in septic injury because IL-10 leads to a loss of cell surface αMβ2 (142). Invading neutrophils in septic injury tend to arrest soon after infiltrating the tissue, whereas in sterile injury these cells migrate toward the focus of damage and adopt a swarming behavior which restricts neutrophil motility to within the boundary of the injury. This behavior is amplified by leukotriene B4 (LTB4) produced by the first invading neutrophils (21, 143). In sterile injury neutrophil recruitment can be promoted by ATP release from necrotic hepatocytes leading to activation of the inflammasome, and presentation of ligands for CXCR2 on the surface of the hepatic sinusoids (21). Alternatively N-formyl peptides released from dying and dead hepatocytes are detected by the formylated peptide receptor-1 on neutrophils which guide them toward the site of injury (21, 144, 145). This enables neutrophils to prioritize their responses to chemoattractant gradients that arise directly from damaged tissue over competing signals from chemokines or LTB4 and remain within the boundaries of the necrotized tissue (146–149). Live cell imaging in mice identified a non-muscle myosin II protein that was essential for neutrophil trafficking, demonstrating that myosin heavy chain 9 (Myh9) was localized in branching lamellipodia and in the uropod where it may enable fast neutrophil migration (150).

During acute liver injury, neutrophils use the receptor for advanced glycation end products (RAGE) to respond to HMGB1 released by necrotic hepatocytes (151). However, this pathway also contributes to sepsis through diminished bacterial killing by neutrophils and reduced NADPH oxidase activation (152). Neutrophils form extracellular traps by a process known as NETosis to enhance antibacterial defenses [reviewed in (153)]. Defects in NET formation have been linked to impaired efferocytosis and contribute to liver injury and sepsis in models of liver disease (154). In murine models of chronic liver disease neutrophils drive hepatocellular damage but are also associated with mechanisms of tissue repair. Myeloperoxidase secreted by neutrophils drives oxidative damage and contributes to the development of NASH in mice (155) and increased levels of myeloperoxidase activity have been detected in patients with NASH (156). The development of obesity-related inflammation in patients with NASH also correlated with an increase in the ratio of neutrophil elastase to its inhibitor α1-antitrypsin, although the ratio reduced as the disease progressed to fibrosis (157). Conversely murine neutrophils can alleviate fibrosis through secretion of MMP8 and MMP9 (158), and depletion of neutrophils improved liver function in a diet-induced model of NASH (159). Following resolution of tissue damage in sterile injury neutrophils migrate out of the tissue and back into the vasculature and, following passage through the lungs where they upregulate CXCR4, return to the bone marrow where they undergo apoptosis (160). It is not currently known if this process contributes to the pathogenesis of other hepatic diseases.

The Contribution of Dendritic Cells to the Development of Liver Disease

In contrast to hepatic macrophages liver dendritic cells are scarce and mostly scattered in the portal region where they capture antigens delivered by via the portal vein (161). Dendritic cells can also translocate from blood to lymph via the hepatic sinusoids to concentrate in regional perihepatic lymph nodes (162). Hepatic dendritic cells comprise plasmacytoid DCs (pDCs) and classical (myeloid) DCs (cDCs) which express high levels of MHC-Class II molecules (e.g., HLA-DR) but are negative for other hematopoietic lineage markers (163). In general hepatic DCs are tolerogenic and inherently anti-inflammatory, but they can gain pro-inflammatory properties in the setting of chronic liver injury (164, 165). Plasmacytoid DCs identified as $lin^{-}CD11c^{int}MHC\text{-}II^{int}PDCA\text{-}1^{+}Siglec\text{-}H^{+}$ in some respects resemble B-cells and represent the most abundant subset in the murine liver under steady-state conditions (163, 166). Human pDCs are characterized by BDCA-2 and CD123 expression, but occur less frequently than in mice (167). This cell population responds to TLR7/8 ligands and mediate antiviral immunity by secreting type I interferons such as IFN-α but are less potent T-cell inductors. Classical DCs comprise two subtypes: cross-presenting $lin^{-}CD11c^{+}CD11b^{-}CD103^{+}CX_3CR1^{-}$ DCs (mainly interacting with $CD8^{+}$ T-cells via MHC-I) and conventional $lin^{-}CD11c^{+}CD11b^{+}CD103^{-}CX_3CR1^{+}$ DCs (presenting MHC-II bound antigens to $CD4^{+}$ T-cells) which correspond to human CD141 (BDCA-3) and CD1c (BDCA-1) DCs respectively (61, 163). In human liver $CD1c^{+}$ DCs prevail in contrast to mice (168). Another recent nomenclature differentiates hepatic DCs based on lipid content with high-lipid liver DCs inducing robust T-cell activation and cytokine secretion whereas low-lipid DC promote immune tolerance in both mice and humans (169).

Several factors contribute to the tolerogenic nature of hepatic DCs. When compared to splenic DCs, hepatic DCs were shown to be relatively immature (less CD40, CD80, CD86, CD83) with a reduced capacity to cross-present antigen to T-cells. Human DCs secrete high levels of IL-10, but less IL12p70 upon LPS-exposure (165) thereby contributing to endotoxin tolerance in the healthy liver (170). According to some reports hepatic DCs also predominantly induce regulatory and IL-4 secreting T-cells (171). During homeostasis low levels of circulating LPS trigger the expression of indoleamine-2,3-dioxygenase in human pDCs which catalyzes the production of immunoregulatory metabolites (172, 173). Following CpG stimulation murine pDC also fail to release abundant class I interferons owing to high NOD2 expression (174). Interestingly, circulating DCs that cross the hepatic sinusoids to reach the afferent lymphatics are educated by the hepatic microenvironment to adopt a regulatory phenotype, emphasizing the inherent tolerogenic phenotype of the hepatic niche (175).

Compared to other myeloid cells such as macrophages and monocytes the role of DCs in the initiation and progression of liver diseases is poorly defined. After switching from a regulatory to a proinflammatory state hepatic DCs can exacerbate acute liver injury in certain murine models (176, 177) whereas in human fatty liver disease there is emerging evidence they are protective by removing cellular debris and restricting DAMP driven activation of innate effector $CD8^{+}$ T-cells (178). $CD103^{+}$ DCs might be central to this response as *Batf3* deficient mice that lack CD103 displayed a more aggressive course in an experimental model of NASH (179). The failure to clear HCV has been associated with a reduced capacity of pDCs to secrete antiviral IFN-α and their ability to stimulate inhibitory T-cell receptors such as PD-1, TIM-3, and CTLA-4 (180–182). Thus, impaired DC activation in HCV infection might favor T-cell unresponsiveness leading to viral immune escape and persistence. DCs are not the only APCs within the liver. The liver's unique metabolic functions and constant exposure to gut antigens and gut-derived microbial products has resulted in a complex system for regulating immune responses in which DCs, endothelial cells and stromal cells may all contribute to presenting antigens and maintaining immune homeostasis (175).

Some studies have suggested that DCs may play a role in driving fibrogenesis beyond their ability to activate immune responses. However, the data are not compelling and most evidence points to DCs being largely dispensable for the progression of fibrosis. Although the expansion of $CD11b^{+}$ DCs has been observed during hepatic fibrogenesis in mice (183, 184), DCs are thought to promote resolution rather than progression of fibrosis. For example depletion of DCs during the regression phase of murine liver fibrosis significantly impairs tissue repair whereas *in vivo* expansion or adoptive transfer of purified DCs enhanced fibrosis reversal. This pro-resolution effect was mediated by MMP9 activity and clearance of activated hepatic stellate cells (185). Moreover, due to their anti-angiogenic properties DCs can counteract the profibrotic effect of VEGF mainly by expressing the VEGF receptor 1 (sFLT1) thus reducing the bioavailability of VEGF (186).

Role of Macrophages in Fibrosis Progression and Resolution

Liver fibrogenesis was previously regarded as a unidirectional process with little chance of resolution once scar tissue has formed. However, evidence now shows that even advanced fibrosis and in some circumstances cirrhosis are at least partially reversible if the cause of liver injury can be eliminated (187). This concept has been demonstrated in both experimental models of chronic liver injury (188–190) and in human liver disease (191). For example in humans successful treatment of chronic viral hepatitis can lead to a marked improvement in liver architecture indicating that the liver has the potential for regeneration and remodeling of scar tissue. A landmark study by Marcellin et al. demonstrated that following 5 years of treatment of chronic Hepatitis B infection with tenofovir disoproxil fumarate, cirrhosis could be reverted in 74% of cases (192).

Kupffer cells and infiltrating monocyte-derived macrophages are crucially involved in this process of tissue remodeling (**Figure 3**) and it is clear that hepatic macrophages can play context-dependent fibrogenic and fibrolytic roles due to their heterogeneity and plasticity. For example hepatocyte-derived HRG, a non-inflammasome activating factor contributing to KC stimulation, favors a profibrotic phenotype of murine hepatic macrophages. This was demonstrated in HRG-deficient knockout mice where liver fibrosis was significantly attenuated in diet and toxin-induced models of liver injury (193). Similarly in humans interleukin-34 and macrophage colony-stimulating factor (M-CSF) promote a profibrotic phenotype in hepatic macrophages in the setting of chronic viral hepatitis (194). KC neutralize circulating endotoxins during homeostasis and release anti-inflammatory mediators such as IL-10 during low-level lipopolysaccharide (LPS) exposure (26). However, dysbiosis and translocation of gut bacteria and bacterial products due to intestinal barrier dysfunction result in the excessive presence of PAMPs within the hepatic microvasculature that reach the liver via the portal vein (195) which, in murine models, drives inflammasome activation of profibrotic hepatic stellate cells (196, 197). In a recent publication the cell-specific innate immune receptor triggering receptor expressed on myeloid cells-1 (TREM-1) was reported to promote hepatic inflammation and fibrosis in mice and humans (198), and inhibition of TREM-1 in mice ameliorated inflammation and macrophage and neutrophil activation in a mouse model of ARLD (199).

Chemokines released by KCs shapes the subsequent phase of hepatic inflammation. The CXC chemokines CXCL1, CXCL2, CXCL8 attract neutrophils whereas CCL2 is the major chemokine that governs influx of bone-marrow-derived monocytes (5). Hepatic stellate cells are another important source of CCL2 and there is a bidirectional relationship between pro-fibrotic effector cells and hepatic macrophages (197) as shown by the ability of HSC to respond to CCL2 and CCL5 produced by hepatic macrophages. Bone-marrow chimeric mice were used to show that activation of CCR2 and CCR5 in HSC drives fibrogenesis through stimulation of HSC migration and collagen production, whereas CCR1 acts solely on monocytes/macrophages (200–202). In humans macrophages exposed to HCV serum synthesize CCL5 and activate hepatic stellate cell confirming the murine data (203). CCL3 deficient mice display reduced HSC proliferation and migration and attenuated fibrogenesis (204). Secretion of CCL3 was shown to be dependent on the expression of the scavenger receptor Stabilin-1 by a specific macrophage population, and genetic deletion of *Stab1* led to diminished anti-fibrotic responses in diet and toxin-induced murine models of liver disease (205).

The release of CCL2 during early hepatic injury in mice augments the intrahepatic pool of macrophages by selectively attracting bone-marrow derived inflammatory $CCR2^{+}CX_3CR1^{low}Ly6C^{high}$ monocytes but not $CCR2^{-}CX_3CR1^{high}Ly6C^{low}$ counterparts (56). The expansion of hepatic macrophages is maintained during iterative episodes of liver injury that drive fibrogenesis (56) and CCR2 directed inhibition of monocyte recruitment during liver injury in murine models reduces liver scarring (56, 200, 206, 207). Targeting CCR2 with either the small molecule inhibitor cenicriviroc (208–210) or the L-enantiomeric RNA oligonucleotide mNOX-E36 (211) achieved similar results. In line with this data from the phase 2b Centaur trial revealed that treatment with cenicriviroc reduces fibrosis in patients with NASH after 1 year of treatment (212). Despite these advances, the profibrotic role of monocytic CCR2 is not fully understood following recent studies demonstrating that CCR2 expressed by monocytes/macrophages is dispensable for liver fibrogenesis (200). This was confirmed following further studies in mice which revealed that CCR1 (which binds CCL3 and CCL4), CCR8 (which binds mainly CCL1) and CCR9 which binds CCL25 are also involved in recruiting monocytes to the site of hepatic injury during fibrogenesis (42, 201, 213).

Both monocyte-derived macrophages and Kupffer cells promote fibrogenesis by secreting TGF-β and galectin-3, which drive transdifferentiation of HSCs into matrix secreting myofibroblasts (56, 214–216). Hepatic macrophages are also implicated in the survival and activation of HSC through secretion of IL-1β and TNF-α [in a NF-κB activation-dependent fashion (183)] or via IL-4 and IL-13 secretion in Th2-dominated rodent injury models such as parasitic infections (217). Oncostatin M (OSM) might also function as a potent regulator of hepatic macrophage/HSC interaction by enhancing the expression of profibrotic and mitogenic genes such as TGF-β and PDGF in bone-marrow derived infiltrating macrophages, with macrophage-depleted livers being largely protected from OSM-induced fibrosis (218). Interestingly, the profibrotic effect of KC-secreted TGF-β is retained following inhibition of CCL2-dependent monocyte in experimental steatohepatitis (102) which might impede the effectiveness of CCL2/CCR2 based therapies to treat liver fibrogenesis.

The first reports of hepatic macrophages driving fibrosis resolution were published alongside data describing the profibrogenic nature of Kupffer cells and monocyte-derived macrophages in liver injury. This apparent paradox was clarified when Duffield and colleagues reported a dual role for macrophages during different phases of chronic liver injury in mice. They used a CCl_4 model to show that mice in which hepatic macrophages were selectively depleted exhibited less matrix deposition at advanced stages of fibrogenesis but more fibrosis when macrophages were depleted during the resolution phase (219). These data suggested the existence of distinct macrophage populations within the liver that fulfill opposing functions according to the disease stage. A subsequent study by the same group confirmed this by reporting the accumulation of macrophages around scar fibers during the resolution phase that were capable of degrading ECM through expression of matrix metalloproteinase protein 13 (MMP13) (220). These scar-associated macrophages are also equipped with MMP9, MMP12 and TRAIL, and contribute to the disruption of scar tissue and induction of fibroblast apoptosis (187). However, these studies did not identify which hepatic macrophage population gave rise to this profibrolytic subset. One of the first lines of evidence that monocyte-derived macrophages might be responsible stems from a paper showing that CCR2 deficiency is protective during fibrogenesis but hinders scar removal during the regression phase following cessation of CCl_4 challenge in rodents. The putative mechanism is a balance between levels of tissue inhibitor of metalloproteinase-1 (TIMP1) and MMP1 and MMP13 mRNA, in the liver (207). This study also determined that profibrotic and pro-resolution macrophages share the same precursor cells; a hypothesis supported by a seminal paper in 2012 showing that in mice Ly6C^{high} inflammatory macrophages undergo a phenotypic switch to an anti-inflammatory and anti-fibrotic "restorative" CD11b^{high}F4/80^{int}Ly6C^{low} subtype (52). The accumulation of Ly6C^{low} macrophages producing matrilytic MMPs peaked at the maximum point of fibrosis resolution whereas the early phase of liver parenchyma damage is dominated by freshly recruited inflammatory CCR2^{+}Ly6C^{high} macrophages. Phagocytosis of cell debris drives macrophage transdifferentiation toward a restorative Ly6C^{low} phenotype (52). The concept of a context dependent hepatic macrophage plasticity was demonstrated using sterile liver inflammation models in which CCR2^{high}CX$_3$CR1^{low} macrophages accumulate early after focal tissue injury in a ring-like structure and then give rise to a reparative CCR2^{low}CX$_3$CR1^{high} phenotype which facilitate wound repair (14). There is also evidence that *in situ* reprogramming of infiltrating macrophages from a profibrotic to an antifibrotic subset is controlled by the CX$_3$CR1/CX$_3$CL1 axis, which promotes macrophage survival and imprints an anti-inflammatory state. Consequently, CX$_3$CR1 knockout mice display enhanced tissue damage and fibrosis after bile duct ligation and CCl_4 exposure (221, 222). Though circulating Gr1^{low} (Ly6C^{low}) CX$_3$CR1^{+} monocytes show patrolling behavior in blood stream (34) there is no data so far to support the idea that these cells are directly recruited to the inflamed liver and thereby perpetuate fibrosis resolution. Never the less, this cannot be excluded since extravasation of CX$_3$CR1^{+} monocytes into affected organs has been demonstrated in models of myocardial infarction and lung injury (223, 224).

Translating findings from rodent models into patients is not straightforward. Most importantly—as outlined above—human liver macrophage subsets lack well-defined surface marker patterns that allow for distinction of resident Kupffer cells from infiltrating monocytes. For example CD68^{+} which is deemed to be a macrophage marker in mice can also be detected on circulating monocytes in human, and although gene profiles show overlap between murine Ly6C^{high} and "classical" human CD14^{++}CD16^{-} monocytes and murine Ly6C^{low} and "non-classical" human CD14^{+}CD16^{++} monocytes (31) there are clear functional differences. In addition, it is difficult to integrate the "intermediate" CD14^{++}CD16^{+} subset into the murine nomenclature (225). In general, CD16^{+} monocytes are enriched in the liver in comparison to peripheral blood even under steady state conditions (46), with increased numbers being observed in patients with cirrhosis (47). CD14^{+}CD16^{-} cells can acquire CD16 expression under the influence of soluble factors present in the diseased liver such as IL-10 and TGF-β, and CD16^{+} monocytes display higher phagocytic capacity and can secrete both pro- and anti-inflammatory cytokines upon LPS stimulation thus resembling both Ly6C^{low} and Ly6C^{high} monocytes/macrophages in mice. Of note, CD16^{+} but not CD16^{-} monocytes can directly activate human HSC (47). Rodent models also lack the highly-crosslinked scar tissue observed for patients with advanced fibrosis, and as a result macrophage-mediated resolution of fibrosis is accelerated in murine models compared to humans. Therefore, further research is warranted to better define disease-specific characteristics of hepatic monocyte and macrophage subsets in human diseases. Despite these differences there are some striking parallels between mice and humans. For example, the CCL2/CCR2 axis plays a similar role in fibrosis and macrophage infiltration to the inflamed liver in mice and humans, and TREM-1 is emerging as an additional shared marker.

MALIGNANCY

Myeloid cell subsets are linked to virtually all steps in the natural course of tumor formation and spreading in the liver. Extensive research has shown a prominent role for tumor associated macrophages (TAM) and MDSC in the development of hepatocellular carcinoma (HCC), an archetypical inflammatory tumor in which chronic inflammation drives liver cancer pathogenesis, invasion, and metastasis (226). In the context of liver carcinogenesis monocytes/macrophages exert dualistic functions in a stage-dependent manner with CCR2^{+} CCL2-responsive monocytes promoting tumor surveillance through the elimination of senescent premalignant hepatocytes in healthy livers (**Figure 4**), whereas in established tumors monocytes/macrophages are reprogrammed to silence NK cells resulting in tumor growth (227, 228). Tumor associated macrophages derived from infiltrating monocytes are a dominant cellular component of human tumor stroma with increased density of TAMs in peritumoral margins being closely linked to poor prognosis (229, 230). Consistent with this the absence of macrophages correlated with improved patient survival (231). In both humans and murine models TAMs drive tumorigenesis by sustaining inflammatory pathways mediated through secretion of cytokines such as TNF-α and IL-6 that suppress hepatocyte apoptosis and induce proliferation in response to tissue damage (232–234). The surface receptor TREM-1 expressed on myeloid cells governs the secretion of proinflammatory mediators and engagement of TREM-1 in hepatic macrophages has been shown to trigger carcinogenesis (235). *Trem1*-deficient mice treated with diethylnitrosamine (DEN) were protected from malignancy due to attenuation of cytokine secretion (e.g., IL-6, IL-1β, TNF, CCL2)

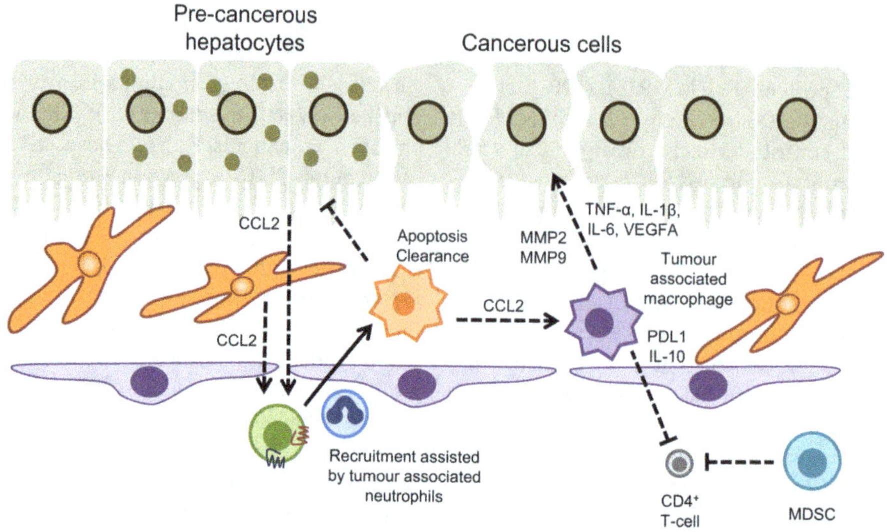

FIGURE 4 | Myeloid cells in hepatic malignancy. Tumor associated macrophages promote cancer cell proliferation and neoangiogenesis, and act in concert with myeloid-derived suppressor cells to dampen T-cell immunosurveillance. Conversely recruitment of monocytes into the tumor microenvironment driven by CCL2 produced by hepatocytes and hepatic stellate cells, and interactions with tumor associated neutrophils promotes apoptosis and clearance of pre-cancerous hepatocytes to prevent HCC.

and ablation of inflammatory signaling pathways (p38, ERK1/2, JNK, MAPK, and NF-κB) in KC (235).

The inflammatory environment present in chronic liver injury facilitates the recruitment and retention of monocyte-derived TAMs which promote tumorigenesis in a MMP2/MMP9 dependent fashion. This was demonstrated by comparing the seeding of injected HCC cells in healthy livers with CCl_4 preconditioned livers where an alternatively-activated macrophage population (M2-like) were enriched in the tumor environment (236). Infiltrating TAMs are frequently reported to resemble alternatively-activated macrophages (237–239) although the dichotomous approach of M1/M2 polarization does not fully reflect the entire spectrum and heterogeneity of tissue macrophages. Nevertheless, reversal of M2-like polarization in experimental HCC has yielded promising results in containing tumor progression (240) with TIM-3 and Wnt ligands identified as critical drivers of alternative activation of TAMs and HCC growth (239, 241). In patients, total immune cell infiltration into HCC correlated with M1-like macrophage populations and a more favorable prognosis (242).

The CCL2/CCR2 axis is a promising novel target in HCC therapy. Antagonism of CCR2 by the compound RDC018 not only reduced TAM infiltration but also restored anti-tumor immune response and ameliorated HCC outcome in murine models of HCC (243). Tumor associated neutrophils (TAN) provide an important source of CCL2 in HCC and can act synergistically with TAM to support liver tumor progression (244). In humans neutrophil extracellular traps can also promote inflammation and development of HCC on the background of NASH, driven by the presence of free fatty acids (245); however our understanding of the precise role played by neutrophils in liver cancer remains elusive. One striking feature of TAM is the induction of an immune suppressive microenvironment that disrupts anti-tumor immunity. For example, release of regulatory cytokines such as TGF-β and IL-10 by TAM impair Th1 and cytotoxic T-cells but promote regulatory T cells and Th2 activity all of which facilitate tumor growth. TAMs also express high levels of PDL1, galectin-9, and indoleamine-pyrrole 2,3-dioxygenase (IDO) that foster T-cell exhaustion and prevent effective anti-tumor immune response (241). In HCC the expression of PDL1 by TAMs correlated with increased tumor burden and the intensity of the protein was associated with high mortality and reduced survival (246). MDSC share many mechanisms with TAM to protect from HCC-targeted T-cell activity, and the net effect of MDSCs in HCC nodules and peritumoral stroma is progression of the tumor (241). Furthermore, MDSC reduce the tissue availability of arginine and cysteine, which are essential for T-cell proliferation and impede NK cell cytotoxicity and development via NKp30 receptor (241).

RATIONAL DESIGN OF THERAPEUTIC STRATEGIES TARGETING MYELOID POPULATIONS

There is a major unmet need for effective therapies to prevent or reverse liver fibrosis particularly in the context of a major increase in fatty liver disease and the continuing high prevalence of alcoholic cirrhosis (247). Macrophages have the dual potential to serve as therapeutic targets and as treatment vehicles for inflammation-induced liver fibrosis and carcinogenesis (248). In principle, macrophages can be targeted at different stages

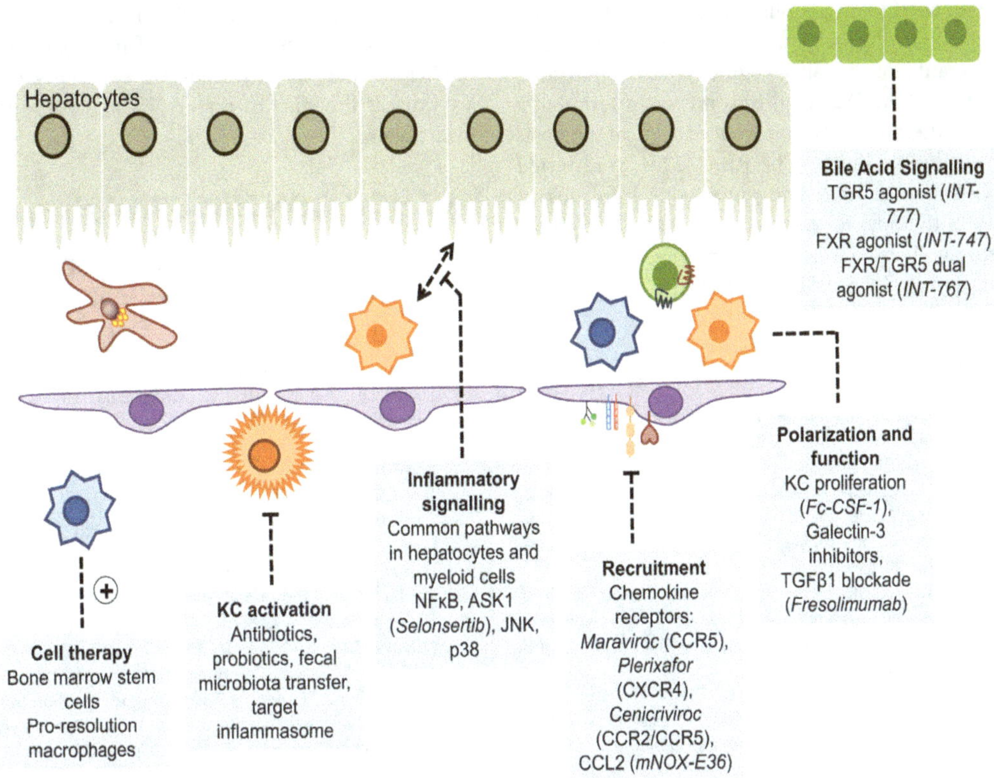

FIGURE 5 | Myeloid cells as therapeutic targets. Approaches that have been adopted to enhance or diminish the role of myeloid cells in liver disease include disruption of the recruitment cascade or inflammatory signaling pathways, and augmented pro-resolution responses through cellular infusions of stem cells or the provision of agonists driving macrophage polarization.

of disease and different subsets of monocyte macrophages can be targeted. Such strategies include (i) attenuation of Kupffer cell activation by anti-inflammatory compounds; (ii) inhibition of macrophage precursor cell (i.e., monocyte) recruitment to the injured liver; (iii) manipulation of macrophage polarization and differentiation to facilitate transition toward a restorative reparative phenotype (iv) infusion of beneficial pro-restorative macrophages (248) (**Figure 5**). Interference with chemokine pathways to restrict influx of inflammatory monocytes is one of the most advanced approaches. As stated earlier, the CCR2/CCR5 antagonist Cenicriviroc has entered phase 2b clinical trials with promising results reported after 12 months treatment of NASH-related fibrosis (212). The current options in targeting macrophages in the context of liver disease have recently been comprehensively summarized (248). Adoptive cell therapy using hematopoietic stem cells or macrophages is an approach that is attracting increasing interest. The first studies reporting efficacy of bone marrow cell transfer in murine models of liver fibrosis were published almost 15 years ago when injection of bone marrow cells was shown to cause MMP9-dependent reduction in ECM deposition in response to CCl_4 (249). In a study by Thomas et al. in 2011 bone-marrow derived macrophages (BMM) were prepared *in vitro* by stimulation with CSF-1 and subsequently injected into the portal vein of mice with long-term CCl_4 induced fibrosis. The infused cells did not conform to the M1/M2 paradigm but expressed IL-10, TWEAK, and MMP13, which are known to suppress inflammation and to promote cell regeneration and fibrolysis. Treatment significantly reduced liver scarring by promoting myofibroblasts apoptosis, MMP-induced degradation of ECM and by stimulating liver regeneration. In contradistinction, non-purified whole bone marrow cells increased liver fiber content (250). Similar results were obtained in another study showing that IL-10 producing $CD11b^+Gr1^+$ myeloid cells account for the tissue remodeling effect of bone marrow transplantation in liver fibrosis (251). BMM also ameliorate oxidative stress and reduce production of the potent profibrotic cytokine IL-13 (252). Interestingly, macrophages derived from pluripotent embryonic stem cells exhibit comparable antifibrotic effects to BMM though these cells tend to resemble resident Kupffer cells rather than infiltrating macrophages (253). A contributing factor to the success of bone marrow derived macrophage transplantation in liver fibrosis could be activation of the sphingosine-1-phosphate receptor (S1PR) that critically controls BMM motility (254). Mice treated with FTY720 which triggers S1PR internalization retained infused c-kit$^+$/sca1$^+$/lin$^-$ hematopoietic stem cells in the liver due to a failure of the cells to egress into the draining lymph. This was associated with reduced scarring in methionine-choline-deficient diet fed and CCl_4 treated mice (255). Further studies are needed to dissect whether S1P/S1PR antagonism also augments the antifibrotic effects of transplanted BMM. Despite the promising experimental findings human cell therapy trials in advanced clinical cirrhosis have so far proven disappointing. The REALISTIC trial tested the efficacy of G-CSF mobilized and autologous infusions of $CD133^+$ stem cell therapy in cirrhosis but failed to show any improvement in liver function with more complications in the treatment group (256). This is perhaps unsurprising given that resolution will only occur if the right cells are infused into the right microenvironment at the right disease stage. This requires the design of more sophisticated precision medicine trials. Such studies are underway (257, 258) but we are only at the start of understanding macrophage therapy for liver diseases.

AUTHOR CONTRIBUTIONS

CW, HZ wrote parts of the manuscript. DA edited and finalized the manuscript.

REFERENCES

1. Jung S. Macrophages and monocytes in 2017: Macrophages and monocytes: of tortoises and hares. *Nat Rev Immunol.* (2018) 18:85–6. doi: 10.1038/nri.2017.158
2. Scott CL, T'Jonck W, Martens L, Todorov H, Sichien D, Soen B, et al. The transcription factor ZEB2 is required to maintain the tissue-specific identities of macrophages. *Immunity.* (2018) 49:312–25. doi: 10.1016/j.immuni.2018.07.004
3. Lavin Y, Winter D, Blecher-Gonen R, David E, Keren-Shaul H, Merad M, et al. Tissue-resident macrophage enhancer landscapes are shaped by the local microenvironment. *Cell.* (2014) 159:1312–26. doi: 10.1016/j.cell.2014.11.018
4. Xue J, Schmidt SV, Sander J, Draffehn A, Krebs W, Quester I, et al. Transcriptome-based network analysis reveals a spectrum model of human macrophage activation. *Immunity.* (2014) 40:274–88. doi: 10.1016/j.immuni.2014.01.006
5. Krenkel O, Tacke F. Liver macrophages in tissue homeostasis and disease. *Nat Rev Immunol.* (2017) 17:306–21. doi: 10.1038/nri.2017.11
6. Tacke F, Zimmermann HW. Macrophage heterogeneity in liver injury and fibrosis. *J Hepatol.* (2014) 60:1090–6. doi: 10.1016/j.jhep.2013.12.025
7. Boulter L, Govaere O, Bird TG, Radulescu S, Ramachandran P, Pellicoro A, et al. Macrophage-derived Wnt opposes Notch signaling to specify hepatic progenitor cell fate in chronic liver disease. *Nat Med.* (2012) 18:572–9. doi: 10.1038/nm.2667
8. Gomez Perdiguero E, Klapproth K, Schulz C, Busch K, Azzoni E, Crozet L, et al. Tissue-resident macrophages originate from yolk-sac-derived erythro-myeloid progenitors. *Nature.* (2015) 518:547–51. doi: 10.1038/nature13989
9. Hoeffel G, Chen J, Lavin Y, Low D, Almeida FF, See P, et al. C-Myb(+) erythro-myeloid progenitor-derived fetal monocytes give rise to adult tissue-resident macrophages. *Immunity.* (2015) 42:665–78. doi: 10.1016/j.immuni.2015.03.011
10. Sheng J, Ruedl C, Karjalainen K. Fetal HSCs versus EMP2s. *Immunity.* (2015) 43:1025. doi: 10.1016/j.immuni.2015.11.023
11. Mass E, Ballesteros I, Farlik M, Halbritter F, Gunther P, Crozet L, et al. Specification of tissue-resident macrophages during organogenesis. *Science.* (2016) 353:aaf4238. doi: 10.1126/science.aaf4238
12. Scott CL, Zheng F, De Baetselier P, Martens L, Saeys Y, De Prijck S, et al. Bone marrow-derived monocytes give rise to self-renewing and fully differentiated Kupffer cells. *Nat Commun.* (2016) 7:10321. doi: 10.1038/ncomms10321
13. Beattie L, Sawtell A, Mann J, Frame TCM, Teal B, de Labastida Rivera F, et al. Bone marrow-derived and resident liver macrophages display unique transcriptomic signatures but similar biological functions. *J Hepatol.* (2016) 65:758–68. doi: 10.1016/j.jhep.2016.05.037
14. Dal-Secco D, Wang J, Zeng Z, Kolaczkowska E, Wong CH, Petri B, et al. A dynamic spectrum of monocytes arising from the *in situ* reprogramming of CCR2+ monocytes at a site of sterile injury. *J Exp Med.* (2015) 212:447–56. doi: 10.1084/jem.20141539
15. Epelman S, Lavine KJ, Randolph GJ. Origin and functions of tissue macrophages. *Immunity.* (2014) 41:21–35. doi: 10.1016/j.immuni.2014.06.013
16. Bieghs V, Wouters K, van Gorp PJ, Gijbels MJ, de Winther MP, Binder CJ, et al. Role of scavenger receptor A and CD36 in diet-induced nonalcoholic steatohepatitis in hyperlipidemic mice. *Gastroenterology.* (2010) 138:2477–86, 2486.e1–3. doi: 10.1053/j.gastro.2010.02.051
17. Iacobini C, Menini S, Ricci C, Scipioni A, Sansoni V, Cordone S, et al. Accelerated lipid-induced atherogenesis in galectin-3-deficient mice: role of lipoxidation via receptor-mediated mechanisms. *Arterioscler Thromb Vasc Biol.* (2009) 29:831–6. doi: 10.1161/ATVBAHA.109.186791
18. Zannetti C, Roblot G, Charrier E, Ainouze M, Tout I, Briat F, et al. Characterization of the inflammasome in human kupffer cells in response to synthetic agonists and pathogens. *J Immunol.* (2016) 197:356–67. doi: 10.4049/jimmunol.1502301
19. Kubes P, Mehal WZ. Sterile inflammation in the liver. *Gastroenterology.* (2012) 143:1158–72. doi: 10.1053/j.gastro.2012.09.008
20. Toki Y, Takenouchi T, Harada H, Tanuma S, Kitani H, Kojima S, et al. Extracellular ATP induces P2X7 receptor activation in mouse Kupffer cells, leading to release of IL-1beta, HMGB1, and PGE2, decreased MHC class I expression and necrotic cell death. *Biochem Biophys Res Commun.* (2015) 458:771–6. doi: 10.1016/j.bbrc.2015.02.011
21. McDonald B, Pittman K, Menezes GB, Hirota SA, Slaba I, Waterhouse CC, et al. Intravascular danger signals guide neutrophils to sites of sterile inflammation. *Science.* (2010) 330:362–6. doi: 10.1126/science.1195491
22. Amaral SS, Oliveira AG, Marques PE, Quintao JL, Pires DA, Resende RR, et al. Altered responsiveness to extracellular ATP enhances acetaminophen hepatotoxicity. *Cell Commun Signal.* (2013) 11:10. doi: 10.1186/1478-811X-11-10
23. Henao-Mejia J, Elinav E, Jin C, Hao L, Mehal WZ, Strowig T, et al. Inflammasome-mediated dysbiosis regulates progression of NAFLD and obesity. *Nature.* (2012) 482:179–85. doi: 10.1038/nature10809
24. Wree A, McGeough MD, Inzaugarat ME, Eguchi A, Schuster S, Johnson CD, et al. NLRP3 inflammasome driven liver injury and fibrosis: roles of IL-17 and TNF in mice. *Hepatology.* (2018) 67:736–49. doi: 10.1002/hep.29523
25. Knolle PA, Uhrig A, Protzer U, Trippler M, Duchmann R, Meyer zum Buschenfelde KH, et al. Interleukin-10 expression is autoregulated at the transcriptional level in human and murine Kupffer cells. *Hepatology.* (1998) 27:93–9. doi: 10.1002/hep.510270116
26. Knolle P, Schlaak J, Uhrig A, Kempf P, Meyer zum Buschenfelde KH, Gerken G. Human Kupffer cells secrete IL-10 in response to lipopolysaccharide (LPS) challenge. *J Hepatol.* (1995) 22:226–9. doi: 10.1016/0168-8278(95)80433-1
27. Heymann F, Peusquens J, Ludwig-Portugall I, Kohlhepp M, Ergen C, Niemietz P, et al. Liver inflammation abrogates immunological tolerance induced by Kupffer cells. *Hepatology.* (2015) 62:279–91. doi: 10.1002/hep.27793
28. You Q, Cheng L, Kedl RM, Ju C. Mechanism of T cell tolerance induction by murine hepatic Kupffer cells. *Hepatology.* (2008) 48:978–90. doi: 10.1002/hep.22395
29. Yan ML, Wang YD, Tian YF, Lai ZD, Yan LN. Inhibition of allogeneic T-cell response by Kupffer cells expressing indoleamine 2,3-dioxygenase. *World J Gastroenterol.* (2010) 16:636–40. doi: 10.3748/wjg.v16.i5.636
30. Wang Y, Song L, Liu M, Ge R, Zhou Q, Liu W, et al. A proteomics landscape of circadian clock in mouse liver. *Nat Commun.* (2018) 9:1553. doi: 10.1038/s41467-018-03898-2
31. Ingersoll MA, Spanbroek R, Lottaz C, Gautier EL, Frankenberger M, Hoffmann R, et al. Comparison of gene expression profiles

between human and mouse monocyte subsets. *Blood.* (2010) 115:e10–9. doi: 10.1182/blood-2009-07-235028
32. Tacke F, Randolph GJ. Migratory fate and differentiation of blood monocyte subsets. *Immunobiology.* (2006) 211:609–18. doi: 10.1016/j.imbio.2006.05.025
33. David BA, Rezende RM, Antunes MM, Santos MM, Freitas Lopes MA, Diniz AB, et al. Combination of mass cytometry and imaging analysis reveals origin, location, and functional repopulation of liver myeloid cells in mice. *Gastroenterology.* (2016) 151:1176–91. doi: 10.1053/j.gastro.2016.08.024
34. Auffray C, Fogg D, Garfa M, Elain G, Join-Lambert O, Kayal S, et al. Monitoring of blood vessels and tissues by a population of monocytes with patrolling behavior. *Science.* (2007) 317:666–70. doi: 10.1126/science.1142883
35. Carlin LM, Stamatiades EG, Auffray C, Hanna RN, Glover L, Vizcay-Barrena G, et al. Nr4a1-dependent Ly6C(low) monocytes monitor endothelial cells and orchestrate their disposal. *Cell.* (2013) 153:362–75. doi: 10.1016/j.cell.2013.03.010
36. Varol C, Mildner A, Jung S. Macrophages: development and tissue specialization. *Ann Rev Immunol.* (2015) 33:643–75. doi: 10.1146/annurev-immunol-032414-112220
37. Poschke I, Kiessling R. On the armament and appearances of human myeloid-derived suppressor cells. *Clin Immunol.* (2012) 144:250–68. doi: 10.1016/j.clim.2012.06.003
38. Hammerich L, Tacke F. Emerging roles of myeloid derived suppressor cells in hepatic inflammation and fibrosis. *World J Gastrointest Pathophysiol.* (2015) 6:43–50. doi: 10.4291/wjgp.v6.i3.43
39. Shetty S, Lalor PF, Adams DH. Liver sinusoidal endothelial cells—gatekeepers of hepatic immunity. *Nat Rev Gastroenterol Hepatol.* (2018) 15:555–67. doi: 10.1038/s41575-018-0020-y
40. Miura K, Yang L, van Rooijen N, Ohnishi H, Seki E. Hepatic recruitment of macrophages promotes nonalcoholic steatohepatitis through CCR2. *Am J Physiol Gastrointest Liver Physiol.* (2012) 302:G1310–21. doi: 10.1152/ajpgi.00365.2011
41. Galastri S, Zamara E, Milani S, Novo E, Provenzano A, Delogu W, et al. Lack of CC chemokine ligand 2 differentially affects inflammation and fibrosis according to the genetic background in a murine model of steatohepatitis. *Clin Sci.* (2012) 123:459–71. doi: 10.1042/CS20110515
42. Heymann F, Hammerich L, Storch D, Bartneck M, Huss S, Russeler V, et al. Hepatic macrophage migration and differentiation critical for liver fibrosis is mediated by the chemokine receptor C-C motif chemokine receptor 8 in mice. *Hepatology.* (2012) 55:898–909. doi: 10.1002/hep.24764
43. Tomita K, Freeman BL, Bronk SF, LeBrasseur NK, White TA, Hirsova P, et al. CXCL10-mediates macrophage, but not other innate immune cells-associated inflammation in murine nonalcoholic steatohepatitis. *Sci Rep.* (2016) 6:28786. doi: 10.1038/srep28786
44. Zhang X, Han J, Man K, Li X, Du J, Chu ES, et al. CXC chemokine receptor 3 promotes steatohepatitis in mice through mediating inflammatory cytokines, macrophages and autophagy. *J Hepatol.* (2016) 64:160–70. doi: 10.1016/j.jhep.2015.09.005
45. Aspinall AI, Curbishley SM, Lalor PF, Weston CJ, Blahova M, Liaskou E, et al. CX(3)CR1 and vascular adhesion protein-1-dependent recruitment of CD16(+) monocytes across human liver sinusoidal endothelium. *Hepatology.* (2010) 51:2030–9. doi: 10.1002/hep.23591
46. Liaskou E, Zimmermann HW, Li KK, Oo YH, Suresh S, Stamataki Z, et al. Monocyte subsets in human liver disease show distinct phenotypic and functional characteristics. *Hepatology.* (2013) 57:385–98. doi: 10.1002/hep.26016
47. Zimmermann HW, Seidler S, Nattermann J, Gassler N, Hellerbrand C, Zernecke A, et al. Functional contribution of elevated circulating and hepatic non-classical CD14CD16 monocytes to inflammation and human liver fibrosis. *PLoS ONE.* (2010) 5:e11049. doi: 10.1371/journal.pone.0011049
48. Zimmermann HW, Bruns T, Weston CJ, Curbishley SM, Liaskou E, Li KK, et al. Bidirectional transendothelial migration of monocytes across hepatic sinusoidal endothelium shapes monocyte differentiation and regulates the balance between immunity and tolerance in liver. *Hepatology.* (2016) 63:233–46. doi: 10.1002/hep.28285
49. Antoniades CG, Quaglia A, Taams LS, Mitry RR, Hussain M, Abeles R, et al. Source and characterization of hepatic macrophages in acetaminophen-induced acute liver failure in humans. *Hepatology.* (2012) 56:735–46. doi: 10.1002/hep.25657
50. Hochst B, Schildberg FA, Sauerborn P, Gabel YA, Gevensleben H, Goltz D, et al. Activated human hepatic stellate cells induce myeloid derived suppressor cells from peripheral blood monocytes in a CD44-dependent fashion. *J Hepatol.* (2013) 59:528–35. doi: 10.1016/j.jhep.2013.04.033
51. Resheq YJ, Li KK, Ward ST, Wilhelm A, Garg A, Curbishley SM, et al. Contact-dependent depletion of hydrogen peroxide by catalase is a novel mechanism of myeloid-derived suppressor cell induction operating in human hepatic stellate cells. *J Immunol.* (2015) 194:2578–86. doi: 10.4049/jimmunol.1401046
52. Ramachandran P, Pellicoro A, Vernon MA, Boulter L, Aucott RL, Ali A, et al. Differential Ly-6C expression identifies the recruited macrophage phenotype, which orchestrates the regression of murine liver fibrosis. *Proc Natl Acad Sci USA.* (2012) 109:E3186–95. doi: 10.1073/pnas.1119964109
53. Wang J, Kubes P. A reservoir of mature cavity macrophages that can rapidly invade visceral organs to affect tissue repair. *Cell.* (2016) 165:668–78. doi: 10.1016/j.cell.2016.03.009
54. Bernal W, Lee WM, Wendon J, Larsen FS, Williams R. Acute liver failure: a curable disease by 2024? *J Hepatol.* (2015) 62(1 Suppl.):S112–20. doi: 10.1016/j.jhep.2014.12.016
55. Bernal W, Wendon J. Acute liver failure. *N Engl J Med.* (2013) 369:2525–34. doi: 10.1056/NEJMra1208937
56. Karlmark KR, Weiskirchen R, Zimmermann HW, Gassler N, Ginhoux F, Weber C, et al. Hepatic recruitment of the inflammatory Gr1+ monocyte subset upon liver injury promotes hepatic fibrosis. *Hepatology.* (2009) 50:261–74. doi: 10.1002/hep.22950
57. Hitchcock JR, Cook CN, Bobat S, Ross EA, Flores-Langarica A, Lowe KL, et al. Inflammation drives thrombosis after Salmonella infection via CLEC-2 on platelets. *J Clin Invest.* (2015) 125:4429–46. doi: 10.1172/JCI79070
58. Erhardt A, Biburger M, Papadopoulos T, Tiegs G. IL-10, regulatory T cells, and Kupffer cells mediate tolerance in concanavalin A-induced liver injury in mice. *Hepatology.* (2007) 45:475–85. doi: 10.1002/hep.21498
59. Zhai Y, Busuttil RW, Kupiec-Weglinski JW. Liver ischemia and reperfusion injury: new insights into mechanisms of innate-adaptive immune-mediated tissue inflammation. *Am J Transplant.* (2011) 11:1563–9. doi: 10.1111/j.1600-6143.2011.03579.x
60. Movita D, van de Garde MD, Biesta P, Kreefft K, Haagmans B, Zuniga E, et al. Inflammatory monocytes recruited to the liver within 24 hours after virus-induced inflammation resemble Kupffer cells but are functionally distinct. *J Virol.* (2015) 89:4809–17. doi: 10.1128/JVI.03733-14
61. Heymann F, Tacke F. Immunology in the liver–from homeostasis to disease. *Nat Rev Gastroenterol Hepatol.* (2016) 13:88–110. doi: 10.1038/nrgastro.2015.200
62. Holt MP, Cheng L, Ju C. Identification and characterization of infiltrating macrophages in acetaminophen-induced liver injury. *J Leukoc Biol.* (2008) 84:1410–21. doi: 10.1189/jlb.0308173
63. Zigmond E, Samia-Grinberg S, Pasmanik-Chor M, Brazowski E, Shibolet O, Halpern Z, et al. Infiltrating monocyte-derived macrophages and resident kupffer cells display different ontogeny and functions in acute liver injury. *J Immunol.* (2014) 193:344–53. doi: 10.4049/jimmunol.1400574
64. Michael SL, Pumford NR, Mayeux PR, Niesman MR, Hinson JA. Pretreatment of mice with macrophage inactivators decreases acetaminophen hepatotoxicity and the formation of reactive oxygen and nitrogen species. *Hepatology.* (1999) 30:186–95. doi: 10.1002/hep.510300104
65. Laskin DL, Gardner CR, Price VF, Jollow DJ. Modulation of macrophage functioning abrogates the acute hepatotoxicity of acetaminophen. *Hepatology.* (1995) 21:1045–50. doi: 10.1002/hep.1840210424
66. Mossanen JC, Krenkel O, Ergen C, Govaere O, Liepelt A, Puengel T, et al. Chemokine (C-C motif) receptor 2-positive monocytes aggravate the early phase of acetaminophen-induced acute liver injury. *Hepatology.* (2016) 64:1667–82. doi: 10.1002/hep.28682
67. Bourdi M, Masubuchi Y, Reilly TP, Amouzadeh HR, Martin JL, George JW, et al. Protection against acetaminophen-induced liver injury and lethality

by interleukin 10: role of inducible nitric oxide synthase. *Hepatology.* (2002) 35:289–98. doi: 10.1053/jhep.2002.30956

68. Yee SB, Bourdi M, Masson MJ, Pohl LR. Hepatoprotective role of endogenous interleukin-13 in a murine model of acetaminophen-induced liver disease. *Chem Res Toxicol.* (2007) 20:734–44. doi: 10.1021/tx600349f
69. Bourdi M, Eiras DP, Holt MP, Webster MR, Reilly TP, Welch KD, et al. Role of IL-6 in an IL-10 and IL-4 double knockout mouse model uniquely susceptible to acetaminophen-induced liver injury. *Chem Res Toxicol.* (2007) 20:208–16. doi: 10.1021/tx060228l
70. Stutchfield BM, Antoine DJ, Mackinnon AC, Gow DJ, Bain CC, Hawley CA, et al. CSF1 restores innate immunity after liver injury in mice and serum levels indicate outcomes of patients with acute liver failure. *Gastroenterology.* (2015) 149:1896–909.e14. doi: 10.1053/j.gastro.2015.08.053
71. Antoniades CG, Khamri W, Abeles RD, Taams LS, Triantafyllou E, Possamai LA, et al. Secretory leukocyte protease inhibitor: a pivotal mediator of anti-inflammatory responses in acetaminophen-induced acute liver failure. *Hepatology.* (2014) 59:1564–76. doi: 10.1002/hep.26933
72. Triantafyllou E, Pop OT, Possamai LA, Wilhelm A, Liaskou E, Singanayagam A, et al. MerTK expressing hepatic macrophages promote the resolution of inflammation in acute liver failure. *Gut.* (2018) 67:333–47. doi: 10.1136/gutjnl-2016-313615
73. Krenkel O, Mossanen JC, Tacke F. Immune mechanisms in acetaminophen-induced acute liver failure. *Hepatobiliary Surg Nutr.* (2014) 3:331–43. doi: 10.3978/j.issn.2304-3881.2014.11.01
74. Campana L, Starkey Lewis PJ, Pellicoro A, Aucott RL, Man J, O'Duibhir E, et al. The STAT3-IL-10-IL-6 pathway is a novel regulator of macrophage efferocytosis and phenotypic conversion in sterile liver injury. *J Immunol.* (2018) 200:1169–87. doi: 10.4049/jimmunol.1701247
75. Ju C, Reilly TP, Bourdi M, Radonovich MF, Brady JN, George JW, et al. Protective role of Kupffer cells in acetaminophen-induced hepatic injury in mice. *Chem Res Toxicol.* (2002) 15:1504–13. doi: 10.1021/tx0255976
76. Bernsmeier C, Pop OT, Singanayagam A, Triantafyllou E, Patel VC, Weston CJ, et al. Patients with acute-on-chronic liver failure have increased numbers of regulatory immune cells expressing the receptor tyrosine kinase MERTK. *Gastroenterology.* (2015) 148:603–15.e14. doi: 10.1053/j.gastro.2014.11.045
77. Khakoo SI, Soni PN, Savage K, Brown D, Dhillon AP, Poulter LW, et al. Lymphocyte and macrophage phenotypes in chronic hepatitis C infection. Correlation with disease activity. *Am J Pathol.* (1997) 150:963–70.
78. McGuinness PH, Painter D, Davies S, McCaughan GW. Increases in intrahepatic CD68 positive cells, MAC387 positive cells, and proinflammatory cytokines (particularly interleukin 18) in chronic hepatitis C infection. *Gut.* (2000) 46:260–9. doi: 10.1136/gut.46.2.260
79. Shrivastava S, Mukherjee A, Ray R, Ray RB. Hepatitis C virus induces interleukin-1beta (IL-1beta)/IL-18 in circulatory and resident liver macrophages. *J Virol.* (2013) 87:12284–90. doi: 10.1128/JVI.01962-13
80. Hosomura N, Kono H, Tsuchiya M, Ishii K, Ogiku M, Matsuda M, et al. HCV-related proteins activate Kupffer cells isolated from human liver tissues. *Digest Dis Sci.* (2011) 56:1057–64. doi: 10.1007/s10620-010-1395-y
81. Boltjes A, Movita D, Boonstra A, Woltman AM. The role of Kupffer cells in hepatitis B and hepatitis C virus infections. *J Hepatol.* (2014) 61:660–71. doi: 10.1016/j.jhep.2014.04.026
82. Broering R, Wu J, Meng Z, Hilgard P, Lu M, Trippler M, et al. Toll-like receptor-stimulated non-parenchymal liver cells can regulate hepatitis C virus replication. *J Hepatol.* (2008) 48:914–22. doi: 10.1016/j.jhep.2008.01.028
83. Boltjes A, van Montfoort N, Biesta PJ, Op den Brouw ML, Kwekkeboom J, van der Laan LJ, et al. Kupffer cells interact with hepatitis B surface antigen *in vivo* and *in vitro*, leading to proinflammatory cytokine production and natural killer cell function. *J Infect Dis.* (2015) 211:1268–78. doi: 10.1093/infdis/jiu599
84. Chang S, Dolganiuc A, Szabo G. Toll-like receptors 1 and 6 are involved in TLR2-mediated macrophage activation by hepatitis C virus core and NS3 proteins. *J Leukoc Biol.* (2007) 82:479–87. doi: 10.1189/jlb.0207128
85. Huang LR, Wohlleber D, Reisinger F, Jenne CN, Cheng RL, Abdullah Z, et al. Intrahepatic myeloid-cell aggregates enable local proliferation of CD8(+) T cells and successful immunotherapy against chronic viral liver infection. *Nat Immunol.* (2013) 14:574–83. doi: 10.1038/ni.2573
86. Liu J, Yu Q, Wu W, Huang X, Broering R, Werner M, et al. TLR2 stimulation strengthens intrahepatic myeloid-derived cell-mediated T cell tolerance through inducing Kupffer cell expansion and IL-10 production. *J Immunol.* (2018) 200:2341–51. doi: 10.4049/jimmunol.1700540
87. Wang S, Chen Z, Hu C, Qian F, Cheng Y, Wu M, et al. Hepatitis B virus surface antigen selectively inhibits TLR2 ligand-induced IL-12 production in monocytes/macrophages by interfering with JNK activation. *J Immunol.* (2013) 190:5142–51. doi: 10.4049/jimmunol.1201625
88. Li M, Sun R, Xu L, Yin W, Chen Y, Zheng X, et al. Kupffer cells support hepatitis B virus-mediated CD8+ T cell exhaustion via hepatitis B core antigen-TLR2 interactions in mice. *J Immunol.* (2015) 195:3100–9. doi: 10.4049/jimmunol.1500839
89. Nebbia G, Peppa D, Schurich A, Khanna P, Singh HD, Cheng Y, et al. Upregulation of the Tim-3/galectin-9 pathway of T cell exhaustion in chronic hepatitis B virus infection. *PLoS ONE.* (2012) 7:e47648. doi: 10.1371/journal.pone.0047648
90. Tian Y, Kuo CF, Akbari O, Ou JH. Maternal-derived hepatitis B virus e antigen alters macrophage function in offspring to drive viral persistence after vertical transmission. *Immunity.* (2016) 44:1204–14. doi: 10.1016/j.immuni.2016.04.008
91. Jiang M, Broering R, Trippler M, Poggenpohl L, Fiedler M, Gerken G, et al. Toll-like receptor-mediated immune responses are attenuated in the presence of high levels of hepatitis B virus surface antigen. *J Viral Hepatitis.* (2014) 21:860–72. doi: 10.1111/jvh.12216
92. Pellicoro A, Ramachandran P, Iredale JP, Fallowfield JA. Liver fibrosis and repair: immune regulation of wound healing in a solid organ. *Nat Rev Immunol.* (2014) 14:181–94. doi: 10.1038/nri3623
93. Ndugga N, Lightbourne TG, Javaherian K, Cabezas J, Verma N, Barritt ASt, et al. Disparities between research attention and burden in liver diseases: implications on uneven advances in pharmacological therapies in Europe and the USA. *BMJ Open.* (2017) 7:e013620. doi: 10.1136/bmjopen-2016-013620
94. Schuster S, Cabrera D, Arrese M, Feldstein AE. Triggering and resolution of inflammation in NASH. *Nat Rev Gastroenterol Hepatol.* (2018) 15:349–64. doi: 10.1038/s41575-018-0009-6
95. Park JW, Jeong G, Kim SJ, Kim MK, Park SM. Predictors reflecting the pathological severity of non-alcoholic fatty liver disease: comprehensive study of clinical and immunohistochemical findings in younger Asian patients. *J Gastroenterol Hepatol.* (2007) 22:491–7. doi: 10.1111/j.1440-1746.2006.04758.x
96. Clementi AH, Gaudy AM, van Rooijen N, Pierce RH, Mooney RA. Loss of Kupffer cells in diet-induced obesity is associated with increased hepatic steatosis, STAT3 signaling, and further decreases in insulin signaling. *Biochim Biophys Acta.* (2009) 1792:1062–72. doi: 10.1016/j.bbadis.2009.08.007
97. Huang W, Metlakunta A, Dedousis N, Zhang P, Sipula I, Dube JJ, et al. Depletion of liver Kupffer cells prevents the development of diet-induced hepatic steatosis and insulin resistance. *Diabetes.* (2010) 59:347–57. doi: 10.2337/db09-0016
98. Hirsova P, Ibrahim SH, Krishnan A, Verma VK, Bronk SF, Werneburg NW, et al. Lipid-induced signaling causes release of inflammatory extracellular vesicles from hepatocytes. *Gastroenterology.* (2016) 150:956–67. doi: 10.1053/j.gastro.2015.12.037
99. Robert O, Boujedidi H, Bigorgne A, Ferrere G, Voican CS, Vettorazzi S, et al. Decreased expression of the glucocorticoid receptor-GILZ pathway in Kupffer cells promotes liver inflammation in obese mice. *J Hepatol.* (2016) 64:916–24. doi: 10.1016/j.jhep.2015.11.023
100. Morinaga H, Mayoral R, Heinrichsdorff J, Osborn O, Franck N, Hah N, et al. Characterization of distinct subpopulations of hepatic macrophages in HFD/obese mice. *Diabetes.* (2015) 64:1120–30. doi: 10.2337/db14-1238
101. Miyachi Y, Tsuchiya K, Komiya C, Shiba K, Shimazu N, Yamaguchi S, et al. Roles for cell-cell adhesion and contact in obesity-induced hepatic myeloid cell accumulation and glucose intolerance. *Cell Rep.* (2017) 18:2766–79. doi: 10.1016/j.celrep.2017.02.039
102. Baeck C, Wehr A, Karlmark KR, Heymann F, Vucur M, Gassler N, et al. Pharmacological inhibition of the chemokine CCL2 (MCP-1) diminishes liver macrophage infiltration and steatohepatitis in chronic hepatic injury. *Gut.* (2012) 61:416–26. doi: 10.1136/gutjnl-2011-300304

103. Weston CJ, Shepherd EL, Claridge LC, Rantakari P, Curbishley SM, Tomlinson JW, et al. Vascular adhesion protein-1 promotes liver inflammation and drives hepatic fibrosis. *J Clin Invest.* (2015) 125:501–20. doi: 10.1172/JCI73722
104. Rivera CA, Adegboyega P, van Rooijen N, Tagalicud A, Allman M, Wallace M. Toll-like receptor-4 signaling and Kupffer cells play pivotal roles in the pathogenesis of non-alcoholic steatohepatitis. *J Hepatol.* (2007) 47:571–9. doi: 10.1016/j.jhep.2007.04.019
105. Garcia-Martinez I, Santoro N, Chen Y, Hoque R, Ouyang X, Caprio S, et al. Hepatocyte mitochondrial DNA drives nonalcoholic steatohepatitis by activation of TLR9. *J Clin Invest.* (2016) 126:859–64. doi: 10.1172/JCI83885
106. Mridha AR, Haczeyni F, Yeh MM, Haigh WG, Ioannou GN, Barn V, et al. TLR9 is up-regulated in human and murine NASH: pivotal role in inflammatory recruitment and cell survival. *Clin Sci.* (2017) 131:2145–59. doi: 10.1042/CS20160838
107. Balmer ML, Slack E, de Gottardi A, Lawson MA, Hapfelmeier S, Miele L, et al. The liver may act as a firewall mediating mutualism between the host and its gut commensal microbiota. *Sci Transl Med.* (2014) 6:237ra66. doi: 10.1126/scitranslmed.3008618
108. Wan J, Benkdane M, Teixeira-Clerc F, Bonnafous S, Louvet A, Lafdil F, et al. M2 Kupffer cells promote M1 Kupffer cell apoptosis: a protective mechanism against alcoholic and nonalcoholic fatty liver disease. *Hepatology.* (2014) 59:130–42. doi: 10.1002/hep.26607
109. Han YH, Kim HJ, Na H, Nam MW, Kim JY, Kim JS, et al. RORalpha induces KLF4-mediated M2 polarization in the liver macrophages that protect against nonalcoholic steatohepatitis. *Cell Rep.* (2017) 20:124–35. doi: 10.1016/j.celrep.2017.06.017
110. Du X, Wu Z, Xu Y, Liu Y, Liu W, Wang T, et al. Increased Tim-3 expression alleviates liver injury by regulating macrophage activation in MCD-induced NASH mice. *Cell Mol Immunol.* (2018). doi: 10.1038/s41423-018-0032-0. [Epub ahead of print].
111. Petrasek J, Bala S, Csak T, Lippai D, Kodys K, Menashy V, et al. IL-1 receptor antagonist ameliorates inflammasome-dependent alcoholic steatohepatitis in mice. *J Clin Invest.* (2012) 122:3476–89. doi: 10.1172/JCI60777
112. Enomoto N, Ikejima K, Bradford BU, Rivera CA, Kono H, Goto M, et al. Role of Kupffer cells and gut-derived endotoxins in alcoholic liver injury. *J Gastroenterol Hepatol.* (2000) 15(Suppl):D20–5. doi: 10.1046/j.1440-1746.2000.02179.x
113. Koop DR, Klopfenstein B, Iimuro Y, Thurman RG. Gadolinium chloride blocks alcohol-dependent liver toxicity in rats treated chronically with intragastric alcohol despite the induction of CYP2E1. *Mol Pharmacol.* (1997) 51:944–50. doi: 10.1124/mol.51.6.944
114. Wang M, Frasch SC, Li G, Feng D, Gao B, Xu L, et al. Role of gp91(phox) in hepatic macrophage programming and alcoholic liver disease. *Hepatol Commun.* (2017) 1:765–79. doi: 10.1002/hep4.1078
115. Ju C, Mandrekar P. Macrophages and alcohol-related liver inflammation. *Alcohol Res.* (2015) 37:251–62.
116. Afford SC, Fisher NC, Neil DA, Fear J, Brun P, Hubscher SG, et al. Distinct patterns of chemokine expression are associated with leukocyte recruitment in alcoholic hepatitis and alcoholic cirrhosis. *J Pathol.* (1998) 186:82–9. doi: 10.1002/(SICI)1096-9896(199809)186:1<82::AID-PATH151>3.0.CO;2-D
117. Luna-Casado L, Diez-Ruiz A, Gutierrez-Gea F, Santos-Perez JL, Rico-Irles J, Wachter H, et al. Increased peripheral mononuclear cells expression of adhesion molecules in alcoholic cirrhosis: its relation to immune activation. *J Hepatol.* (1997) 27:477–83. doi: 10.1016/S0168-8278(97)80351-0
118. Fisher NC, Neil DA, Williams A, Adams DH. Serum concentrations and peripheral secretion of the beta chemokines monocyte chemoattractant protein 1 and macrophage inflammatory protein 1alpha in alcoholic liver disease. *Gut.* (1999) 45:416–20. doi: 10.1136/gut.45.3.416
119. McClain CJ, Barve S, Deaciuc I, Kugelmas M, Hill D. Cytokines in alcoholic liver disease. *Semin Liver Dis.* (1999) 19:205–19. doi: 10.1055/s-2007-1007110
120. Gobejishvili L, Barve S, Joshi-Barve S, Uriarte S, Song Z, McClain C. Chronic ethanol-mediated decrease in cAMP primes macrophages to enhanced LPS-inducible NF-kappaB activity and TNF expression: relevance to alcoholic liver disease. *Am J Physiol Gastrointest Liver Physiol.* (2006) 291:G681–8. doi: 10.1152/ajpgi.00098.2006
121. Zhang Z, Bagby GJ, Stoltz D, Oliver P, Schwarzenberger PO, Kolls JK. Prolonged ethanol treatment enhances lipopolysaccharide/phorbol myristate acetate-induced tumor necrosis factor-alpha production in human monocytic cells. *Alcohol Clin Exp Res.* (2001) 25:444–9. doi: 10.1111/j.1530-0277.2001.tb02233.x
122. Mandrekar P, Ambade A, Lim A, Szabo G, Catalano D. An essential role for monocyte chemoattractant protein-1 in alcoholic liver injury: regulation of proinflammatory cytokines and hepatic steatosis in mice. *Hepatology.* (2011) 54:2185–97. doi: 10.1002/hep.24599
123. Nagy LE. The role of innate immunity in alcoholic liver disease. *Alcohol Res.* (2015) 37:237–50.
124. Cameron RG, Blendis LM, Neuman MG. Accumulation of macrophages in primary sclerosing cholangitis. *Clin Biochem.* (2001) 34:195–201. doi: 10.1016/S0009-9120(01)00215-6
125. Guicciardi ME, Trussoni CE, Krishnan A, Bronk SF, Lorenzo Pisarello MJ, O'Hara SP, et al. Macrophages contribute to the pathogenesis of sclerosing cholangitis in mice. *J Hepatol.* (2018) 69:676–86. doi: 10.1016/j.jhep.2018.05.018
126. Calmus Y, Poupon R. Shaping macrophages function and innate immunity by bile acids: mechanisms and implication in cholestatic liver diseases. *Clin Res Hepatol Gastroenterol.* (2014) 38:550–6. doi: 10.1016/j.clinre.2014.07.007
127. Gong Z, Zhou J, Zhao S, Tian C, Wang P, Xu C, et al. Chenodeoxycholic acid activates NLRP3 inflammasome and contributes to cholestatic liver fibrosis. *Oncotarget.* (2016) 7:83951–63. doi: 10.18632/oncotarget.13796
128. Haselow K, Bode JG, Wammers M, Ehlting C, Keitel V, Kleinebrecht L, et al. Bile acids PKA-dependently induce a switch of the IL-10/IL-12 ratio and reduce proinflammatory capability of human macrophages. *J Leukoc Biol.* (2013) 94:1253–64. doi: 10.1189/jlb.0812396
129. Keitel V, Donner M, Winandy S, Kubitz R, Haussinger D. Expression and function of the bile acid receptor TGR5 in Kupffer cells. *Biochem Biophys Res Commun.* (2008) 372:78–84. doi: 10.1016/j.bbrc.2008.04.171
130. Pean N, Doignon I, Garcin I, Besnard A, Julien B, Liu B, et al. The receptor TGR5 protects the liver from bile acid overload during liver regeneration in mice. *Hepatology.* (2013) 58:1451–60. doi: 10.1002/hep.26463
131. Guo C, Xie S, Chi Z, Zhang J, Liu Y, Zhang L, et al. Bile acids control inflammation and metabolic disorder through inhibition of NLRP3 inflammasome. *Immunity.* (2016) 45:802–16. doi: 10.1016/j.immuni.2016.09.008
132. Biagioli M, Carino A, Cipriani S, Francisci D, Marchiano S, Scarpelli P, et al. The bile acid receptor GPBAR1 regulates the M1/M2 phenotype of intestinal macrophages and activation of GPBAR1 rescues mice from murine colitis. *J Immunol.* (2017) 199:718–33. doi: 10.4049/jimmunol.1700183
133. Hegade VS, Speight RA, Etherington RE, Jones DE. Novel bile acid therapeutics for the treatment of chronic liver diseases. *Therap Adv Gastroenterol.* (2016) 9:376–91. doi: 10.1177/1756283X16630712
134. Nathan C. Neutrophils and immunity: challenges and opportunities. *Nat Rev Immunol.* (2006) 6:173–82. doi: 10.1038/nri1785
135. Segal AW. How neutrophils kill microbes. *Ann Rev Immunol.* (2005) 23:197–223. doi: 10.1146/annurev.immunol.23.021704.115653
136. Deniset JF, Kubes P. Neutrophil heterogeneity: bona fide subsets or polarization states? *J Leukoc Biol.* (2018) 103:829–38. doi: 10.1002/JLB.3RI0917-361R
137. Kubes P. The enigmatic neutrophil: what we do not know. *Cell Tiss Res.* (2018) 371:399–406. doi: 10.1007/s00441-018-2790-5
138. Wong J, Johnston B, Lee SS, Bullard DC, Smith CW, Beaudet AL, et al. A minimal role for selectins in the recruitment of leukocytes into the inflamed liver microvasculature. *J Clin Invest.* (1997) 99:2782–90. doi: 10.1172/JCI119468
139. McDonald B, McAvoy EF, Lam F, Gill V, de la Motte C, Savani RC, et al. Interaction of CD44 and hyaluronan is the dominant mechanism for neutrophil sequestration in inflamed liver sinusoids. *J Exp Med.* (2008) 205:915–27. doi: 10.1084/jem.20071765
140. Moles A, Murphy L, Wilson CL, Chakraborty JB, Fox C, Park EJ, et al. A TLR2/S100A9/CXCL-2 signaling network is necessary for neutrophil recruitment in acute and chronic liver injury in the mouse. *J Hepatol.* (2014) 60:782–91. doi: 10.1016/j.jhep.2013.12.005

141. McDonald B, Jenne CN, Zhuo L, Kimata K, Kubes P. Kupffer cells and activation of endothelial TLR4 coordinate neutrophil adhesion within liver sinusoids during endotoxemia. *Am J Physiol Gastrointest Liver Physiol.* (2013) 305:G797–806. doi: 10.1152/ajpgi.00058.2013
142. Menezes GB, Lee WY, Zhou H, Waterhouse CC, Cara DC, Kubes P. Selective down-regulation of neutrophil Mac-1 in endotoxemic hepatic microcirculation via IL-10. *J Immunol.* (2009) 183:7557–68. doi: 10.4049/jimmunol.0901786
143. Lammermann T, Afonso PV, Angermann BR, Wang JM, Kastenmuller W, Parent CA, et al. Neutrophil swarms require LTB4 and integrins at sites of cell death *in vivo*. *Nature.* (2013) 498:371–5. doi: 10.1038/nature12175
144. Ng LG, Qin JS, Roediger B, Wang Y, Jain R, Cavanagh LL, et al. Visualizing the neutrophil response to sterile tissue injury in mouse dermis reveals a three-phase cascade of events. *J Invest Dermatol.* (2011) 131:2058–68. doi: 10.1038/jid.2011.179
145. Zhang Q, Raoof M, Chen Y, Sumi Y, Sursal T, Junger W, et al. Circulating mitochondrial DAMPs cause inflammatory responses to injury. *Nature.* (2010) 464:104–7. doi: 10.1038/nature08780
146. Volmering S, Block H, Boras M, Lowell CA, Zarbock A. The neutrophil Btk signalosome regulates integrin activation during sterile inflammation. *Immunity.* (2016) 44:73–87. doi: 10.1016/j.immuni.2015.11.011
147. Heit B, Robbins SM, Downey CM, Guan Z, Colarusso P, Miller BJ, et al. PTEN functions to 'prioritize' chemotactic cues and prevent 'distraction' in migrating neutrophils. *Nat Immunol.* (2008) 9:743–52. doi: 10.1038/ni.1623
148. Foxman EF, Campbell JJ, Butcher EC. Multistep navigation and the combinatorial control of leukocyte chemotaxis. *J Cell Biol.* (1997) 139:1349–60. doi: 10.1083/jcb.139.5.1349
149. Heit B, Tavener S, Raharjo E, Kubes P. An intracellular signaling hierarchy determines direction of migration in opposing chemotactic gradients. *J Cell Biol.* (2002) 159:91–102. doi: 10.1083/jcb.200202114
150. Zehrer A, Pick R, Salvermoser M, Boda A, Miller M, Stark K, et al. A fundamental role of Myh9 for neutrophil migration in innate immunity. *J Immunol.* (2018) 201:1748–64. doi: 10.4049/jimmunol.1701400
151. Huebener P, Pradere JP, Hernandez C, Gwak GY, Caviglia JM, Mu X, et al. The HMGB1/RAGE axis triggers neutrophil-mediated injury amplification following necrosis. *J Clin Invest.* (2015) 125:539–50. doi: 10.1172/JCI 76887
152. Tadie JM, Bae HB, Banerjee S, Zmijewski JW, Abraham E. Differential activation of RAGE by HMGB1 modulates neutrophil-associated NADPH oxidase activity and bacterial killing. *Am J Physiol Cell Physiol.* (2012) 302:C249–56. doi: 10.1152/ajpcell.00302.2011
153. Honda M, Kubes P. Neutrophils and neutrophil extracellular traps in the liver and gastrointestinal system. *Nat Rev Gastroenterol Hepatol.* (2018) 15:206–21. doi: 10.1038/nrgastro.2017.183
154. Bukong TN, Cho Y, Iracheta-Vellve A, Saha B, Lowe P, Adejumo A, et al. Abnormal neutrophil traps and impaired efferocytosis contribute to liver injury and sepsis severity after binge alcohol use. *J Hepatol.* (2018). 69:1145–54. doi: 10.1016/j.jhep.2018.07.005
155. Rensen SS, Bieghs V, Xanthoulea S, Arfianti E, Bakker JA, Shiri-Sverdlov R, et al. Neutrophil-derived myeloperoxidase aggravates non-alcoholic steatohepatitis in low-density lipoprotein receptor-deficient mice. *PLoS ONE.* (2012) 7:e52411. doi: 10.1371/journal.pone.0052411
156. Rensen SS, Slaats Y, Nijhuis J, Jans A, Bieghs V, Driessen A, et al. Increased hepatic myeloperoxidase activity in obese subjects with nonalcoholic steatohepatitis. *Am J Pathol.* (2009) 175:1473–82. doi: 10.2353/ajpath.2009.080999
157. Zang S, Ma X, Zhuang Z, Liu J, Bian D, Xun Y, et al. Increased ratio of neutrophil elastase to alpha1-antitrypsin is closely associated with liver inflammation in patients with nonalcoholic steatohepatitis. *Clin Exp Pharmacol Physiol.* (2016) 43:13–21. doi: 10.1111/1440-1681.12499
158. Saijou E, Enomoto Y, Matsuda M, Yuet-Yin Kok C, Akira S, Tanaka M, et al. Neutrophils alleviate fibrosis in the CCl4-induced mouse chronic liver injury model. *Hepatol Commun.* (2018) 2:703–17. doi: 10.1002/hep4.1178
159. Ou R, Liu J, Lv M, Wang J, Wang J, Zhu L, et al. Neutrophil depletion improves diet-induced non-alcoholic fatty liver disease in mice. *Endocrine.* (2017) 57:72–82. doi: 10.1007/s12020-017-1323-4
160. Wang J, Hossain M, Thanabalasuriar A, Gunzer M, Meininger C, Kubes P. Visualizing the function and fate of neutrophils in sterile injury and repair. *Science.* (2017) 358:111–6. doi: 10.1126/science.aam9690
161. Thomson AW, O'Connell PJ, Steptoe RJ, Lu L. Immunobiology of liver dendritic cells. *Immunol Cell Biol.* (2002) 80:65–73. doi: 10.1046/j.0818-9641.2001.01058.x
162. Kudo S, Matsuno K, Ezaki T, Ogawa M. A novel migration pathway for rat dendritic cells from the blood: hepatic sinusoids-lymph translocation. *J Exp Med.* (1997) 185:777–84. doi: 10.1084/jem.185.4.777
163. Rahman AH, Aloman C. Dendritic cells and liver fibrosis. *Biochim Biophys Acta.* (2013) 1832:998–1004. doi: 10.1016/j.bbadis.2013.01.005
164. Lukacs-Kornek V, Schuppan D. Dendritic cells in liver injury and fibrosis: shortcomings and promises. *J Hepatol.* (2013) 59:1124–6. doi: 10.1016/j.jhep.2013.05.033
165. Goddard S, Youster J, Morgan E, Adams DH. Interleukin-10 secretion differentiates dendritic cells from human liver and skin. *Am J Pathol.* (2004) 164:511–9. doi: 10.1016/S0002-9440(10)63141-0
166. Zhang J, Raper A, Sugita N, Hingorani R, Salio M, Palmowski MJ, et al. Characterization of Siglec-H as a novel endocytic receptor expressed on murine plasmacytoid dendritic cell precursors. *Blood.* (2006) 107:3600–8. doi: 10.1182/blood-2005-09-3842
167. Lai WK, Curbishley SM, Goddard S, Alabraba E, Shaw J, Youster J, et al. Hepatitis C is associated with perturbation of intrahepatic myeloid and plasmacytoid dendritic cell function. *J Hepatol.* (2007) 47:338–47. doi: 10.1016/j.jhep.2007.03.024
168. Collin M, McGovern N, Haniffa M. Human dendritic cell subsets. *Immunology.* (2013) 140:22–30. doi: 10.1111/imm.12117
169. Ibrahim J, Nguyen AH, Rehman A, Ochi A, Jamal M, Graffeo CS, et al. Dendritic cell populations with different concentrations of lipid regulate tolerance and immunity in mouse and human liver. *Gastroenterology.* (2012) 143:1061–72. doi: 10.1053/j.gastro.2012.06.003
170. Strauss O, Dunbar PR, Bartlett A, Phillips A. The immunophenotype of antigen presenting cells of the mononuclear phagocyte system in normal human liver–a systematic review. *J Hepatol.* (2015) 62:458–68. doi: 10.1016/j.jhep.2014.10.006
171. Zhu J, Yamane H, Paul WE. Differentiation of effector CD4 T cell populations (*). *Ann Rev Immunol.* (2010) 28:445–89. doi: 10.1146/annurev-immunol-030409-101212
172. Jurgens B, Hainz U, Fuchs D, Felzmann T, Heitger A. Interferon-gamma-triggered indoleamine 2,3-dioxygenase competence in human monocyte-derived dendritic cells induces regulatory activity in allogeneic T cells. *Blood.* (2009) 114:3235–43. doi: 10.1182/blood-2008-12-195073
173. Frumento G, Rotondo R, Tonetti M, Damonte G, Benatti U, Ferrara GB. Tryptophan-derived catabolites are responsible for inhibition of T and natural killer cell proliferation induced by indoleamine 2,3-dioxygenase. *J Exp Med.* (2002) 196:459–68. doi: 10.1084/jem.20020121
174. Castellaneta A, Sumpter TL, Chen L, Tokita D, Thomson AW. NOD2 ligation subverts IFN-alpha production by liver plasmacytoid dendritic cells and inhibits their T cell allostimulatory activity via B7-H1 up-regulation. *J Immunol.* (2009) 183:6922–32. doi: 10.4049/jimmunol.0900582
175. Thomson AW, Knolle PA. Antigen-presenting cell function in the tolerogenic liver environment. *Nat Rev Immunol.* (2010) 10:753–66. doi: 10.1038/nri2858
176. Wang J, Cao X, Zhao J, Zhao H, Wei J, Li Q, et al. Critical roles of conventional dendritic cells in promoting T cell-dependent hepatitis through regulating natural killer T cells. *Clin Exp Immunol.* (2017) 188:127–37. doi: 10.1111/cei.12907
177. Connolly MK, Ayo D, Malhotra A, Hackman M, Bedrosian AS, Ibrahim J, et al. Dendritic cell depletion exacerbates acetaminophen hepatotoxicity. *Hepatology.* (2011) 54:959–68. doi: 10.1002/hep.24429
178. Henning JR, Graffeo CS, Rehman A, Fallon NC, Zambirinis CP, Ochi A, et al. Dendritic cells limit fibroinflammatory injury in nonalcoholic steatohepatitis in mice. *Hepatology.* (2013) 58:589–602. doi: 10.1002/hep.26267
179. Heier EC, Meier A, Julich-Haertel H, Djudjaj S, Rau M, Tschernig T, et al. Murine CD103(+) dendritic cells protect against steatosis progression towards steatohepatitis. *J Hepatol.* (2017) 66:1241–50. doi: 10.1016/j.jhep.2017.01.008

180. Velazquez VM, Hon H, Ibegbu C, Knechtle SJ, Kirk AD, Grakoui A. Hepatic enrichment and activation of myeloid dendritic cells during chronic hepatitis C virus infection. *Hepatology.* (2012) 56:2071–81. doi: 10.1002/hep.25904
181. Cervantes-Barragan L, Lewis KL, Firner S, Thiel V, Hugues S, Reith W, et al. Plasmacytoid dendritic cells control T-cell response to chronic viral infection. *Proc Natl Acad Sci USA.* (2012) 109:3012–7. doi: 10.1073/pnas.1117359109
182. Lee J, Suh WI, Shin EC. T-cell dysfunction and inhibitory receptors in hepatitis C virus infection. *Immune Netw.* (2010) 10:120–5. doi: 10.4110/in.2010.10.4.120
183. Pradere JP, Kluwe J, De Minicis S, Jiao JJ, Gwak GY, Dapito DH, et al. Hepatic macrophages but not dendritic cells contribute to liver fibrosis by promoting the survival of activated hepatic stellate cells in mice. *Hepatology.* (2013) 58:1461–73. doi: 10.1002/hep.26429
184. Connolly MK, Bedrosian AS, Mallen-St Clair J, Mitchell AP, Ibrahim J, Stroud A, et al. In liver fibrosis, dendritic cells govern hepatic inflammation in mice via TNF-alpha. *J Clin Invest.* (2009) 119:3213–25. doi: 10.1172/JCI37581
185. Jiao J, Sastre D, Fiel MI, Lee UE, Ghiassi-Nejad Z, Ginhoux F, et al. Dendritic cell regulation of carbon tetrachloride-induced murine liver fibrosis regression. *Hepatology.* (2012) 55:244–55. doi: 10.1002/hep.24621
186. Blois SM, Piccioni F, Freitag N, Tirado-Gonzalez I, Moschansky P, Lloyd R, et al. Dendritic cells regulate angiogenesis associated with liver fibrogenesis. *Angiogenesis.* (2014) 17:119–28. doi: 10.1007/s10456-013-9382-5
187. Ramachandran P, Iredale JP, Fallowfield JA. Resolution of liver fibrosis: basic mechanisms and clinical relevance. *Semin Liver Dis.* (2015) 35:119–31. doi: 10.1055/s-0035-1550057
188. Yoshiji H, Kuriyama S, Yoshii J, Ikenaka Y, Noguchi R, Nakatani T, et al. Tissue inhibitor of metalloproteinases-1 attenuates spontaneous liver fibrosis resolution in the transgenic mouse. *Hepatology.* (2002) 36:850–60. doi: 10.1053/jhep.2002.35625
189. Iredale JP, Benyon RC, Pickering J, McCullen M, Northrop M, Pawley S, et al. Mechanisms of spontaneous resolution of rat liver fibrosis. Hepatic stellate cell apoptosis and reduced hepatic expression of metalloproteinase inhibitors. *J Clin Invest.* (1998) 102:538–49. doi: 10.1172/JCI1018
190. Issa R, Williams E, Trim N, Kendall T, Arthur MJ, Reichen J, et al. Apoptosis of hepatic stellate cells: involvement in resolution of biliary fibrosis and regulation by soluble growth factors. *Gut.* (2001) 48:548–57. doi: 10.1136/gut.48.4.548
191. Ellis EL, Mann DA. Clinical evidence for the regression of liver fibrosis. *J Hepatol.* (2012) 56:1171–80. doi: 10.1016/j.jhep.2011.09.024
192. Marcellin P, Gane E, Buti M, Afdhal N, Sievert W, Jacobson IM, et al. Regression of cirrhosis during treatment with tenofovir disoproxil fumarate for chronic hepatitis B: a 5-year open-label follow-up study. *Lancet.* (2013) 381:468–75. doi: 10.1016/S0140-6736(12)61425-1
193. Bartneck M, Fech V, Ehling J, Govaere O, Warzecha KT, Hittatiya K, et al. Histidine-rich glycoprotein promotes macrophage activation and inflammation in chronic liver disease. *Hepatology.* (2016) 63:1310–24. doi: 10.1002/hep.28418
194. Preisser L, Miot C, Le Guillou-Guillemette H, Beaumont E, Foucher ED, Garo E, et al. IL-34 and macrophage colony-stimulating factor are overexpressed in hepatitis C virus fibrosis and induce profibrotic macrophages that promote collagen synthesis by hepatic stellate cells. *Hepatology.* (2014) 60:1879–90. doi: 10.1002/hep.27328
195. Wiest R, Lawson M, Geuking M. Pathological bacterial translocation in liver cirrhosis. *J Hepatol.* (2014) 60:197–209. doi: 10.1016/j.jhep.2013.07.044
196. Aoyama T, Paik YH, Seki E. Toll-like receptor signaling and liver fibrosis. *Gastroenterol Res Pract.* (2010) 2010:8. doi: 10.1155/2010/192543
197. Seki E, De Minicis S, Osterreicher CH, Kluwe J, Osawa Y, Brenner DA, et al. TLR4 enhances TGF-beta signaling and hepatic fibrosis. *Nat Med.* (2007) 13:1324–32. doi: 10.1038/nm1663
198. Nguyen-Lefebvre AT, Ajith A, Portik-Dobos V, Horuzsko DD, Arbab AS, Dzutsev A, et al. The innate immune receptor TREM-1 promotes liver injury and fibrosis. *J Clin Invest.* (2018) 128:4870–83. doi: 10.1172/JCI98156
199. Tornai D, Furi I, Shen ZT, Sigalov AB, Coban S, Szabo G. Inhibition of triggering receptor expressed on myeloid cells 1 ameliorates inflammation and macrophage and neutrophil activation in alcoholic liver disease in mice. *Hepatol Commun.* (2019) 3:99–115. doi: 10.1002/hep4.1269
200. Seki E, de Minicis S, Inokuchi S, Taura K, Miyai K, van Rooijen N, et al. CCR2 promotes hepatic fibrosis in mice. *Hepatology.* (2009) 50:185–97. doi: 10.1002/hep.22952
201. Seki E, De Minicis S, Gwak GY, Kluwe J, Inokuchi S, Bursill CA, et al. CCR1 and CCR5 promote hepatic fibrosis in mice. *J Clin Invest.* (2009) 119:1858–70. doi: 10.1172/JCI37444
202. Berres ML, Koenen RR, Rueland A, Zaldivar MM, Heinrichs D, Sahin H, et al. Antagonism of the chemokine Ccl5 ameliorates experimental liver fibrosis in mice. *J Clin Invest.* (2010) 120:4129–40. doi: 10.1172/JCI 41732
203. Sasaki R, Devhare PB, Steele R, Ray R, Ray RB. Hepatitis C virus-induced CCL5 secretion from macrophages activates hepatic stellate cells. *Hepatology.* (2017) 66:746–57. doi: 10.1002/hep.29170
204. Heinrichs D, Berres ML, Nellen A, Fischer P, Scholten D, Trautwein C, et al. The chemokine CCL3 promotes experimental liver fibrosis in mice. *PLoS ONE.* (2013) 8:e66106. doi: 10.1371/journal.pone.0066106
205. Rantakari P, Patten DA, Valtonen J, Karikoski M, Gerke H, Dawes H, et al. Stabilin-1 expression defines a subset of macrophages that mediate tissue homeostasis and prevent fibrosis in chronic liver injury. *Proc Natl Acad Sci USA.* (2016) 113:9298–303. doi: 10.1073/pnas.1604780113
206. Imamura M, Ogawa T, Sasaguri Y, Chayama K, Ueno H. Suppression of macrophage infiltration inhibits activation of hepatic stellate cells and liver fibrogenesis in rats. *Gastroenterology.* (2005) 128:138–46. doi: 10.1053/j.gastro.2004.10.005
207. Mitchell C, Couton D, Couty JP, Anson M, Crain AM, Bizet V, et al. Dual role of CCR2 in the constitution and the resolution of liver fibrosis in mice. *Am J Pathol.* (2009) 174:1766–75. doi: 10.2353/ajpath.2009.080632
208. Krenkel O, Puengel T, Govaere O, Abdallah AT, Mossanen JC, Kohlhepp M, et al. Therapeutic inhibition of inflammatory monocyte recruitment reduces steatohepatitis and liver fibrosis. *Hepatology.* (2018) 67:1270–83. doi: 10.1002/hep.29544
209. Lefebvre E, Moyle G, Reshef R, Richman LP, Thompson M, Hong F, et al. Antifibrotic effects of the dual CCR2/CCR5 antagonist cenicriviroc in animal models of liver and kidney fibrosis. *PLoS ONE.* (2016) 11:e0158156. doi: 10.1371/journal.pone.0158156
210. Kruger AJ, Fuchs BC, Masia R, Holmes JA, Salloum S, Sojoodi M, et al. Prolonged cenicriviroc therapy reduces hepatic fibrosis despite steatohepatitis in a diet-induced mouse model of nonalcoholic steatohepatitis. *Hepatol Commun.* (2018) 2:529–45. doi: 10.1002/hep4.1160
211. Baeck C, Wei X, Bartneck M, Fech V, Heymann F, Gassler N, et al. Pharmacological inhibition of the chemokine C-C motif chemokine ligand 2 (monocyte chemoattractant protein 1) accelerates liver fibrosis regression by suppressing Ly-6C(+) macrophage infiltration in mice. *Hepatology.* (2014) 59:1060–72. doi: 10.1002/hep.26783
212. Friedman SL, Ratziu V, Harrison SA, Abdelmalek MF, Aithal GP, Caballeria J, et al. A randomized, placebo-controlled trial of cenicriviroc for treatment of nonalcoholic steatohepatitis with fibrosis. *Hepatology.* (2018) 67:1754–67. doi: 10.1002/hep.29477
213. Chu PS, Nakamoto N, Ebinuma H, Usui S, Saeki K, Matsumoto A, et al. C-C motif chemokine receptor 9 positive macrophages activate hepatic stellate cells and promote liver fibrosis in mice. *Hepatology.* (2013) 58:337–50. doi: 10.1002/hep.26351
214. Bataller R, Brenner DA. Liver fibrosis. *J Clin Invest.* (2005) 115:209–18. doi: 10.1172/JCI24282
215. Li H, Zheng HW, Chen H, Xing ZZ, You H, Cong M, et al. Hepatitis B virus particles preferably induce Kupffer cells to produce TGF-beta1 over pro-inflammatory cytokines. *Digest Liver Dis.* (2012) 44:328–33. doi: 10.1016/j.dld.2011.11.005
216. Henderson NC, Mackinnon AC, Farnworth SL, Poirier F, Russo FP, Iredale JP, et al. Galectin-3 regulates myofibroblast activation and hepatic fibrosis. *Proc Natl Acad Sci USA.* (2006) 103:5060–5. doi: 10.1073/pnas.0511167103
217. Wynn TA, Barron L. Macrophages: master regulators of inflammation and fibrosis. *Semin Liver Dis.* (2010) 30:245–57. doi: 10.1055/s-0030-12 55354
218. Matsuda M, Tsurusaki S, Miyata N, Saijou E, Okochi H, Miyajima A, et al. Oncostatin M causes liver fibrosis by regulating cooperation between hepatic stellate cells and macrophages in mice. *Hepatology.* (2018) 67:296–312. doi: 10.1002/hep.29421

219. Duffield JS, Forbes SJ, Constandinou CM, Clay S, Partolina M, Vuthoori S, et al. Selective depletion of macrophages reveals distinct, opposing roles during liver injury and repair. *J Clin Invest.* (2005) 115:56–65. doi: 10.1172/JCI200522675
220. Fallowfield JA, Mizuno M, Kendall TJ, Constandinou CM, Benyon RC, Duffield JS, et al. Scar-associated macrophages are a major source of hepatic matrix metalloproteinase-13 and facilitate the resolution of murine hepatic fibrosis. *J Immunol.* (2007) 178:5288–95. doi: 10.4049/jimmunol.178.8.5288
221. Aoyama T, Inokuchi S, Brenner DA, Seki E. CX3CL1-CX3CR1 interaction prevents carbon tetrachloride-induced liver inflammation and fibrosis in mice. *Hepatology.* (2010) 52:1390–400. doi: 10.1002/hep.23795
222. Karlmark KR, Zimmermann HW, Roderburg C, Gassler N, Wasmuth HE, Luedde T, et al. The fractalkine receptor CX(3)CR1 protects against liver fibrosis by controlling differentiation and survival of infiltrating hepatic monocytes. *Hepatology.* (2010) 52:1769–82. doi: 10.1002/hep.23894
223. Nahrendorf M, Swirski FK, Aikawa E, Stangenberg L, Wurdinger T, Figueiredo JL, et al. The healing myocardium sequentially mobilizes two monocyte subsets with divergent and complementary functions. *J Exp Med.* (2007) 204:3037–47. doi: 10.1084/jem.20070885
224. Landsman L, Varol C, Jung S. Distinct differentiation potential of blood monocyte subsets in the lung. *J Immunol.* (2007) 178:2000–7. doi: 10.4049/jimmunol.178.4.2000
225. Ziegler-Heitbrock L, Hofer TP. Toward a refined definition of monocyte subsets. *Front Immunol.* (2013) 4:23. doi: 10.3389/fimmu.2013.00023
226. Thorgeirsson SS, Grisham JW. Molecular pathogenesis of human hepatocellular carcinoma. *Nat Genet.* (2002) 31:339–46. doi: 10.1038/ng0802-339
227. Kang TW, Yevsa T, Woller N, Hoenicke L, Wuestefeld T, Dauch D, et al. Senescence surveillance of pre-malignant hepatocytes limits liver cancer development. *Nature.* (2011) 479:547–51. doi: 10.1038/nature10599
228. Eggert T, Wolter K, Ji J, Ma C, Yevsa T, Klotz S, et al. Distinct functions of senescence-associated immune responses in liver tumor surveillance and tumor progression. *Cancer Cell.* (2016) 30:533–47. doi: 10.1016/j.ccell.2016.09.003
229. Ding T, Xu J, Wang F, Shi M, Zhang Y, Li SP, et al. High tumor-infiltrating macrophage density predicts poor prognosis in patients with primary hepatocellular carcinoma after resection. *Hum Pathol.* (2009) 40:381–9. doi: 10.1016/j.humpath.2008.08.011
230. Zhu XD, Zhang JB, Zhuang PY, Zhu HG, Zhang W, Xiong YQ, et al. High expression of macrophage colony-stimulating factor in peritumoral liver tissue is associated with poor survival after curative resection of hepatocellular carcinoma. *J Clin Oncol.* (2008) 26:2707–16. doi: 10.1200/JCO.2007.15.6521
231. Foerster F, Hess M, Gerhold-Ay A, Marquardt JU, Becker D, Galle PR, et al. The immune contexture of hepatocellular carcinoma predicts clinical outcome. *Sci Rep.* (2018) 8:5351. doi: 10.1038/s41598-018-21937-2
232. Pikarsky E, Porat RM, Stein I, Abramovitch R, Amit S, Kasem S, et al. NF-kappaB functions as a tumour promoter in inflammation-associated cancer. *Nature.* (2004) 431:461–6. doi: 10.1038/nature 02924
233. Maeda S, Kamata H, Luo JL, Leffert H, Karin M. IKKbeta couples hepatocyte death to cytokine-driven compensatory proliferation that promotes chemical hepatocarcinogenesis. *Cell.* (2005) 121:977–90. doi: 10.1016/j.cell.2005.04.014
234. Wan S, Zhao E, Kryczek I, Vatan L, Sadovskaya A, Ludema G, et al. Tumor-associated macrophages produce interleukin 6 and signal via STAT3 to promote expansion of human hepatocellular carcinoma stem cells. *Gastroenterology.* (2014) 147:1393–404. doi: 10.1053/j.gastro.2014.08.039
235. Wu J, Li J, Salcedo R, Mivechi NF, Trinchieri G, Horuzsko A. The proinflammatory myeloid cell receptor TREM-1 controls Kupffer cell activation and development of hepatocellular carcinoma. *Cancer Res.* (2012) 72:3977–86. doi: 10.1158/0008-5472.CAN-12-0938
236. Delire B, Henriet P, Lemoine P, Leclercq IA, Starkel P. Chronic liver injury promotes hepatocarcinoma cell seeding and growth, associated with infiltration by macrophages. *Cancer Sci.* (2018) 109:2141–52. doi: 10.1111/cas.13628
237. Yeung OW, Lo CM, Ling CC, Qi X, Geng W, Li CX, et al. Alternatively activated (M2) macrophages promote tumour growth and invasiveness in hepatocellular carcinoma. *J Hepatol.* (2015) 62:607–16. doi: 10.1016/j.jhep.2014.10.029
238. Takai H, Ashihara M, Ishiguro T, Terashima H, Watanabe T, Kato A, et al. Involvement of glypican-3 in the recruitment of M2-polarized tumor-associated macrophages in hepatocellular carcinoma. *Cancer Biol Ther.* (2009) 8:2329–38. doi: 10.4161/cbt.8.24.9985
239. Yang Y, Ye YC, Chen Y, Zhao JL, Gao CC, Han H, et al. Crosstalk between hepatic tumor cells and macrophages via Wnt/beta-catenin signaling promotes M2-like macrophage polarization and reinforces tumor malignant behaviors. *Cell Death Dis.* (2018) 9:793. doi: 10.1038/s41419-018-0818-0
240. Ye Y, Xu Y, Lai Y, He W, Li Y, Wang R, et al. Long non-coding RNA cox-2 prevents immune evasion and metastasis of hepatocellular carcinoma by altering M1/M2 macrophage polarization. *J Cell Biochem.* (2018) 119:2951–63. doi: 10.1002/jcb.26509
241. Yan W, Liu X, Ma H, Zhang H, Song X, Gao L, et al. Tim-3 fosters HCC development by enhancing TGF-beta-mediated alternative activation of macrophages. *Gut.* (2015) 64:1593–604. doi: 10.1136/gutjnl-2014-307671
242. Rohr-Udilova N, Klinglmuller F, Schulte-Hermann R, Stift J, Herac M, Salzmann M, et al. Deviations of the immune cell landscape between healthy liver and hepatocellular carcinoma. *Sci Rep.* (2018) 8:6220. doi: 10.1038/s41598-018-24437-5
243. Li X, Yao W, Yuan Y, Chen P, Li B, Li J, et al. Targeting of tumour-infiltrating macrophages via CCL2/CCR2 signalling as a therapeutic strategy against hepatocellular carcinoma. *Gut.* (2017) 66:157–67. doi: 10.1136/gutjnl-2015-310514
244. Zhou SL, Zhou ZJ, Hu ZQ, Huang XW, Wang Z, Chen EB, et al. Tumor-associated neutrophils recruit macrophages and T-regulatory cells to promote progression of hepatocellular carcinoma and resistance to sorafenib. *Gastroenterology.* (2016) 150:1646–58e17. doi: 10.1053/j.gastro.2016.02.040
245. van der Windt DJ, Sud V, Zhang H, Varley PR, Goswami J, Yazdani HO, et al. Neutrophil extracellular traps promote inflammation and development of hepatocellular carcinoma in nonalcoholic steatohepatitis. *Hepatology.* (2018). 68:1347–60. doi: 10.1002/hep.29914
246. Kuang DM, Zhao Q, Peng C, Xu J, Zhang JP, Wu C, et al. Activated monocytes in peritumoral stroma of hepatocellular carcinoma foster immune privilege and disease progression through PD-L1. *J Exp Med.* (2009) 206:1327–37. doi: 10.1084/jem.20082173
247. Lens S, Alvarado-Tapias E, Marino Z, Londono MC, E LL, Martinez J, et al. Effects of all-oral anti-viral therapy on HVPG and systemic hemodynamics in patients with hepatitis C virus-associated cirrhosis. *Gastroenterology.* (2017) 153:1273–83e1. doi: 10.1053/j.gastro.2017.07.016
248. Tacke F. Targeting hepatic macrophages to treat liver diseases. *J Hepatol.* (2017) 66:1300–12. doi: 10.1016/j.jhep.2017.02.026
249. Sakaida I, Terai S, Yamamoto N, Aoyama K, Ishikawa T, Nishina H, et al. Transplantation of bone marrow cells reduces CCl4-induced liver fibrosis in mice. *Hepatology.* (2004) 40:1304–11. doi: 10.1002/hep.20452
250. Thomas JA, Pope C, Wojtacha D, Robson AJ, Gordon-Walker TT, Hartland S, et al. Macrophage therapy for murine liver fibrosis recruits host effector cells improving fibrosis, regeneration, and function. *Hepatology.* (2011) 53:2003–15. doi: 10.1002/hep.24315
251. Suh YG, Kim JK, Byun JS, Yi HS, Lee YS, Eun HS, et al. CD11b(+) Gr1(+) bone marrow cells ameliorate liver fibrosis by producing interleukin-10 in mice. *Hepatology.* (2012) 56:1902–12. doi: 10.1002/hep.25817
252. de Souza VCA, Pereira TA, Teixeira VW, Carvalho H, de Castro M, D'Assuncao C G, et al. Bone marrow-derived monocyte infusion improves hepatic fibrosis by decreasing osteopontin, TGF-beta1, IL-13 and oxidative stress. *World J Gastroenterol.* (2017) 23:5146–57. doi: 10.3748/wjg.v23.i28.5146
253. Haideri SS, McKinnon AC, Taylor AH, Kirkwood P, Starkey Lewis PJ, O'Duibhir E, et al. Injection of embryonic stem cell derived macrophages ameliorates fibrosis in a murine model of liver injury. *NPJ Regen Med.* (2017) 2:14. doi: 10.1038/s41536-017-0017-0

254. Yang L, Han Z, Tian L, Mai P, Zhang Y, Wang L, et al. Sphingosine 1-phosphate receptor 2 and 3 mediate bone marrow-derived monocyte/macrophage motility in cholestatic liver injury in mice. *Sci. Rep.* (2015) 5:13423. doi: 10.1038/srep13423
255. King A, Houlihan DD, Kavanagh D, Haldar D, Luu N, Owen A, et al. Sphingosine-1-phosphate prevents egress of hematopoietic stem cells from liver to reduce fibrosis. *Gastroenterology.* (2017) 153:233–48e16. doi: 10.1053/j.gastro.2017.03.022
256. Newsome PN, Fox R, King AL, Barton D, Than NN, Moore J, et al. Granulocyte colony-stimulating factor and autologous CD133-positive stem-cell therapy in liver cirrhosis (REALISTIC): an open-label, randomised, controlled phase 2 trial. *Lancet Gastroenterol Hepatol.* (2018) 3:25–36. doi: 10.1016/S2468-1253(17)30326-6
257. Thomas JA, Ramachandran P, Forbes SJ. Studies of macrophage therapy for cirrhosis - From mice to men. *J Hepatol.* (2018) 68:1090–1. doi: 10.1016/j.jhep.2017.11.043
258. Fraser AR, Pass C, Burgoyne P, Atkinson A, Bailey L, Laurie A, et al. Development, functional characterization and validation of methodology for GMP-compliant manufacture of phagocytic macrophages: A novel cellular therapeutic for liver cirrhosis. *Cytotherapy.* (2017) 19:1113–24. doi: 10.1016/j.jcyt.2017.05.009

9

Macrophage Phenotype and Function in Liver Disorder

Lang Dou [1,2,3], *Xiaomin Shi* [1,2,3], *Xiaoshun He* [1,2,3] *and Yifang Gao* [1,2,3]*

[1] *Organ Transplantation Center, The First Affiliated Hospital, Sun Yat-sen University, Guangzhou, China,* [2] *Guangdong Provincial Key Laboratory of Organ Donation and Transplant Immunology, The First Affiliated Hospital, Sun Yat-sen University, Guangzhou, China,* [3] *Guangdong Provincial International Cooperation Base of Science and Technology (Organ Transplantation), The First Affiliated Hospital, Sun Yat-sen University, Guangzhou, China*

Correspondence:
Yifang Gao
gaoyf26@sysu.edu.cn

Hepatic macrophages are a remarkably heterogeneous population consisting of self-renewing tissue-resident phagocytes, termed Kupffer cells (KCs), and recruited macrophages derived from peritoneal cavity as well as the bone marrow. KCs are located in the liver sinusoid where they scavenge the microbe from the portal vein to maintain liver homeostasis. Liver injury may trigger hepatic recruitment of peritoneal macrophages and monocyte-derived macrophages. Studies describing macrophage accumulation have shown that hepatic macrophages are involved in the initiation and progression of various liver diseases. They act as tolerogenic antigen-presenting cells to inhibit T-cell activation by producing distinct sets of cytokines, chemokines, and mediators to maintain or resolve inflammation. Furthermore, by releasing regenerative growth factors, matrix metalloproteinase arginase, they promote tissue repair. Recent experiments found that KCs and recruited macrophages may play different roles in the development of liver disease. Given that hepatic macrophages are considerably plastic populations, their phenotypes and functions are likely switching along disease progression. In this review, we summarize current knowledge about the role of tissue-resident macrophages and recruited macrophages in pathogenesis of alcoholic liver disease (ALD), non-alcoholic steatohepatitis (NASH), viral hepatitis, and hepatocellular carcinoma (HCC).

Keywords: hepatic macrophages, Kupffer cells, alcoholic liver disease, hepatocellular carcinoma, viral hepatitis, non-alcoholic steatohepatitis

INTRODUCTION

Hepatic macrophages, consisting of Kupffer cells (KCs) and recruited macrophages, are the largest population of innate immune cells in the liver. In the healthy rodent liver, macrophages comprise around 20–25% of non-parenchymal cells (1, 2); the high occupancy implies that the hepatic macrophages play a vital role in maintaining liver function and homeostasis. KCs, self-renewing tissue-resident phagocytes, are located in the liver sinusoids. During homeostasis, distinct Fc and scavenger receptors are expressed on the KC surface, which allows them to recognize modified self-molecules, resulting in clearing of apoptotic cells, cell debris, and immune complex (3, 4). Additionally, KCs are involved in controlling the iron (5), cholesterol (6), and bilirubin (7) balance of the blood. KCs also express a wide range of pattern recognition receptors (PRRs), including toll-like receptors (TLRs) (8), nucleotide oligomerization (NOD)-like receptors (9), and retinoic acid-inducible gene I (RIG-I)-like receptors (10). These receptors assist KCs to recognize and eliminate invading foreign pathogens.

Hepatic macrophages form highly heterogeneous populations, and several markers have been used to distinguish between KCs and recruited macrophages. In mice, KCs were found to express a unique maker C-Type Lectin Domain Family 4 Member F (CLEC4F) and can be characterized as CD11b+, F4/80+, TIM4+, and CLEC4F+ cell populations (11). The bone-marrow-derived macrophages are CD11b+, F4/80+, CCR2+, and CX3CR1+. MacParland et al. showed that human hepatic macrophages could be classified as CD68+ MACRO+ KCs and CD68+ MACRO− recruited macrophages in the steady state using single-cell analysis (12). According to activation programs, hepatic macrophages can be broadly divided into classically activated pro-inflammatory and alternatively activated anti-inflammatory phenotypes (13, 14). Pro-inflammatory macrophage stimuli lipopolysaccharide (LPS) and interferon (IFN)-γ activate signal transducers and activators of transcription (STAT)1, myeloid differentiation factor 88 (MyD88), Toll-interleukin 1 receptor domain containing adaptor protein (MaL/Tirap), and IFN regulatory factor (IRF)-dependent pathways, resulting in the release of interleukin (IL)-1β, IL-6, tumor necrosis factor (TNF), reactive oxygen species (ROS), and nitric oxide synthase (14–16). These macrophages are likely to contribute to hepatic inflammation and damage in distinct liver diseases. Anti-inflammatory macrophages exhibit high phagocytic capacity and produce high levels of arginase 1 as well as IL-10 via activating Janus kinase (JAK)1 and JAK3; they are featured by immunoregulation and tissue remodeling (14, 16).

It has been suggested that hepatic macrophages have two origins (17, 18): recruited macrophages derived from the hematopoietic stem cells and tissue-resident macrophages from the yolk sac. HSC-derived macrophages differentiate from circulating myeloid precursor cells from the bone marrow; this process is mediated by colony-stimulating factor (CSF)-1 (17, 18). The majority of KCs are believed to develop from the yolk sac before the appearance of HSCs (18). However, this theory has been challenged by a recent study that revealed a common progenitor for tissue-resident macrophages, called premacrophages, which were generated early in development and had colonized the whole embryo from embryonic day 9.5. Tissue-specific sets of transcriptional regulators control the differentiation of premacrophages into tissue-resident macrophages, whereby the development of KCs is regulated by Id3, a transcription factor inhibitor of DNA binding 3, and inactivation of Id3 causes KC deficiency in adults (19).

Hepatic recruited macrophages are derived from not only circulating monocytes but also macrophages of different compartments. Circulating monocytes are classified into CD11b+Ly6C^{hi} (20) and CD11b+Ly6C^{low} (21) in mice. CD11b+Ly6C^{hi} subsets can infiltrate into the liver during inflammation (20), whereas the Ly6C^{low} monocytes serve as sentinels to scavenge microparticles and cell debris in the capillaries (21). Monocytes may downregulate Ly6C expression after infiltration and before differentiation (22). Recent findings suggest that self-reviewing peritoneal cavity macrophages, characterized by F4/80^{hi}GATA6+, can rapidly migrate to the liver through the mesothelium in response to a sterile injury (23). This result suggests that the composition of hepatic macrophages may be more complicated than expected. Numerous studies have shown that hepatic macrophages are involved in the progression of inflammation and fibrosis and, therefore, hold the key to controlling the pathogenesis of liver disease (14, 15, 24). In this review, we will summarize current knowledge about hepatic macrophages in pathogenesis of alcoholic liver disease (ALD), non-alcoholic steatohepatitis (NASH), hepatitis B virus/hepatitis C virus (HBV/HCV), and hepatocellular carcinoma (HCC) with a particular focus on KCs and monocyte-derived macrophages.

HEPATIC MACROPHAGES IN ALD

Chronic alcohol consumption, the primary cause of ALD, results in a broad range of disorders, including liver steatosis, alcoholic hepatitis, chronic hepatitis, HCC, liver fibrosis, and/or cirrhosis (25–27). It has been documented that hepatic macrophages accumulate within the portal tracts of ALD patients (28), whereas the depletion of hepatic macrophages via the administration of gadolinium chloride ($GdCl_3$) prevents alcohol-induced liver inflammation in the rat (29). These results suggest that hepatic macrophages play a central role in the pathogenesis of ALD.

One hypothesis for this effect is that ethanol ingestion disrupts the intestinal barrier, which increases the permeability of the gut, thereby enhancing the migration of Gram-negative bacteria into the portal circulation (30, 31) and leading to ALD pathogenesis. The ligation of LPS with the CD14/TLR4 receptor complex on KCs triggers the downstream IL-1 receptor-associated kinase (IRAK) and inhibitor of nuclear factor kappa-B kinase (IKK) pathways, resulting in the release of the inflammatory cytokines IL-6 and TNF-α and chemokines, such as monocyte chemoattractant protein (MCP-1) (32) (**Figure 1A**). These mediators augment inflammation and alcohol-induced liver injury in ALD (32). Compared with wild-type (WT) mice, alcohol-fed mice are more sensitive to LPS and produce more MCP-1 (33) and TNF-α (34) post stimulation. Recent studies showed that a small non-coding RNA, termed microRNA (miRNA), is involved in regulating macrophage infiltration, activation, and ALD progression (**Figure 1A**). Unbiased analysis of miRNA revealed that miR181b-3p released by KCs regulated TLR4 signaling during ethanol consumption (35). In ethanol-fed rats, the overexpression of miR181b-3p inhibited importin α5 expression and suppressed LPS-induced TNF-α expression in KCs (35). In a study in mice, chronic alcohol feeding promoted miR-155 production by KCs via the nuclear factor kappa-light-chain-enhancer of activated B cells (NF-κB) pathway (36). A later study revealed that macrophage infiltration induced by chronic alcohol consumption was reduced in miR-155-deficient mice (37). In the same study, knockout of miR-155 also alleviated the inflammation and steatosis triggered by chronic alcohol ingestion (37).

During ALD, hepatocytes injured by alcohol consumption can activate KCs. Acute and chronic ethanol exposure stimulates KCs via danger-associated molecular patterns produced by injured hepatocytes (38) (**Figure 1A**). Additionally, Verma et al. found that ethanol exposure stimulated hepatocytes to produce considerably more CD40L-containing extracellular

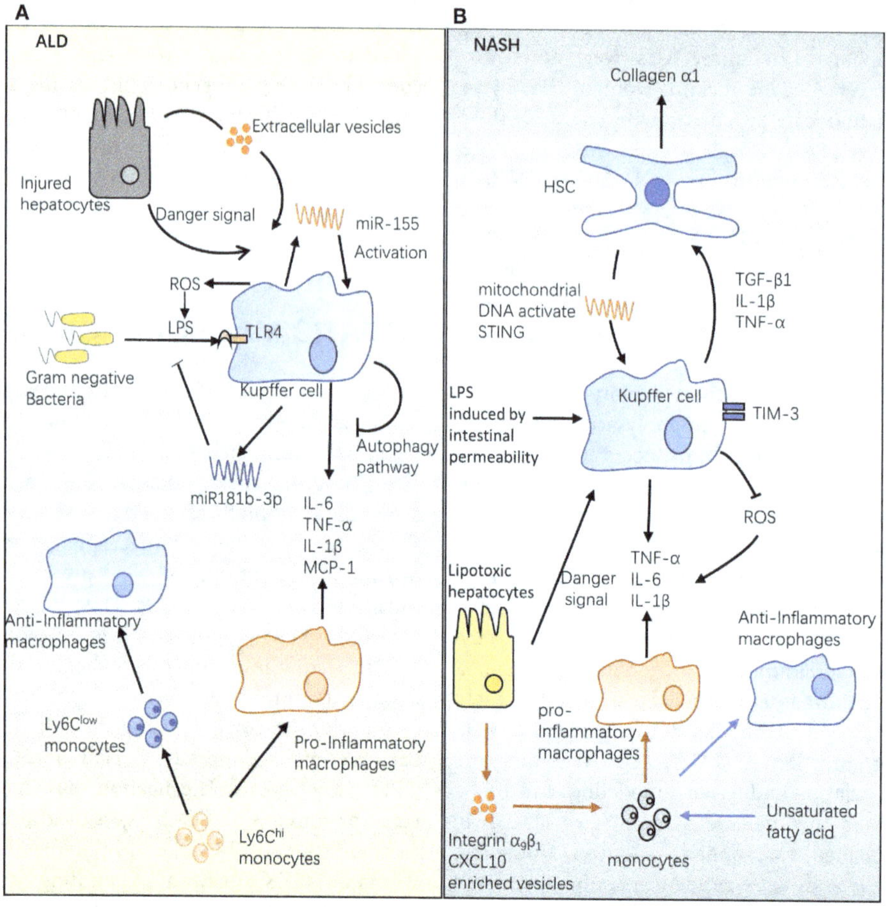

FIGURE 1 | Hepatic macrophages in alcoholic liver disease (ALD) and non-alcoholic steatohepatitis (NASH). **(A)** The role of hepatic macrophages in ALD. Chronic alcohol consumption disrupts the intestinal barrier, which increases the permeability of the gut and allows Gram-negative bacteria to migrate into the portal circulation. Lipopolysaccharide (LPS) expressed on Gram-negative bacteria activates Kupffer cells (KCs) and promotes interleukin (IL)-6, tumor necrosis factor (TNF)-α, IL-1β, and monocyte chemoattractant protein (MCP)-1 release. Hepatocytes injured by alcohol consumption activate KCs via danger signal and CD40-containing extracellular vesicles. Chronic alcohol ingestion induces microRNA (miR)-155 and miR181b-3p expression; the former activates KCs and promotes inflammatory production, while the latter regulates LPS-induced inflammation. The Ly6C^{hi} monocyte can differentiate into pro-inflammatory and anti-inflammatory macrophages during ALD, and the ratio of these two populations may mediate ALD development. **(B)** The role of hepatic macrophages in NASH. High levels of LPS induced by increasing intestinal permeability and/or danger signal from lipotoxic hepatocytes stimulate KCs; activated KCs produce the survival signals, transforming growth factor β, IL-1β, and TNF-α, which stimulate hepatic stellate cells and increase generation of hepatic collagen α1, ultimately triggering fibrosis. Mitochondrial DNA from hepatocytes of high-fat diet (HFD)-fed mice activates KCs and promotes cytokine release, steatosis, and inflammation. Conversely, TIM-3 expressed on hepatic macrophages protects animals from HFD-induced NASH by inhibiting reactive oxygen species production. An HFD augments the infiltration of bone-marrow-derived monocytes into the liver and further differentiates them into protective anti-inflammatory macrophages.

vesicles in a caspase-3-dependent manner, ultimately triggering macrophage activation and production of MCP-1, TNF-α, and ROS (39) (**Figure 1A**). Genetic knockout of CD40 (CD40-/-) or the caspase-activating TNF-related apoptosis-inducing ligand (TRAIL) receptor (TR-/-) protected mice from alcohol-induced injury (39). Notably, during alcohol exposure, KCs are a major source of ROS, which is essential for LPS sensitization (40) and inflammatory cytokine production (41) (**Figure 1A**). In a chronic-plus-binge ethanol-feeding model, KCs show extracellular signal-regulated kinase 1/2 (ERK1/2) signaling attenuation and TNF-α production impairment, when they are pretreated with ROS generation inhibitor NADPH oxidase (40, 41). It has been documented that the cannabinoid receptor 2 (CB2) expressed on KCs protects mice from ALD via an autophagy pathway (**Figure 1A**). This effect is supported by the findings that mice with specifically targeted deletion of the CB2 receptor ($CB2^{Mye-/-}$) or autophagy gene ATG5 ($ATG5^{Mye-/-}$) had exacerbated liver inflammation and alcohol-induced steatosis (42). Upon exposure to LPS, KCs isolated from $CB2^{Mye-/-}$ mice showed a pro-inflammatory phenotype that is characterized by an increased expression of chemokines IL-1β, IL-1α, IL-6, TNF-α, and CCL3 (42). These data suggest that KCs are activated toward a pro-inflammatory phenotype that increases liver inflammation and damage during ALD.

The role of recruited macrophages in ALD is less well studied. Chronic alcohol administration increases the population of recruited macrophages in the mouse liver (43). In an animal model, ethanol feeding promoted the differentiation of $Ly6C^{hi}$ monocytes into tissue-damaging pro-inflammatory macrophages (43). Moreover, phagocytosis of apoptotic hepatocytes allows $Ly6C^{hi}$ monocytes/macrophages to switch to $Ly6C^{low}$ monocytes/macrophages, which then differentiate into tissue-protective macrophages (43) (**Figure 1A**). It has been suggested that the ratio of these two subsets determines the role of recruited macrophages in the pathogenesis of ALD (43).

HEPATIC MACROPHAGES CONTRIBUTE TO NASH

About 20% of patients who suffer from non-alcoholic fatty liver disease will develop NASH, which is defined by the existence of progressive fibrosis and steatosis with inflammation, ultimately leading to HCC and cirrhosis. To date, the pathogenesis of NASH is still obscure, but several risk factors are known to be involved in the process, ranging from oxidative stress, insulin resistance, cytokines, and epigenetic modification to microbiota alteration and environmental elements (44).

One connection between KCs and NASH is the presence of hepatic stellate cells (HSCs). NASH augments endotoxin influx by increasing intestinal permeability; the high level of endotoxin and/or danger signal from lipotoxic hepatocytes can stimulate KCs (45) (**Figure 1B**). Activated KCs produce transforming growth factor (TGF)-β1, which stimulates HSCs and increases the generation of hepatic collagen-α1(I), eventually triggering fibrosis (46) (**Figure 1B**). In comparison with that in controls, collagen-α1(I) messenger RNA (mRNA) was substantially increased in carbon tetrachloride (CCl_4)-treated mice, and this increase was abolished in TGF-β1-knockout mice (47). In addition, IL-1β and TNF-α production by stimulated KCs was required to maintain HSC survival via the NF-κB pathway (48) (**Figure 1B**). In a low-serum media model, hepatic macrophages protected HSCs from apoptosis, and, in the same model, neutralization of IL-1 and TNF inhibited the protective effects of hepatic macrophages. Additionally, suppression of NF-κB by sulfasalazine induces apoptosis of HSC in humans and rats (49). Furthermore, the depletion of macrophages by clodronate liposome reduced IL-1β and TNF-α mRNA in the fibrotic liver (48). Recent research has shown that mitochondrial DNA from hepatocytes of high-fat diet (HFD)-fed mice activates KCs and induces steatosis and inflammation via the stimulator of IFN genes (STING) pathway (50) (**Figure 1B**). In a mouse model of NASH, fibrosis, inflammation, and steatosis were diminished in the livers of STING-deficient mice (50). The STING agonist, dimethylxanthenone-4-acetic acid, augmented the TNF-α and IL-6 produced by KCs from WT mice, and this increase was attenuated in STING-deficient mice (50). The current literature suggests that activated hepatic macrophages promote the progression of NASH. In contrast, Du et al. found that the expression of TIM-3 on hepatic macrophages is dramatically increased in a methionine- and choline-deficient diet (MCD)-induced NASH model (51). In the same study, TIM-3 deficiency increased the release of ROS by hepatic macrophages and promoted MCD-induced liver fibrosis, as well as steatosis (51) (**Figure 1B**). These results suggest a mechanism by which hepatic macrophages can inhibit NASH development.

RECRUITED MACROPHAGES: FRIEND OR FOE IN NASH PROGRESSION? (51)

Odegaard et al. demonstrated that, in lethally irradiated mice, an HFD promotes the recruitment of bone-marrow-derived monocytes to the liver; these cells then differentiate into anti-inflammatory macrophages, which provide a protective effect against diet-induced insulin resistance via the peroxisome proliferator-activated receptor δ (PPARδ) pathway (52) (**Figure 1B**). The adoptive transfer of PPARδ-/- bone marrow into WT mice failed to activate alternative macrophages or attenuate the induced glucose intolerance caused by the HFD (52). In agreement with these finds, Oliver et al. demonstrated that in an overdose of acetaminophen-induced acute liver damage model, high-fructose, high-fat, and high-cholesterol (FFC)-diet-fed mice shows attenuated liver injury than normal-diet-fed mice (53). In the same model, adopting bone-marrow-derived macrophages (BMDMs) from normal-diet-fed mice into FFC-diet-fed mice increases liver damage (53). Single-cell RNA sequencing reveals that these BMDMs from FFC-diet-fed mice downregulate *S100a8/S100a9*, genes encoding inflammatory marker calprotectin, compared with normal-diet-fed mice (53). Additionally, FFC diet also suppresses the TLR4-dependent inflammatory capacity of BMDMs in the mouse NASH model (53). BMDMs from FFC-diet-fed mice are insensitive to LPS stimulation, reflected by less IL-6 and TNF-α production compared with their normal-diet-fed counterparts (53). In contrast, growing evidence has demonstrated that NASH niche favors pro-inflammatory macrophage/monocyte infiltration, and these infiltrated cells increase liver damage and inflammation (54). The fatty acid palmitate can stimulate death receptor 5 on hepatocytes, resulting in release of extracellular vehicles (EVs) (54). The EVs released from lipotoxic hepatocytes have been shown to promote BMDMs toward the pro-inflammatory phenotype characterized by increasing expression of *Il1b* and *Il6* mRNAs (54). Moreover, hepatocyte-lipotoxicity-induced EVs are enriched with integrin $\alpha_9\beta_1$ (55) and/or CXCL10 (56), which augment pro-inflammatory macrophage infiltration and enhance hepatic fibrosis (**Figure 1B**). Integrin $\alpha_9\beta_1$ is required for monocytes to attach liver sinusoidal endothelial; blockade of this interaction by anti-integrin $\alpha_9\beta_1$ antibody decreases FFC-diet-induced liver fibrosis and injury in NASH mice (55). During hepatic injury, pro-inflammatory macrophages/monocytes are attracted to liver via the CXCL10–CXCR3 axis (57). Compared with those in WT mice, FFC-diet-induced liver injury and inflammation are alleviated in CXCL10–/– mice (56). In a randomized trial, targeting pro-inflammatory monocytes/macrophages by cenicriviroc, a dual antagonist of CCR2 and CCR5, improves hepatic fibrosis in NASH patients (58). One crucial signal that controls the fate of these monocyte-derived macrophages is the type of fatty acids to which the macrophage is exposed. Exposure by saturated fatty acid causes hepatocyte lipotoxicity that then promotes pro-inflammatory macrophage differentiation, whereas stimulation by unsaturated fatty acids activates PPARδ to enhance anti-inflammatory differentiation in NASH (**Figure 1B**) (52, 59). Taken together, monocytes/macrophages are recruited to the liver during NASH; in response to different compositions of fatty acids, these cells can be differentiated into tissue damage pro-inflammatory macrophages and/or tissue repair anti-inflammatory macrophages; the ratio of two macrophage subsets may determine the role of hepatic macrophage in the pathogenesis of NASH.

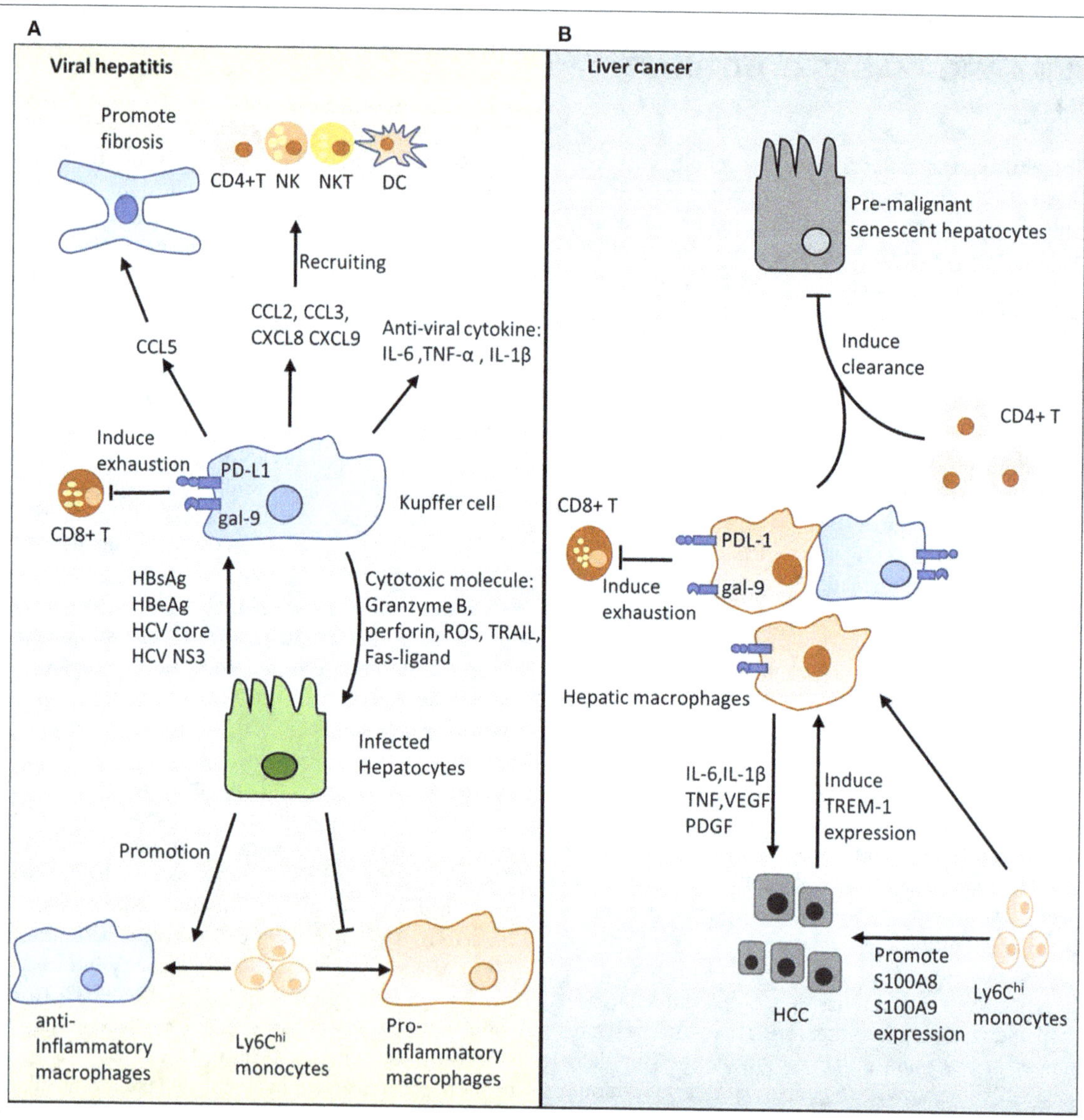

FIGURE 2 | The role of hepatic macrophages in viral hepatitis and hepatocellular carcinoma (HCC). **(A)** Hepatic macrophages and hepatitis B virus (HBV)/hepatitis C virus (HCV). Interleukin (IL)-6, tumor necrosis factor (TNF)-α, and IL-1β produced by Kupffer cells (KCs) show strong antiviral activities. Additionally, KCs may remove infected hepatocytes by producing cytotoxic molecules, including granzyme B, perforin, reactive oxygen species, TNF-related apoptosis-inducing ligand, and Fas-ligand. KCs produce distinct chemokines, including CC- chemokine ligand (CCL)2, CCL3, CXC-chemokine ligand (CXCL)8, and CXCL9, and, together, these chemokines recruit natural killer cells, natural killer T cells, dendritic cells, and CD4+ T cells to infected sites and enhance infection clearance. HCV stimulation induces hepatic macrophages to generate CCL5, which in turn activates hepatic stellate cells and eventually triggers live inflammation and fibrosis. KCs mediate T-cell dysfunction via PD-1/PD-L1 and TIM-3/galectin-9 pathways. Increased HBV inoculum suppresses polarization of pro-inflammation macrophages. **(B)** Hepatic macrophages contribute to HCC. Hepatic macrophages produce IL-6, IL-1β, TNF, vascular endothelial growth factor, and platelet-derived growth factor to promote tumor growth and angiogenesis during HCC. KCs suppress antitumor activity by inducing T-cell dysfunction through PD-L1/PD-1 and galectin-9/TIM-3 in the HCC setting. In contrast, hepatic macrophages assist CD4+ T cells in removing the premalignant senescent hepatocytes that enhance HCC progression. Ly6C^{hi} monocytes increase the expression of S100A8 and S100A9 on cancer cells and promote tumor migration and invasion.

THE ROLE OF HEPATIC MACROPHAGES IN VIRAL HEPATITIS

The role of hepatic macrophages in the progression of viral hepatitis is still controversial. Activated KCs, characterized by the upregulation of CD33 and CD163, accumulate in the portal tract during chronic HBV/HCV infection, highlighting the importance of these cells in fighting viral hepatitis (60, 61). KCs are the primary source of IL-1β, TNF-α, and IL-6; these inflammatory cytokines exhibit strong antiviral activity during an infection (62) (**Figure 2A**). Additionally, it has been shown that KCs may eliminate infected hepatocytes by releasing cytotoxic molecules, such as granzyme B, perforin, ROS, TRAIL, and Fas ligand (63, 64) (**Figure 2A**). Furthermore, the supernatant from differentiated pro-inflammatory macrophages contains reasonable amounts of IL-1β and IL-6, which inhibit the progression of HBV by decreasing levels of hepatitis B surface antigen (HBsAg) and hepatitis B early antigen (HBeAg) (65).

Several studies have indicated that, in humans, HBV/HCV can directly stimulate hepatic macrophages to trigger inflammatory cytokine secretion, thereby enhancing antiviral activity (15, 66) (**Figure 2A**). *In vitro* stimulation with HBsAg and HBeAg promoted primary human non-parenchymal liver cells to produce IL-6, IL-8, TNF-α, and IL-1β via the NF-κB pathway (67, 68). Similarly, culturing with HCV enhanced the production of IL-1β and IL-18 by KCs and monocyte-derived macrophages (69, 70). It has been documented that HCV core proteins and nonstructural protein 3 trigger monocyte-derived macrophage activation via TLR1, TLR2, and TLR6 signaling (71). In agreement with these findings, immunofluorescence analysis showed that IL-1β and CD68 are co-localized in liver tissues of chronic HCV patients (72). Apart from inflammatory cytokines, activated KCs also produce CCL2 (73), CCL3 (74), CXCL8 (67), and CXCL9 (74, 75). Together, these chemokines recruit natural killer (NK), NKT, dendritic cells (DC), and CD4+ T cells to infected sites to accelerate infection clearance (74, 75). Although uptake of HBV/HCV by KCs *ex vivo* has not been reported, accumulating evidence from *in vitro* experiments suggests that KCs are involved in HBV/HCV clearance via producing inflammatory cytokines and activating other immune cells.

In contrast, it has been shown that hepatic macrophages are involved in the development of HBV/HCV-induced fibrosis. Incubation with HBV significantly enhanced the generation of the pro-fibrotic growth factor TGF-β1 by primary rat KCs (76). Sasaki et al. found that HCV stimulation induced hepatic macrophages to produce CCL5, which in turn activated HSCs and triggered live inflammation as well as fibrosis (77) (**Figure 2A**). In the same study, neutralizing CCL5 with an antibody suppressed HSC activation (77). Furthermore, stimulation with the HCV core protein induces programmed death ligand 1 (PD-L1) expression by KCs (78). Similarly, high galectin-9 expression is seen on the KCs of patients with chronic HBV infections (79). Activation of the programmed cell death protein 1 (PD-1)/PD-L1 and TIM-3/galectin-9 pathways in T cells evokes T-cell dysfunction and, thereby, favors the establishment of a chronic infection (78, 79) (**Figure 2A**).

One hypothesis for these phenomena is that the phenotype of the hepatic macrophages may be shaped by HBV/HCV as the infection progresses. During the early phase of infection, hepatic macrophages are dominated by pro-inflammatory subsets that inhibit virus development by producing cytokines with antiviral activity. In contrast, the chronic hepatitis infection environment suppresses hepatic macrophages polarizing toward the pro-inflammatory phenotype and pushes cells toward the immunoregulation phenotype. Thus, hepatic macrophages show weak antiviral and strong pathological activities in the chronic hepatitis (14). This finding is supported by a recent study showing that an increase in the HBV inoculum attenuated the polarization of monocytes into pro-inflammatory macrophages, evidenced by decreased IL-6 production (65) (**Figure 2A**). In the same study, exposure to the HBV virus enhanced monocyte anti-inflammatory differentiation, evidenced by increased IL-10 production (65) (**Figure 2A**). It is likely that a high virus titer suppresses the antiviral activity of hepatic macrophages and polarizes hepatic macrophages toward a tolerogenic phenotype. In agreement with this hypothesis, Faure-Dupuy et al. demonstrated that exposure to HBV attenuated cytokine release by pro-inflammatory hepatic macrophages and enhanced cytokine production by anti-inflammatory hepatic macrophages (65). This modulation suppresses the antiviral surveillance and favors the establishment of an infection (65). Taken together, a high HBV/HCV titer not only inhibits pro-inflammatory macrophage polarization but also promotes macrophages differentiating toward a tolerogenic phenotype, which favors HBV/HCV development by releasing immunoregulation cytokine IL-10.

HEPATIC MACROPHAGES AND HCC

Hepatic macrophages play a crucial role in the pathogenesis of HCC, as evidenced by the accumulation of hepatic macrophages in resections of HCC patients (80) and the liver tissue of chemically induced HCC mice (81). The majority of studies suggest that hepatic macrophages are pro-inflammatory and pro-tumorigenic cells, which inhibit antitumor immunity and favor the establishment of tumors (82–84). Having a large population of hepatic macrophages is associated with poor survival in HCC patients (80, 85). During HCC, hepatic macrophages produce the pro-angiogenic factors, TGF-β, vascular endothelial growth factor (VEGF), and platelet-derived growth factor (PDGF), which, together, promote tumor growth (84, 86) (**Figure 2B**). Additionally, it has been documented that hepatic macrophages release different mediators, including IL-6, IL-1β, CCL2, VEGF A (VEGFA), and TNF, to augment tumor cell proliferation in HCC (83, 86) (**Figure 2B**). The evidence for liver macrophage inhibition of HCC growth is limited. The most convincing evidence probably comes from a study of 302 HCC patients, which demonstrated that a high number of CD68+ macrophages is associated with better overall survival (87). Moreover, Kang et al. showed that hepatic macrophages assisted CD4+ T cells

TABLE 1 | Pharmacological agents targeting macrophages in alcoholic liver disease, non-alcoholic steatohepatitis, viral hepatitis, or hepatocellular carcinoma.

Target	Agent	Mechanism of action	Phase	Clinical trial number
ALCOHOLIC LIVER DISEASE				
Gut bacteria	Combined vancomycin and gentamycin and meropenem	Inhibiting macrophage activation by gut bacteria eradication	Ongoing	NCT03157388
NON-ALCOHOLIC STEATOHEPATITIS				
Galectin 3	GR-MD-02	Galectin 3 antagonist on macrophages	Phase 2	NCT02462967
CCR2/CCR5	Cenicriviroc	CCR2/CCR5 antagonist (inhibits monocyte/macrophage infiltration)	Phase 2	NCT02217475
PPARα/δ	Elafibranor	Dual PPARα/δ agonist, PPARδ agonist promotes anti-inflammatory differentiation	Phase 3	NCT02704403
VIRAL HEPATITIS				
GM-CSF	Entecavir plus GM-CSF	GM-CSF promotes macrophage differentiation	Ongoing	NCT03164889
GM-CSF	Y peginterferon alpha-2b plus GM-CSF	GM-CSF promotes macrophage differentiation	Phase 2	NCT02332473
HEPATOCELLULAR CARCINOMA				
CSF1R	Chiauranib	Multi-target inhibitor that suppresses angiogenesis-related kinases, mitosis-related kinase Aurora B, and CSF1R. Blockade of CSF1R decreases the macrophage differentiation.	Phase 1	NCT03245190
CCR2/5	Nivolumab plus CCR2/5 inhibitor	CCR2/CCR5 antagonist (inhibits monocyte/macrophage infiltration)	Phase 2	NCT04123379

CCR2, CC chemokine receptor 2, CSF1R, colony-stimulating factor 1 receptor, GM-CSF, granulocyte-macrophage colony-stimulating factor.

in cleaning the premalignant senescent hepatocytes that promote HCC development in an animal model (88). Therefore, two clinical studies with similar clinical–pathologic characteristics but varied in the number of patients have led to contradictory results (80, 87). It is possible that different therapeutic strategies, in particular, post-recurrence therapies, may have been used in these studies (80, 87). CD68 was used to identify tumor-associated macrophages (TAMs) (80, 87). It is widely accepted that TAMs form heterogeneous populations; therefore, the TAM subset contributions to tumor growth progression or inhibition remain to be investigated. This may help to further evaluate the discrepancy between these two studies.

Studies have found that KCs suppress antitumor activity by inducing T-cell tolerance and dysfunction in an HCC setting. KCs have been demonstrated to function as incomplete antigen-presenting cells (APCs) to induce T-cell tolerance (89). This idea is further supported by a recent study which showed that human KCs might exhibit a tolerogenic phenotype (12); they accumulate at the peritumoral stroma expressing high levels of PD-L1 (90, 91) and galectin-9 (92), thereby inhibiting the antitumor response by activating PD-L1/PD-1 and galectin-9/TIM-3 signaling in T cells (**Figure 2B**). Moreover, the triggering receptor expressed on myeloid cells-1 (TREM-1) is an activating receptor that is widely expressed on monocytes, macrophages, and neutrophils (93). Cancer cell stimulation has been shown to directly increase the expression TREM-1 on KCs, which, in turn, promotes KC activation and HCC progression (93, 94) (**Figure 2B**). In the same study, *Trem1* deficiency diminished IL-1β, IL-6, TNF, CCL2, and CXCL10 release by KCs and suppressed HCC growth (94). Taken together, interaction between T cells and KCs hinders antitumor response by promoting T-cell exhaustion in HCC.

The role of recruited macrophages in HCC development is highlighted by the importance of the CCL2/CCR2 signaling axis, which is crucial for Ly6C^{hi} monocyte recruitment to inflammatory sites (95). It has been suggested that monocyte recruitment during HCC depends on KCs (96), senescent hepatocytes (97), and tumor-associated neutrophils (98). Conditional media from Ly6C^{hi} monocytes increased the expression of S100A8 and S100A9 in cancer cells and promoted tumor migration and invasion in an experimental liver metastasis model (99) (**Figure 2B**). In a preclinical model of HCC, blocking CCL2/CCR2 signaling with a CCR2 antagonist reduced Ly6C^{hi} monocyte numbers in the peripheral blood and suppressed anti-inflammatory macrophage polarization in the liver, ultimately inhibiting tumor growth (100). Indeed, a large number of studies have shown that the CCL2/CCR2 pathway involves the recruitment of myeloid-derived suppressor cells (MDSCs) during inflammation, and Ly6C^{hi} monocytes have been shown to be the precursor of MDSCs (101, 102); therefore, the antitumor effect triggered by blocking the CCL2/CCR2 pathway may be partially due to MDSC depletion. To sum up, during HCC progression, macrophages and MDSCs are recruited to the liver via the CCL2/CCR2 axis; these cells have been shown to promote tumor proliferation and metastasis.

PERSPECTIVE

A tremendous amount of research over the last few decades has revealed that hepatic macrophages play a central role in the pathogenesis of liver disease. Several strategies have been employed to specifically target hepatic macrophages in different liver diseases (**Table 1**). Notably, CD11b, F4/80, and Ly6C in mice and CD14, HLA-DR, and CD68 in humans have been widely used to identify KCs; however, these markers may be inadequate to distinguish KCs from recruited macrophages. It has been shown that murine KCs express a unique marker, CLEC4F (11). Meanwhile, single-cell RNA-seq analysis showed that KCs are CD68+ Macro+ in healthy humans (12). Therefore, adding these new markers to the conventional hepatic macrophage identification panel should be considered for precise future investigations into the role of liver macrophage subsets in the development of the liver disease. The recently developed mass cytometry Cyto F technique has been used to study hepatic macrophage in liver disease (55); this technique can simultaneously label up to 350 markers on a single cell, therefore providing a powerful platform to investigate in depth the heterogeneity of hepatic macrophages under different liver diseases as well as pharmaceutical intervention conditions.

During inflammation, circulating monocytes infiltrate the liver and are involved in the progression of various liver diseases. The phenotypes and roles of monocyte-derived hepatic macrophages are highly dependent on local stimuli during liver disease (103). For example, during fibrosis, a novel monocyte-derived TREM2+ CD9+ scar-associated macrophage has been discovered; this population is expanded in cirrhotic livers and exhibited a pro-fibrogenic phenotype (104). The current M1–M2 model has limitations; this concept cannot define all cell phenotypes, especially macrophages during chronic inflammation and chronic infection liver disease (16). A recent study suggested an extension to the M1–M2 model by showing that, other than M1 and M2 macrophages, human macrophages can be polarized into distinct phenotypes in response to various stimuli (103). Therefore, it is important to precisely describe macrophage populations based on their origins, stimuli, and identification markers (105).

Self-renewing peritoneal macrophages have been shown to migrate to the liver in response to sterile injury (23). Additionally, the spleen is thought to be a reservoir for inflammatory monocytes, which infiltrate the liver and differentiate into hepatic macrophages during liver injury (106). These studies suggest that recruited macrophages are a highly heterogeneous population, composed of subsets with different origins and functions (23, 107). Currently, monocyte-derived recruited macrophages are extensively studied; however, the contributions of peritoneal cavity and spleen-derived recruited macrophages to the pathogenesis of distinct liver diseases are obscured and remain to be explored in the future.

AUTHOR CONTRIBUTIONS

LD wrote the first draft of the manuscript. YG, XH, and XS contributed to manuscript revision and read and approved the submitted version.

REFERENCES

1. Lopez BG, Tsai MS, Baratta JL, Longmuir KJ, Robertson RT. Characterization of Kupffer cells in livers of developing mice. *Comp Hepatol.* (2011) 10:2. doi: 10.1186/1476-5926-10-2
2. Dong Z, Wei H, Sun R, Tian Z. The roles of innate immune cells in liver injury and regeneration. *Cell Mol Immunol.* (2007) 4:241–52.
3. Jenne CN, Kubes P. Immune surveillance by the liver. *Nat Immunol.* (2013) 14:996–1006. doi: 10.1038/ni.2691
4. Parker GA, Picut CA. Liver immunobiology. *Toxicol Pathol.* (2005) 33:52–62. doi: 10.1080/01926230590522365
5. Gammella E, Buratti P, Cairo G, Recalcati S. Macrophages: central regulators of iron balance. *Metallomics.* (2014) 6:1336–45. doi: 10.1039/C4MT00104D
6. Wang Y, van der Tuin S, Tjeerdema N, van Dam AD, Rensen SS, Hendrikx T, et al. Plasma cholesteryl ester transfer protein is predominantly derived from Kupffer cells. *Hepatology.* (2015) 62:1710–22. doi: 10.1002/hep.27985
7. Naito M, Hasegawa G, Ebe Y, Yamamoto T. Differentiation and function of Kupffer cells. *Med Electron Microsc.* (2004) 37:16–28. doi: 10.1007/s00795-003-0228-x
8. Nakamoto N, Kanai T. Role of toll-like receptors in immune activation and tolerance in the liver. *Front Immunol.* (2014) 5:221. doi: 10.3389/fimmu.2014.00221
9. Kanneganti T-D, Lamkanfi M, Núñez G. Intracellular NOD-like receptors in host defense and disease. *Immunity.* (2007) 27:549–59. doi: 10.1016/j.immuni.2007.10.002
10. Terpstra V, van Berkel TJC. Scavenger receptors on liver Kupffer cells mediate the *in vivo* uptake of oxidatively damaged red blood cells in mice. *Blood.* (2000) 95:2157. doi: 10.1182/blood.V95.6.2157
11. Scott CL, Zheng F, De Baetselier P, Martens L, Saeys Y, De Prijck S, et al. Bone marrow-derived monocytes give rise to self-renewing and fully differentiated Kupffer cells. *Nat Commun.* (2016) 7:10321. doi: 10.1038/ncomms10321
12. MacParland SA, Liu JC, Ma XZ, Innes BT, Bartczak AM, Gage BK, et al. Single cell RNA sequencing of human liver reveals distinct intrahepatic macrophage populations. *Nat Commun.* (2018) 9:4383. doi: 10.1038/s41467-018-06318-7
13. Mills CD, Kincaid K, Alt JM, Heilman MJ, Hill AM. M-1/M-2 macrophages and the Th1/Th2 paradigm. *J Immunol.* (2000) 164:6166–73. doi: 10.4049/jimmunol.164.12.6166
14. Krenkel O, Tacke F. Liver macrophages in tissue homeostasis and disease. *Nat Rev Immunol.* (2017) 17:306–21. doi: 10.1038/nri.2017.11
15. Tacke F. Targeting hepatic macrophages to treat liver diseases. *J Hepatol.* (2017) 66:1300–12. doi: 10.1016/j.jhep.2017.02.026
16. Martinez FO, Gordon S. The M1 and M2 paradigm of macrophage activation: time for reassessment. *F1000prime Rep.* (2014) 6:13. doi: 10.12703/P6-13
17. van Furth R, Cohn ZA. The origin and kinetics of mononuclear phagocytes. *J Exp Med.* (1968) 128:415–35. doi: 10.1084/jem.128.3.415
18. Schulz C, Gomez Perdiguero E, Chorro L, Szabo-Rogers H, Cagnard N, Kierdorf K, et al. A lineage of myeloid cells independent of Myb and hematopoietic stem cells. *Science.* (2012) 336:86–90. doi: 10.1126/science.1219179
19. Mass E, Ballesteros I, Farlik M, Halbritter F, Gunther P, Crozet L, et al. Specification of tissue-resident macrophages during organogenesis. *Science.* (2016) 353:aaf4238. doi: 10.1126/science.aaf4238
20. Brempelis KJ, Crispe IN. Infiltrating monocytes in liver injury and repair. *Clin Transl Immunol.* (2016) 5:e113. doi: 10.1038/cti.2016.62
21. Carlin LM, Stamatiades EG, Auffray C, Hanna RN, Glover L, Vizcay-Barrena G, et al. Nr4a1-dependent Ly6C(low) monocytes monitor endothelial cells and orchestrate their disposal. *Cell.* (2013) 153:362–375. doi: 10.1016/j.cell.2013.03.010
22. Ramachandran P, Pellicoro A, Vernon MA, Boulter L, Aucott RL, Ali A, et al. Differential Ly-6C expression identifies the recruited macrophage phenotype, which orchestrates the regression of murine liver fibrosis. *Proc Natl Acad Sci USA.* (2012) 109:E3186–95. doi: 10.1073/pnas.1119964109
23. Wang J, Kubes P. A reservoir of mature cavity macrophages that can rapidly invade visceral organs to affect tissue repair. *Cell.* (2016) 165:668–78. doi: 10.1016/j.cell.2016.03.009
24. Guillot A, Tacke F. Liver macrophages: old dogmas and new insights. *Hepatol Commun.* (2019) 3:730–43. doi: 10.1002/hep4.1356
25. Gao B, Bataller R. Alcoholic liver disease: pathogenesis and new therapeutic targets. *Gastroenterology.* (2011) 141:1572–85. doi: 10.1053/j.gastro.2011.09.002

26. Dunn W, Shah VH. Pathogenesis of alcoholic liver disease. *Clin Liver Dis.* (2016) 20:445–56. doi: 10.1016/j.cld.2016.02.004
27. Deng Q-G, She H, Cheng JH, French SW, Koop DR, Xiong S, et al. Steatohepatitis induced by intragastric overfeeding in mice. *Hepatology.* (2005) 42:905–14. doi: 10.1002/hep.20877
28. Karakucuk I, Dilly SA, Maxwell JD. Portal tract macrophages are increased in alcoholic liver disease. *Histopathology.* (1989) 14:245–53. doi: 10.1111/j.1365-2559.1989.tb02143.x
29. Koop DR, Klopfenstein B, Iimuro Y, Thurman RG. Gadolinium chloride blocks alcohol-dependent liver toxicity in rats treated chronically with intragastric alcohol despite the induction of CYP2E1. *Mol Pharmacol.* (1997) 51:944–50. doi: 10.1124/mol.51.6.944
30. Schnabl B, Brenner DA. Interactions between the intestinal microbiome and liver diseases. *Gastroenterology.* (2014) 146:1513–24. doi: 10.1053/j.gastro.2014.01.020
31. Enomoto N, Ikejima K, Yamashina S, Hirose M, Shimizu H, Kitamura T, et al. Kupffer cell sensitization by alcohol involves increased permeability to gut-derived endotoxin. *Alcohol Clin Exp Res.* (2001) 25(6 Suppl):51S–4S. doi: 10.1111/j.1530-0277.2001.tb02418.x
32. Ju C, Mandrekar P. Macrophages and alcohol-related liver inflammation. *Alcohol Res.* (2015) 37:251–62.
33. Mandrekar P, Ambade A, Lim A, Szabo G, Catalano D. An essential role for monocyte chemoattractant protein-1 in alcoholic liver injury: regulation of proinflammatory cytokines and hepatic steatosis in mice. *Hepatology.* (2011) 54:2185–97. doi: 10.1002/hep.24599
34. Nagy LE. Recent insights into the role of the innate immune system in the development of alcoholic liver disease. *Exp Biol Med.* (2003) 228:882–90. doi: 10.1177/153537020322800803
35. Saikia P, Bellos D, McMullen MR, Pollard KA, de la Motte C, Nagy LE. MicroRNA 181b-3p and its target importin α5 regulate toll-like receptor 4 signaling in Kupffer cells and liver injury in mice in response to ethanol. *Hepatology.* (2017) 66:602–15. doi: 10.1002/hep.29144
36. Bala S, Marcos M, Kodys K, Csak T, Catalano D, Mandrekar P, et al. Up-regulation of microRNA-155 in macrophages contributes to increased tumor necrosis factor α (TNFα) production via increased mRNA half-life in alcoholic liver disease. *J Biol Chem.* (2011) 286:1436–44. doi: 10.1074/jbc.M110.145870
37. Bala S, Csak T, Saha B, Zatsiorsky J, Kodys K, Catalano D, et al. The pro-inflammatory effects of miR-155 promote liver fibrosis and alcohol-induced steatohepatitis. *J Hepatol.* (2016) 64:1378–87. doi: 10.1016/j.jhep.2016.01.035
38. Petrasek J, Iracheta-Vellve A, Saha B, Satishchandran A, Kodys K, Fitzgerald KA, et al. Metabolic danger signals, uric acid and ATP, mediate inflammatory cross-talk between hepatocytes and immune cells in alcoholic liver disease. *J Leukoc Biol.* (2015) 98:249–56. doi: 10.1189/jlb.3AB1214-590R
39. Verma VK, Li H, Wang R, Hirsova P, Mushref M, Liu Y, et al. Alcohol stimulates macrophage activation through caspase-dependent hepatocyte derived release of CD40L containing extracellular vesicles. *J Hepatol.* (2016) 64:651–60. doi: 10.1016/j.jhep.2015.11.020
40. Thakur V, Pritchard MT, McMullen MR, Wang Q, Nagy LE. Chronic ethanol feeding increases activation of NADPH oxidase by lipopolysaccharide in rat Kupffer cells: role of increased reactive oxygen in LPS-stimulated ERK1/2 activation and TNF-alpha production. *J Leukoc Biol.* (2006) 79:1348–56. doi: 10.1189/jlb.1005613
41. Kono H, Rusyn I, Yin M, Gabele E, Yamashina S, Dikalova A, et al. NADPH oxidase-derived free radicals are key oxidants in alcohol-induced liver disease. *J Clin Invest.* (2000) 106:867–72. doi: 10.1172/JCI9020
42. Denaës T, Lodder J, M.-Chobert N, Ruiz I, J.-Pawlotsky M, Lotersztajn S, et al. The cannabinoid receptor 2 protects against alcoholic liver disease via a macrophage autophagy-dependent pathway. *Sci Rep.* (2016) 6:28806. doi: 10.1038/srep28806
43. Wang M, You Q, Lor K, Chen F, Gao B, Ju C. Chronic alcohol ingestion modulates hepatic macrophage populations and functions in mice. *J Leukoc Biol.* (2014) 96:657–65. doi: 10.1189/jlb.6A0114-004RR
44. Machado MV, Diehl AM. Pathogenesis of nonalcoholic steatohepatitis. *Gastroenterology.* (2016) 150:1769–77. doi: 10.1053/j.gastro.2016.02.066
45. Kazankov K, Jorgensen SMD, Thomsen KL, Moller HJ, Vilstrup H, George J, et al. The role of macrophages in nonalcoholic fatty liver disease and nonalcoholic steatohepatitis. *Nat Rev Gastroenterol Hepatol.* (2019) 16:145–59. doi: 10.1038/s41575-018-0082-x
46. Hellerbrand C, Stefanovic B, Giordano F, Burchardt ER, Brenner DA. The role of TGFβ1 in initiating hepatic stellate cell activation *in vivo*. *J Hepatol.* (1999) 30:77–87. doi: 10.1016/S0168-8278(99)80010-5
47. Nakamura T, Sakata R, Ueno T, Sata M, Ueno H. Inhibition of transforming growth factor β prevents progression of liver fibrosis and enhances hepatocyte regeneration in dimethylnitrosamine-treated rats. *Hepatology.* (2000) 32:247–55. doi: 10.1053/jhep.2000.9109
48. Pradere J-P, Kluwe J, De Minicis S, Jiao J-J, G.-Gwak Y, Dapito DH, et al. Hepatic macrophages but not dendritic cells contribute to liver fibrosis by promoting the survival of activated hepatic stellate cells in mice. *Hepatology.* (2013) 58:1461–73. doi: 10.1002/hep.26429
49. Oakley F, Meso M, Iredale JP, Green K, Marek CJ, Zhou X, et al. Inhibition of inhibitor of κB kinases stimulates hepatic stellate cell apoptosis and accelerated recovery from rat liver fibrosis. *Gastroenterology.* (2005) 128:108–20. doi: 10.1053/j.gastro.2004.10.003
50. Yu Y, Liu Y, An W, Song J, Zhang Y, Zhao X. STING-mediated inflammation in Kupffer cells contributes to progression of nonalcoholic steatohepatitis. *J Clin Invest.* (2019) 129:546–55. doi: 10.1172/JCI121842
51. Du X, Wu Z, Xu Y, Liu Y, Liu W, Wang T, et al. Increased Tim-3 expression alleviates liver injury by regulating macrophage activation in MCD-induced NASH mice. *Cell Mol Immunol.* (2018) 16:878–86. doi: 10.1038/s41423-018-0032-0
52. Odegaard JI, Ricardo-Gonzalez RR, Red Eagle A, Vats D, Morel CR, Goforth MH, et al. Alternative M2 activation of Kupffer cells by PPARdelta ameliorates obesity-induced insulin resistance. *Cell Metab.* (2008) 7:496–507. doi: 10.1016/j.cmet.2008.04.003
53. Krenkel O, Hundertmark J, Abdallah AT, Kohlhepp M, Puengel T, Roth T, et al. Myeloid cells in liver and bone marrow acquire a functionally distinct inflammatory phenotype during obesity-related steatohepatitis. *Gut.* (2019). doi: 10.1136/gutjnl-2019-318382. [Epub ahead of print].
54. Hirsova P, Ibrahim SH, Krishnan A, Verma VK, Bronk SF, Werneburg NW, et al. Lipid-induced signaling causes release of inflammatory extracellular vesicles from hepatocytes. *Gastroenterology.* (2016) 150:956–67. doi: 10.1053/j.gastro.2015.12.037
55. Guo Q, Furuta K, Lucien F, Gutierrez Sanchez LH, Hirsova P, Krishnan A, et al. Integrin β1-enriched extracellular vesicles mediate monocyte adhesion and promote liver inflammation in murine NASH. *J Hepatol.* (2019) 71:1193–205. doi: 10.1016/j.jhep.2019.07.019
56. Ibrahim SH, Hirsova P, Tomita K, Bronk SF, Werneburg NW, Harrison SA, et al. Mixed lineage kinase 3 mediates release of C-X-C motif ligand 10-bearing chemotactic extracellular vesicles from lipotoxic hepatocytes. *Hepatology.* (2016) 63:731–44. doi: 10.1002/hep.28252
57. Xuan W, Qu Q, Zheng B, Xiong S, Fan G-H. The chemotaxis of M1 and M2 macrophages is regulated by different chemokines. *J Leukoc Biol.* (2015) 97:61–9. doi: 10.1189/jlb.1A0314-170R
58. Friedman SL, Ratziu V, Harrison SA, Abdelmalek MF, Aithal GP, Caballeria J, et al. A randomized, placebo-controlled trial of cenicriviroc for treatment of nonalcoholic steatohepatitis with fibrosis. *Hepatology.* (2018) 67:1754–67. doi: 10.1002/hep.29477
59. Shi H, Kokoeva MV, Inouye K, Tzameli I, Yin H, Flier JS. TLR4 links innate immunity and fatty acid-induced insulin resistance. *J Clin Invest.* (2006) 116:3015–25. doi: 10.1172/JCI28898
60. McGuinness PH, Painter D, Davies S, McCaughan GW. Increases in intrahepatic CD68 positive cells, MAC387 positive cells, and proinflammatory cytokines (particularly interleukin 18) in chronic hepatitis C infection. *Gut.* (2000) 46:260–9. doi: 10.1136/gut.46.2.260
61. Bility MT, Cheng L, Zhang Z, Luan Y, Li F, Chi L, et al. Hepatitis B virus infection and immunopathogenesis in a humanized mouse model: induction of human-specific liver fibrosis and M2-like macrophages. *PLoS Pathog.* (2014) 10:e1004032. doi: 10.1371/journal.ppat.1004032
62. Isorce N, Testoni B, Locatelli M, Fresquet J, Rivoire M, Luangsay S, et al. Antiviral activity of various interferons and pro-inflammatory cytokines in non-transformed cultured hepatocytes infected with hepatitis B virus. *Antiviral Res.* (2016) 130:36–45. doi: 10.1016/j.antiviral.2016.03.008
63. Tang TJ, Kwekkeboom J, Laman JD, Niesters HG, Zondervan PE, de Man RA, et al. The role of intrahepatic immune effector cells in inflammatory liver injury and viral control during chronic hepatitis B infection. *J Viral Hepat.* (2003) 10:159–67. doi: 10.1046/j.1365-2893.2003.00412.x

64. Kolios G, Valatas V, Kouroumalis E. Role of Kupffer cells in the pathogenesis of liver disease. *World J Gastroenterol.* (2006) 12:7413–20. doi: 10.3748/wjg.v12.i46.7413
65. Faure-Dupuy S, Delphin M, Aillot L, Dimier L, Lebossé F, Fresquet J, et al. Hepatitis B Virus-induced modulation of liver macrophage function promotes hepatocyte infection. *J Hepatol.* (2019) 71:1086–98. doi: 10.1016/j.jhep.2019.06.032
66. Boltjes A, Movita D, Boonstra A, Woltman AM. The role of Kupffer cells in hepatitis B and hepatitis C virus infections. *J Hepatol.* (2014) 61:660–71. doi: 10.1016/j.jhep.2014.04.026
67. Hösel M, Quasdorff M, Wiegmann K, Webb D, Zedler U, Broxtermann M, et al. Not interferon, but interleukin-6 controls early gene expression in hepatitis B virus infection. *Hepatology.* (2009) 50:1773–82. doi: 10.1002/hep.23226
68. Tan AT, Koh S, Goh W, Zhe HY, Gehring AJ, Lim SG, et al. A longitudinal analysis of innate and adaptive immune profile during hepatic flares in chronic hepatitis B. *J Hepatol.* (2010) 52:330–9. doi: 10.1016/j.jhep.2009.12.015
69. Shrivastava S, Mukherjee A, Ray R, Ray RB. Hepatitis C virus induces interleukin-1β (IL-1β)/IL-18 in circulatory and resident liver macrophages. *J Virol.* (2013) 87:12284–90. doi: 10.1128/JVI.01962-13
70. Hosomura N, Kono H, Tsuchiya M, Ishii K, Ogiku M, Matsuda M, et al. HCV-related proteins activate Kupffer cells isolated from human liver tissues. *Dig Dis Sci.* (2011) 56:1057–64. doi: 10.1007/s10620-010-1395-y
71. Chang S, Dolganiuc A, Szabo G. Toll-like receptors 1 and 6 are involved in TLR2-mediated macrophage activation by hepatitis C virus core and NS3 proteins. *J Leukoc Biol.* (2007) 82:479–87. doi: 10.1189/jlb.0207128
72. Negash AA, Ramos HJ, Crochet N, Lau DTY, Doehle B, Papic N, et al. IL-1β production through the NLRP3 inflammasome by hepatic macrophages links hepatitis C virus infection with liver inflammation and disease. *PLoS Pathog.* (2013) 9:e1003330. doi: 10.1371/journal.ppat.1003330
73. Heydtmann M. Macrophages in hepatitis B and hepatitis C virus infections. *J Virol.* (2009) 83:2796–802. doi: 10.1128/JVI.00996-08
74. Salazar-Mather TP, Hokeness KL. Cytokine and chemokine networks: pathways to antiviral defense. *Curr Top Microbiol Immunol.* (2006) 303:29–46. doi: 10.1007/978-3-540-33397-5_2
75. Yoneyama H, Ichida T. Recruitment of dendritic cells to pathological niches in inflamed liver. *Med Mol Morphol.* (2005) 38:136–41. doi: 10.1007/s00795-005-0289-0
76. Li H, Zheng H-W, Chen H, Xing Z-Z, You H, Cong M, et al. Hepatitis B virus particles preferably induce Kupffer cells to produce TGF-β1 over pro-inflammatory cytokines. *Dig Liver Dis.* (2012) 44:328–33. doi: 10.1016/j.dld.2011.11.005
77. Sasaki R, Devhare PB, Steele R, Ray R, Ray RB. Hepatitis C virus–induced CCL5 secretion from macrophages activates hepatic stellate cells. *Hepatology.* (2017) 66:746–57. doi: 10.1002/hep.29170
78. Tu Z, Pierce RH, Kurtis J, Kuroki Y, Crispe IN, Orloff MS. Hepatitis C virus core protein subverts the antiviral activities of human Kupffer cells. *Gastroenterology.* (2010) 138:305–14. doi: 10.1053/j.gastro.2009.09.009
79. Nebbia G, Peppa D, Schurich A, Khanna P, Singh HD, Cheng Y, et al. Upregulation of the Tim-3/galectin-9 pathway of T cell exhaustion in chronic hepatitis B virus infection. *PLoS ONE.* (2012) 7:e47648. doi: 10.1371/journal.pone.0047648
80. Ding T, Xu J, Wang F, Shi M, Zhang Y, Li S-P, et al. High tumor-infiltrating macrophage density predicts poor prognosis in patients with primary hepatocellular carcinoma after resection. *Hum Pathol.* (2009) 40:381–9. doi: 10.1016/j.humpath.2008.08.011
81. Schneider C, Teufel A, Yevsa T, Staib F, Hohmeyer A, Walenda G, et al. Adaptive immunity suppresses formation and progression of diethylnitrosamine-induced liver cancer. *Gut.* (2012) 61:1733–43. doi: 10.1136/gutjnl-2011-301116
82. Ritz T, Krenkel O, Tacke F. Dynamic plasticity of macrophage functions in diseased liver. *Cell Immunol.* (2018) 330:175–82. doi: 10.1016/j.cellimm.2017.12.007
83. Wan S, Kuo N, Kryczek I, Zou W, Welling TH. Myeloid cells in hepatocellular carcinoma. *Hepatology.* (2015) 62:1304–12. doi: 10.1002/hep.27867
84. Capece D, Fischietti M, Verzella D, Gaggiano A, Cicciarelli G, Tessitore A, et al. The inflammatory microenvironment in hepatocellular carcinoma: a pivotal role for tumor-associated macrophages. *Biomed Res Int.* (2013) 2013:187204. doi: 10.1155/2013/187204
85. Yeung OW, Lo CM, Ling CC, Qi X, Geng W, Li CX, et al. Alternatively activated (M2) macrophages promote tumour growth and invasiveness in hepatocellular carcinoma. *J Hepatol.* (2015) 62:607–16. doi: 10.1016/j.jhep.2014.10.029
86. Ju C, Tacke F. Hepatic macrophages in homeostasis and liver diseases: from pathogenesis to novel therapeutic strategies. *Cell Mol Immunol.* (2016) 13:316–27. doi: 10.1038/cmi.2015.104
87. Li Y-W, Qiu S-J, Fan J, Gao Q, Zhou J, Xiao Y-S, et al. Tumor-infiltrating macrophages can predict favorable prognosis in hepatocellular carcinoma after resection. *J Cancer Res Clin Oncol.* (2008) 135:439. doi: 10.1007/s00432-008-0469-0
88. Kang TW, Yevsa T, Woller N, Hoenicke L, Wuestefeld T, Dauch D, et al. Senescence surveillance of pre-malignant hepatocytes limits liver cancer development. *Nature.* (2011) 479:547–51. doi: 10.1038/nature10599
89. You Q, Cheng L, Kedl RM, Ju C. Mechanism of T cell tolerance induction by murine hepatic Kupffer cells. *Hepatology.* (2008) 48:978–90. doi: 10.1002/hep.22395
90. Kuang DM, Zhao Q, Peng C, Xu J, Zhang JP, Wu C, et al. Activated monocytes in peritumoral stroma of hepatocellular carcinoma foster immune privilege and disease progression through PD-L1. *J Exp Med.* (2009) 206:1327–37. doi: 10.1084/jem.20082173
91. Wu K, Kryczek I, Chen L, Zou W, Welling TH. Kupffer cell suppression of CD8+ T cells in human hepatocellular carcinoma is mediated by B7-H1/programmed death-1 interactions. *Cancer Res.* (2009) 69:8067–75. doi: 10.1158/0008-5472.CAN-09-0901
92. Li H, Wu K, Tao K, Chen L, Zheng Q, Lu X, et al. Tim-3/galectin-9 signaling pathway mediates T-cell dysfunction and predicts poor prognosis in patients with hepatitis B virus-associated hepatocellular carcinoma. *Hepatology.* (2012) 56:1342–51. doi: 10.1002/hep.25777
93. Ho CC, Liao WY, Wang CY, Lu YH, Huang HY, Chen HY, et al. TREM-1 expression in tumor-associated macrophages and clinical outcome in lung cancer. *Am J Respir Crit Care Med.* (2008) 177:763–70. doi: 10.1164/rccm.200704-641OC
94. Wu J, Li J, Salcedo R, Mivechi NF, Trinchieri G, Horuzsko A. The proinflammatory myeloid cell receptor TREM-1 controls Kupffer cell activation and development of hepatocellular carcinoma. *Cancer Res.* (2012) 72:3977. doi: 10.1158/0008-5472.CAN-12-0938
95. Shi C, Pamer EG. Monocyte recruitment during infection and inflammation. *Nat Rev Immunol.* (2011) 11:762–74. doi: 10.1038/nri3070
96. Elsegood CL, Chan CW, Degli-Esposti MA, Wikstrom ME, Domenichini A, Lazarus K, et al. Kupffer cell–monocyte communication is essential for initiating murine liver progenitor cell–mediated liver regeneration. *Hepatology.* (2015) 62:1272–84. doi: 10.1002/hep.27977
97. Eggert T, Wolter K, Ji J, Ma C, Yevsa T, Klotz S, et al. Distinct functions of senescence-associated immune responses in liver tumor surveillance and tumor progression. *Cancer Cell.* (2016) 30:533–47. doi: 10.1016/j.ccell.2016.09.003
98. Zhou S-L, Zhou Z-J, Hu Z-Q, Huang X-W, Wang Z, Chen E-B, et al. Tumor-associated neutrophils recruit macrophages and T-regulatory cells to promote progression of hepatocellular carcinoma and resistance to Sorafenib. *Gastroenterology.* (2016) 150:1646–58.e17. doi: 10.1053/j.gastro.2016.02.040
99. Lim SY, Yuzhalin AE, Gordon-Weeks AN, Muschel RJ. Tumor-infiltrating monocytes/macrophages promote tumor invasion and migration by upregulating S100A8 and S100A9 expression in cancer cells. *Oncogene.* (2016) 35:5735–45. doi: 10.1038/onc.2016.107
100. Li X, Yao W, Yuan Y, Chen P, Li B, Li J, et al. Targeting of tumour-infiltrating macrophages via CCL2/CCR2 signalling as a therapeutic strategy against hepatocellular carcinoma. *Gut.* (2017) 66:157. doi: 10.1136/gutjnl-2015-310514

101. Lesokhin AM, Hohl TM, Kitano S, Cortez C, Hirschhorn-Cymerman D, Avogadri F, et al. Monocytic CCR2(+) myeloid-derived suppressor cells promote immune escape by limiting activated CD8 T-cell infiltration into the tumor microenvironment. *Cancer Res.* (2012) 72:876–86. doi: 10.1158/0008-5472.CAN-11-1792

102. Zhao Y, Wu T, Shao S, Shi B, Zhao Y. Phenotype, development, and biological function of myeloid-derived suppressor cells. *Oncoimmunology.* (2015) 5:e1004983. doi: 10.1080/2162402X.2015.1004983

103. Xue J, Schmidt SV, Sander J, Draffehn A, Krebs W, Quester I, et al. Transcriptome-based network analysis reveals a spectrum model of human macrophage activation. *Immunity.* (2014) 40:274–88. doi: 10.1016/j.immuni.2014.01.006

104. Ramachandran P, Dobie R, Wilson-Kanamori JR, Dora EF, Henderson EP, Luu NT, et al. Resolving the fibrotic niche of human liver cirrhosis at single-cell level. *Nature.* (2019) 575:512–8. doi: 10.1038/s41586-019-1631-3

105. Murray PJ, Allen JE, Biswas SK, Fisher EA, Gilroy DW, Goerdt S, et al. Macrophage activation and polarization: nomenclature and experimental guidelines. *Immunity.* (2014) 41:14–20. doi: 10.1016/j.immuni.2014.06.008

106. Mandal M, Gardner CR, Sun R, Choi H, Lad S, Mishin V, et al. The spleen as an extramedullary source of inflammatory cells responding to acetaminophen-induced liver injury. *Toxicol Appl Pharmacol.* (2016) 304:110–20. doi: 10.1016/j.taap.2016.04.019

107. Jenkins SJ, Ruckerl D, Cook PC, Jones LH, Finkelman FD, van Rooijen N, et al. Local macrophage proliferation, rather than recruitment from the blood, is a signature of TH2 inflammation. *Science.* (2011) 332:1284–8. doi: 10.1126/science.1204351

10

Macrophages in the Aging Liver and Age-Related Liver Disease

*Elizabeth C. Stahl, Martin J. Haschak, Branimir Popovic and Bryan N. Brown**

Department of Bioengineering, Pittsburgh Liver Research Center, McGowan Institute for Regenerative Medicine, University of Pittsburgh, Pittsburgh, PA, United States

Correspondence:
Bryan N. Brown
brownb@upmc.edu

The number of individuals aged 65 or older is projected to increase globally from 524 million in 2010 to nearly 1. 5 billion in 2050. Aged individuals are particularly at risk for developing chronic illness, while being less able to regenerate healthy tissue and tolerate whole organ transplantation procedures. In the liver, these age-related diseases include non-alcoholic fatty liver disease, alcoholic liver disease, hepatitis, fibrosis, and cirrhosis. Hepatic macrophages, a population comprised of both Kupffer cells and infiltrating monocyte derived macrophages, are implicated in several chronic liver diseases and also play important roles in the homeostatic functions of the liver. The effects of aging on hepatic macrophage population dynamics, polarization, and function are not well understood. Studies performed on macrophages derived from other aged sources, such as the bone marrow, peritoneal cavity, lungs, and brain, demonstrate general reductions in autophagy and phagocytosis, dysfunction in cytokine signaling, and altered morphology and distribution, likely mediated by epigenetic changes and mitochondrial defects, that may be applicable to hepatic macrophages. This review highlights recent findings in macrophage developmental biology and function, particularly in the liver, and discusses the role of macrophages in various age-related liver diseases. A better understanding of the biology of aging that influences hepatic macrophages and thus the progression of chronic liver disease will be crucial in order to develop new interventions and treatments for liver disease in aging populations.

Keywords: Kupffer cell, monocyte-derived macrophage, chronic liver disease, inflammation, fibrosis, senescence, mitochondria

INTRODUCTION TO MACROPHAGES IN THE LIVER

The liver is an important immunological organ, serving as a surveillance system for gut-derived pathogens and producing several key immune components—complement, acute phase, and coagulation proteins (1, 2). While hepatocytes and certain non-parenchymal cells possess some inherent immunological properties [see reviews (3) and (4)], multiple populations of $CD45^+$ immune cells are transiently or permanently located in the liver.

The healthy liver is home to several populations of lymphocytes, including natural killer (NK) cells, NK T-cells, B-cells, mucosal associated T-cells and γδ-T-cells (5–8). In humans, 40% of the resident lymphocyte population are composed of NK cells, while in mice 40% of the resident lymphocytes are NK T-cells.

Innate immune cells also have a large presence in the liver. The majority of immune cells in the liver are myeloid derived cells (9). Dendritic cell (DC) populations, including both myeloid and plasmacytoid DCs, are present in the liver and can activate T-cells under appropriate conditions (10). Myeloid-derived suppressor cells (MDSC) are also present and suppress T-cell activation (11). Macrophages derived from circulating monocytes have been identified as a motile population of myeloid cells infiltrating the liver during inflammation and at varying levels during homeostasis (12–14). The resident macrophage, known as the Kupffer cell (KC), is the most highly represented immune cell, comprising nearly one-third of non-parenchymal cells in the liver (15).

Macrophages play a key role in the homeostatic functions of the liver as well as in disease states and are among the most widely studied immune cells in the liver (15). The prevalence and severity of many chronic liver diseases increases with age, including alcoholic hepatitis, non-alcoholic steatohepatitis, cirrhosis, and hepatocellular carcinoma (16). However, mechanisms underlying changes in the liver structure and cellular function, including hepatocytes and resident immune cell populations, are not well understood. This review will cover the developmental origin and function of macrophages in the liver, as well as their implications in several age-related liver diseases, in order to better understand and expose gaps in the knowledge of the biology of liver aging and disease. As most of the experimental data has been collected from murine animal models, this review focuses largely on preclinical studies in mice and extends these findings to chronic liver disease in humans.

Development and Polarization of Macrophages

Macrophage development begins in the extraembryonic yolk sac from erythro-myeloid progenitors, a process known as primitive hematopoiesis, prior to the appearance of hematopoietic stem cells or monocytic precursors (17, 18). After this transient wave of primitive hematopoiesis, hematopoietic stem cells appear in the aorto-gonado-mesonephric region and migrate to the fetal liver, marking the start of definitive hematopoiesis and development of naïve macrophages through monocytic precursors (17). Definitive hematopoiesis remains in the fetal liver until approximately E18 in mice or 12 weeks post-conception in humans, after which hematopoietic stem cells migrate from the fetal liver to the bone marrow niche, where they will remain throughout adulthood (19).

Macrophages can be subdivided into tissue resident or monocyte derived populations. The number of resident macrophages varies considerably based on the tissue, and approximately 80% of total tissue resident macrophages are located in the liver (20). Resident macrophages can be colonized from a single developmental source, such as microglia and Kupffer cells, which are derived from yolk sac primitive macrophages. Alternatively, resident macrophages may be repopulated several times during development, such as Langerhans cells in the skin, which are originally derived from yolk-sac macrophages and later replaced by fetal liver monocytes (13, 21). Macrophage populations in the gut, spleen, and lungs are continuously replenished by monocyte input throughout adulthood (12, 13).

During inflammation, both resident and monocyte-derived macrophages participate in migration, expansion, and signaling depending on the tissue type and stimulus. Resident tissue macrophages, including Kupffer cells, peritoneal macrophages, and pleural macrophages, have been shown to undergo rapid proliferation in response to Th2 cytokines, such as interleukin-4 (22). Infiltrating macrophages can be derived from either classical ($CD14^+CD16^-$ human, $Ly6C^{hi}$ mouse) or non-classical ($CD14^+CD16^+$ human, $Ly6C^{lo}$ mouse) monocytes, which extravasate into tissue sites under chemokine concentration gradient guidance (17, 23). Following extravasation, monocytes differentiate into macrophages whose functionality are largely based on the integration of the various signaling molecules present in the local microenvironment (24, 25).

In addition to developmental heterogeneity, macrophages are extraordinarily dynamic cells that exhibit various phenotypes ranging from a pro-inflammatory, classically activated "M1" polarization state to an anti-inflammatory, alternatively activated "M2" polarization state, as shown in **Figure 1** (26, 27). M1/M2 polarization refers to extreme phenotypes that can be simulated *in vitro* with the addition of various stimuli (lipopolysaccharide and/or interferon-gamma for M1 activation; interleukin-4 for M2 activation), but the scenario *in vivo* is often more complex and thus polarization is a spectrum of phenotypes, including but not limited to M2a, M2b, and M2c sub-groups (27, 28).

In general, M1 polarization leads to production of canonical pro-inflammatory cytokines (IL-1, IL-6, IL-12, IL-18, TNF, IL-23, IL-27), reactive oxygen species such as nitric oxide, and chemokines (CCL2, CCL5, CXCL9, CXCL10, CXCL11, IL-8) (27). Macrophage pro-inflammatory cytokine maturation can occur through inflammasome-independent or inflammasome-dependent mechanisms (29, 30). Inflammasome formation is induced by damage-associated molecular patterns (DAMPs) and pathogen-associated molecular patterns (PAMPs) binding to nod-like receptors, including NLRP3 and NLRP1, or to Pyrin receptor family members such as Pyrin and AIM2 on the surface of macrophages (31). Docking proteins, including apoptosis-associated speck-like protein, assemble and recruit pro-caspase 1, where proximity-based autoproteolytic cleavage catalyzes the activation of caspase-1 (29, 32) Caspase-1 activation subsequently catalyzes the cleavage of the pro-forms of IL-1β and IL-18 into activated forms. Caspase-1 may also induce pyroptosis, a programmed cell death pathway characterized by cellular lysis and endogenous DAMP release into the environment, to induce additional inflammatory cell recruitment (33).

M2-polarized macrophages typically appear following M1-polarized macrophages in an injury setting and serve as a counterbalance to resolve inflammation and promote tissue repair (34). The M2 polarization state leads to secretion of cytokines commonly associated with anti-inflammatory properties, such as IL-10, as well as various matrix-modulatory factors including transforming growth factor-β (TGF-β) and matrix metalloproteases (MMPs) (35). The overproduction of remodeling growth factors can lead to excessive deposition of matrix proteins (i.e., fibrosis), or excessive angiogenesis and immunosuppression in the case of tumor-associated macrophages (TAMs) (36). Therefore, the temporal regulation of M1 and M2 macrophage responses are extremely important for appropriate outcomes following

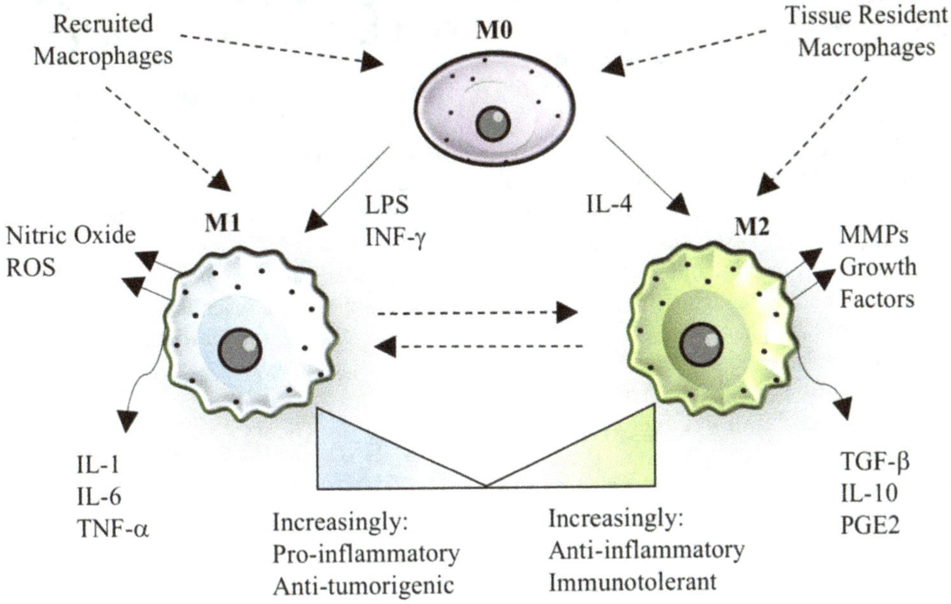

FIGURE 1 | Macrophage polarization. The paradigm of macrophage polarization begins with a quiescent or patrolling M0 cell, that may be derived from either circulating monocytes or tissue-resident populations. The transition from M0 to M1 can be stimulated by lipopolysaccharide (LPS) or interferon-gamma, resulting in a cell that has pro-inflammatory and anti-tumorigenic properties. M1 macrophages also produce nitric oxide and other reactive oxygen species (ROS). The transition from M0 to M2 can be stimulated by interleukin-4, resulting in a cell that has anti-inflammatory or immunotolerant properties. M2 macrophages also produce matrix metalloproteinases (MMPs) and growth factors that aid in tissue regeneration. M1 and M2 phenotypes are dynamic and exist on a spectrum, where recruited macrophages tend to be more "M1-like" in the case of bacterial infection, and tissue-resident macrophages tend to be more "M2-like" during homeostasis. In specific instances, such as helminth infection, recruited macrophages take on an M2 phenotype, demonstrating the versatility and adaptability of the macrophage polarization spectrum in response to the signals in a given context.

injury and infection and are often dysregulated in chronic disease.

The Origin and Function of the Kupffer Cell

The Kupffer cell is a primitive cell, appearing early during embryogenesis (E9.5-E12.5 in mice), derived primarily from the yolk sac (14, 37, 38). Importantly, the KC population is maintained through self-proliferation, with minimal input from circulating monocytes during homeostasis (12–14, 22).

The tissue-resident Kupffer cell is the key detector of commensal or pathogenic microbial signals, danger signals, and tumor cells moving through the hepatic circulation (15, 39, 40). KCs are located along the hepatic sinusoids allowing for the low-pressure blood supply come into contact with both KCs and hepatocytes through the fenestrated endothelium (2). KCs express the complement receptor CRIg, which binds complement fragments C3b and iC3b, allowing phagocytosis of complement C3-opsonized particles even under low-pressure blood flow (41, 42). Bacterial clearance by KCs is crucial for host defense as 80% of blood-borne bacteria accumulate in the liver and are destroyed there (15, 39, 40).

PAMPs and DAMPs are present in relatively high concentrations in blood entering the liver from the gut, via the portal vein, and engage with pattern recognition receptors (PRRs), including Toll-like receptors, on the surface of macrophages and hepatocytes (43–45). With low levels of bacterial endotoxins, KCs promote immune tolerance by secreting anti-inflammatory factors including IL-10, TGF-β, and prostaglandin-E2 (PGE2), thereby inducing regulatory T-cells (46, 47). In the presence of higher concentrations of damage or pathogen-associated signaling molecules, KCs can become polarized toward an M1 phenotype and produce a variety of inflammatory cytokines including IL-1, IL-6, IL-12, TNF-α (15, 39, 40). Several liver diseases are influenced by KC activation and expansion, but their individual role has been difficult to dissect from more recently identified macrophage populations in the liver.

The Origin and Function of Other Hepatic Macrophage Populations

Within the past decade, the heterogeneity of hepatic macrophages, i.e., Kupffer cells and monocyte-derived macrophages (mMØs), has become an emerging topic in hepatology. Fate tracing experiments in the brain first determined that resident microglia are established prenatally and maintained independently from monocyte input, which was later translated to the liver (48). Holt et al. were among the first to identify two populations of macrophages in the liver (49). Through bone marrow chimera experiments, cells expressing $F4/80^{hi}CD11b^{lo}$ were identified as KCs, while cells expressing $F4/80^{lo}CD11b^{hi}$ were found to be derived from circulating monocytic progenitors (49). Shortly after, Klein et al. classified two macrophage populations in the liver: KCs as immobile, "sessile" macrophages and mMØs as motile cells (50).

In most cases, murine mMØs in the liver are derived from an influx of bone marrow derived, Ly6C^{hi} monocytes, primarily driven by monocyte chemoattractant protein, which can be produced by KCs, stellate cells, or hepatocytes (also known as CCR2-CCL2 interactions) (51, 52). Secondary pathways of monocyte recruitment to the liver are CXCR3-CXCL10, CCR1-CCL5, and CCR8-CCL1 dependent (53–55). Murine mMØs may also be derived from Ly6C^{lo} monocytes trafficking from the spleen, which express CD11b, but are thought to take on a more patrolling or regulatory macrophage phenotype (56). Phagocytes from the peritoneal cavity, which express F4/80, CD11b, and GATA6, have been shown to cross into the liver after subcapsular liver lesion (57), but it remains unclear if this infiltration occurs in other liver injury settings.

Kinoshita et al. determined that murine mMØs and KCs could be distinguished by CD11b and CD68 expression, respectively (40). The CD11b^{hi} mMØs were radiosensitive and particularly efficient at producing IL-12, protecting the host against tumor xenografts, while the CD68^{hi} KCs were radioresistant and highly efficient at phagocytosis, protecting the host against bacterial challenge (40). The use of these differentiating markers has been expanded to several disease models, identifying a damaging role of TNF/FasL production by CD11b^{+} mMØs in carbon-tetrachloride acute liver injury and hepatitis in hypercholesterolemic mice (58, 59). The CD11b^{+} mMØs were also found to accumulate in the liver following repeated lipopolysaccharide injections, but suppressed TNF efflux into the systemic circulation, thereby reducing lethal septicemia (60). In addition, the CD11b^{+} mMØs were recruited during diet-induced steatohepatitis in FGF5 deficient mice and following partial hepatectomy, where they were crucial for liver regeneration (61, 62). Others have observed that monocyte derived cells protect the liver from iron toxicity in hemolytic anemia by ingesting senescent and dying erythrocytes (63).

More recently, the C-type lectin, Clec4f, has been identified as a selective murine KC marker (64). Interesting, ablating KCs via Clec4f-driven diphtheria toxin causes an influx of mMØs, which can differentiate into nearly identical KCs when this "niche" is made available. Only 12 genes remained differentially expressed between monocyte derived KCs and embryonically derived KCs, including *CD209f, CD163, C2, CCR3, Timd4,* and *Snrpn* at the time points examined (64).

Taken together, KCs and mMØs play heterogenous roles in various liver disease states and cannot be considered wholly harmful or beneficial without deciphering the given context. Importantly, infiltrating monocytes may also differentiate into dendritic cells, which play distinct immunostimulatory and antigen presentation roles in the liver (65). The heterogeneity of hepatic macrophages is less well defined in humans as compared to murine animal models. The role of these diverse hepatic macrophage populations in a given disease context is just beginning to be understood and has not yet been examined in the natural aging process, a major risk factor for several chronic liver diseases.

CELLULAR MANIFESTATIONS OF AGING ON HEPATOCYTES AND MACROPHAGES

The process of aging is closely associated with a number of degenerative modifications in the liver, where hepatic structure and cell function are observed to decline. Both hepatocytes and macrophages exhibit deficits in mitochondrial function, linked to a decline in autophagy and production of pro-inflammatory molecules (66, 67). While the effects of aging on hepatic macrophages have not been well characterized on a cellular and molecular level, several studies have examined macrophages from alternative tissue sources and may offer some insight about hepatic macrophages.

Changes in Hepatic Structure and Hepatocyte Function

Several studies have shown that the volume of blood in the liver decreases in elderly individuals, leading to a total volume loss of 20–40% (68). In addition, the thickness of liver sinusoidal endothelial cells fenestrations increases, limiting the exchange of molecules to and from the liver (69). At the serum level, aging is associated with reductions in albumin and bilirubin, increases in alkaline phosphatase, and minimal changes in aminotransferase levels (70). The metabolism of cholesterol in the liver also decreases, leading to increased blood cholesterol and neutral fat levels over time (70). However, recent investigations suggest the most essential change in liver aging is loss of the functional liver cell mass (71).

Changes in the morphology of hepatocytes may be related to increased polyploidy, accumulation of lipofuscin in the cytoplasm, and declining surface area of endoplasmic reticulum and number of mitochondria, ultimately negatively affecting the function of hepatocytes (66, 72, 73). The decline in hepatocyte mitochondrial function has been suggested to enhance the vulnerability of aged livers to acute injury and to cause delays in liver regeneration (74). The oxidative capacity of the liver also declines with aging, and therefore medications that require oxidation, such as benzodiazepines, may accumulate in toxic levels and are not prescribed to elderly individuals (75). In addition, aging livers are known to accumulate a multiprotein C/EBPalpha-Brm-HDAC1 complex that silences elongation factor 2 (E2F)-dependent promoters, thereby reducing proliferation and regenerative capacity of hepatocytes (76).

Senescent cells accumulate in the liver during aging and in chronic liver disease; and may include hepatocytes, cholangiocytes, stellate cells, and immune cells [reviewed here: (77)]. Cells become senescent as a result of replicative exhaustion (telomere shortening), DNA damage, or oxidative stress, among other mechanisms (78). Senescent cells are characterized by the expression of cell cycle inhibitors p21, p16, and p53, which prevent replication and apoptosis, as well as secretion of pro-inflammatory cytokines that signal for their removal but can lead to tissue damage when chronically expressed (79, 80). Senescent hepatocytes accumulate with age and appear as an almost "universal phenomenon" in chronic liver diseases including hepatitis B and C infection, alcoholic and non-alcoholic liver disease, and genetic haemochromatosis (77). Senescent hepatocytes undergo metabolic changes, such as increased transport of conjugated bilirubin into the hepatic sinusoids and insulin resistance through dysregulated glucose transporter expression and Akt signaling among others, which dysregulates normal function (81). Interestingly, the length of telomeres was found to be conserved in aged hepatocytes and bile duct cholangiocytes but decreased in aged Kupffer cells and stellate cells, suggesting cell-specific mechanisms of senescent phenotype acquisition in the liver (82).

Overall, the effects of aging on non-parenchymal cell subsets, particularly hepatic macrophages, is an understudied area. Hilmer et al. determined that the number and basal activity of Kupffer cells was increased with old age in a rat model (83), however this work was performed before the heterogeneity of liver macrophages was fully contemplated. Similarly, Singh et al. identified a change in liver macrophage distribution with aging, where old mice had more F4/80^{+} macrophages located in large lymphoid structures (also containing T-cells and B-cells), and a reduction in the number of spindle shaped macrophages throughout the parenchyma (84).

Recent work by Maeso-Diaz et al. characterized molecular changes in LSECs, stellate cells, and hepatic macrophages in the livers of aged rats (85). The authors found a significant deregulation of LSEC phenotype with aging as demonstrated by downregulation of vasodilatory pathways (nitric oxide, heme oxygenase), increase in oxidative stress, and decrease in angiocrine markers (stabilin-2, CD32b, and VEGFR2), in addition to increased portal pressure and vascular resistance (85). Aged stellate cells had increased markers of activation (alpha smooth muscle actin and collagen I), increased intracellular lipid stores, and alterations in retinoid metabolism (85). Finally, the authors noted an increase in recruitment of proinflammatory cells in aged livers, including increased IL-6 expression in isolated hepatic macrophages, but no change in the traditional macrophage polarization markers (85). Human livers showed similar trends in downregulation of endothelial markers, but substantial work remains to extend and decode these findings in both aged murine and human systems.

Declines in Cell Intrinsic Macrophage Function With Aging

The process of aging has been shown to affect macrophage polarization and function in multiple tissues and disease models, with compelling underlying mechanisms that may be broadly applicable to hepatic macrophages, as summarized in **Figure 2**.

Autophagy, or the intracellular degradation of damaged proteins and organelles in autophagosomes, is one such process which has been shown to become dysregulated with increasing age in macrophage populations (86). Deletion of autophagy genes *Atg5* and *Atg7* in bone marrow-derived macrophages results in decreased antigen presentation capacity, impaired maturation, altered mitochondrial metabolism, downregulation of surface receptors such as toll-like receptor 4 (TLR4), and increased secretion of pro-inflammatory cytokines (86, 87). The

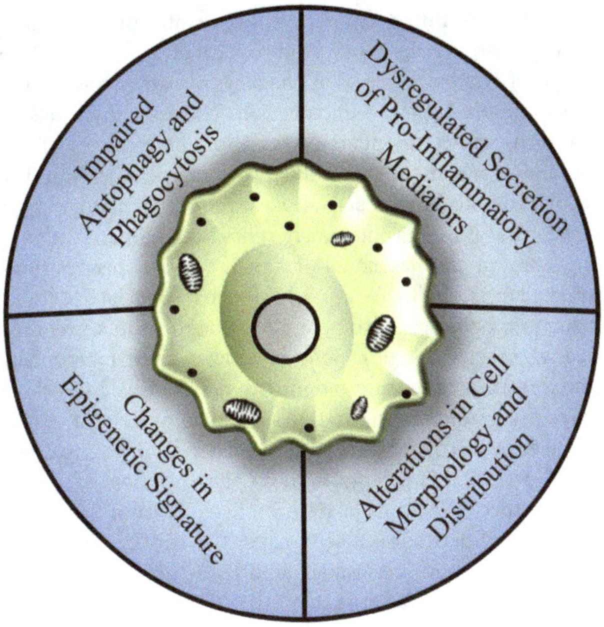

FIGURE 2 | Mechanisms of age-associated decline in macrophage function. Macrophages from various tissue sources, including the bone marrow, peritoneal cavity, lungs, and brain, show an array of dysfunction including a general reduction in autophagy and phagocytosis, dysregulation of pro-inflammatory cytokine production associated with changes in toll-like receptor expression, and alterations in cell morphology and distribution that may be related to repopulation of tissues by infiltrating monocyte populations, largely mediated by changes in epigenetic signature and mitochondrial dysfunction.

phenotype of autophagy deficient bone marrow macrophages closely mimics the phenotype of macrophages isolated from aged individuals (86), which may be driven by the hypermethylation of autophagy associated genes (88). It remains to be seen if restoring autophagic flux to aged macrophages can improve their function and polarization status, however caloric restriction has been shown to improve both longevity and autophagic capacity in animal models (89).

Phagocytic clearance of extracellular pathogens and antigen presentation tends to be attenuated in aged macrophage populations as well (90). While no difference in phagocytic capacity was found between young and aged bone marrow derived macrophages, peritoneal macrophages exhibit an age-associated decline in phagocytic capacity and antigen presentation (90). This reduction in phagocytic ability was driven by age-related alterations in the local microenvironment, as young peritoneal macrophages transplanted into aged peritoneal space exhibited reduced phagocytic and antigen presentation capabilities (90). Alveolar macrophages isolated from aged individuals have been shown to exhibit reduced phagocytic capacity as well as attenuated expression of genes associated with macrophage proliferation (91). This reduction both in cell number and phagocytic ability contributes to the age-related mortality risk following pathogen infection, such as in the case of an influenza lung infection model (91). In the liver, there have been mixed reports on the maintenance of Kupffer cell phagocytosis, where one study reported a deficit (92) and another reported an increase in phagocytosis with aging (83).

Furthermore, the reduction in expression levels of autophagosome components prevents the endocytosis of both inflammasome components and damaged mitochondria and can thereby promote chronic activation of pro-inflammatory signals in aged cells (87). This phenomenon has been termed "inflamm-aging," one of the hallmarks of aging, and has been strongly correlated to morbidity (93). In addition to dysregulated cytokine production, aging can promote alterations in the secretion of oxidative species (94–96). Bone marrow-derived macrophages isolated from aged murine and human donors have been shown to produce greater concentrations of nitric oxide and reactive oxidative species than macrophages isolated from young donors (96). However, this upregulation in the secretion of reactive oxidative species was not observed following pro-inflammatory stimulation of peritoneal macrophages (94, 95). Further studies will be necessary to fully understand tissue-specific changes in respiratory burst characteristics.

The morphology of macrophages can also be influenced by the aging process. Microglia have been shown to increase cell soma volume while reducing the length of cellular processes in aged brains (97). These morphological changes reduce the capability of the microglia to interact with neural cells and perform routine surveillance of the local microenvironment (97). While microglial population sizes increase to account for this reduction in cell process size (17), the population expansion tends to occur in a non-homogenous manner, disrupting the uniform microglial distributions commonly observed in young animals (97). In addition, aged microglia exhibit enhanced secretion of reactive oxidative species following central nervous system injury through upregulation of NADPH oxidase 2 (NOX2) (98), and secrete elevated concentrations of IL-1β mediated by hypomethylation of CpG sires in the IL-1β proximal promoter (99).

Infiltration of monocyte-derived macrophages to multiple tissue sites has been observed in age-related diseases, including Alzheimer's disease (100), which leads to increased inflammation and phagocytosis. In the cardiovascular system, the tissue resident macrophage population (yolk-sac derived, M2-like) is replaced by bone marrow-derived macrophages over time (101, 102). This shift in macrophage populations contributes to deleterious outcomes following cardiac injury, such as chronic inflammation, fibrotic scar deposition, and reduced re-vascularization of ischemic tissue following injury (101, 103). It remains unclear whether age-related changes in macrophage responses are a primary result of shifting cell origins and polarization states driven by the microenvironment or by cell intrinsic functions, although both are likely in play.

The Role of the Aged Microenvironment on Macrophage Function

While cell intrinsic properties, such as mitochondrial capacity and autophagy, may drive changes in age-associated macrophage polarization, this only represents a partial view of the complex innate and adaptive immune dysfunction which occurs with age. For example, age-related alterations in the T cell compartment, which are numerous [reviewed here (104, 105)], can shift the relative Th1 and Th2 cytokine concentrations and directly impact macrophage polarization (106, 107).

Non-immune cell types can also contribute to the age-associated immune dysfunction. With age, increasingly large numbers of pre-adipocytes differentiate into mature adipocytes, with enhanced secretion of leptin, TNF-α, and IL-6, and reduced secretion of adiponectin—a factor commonly associated with M2 macrophage polarization, thereby promoting M1 phenotypes (108–110). Numerous DAMPs, which have been shown to promote inflammasome formation and activation, also have age-related increases in concentration, including cholesterol (111), amyloid-β (112, 113), hydroxyapatite crystals (114), purine catabolic end products such as uric acid (115), and ATP (116). Radical oxidative species, which tend to exhibit an increase in production and secretion with increasing age, have also been shown to play an important role in inflammasome activation through oxidation of proteins, lipids, and DNA, leading to inflammatory cytokine secretion into the aged microenvironment (29, 117, 118). More recently, the effect of the aging gut microbiome on macrophage function has been considered (119). Raising mice under germ-free conditions preserves the bactericidal capacity of alveolar macrophages and reduces secretion of IL-6 in old age, mediated by reduced dysbiosis and improved gut permeability (119).

While this is only a brief consideration of additional factors that have been observed to influence macrophage function, it serves to highlight the complexity and tissue specificity that defines age-related immunomodulation. The mechanisms governing the acquisition of age-related dysfunction in infiltrating and tissue resident macrophage populations continues to be an active area of research, and it will be essential for investigators to utilize an array of cell markers and descriptive methods to appropriately place cells along the spectrum of polarization states.

THE ROLE OF MACROPHAGES IN AGE-RELATED LIVER DISEASE

Aging is a major risk factor for the development and prognosis of several chronic liver diseases and conditions, including nonalcoholic fatty liver disease, alcoholic liver disease, hepatitis C, and an increased susceptibility to develop fibrosis and cirrhosis (16). The reduced capacity of aged livers to regenerate and to tolerate transplantation leads to increased risk of mortality from chronic liver diseases, as demonstrated in **Figure 3**.

Both Kupffer cells and infiltrating monocytes are implicated to various levels in the etiology of chronic liver disease, however the distinction between these two cell populations is less clear in human clinical liver samples compared to animal studies. Importantly, most animal models of chronic liver disease are induced in young, healthy animals through genetic manipulation or by administering specific diets or chemical

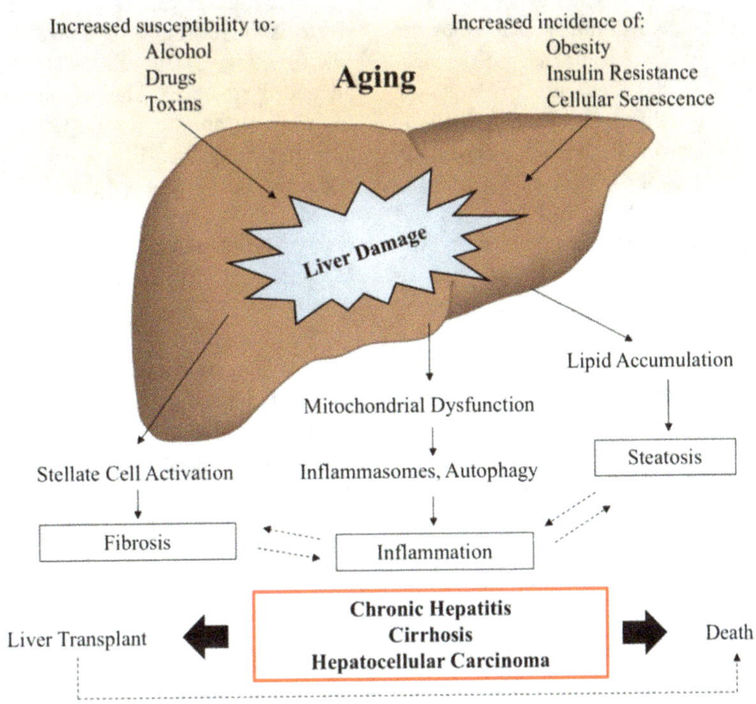

FIGURE 3 | Aging and liver disease. With increasing age, the liver becomes more susceptible to damage from alcohol, drugs, and toxins, while the prevalence of metabolic disease, obesity, and cellular senescence are known to increase. These insults lead to the activation of signaling pathways driving liver pathology, such as inflammation, steatosis, and fibrosis, which are often involved in positive feedback loops, further exacerbating the symptoms of liver disease. In a subset of patients, liver disease will progress to chronic hepatitis, cirrhosis, and hepatocellular carcinoma, also known as end stage liver disease, for which transplant is the only viable therapy. Studies suggest that elderly patients have decreased survival post-transplantation, demonstrating the need for additional therapies to intervene and prevent the onset of age-related liver disease symptoms.

toxins. Findings from these animal studies are important to identify novel mechanisms regulating liver disease but may not prove relevant or all-encompassing when translating the findings to older, human populations, as evidenced by the moderate success of several anti-fibrotic therapies in clinical trials (120). Distinguishing between the biology of aging and age-associated pathologies can be a difficult task but is an important effort in the field of hepatology. Additional studies are needed to assess the effect of aging on the liver prior to the onset of age-associated pathologies in order to dissect mechanisms of aging from the manifestation of the pathology itself.

Liver Fibrosis

Aging is a major risk factor for the progression of liver fibrosis, particularly in hepatitis, which can advance to portal hypertension and cirrhosis (121). Fibrosis occurs when excessive connective tissue is deposited following acute or chronic liver damage, and is often the starting point of architectural distortion and dysfunction that prevents normal functioning of the liver (122). Age-related dysfunction in hepatic macrophages and stellate cells are heavily implicated in development of fibrosis and may be related to oxidative stress and macrophage polarization, but these mechanisms are not well understood (123).

In general, an increase in M1-polarized macrophages appears at the early stages of liver disease and promotes or exacerbates fibrosis, cirrhosis, and eventual liver failure. In clinical studies, the progression from hepatitis to fibrosis and eventually cirrhosis was associated with enrichment of $CD14^{+}CD16^{+}$ non-classical monocytes in the liver, which have been shown to activate stellate cells *in vitro* based on TGF-beta release (124). These cells may be derived from classical $CD14^{+}CD16^{-}$ monocytes or infiltrate directly (125). Activation of the CCL2-CCR2 axis is associated with monocyte infiltration in both rodent models and patients with fibrosis and liver disease (126). A recent study found that the acquisition of M1 phenotypes in liver fibrosis may be regulated by interferon regulatory factor 5 (IRF5), which is significantly induced in liver macrophages in both mouse and human subjects developing fibrosis, and may represent a novel target for therapeutic intervention (127).

Alcoholic Liver Disease

Elderly individuals are more likely to feel socially isolated and depressed, resulting in a rising alcohol consumption rate and prevalence of alcoholic liver disease in this population (128). Alcohol and its breakdown products are toxic to the liver, which can cause a disorder in lipid metabolism by increasing the synthesis of fatty acids and suppressing mitochondrial β-oxidation (129). The risk of alcohol toxicity is further increased in elderly populations due to alterations in metabolism or by the intake of certain medications (130).

Alcoholic liver disease can be classified into three stages: accumulation of extra fat in the liver (steatosis), alcoholic hepatitis, and cirrhosis. Macrophages were found to increase in both the early and late stages of alcoholic liver disease. Increased gut permeability and high levels of endotoxin in the portal blood results in activation of Kupffer cells (131). In addition, $Ly6C^+$ macrophages were found to accumulate in murine models of alcoholic liver injury, regulated by CCL2 chemokine signaling (132). Clinical symptoms of alcoholic liver disease among the elderly are similar to younger counterparts, yet the prevalence of advancing to irreversible stages of the disease is greater in older individuals (133). Oxidative stress and production of TNF by hepatic macrophages, as a result of steatosis or leaky gut, causes progression to later stages (130). Furthermore, the expression of M1 pro-inflammatory genes was found to be higher in peritoneal macrophages from patients with alcohol-related cirrhosis and ascites compared to hepatitis-C related cirrhosis, suggesting systemic differences in macrophage polarization (134). Reducing leaky gut and inflammation have been identified as potential therapeutic targets for treating alcoholic liver disease (135).

Non-alcoholic Fatty Liver Disease

Non-alcoholic fatty liver disease (NAFLD) and non-alcoholic steatohepatitis (NASH) are leading causes of chronic liver disease globally and are projected to become the leading indication for liver transplantation in the United States (136–138). NAFLD often presents with metabolic syndrome, such as obesity and excessive visceral fat, hyperlipidemia, hypertension, insulin resistance and an increased secretion of pro-inflammatory cytokines (139). All of these components of metabolic syndrome are generally observed in elderly populations and many studies find increased rates of NAFLD among elderly people compared with their younger counterparts (140–142).

The mechanism for developing age-related steatosis is not fully understood but has been attributed to hepatocyte senescence driving a reduction in mitochondrial metabolism (143), decreased transport of insulin across the sinusoidal endothelium (144), reduction in autophagic flux (145), or chronic low-level inflammation (146, 147), leading to the build-up of toxic free fatty acids in the liver. Lifestyle choices, such as high fat diet (HFD), may also lead to the development of NAFLD in aged individuals. Work by Fontana et al. found that mice were equally susceptible to steatosis following HFD regardless of age. However, the older mice exhibited more severe hepatocellular injury and inflammation following administration of HFD that was attributed to increased M1 macrophage polarization in both the liver and white adipose tissues (148).

As in other chronic liver diseases, macrophages accumulate in the livers of NAFLD patients (149). Experimental mouse models have shown an accumulation of $Ly6C^+$ monocytes is a critical step in the development of progressive fibrosis from steatohepatitis in a CCL2-dependent mechanism (131). In addition, lipids and free fatty acids contribute to DAMP-induced Kupffer cell activation (150). Patients with low-grade steatosis were found to have higher mRNA expression of M2 markers, CD206 and CD163, compared to patients with advanced steatosis. The M2 macrophages were hypothesized to promote apoptosis of M1 polarized hepatic macrophages and protect against disease progression of NAFLD or alcoholic hepatitis (149). Interestingly, soluble CD163 (sCD163), a marker of M1 macrophage polarization, increases systemically with severity of NAFLD in human patients (151), again suggesting that M1 polarization is associated with more advanced stages of the disease.

Traditional treatments for NAFLD are more challenging for elderly populations as they require lifestyle changes in exercise, diet, and medication or liver transplantation (152, 153). Findings from a recent clinical trial using a CCR2/CCR5 antagonist to block inflammation resulted in twice as many subjects achieving improvement in fibrosis and no worsening of steatohepatitis compared with placebo (154, 155). Subgroup analysis showed the therapy to be similarly effective in patients below and above 56 years of age, demonstrating promise in the context of age-associated disease.

CONCLUSION

The decline in mitochondrial capacity with aging has emerged as a key mechanism underlying several of the observed changes in the function of both hepatocytes and macrophages, likely contributing to the increased prevalence and severity of chronic liver diseases in elderly populations. In general, the accumulation of infiltrating or M1-polarized monocytes/macrophages tends to exacerbate liver disease and contribute to fibrosis, cirrhosis, and liver failure. However, very few, if any, studies have systematically identified changes in the hepatic macrophage populations of aging livers in either animal models or human patients, representing a hugely understudied area of research.

Liver transplantation is the standard treatment for patients with end stage liver disease. The number of elderly people with liver cirrhosis requiring transplantation has grown over the past 20 years and is expected to increase further (66). Overall survival rates after 1 year are approximately 90% and 10-year survival rates may be more than 70% for recipients (156). However, some studies have found a reduced survival rate in transplant recipients over 60 years of age (from 90 to 64% 1 year survival rate), primarily due to kidney dysfunction and cardiopulmonary disease complications (157). Survival rates improve for elderly patients with few comorbidities (158), thus age alone is not an exclusion criterion from liver transplantation, but all disease risk factors must be considered to devise effective treatment strategies for these age-related chronic liver diseases.

Therapies that suppress M1-polarization or infiltration of macrophages might reduce the progression of liver disease from manageable early stages to chronic end-stages requiring liver transplantation. In the context of aging specifically, promoting M2-gene expression might delay the advancement of liver disease to later stages. However, M2 macrophages have been associated with tumor progression, including clinical hepatocellular carcinoma (HCC) specimens (159). Thus, modulating macrophage polarization has been considered a double-edged sword, and the appearance of liver fibrosis or HCC would need to be closely monitored. Treating the primary drivers of age-associated liver diseases such as alcohol consumption, visceral and ectopic fat accumulation, or deficits in mitochondrial capacity and other age-related mechanisms, will be just as important as targeting the inflammatory symptoms to combat these age-related liver diseases.

Elderly populations continue to increase globally and are particularly at risk for succumbing to liver failure due to the declines in regenerative capacity, reduced survival post-liver transplantation, and tendencies to develop inflammation and fibrosis. Between 1999 and 2016, deaths in the United States from cirrhosis increased by 65% and deaths from HCC doubled (160). A better understanding of the biology of liver aging that influences the onset and progression of chronic liver disease will be crucial in order to develop new interventions and treatments for our aging populations.

AUTHOR CONTRIBUTIONS

ES, MH, BP, and BB contributed to the writing and editing of the manuscript and figure preparation.

ACKNOWLEDGMENTS

Contract grant sponsor: National Institute of Health; contract grant numbers: T32-EB001026 (ES, MH), F31 DK112633 (ES), R01 AG055564 (BB). The content is solely the responsibility of the authors and does not necessarily reflect the official views of the National Institutes of Health. Thank you also to the Pittsburgh Liver Research Center for their support.

REFERENCES

1. Crispe IN. The liver as a lymphoid organ. *Annu Rev Immunol.* (2009) 27:147–63. doi: 10.1146/annurev.immunol.021908.132629
2. Robinson MW, Harmon C, O'Farrelly C. Liver immunology and its role in inflammation and homeostasis. *Cell Mol Immunol.* (2016) 13:267–76. doi: 10.1038/cmi.2016.3
3. Zhou Z, Xu MJ, Gao B. Hepatocytes: a key cell type for innate immunity. *Cell Mol Immunol.* (2016) 13:301–15. doi: 10.1038/cmi.2015.97
4. Knolle PA, Wohlleber D. Immunological functions of liver sinusoidal endothelial cells. *Cell Mol Immunol.* (2016) 13:347–53. doi: 10.1038/cmi.2016.5
5. Doherty DG, Norris S, Madrigal-Estebas L, McEntee G, Traynor O, Hegarty JE, et al. The human liver contains multiple populations of NK cells, T cells, and CD3+CD56+ natural T cells with distinct cytotoxic activities and Th1, Th2, and Th0 cytokine secretion patterns. *J Immunol.* (1999) 163:2314–21.
6. Kenna T, Golden-Mason L, Porcelli SA, Koezuka Y, Hegarty JE, O'Farrelly C, et al. NKT cells from normal and tumor-bearing human livers are phenotypically and functionally distinct from murine NKT cells. *J Immunol.* (2003) 171:1775–9. doi: 10.4049/jimmunol.171.4.1775
7. Kenna T, Golden-Mason L, Norris S, Hegarty JE, O'Farrelly C, Doherty DG. Distinct subpopulations of gamma delta T cells are present in normal and tumor-bearing human liver. *Clin Immunol.* (2004) 113:56–63. doi: 10.1016/j.clim.2004.05.003
8. Dusseaux M, Martin E, Serriari N, Peguillet I, Premel V, Louis D, et al. Human MAIT cells are xenobiotic-resistant, tissue-targeted, CD161hi IL-17-secreting T cells. *Blood* (2011) 117:1250–9. doi: 10.1182/blood-2010-08-303339
9. Gao B, Jeong WI, Tian Z. Liver: an organ with predominant innate immunity. *Hepatology* (2008) 47:729–36. doi: 10.1002/hep.22034
10. Thomson AW, Knolle PA. Antigen-presenting cell function in the tolerogenic liver environment. *Nat Rev Immunol.* (2010) 10:753–66. doi: 10.1038/nri2858
11. Chen S, Akbar SM, Abe M, Hiasa Y, Onji M. Immunosuppressive functions of hepatic myeloid-derived suppressor cells of normal mice and in a murine model of chronic hepatitis B virus. *Clin Exp Immunol.* (2011) 166:134–42. doi: 10.1111/j.1365-2249.2011.04445.x
12. Schulz C, Gomez Perdiguero E, Chorro L, Szabo-Rogers H, Cagnard N, Kierdorf K, et al. A lineage of myeloid cells independent of Myb and hematopoietic stem cells. *Science* (2012) 336:86–90. doi: 10.1126/science.1219179
13. Yona S, Kim KW, Wolf Y, Mildner A, Varol D, Breker M, et al. Fate mapping reveals origins and dynamics of monocytes and tissue macrophages under homeostasis. *Immunity* (2013) 38:79–91. doi: 10.1016/j.immuni.2012.12.001
14. Gomez Perdiguero E, Klapproth K, Schulz C, Busch K, Azzoni E, Crozet L, et al. Tissue-resident macrophages originate from yolk-sac-derived erythro-myeloid progenitors. *Nature* (2015) 518:547–51. doi: 10.1038/nature13989
15. Bilzer M, Roggel F, Gerbes AL. Role of Kupffer cells in host defense and liver disease. *Liver Int.* (2006) 26:1175–86. doi: 10.1111/j.1478-3231.2006.01342.x
16. Sheedfar F, Di Biase S, Koonen D, Vinciguerra M. Liver diseases and aging: friends or foes? *Aging Cell* (2013) 12:950–4. doi: 10.1111/acel.12128
17. Dey A, Allen J, Hankey-Giblin PA. Ontogeny and polarization of macrophages in inflammation: blood monocytes versus tissue macrophages. *Front Immunol.* (2014) 5:683. doi: 10.3389/fimmu.2014.00683
18. van de Laar L, Saelens W, De Prijck S, Martens L, Scott CL, Van Isterdael G, et al. Yolk Sac macrophages, fetal liver, and adult monocytes can colonize an empty niche and develop into functional tissue-resident macrophages. *Immunity* (2016) 44:755–68. doi: 10.1016/j.immuni.2016.02.017
19. Wang LD, Wagers AJ. Dynamic niches in the origination and differentiation of haematopoietic stem cells. *Nat Rev Mol Cell Biol.* (2011) 12:643–55. doi: 10.1038/nrm3184
20. Kakinuma Y, Kimura T, Watanabe Y. Possible involvement of liver resident macrophages (kupffer cells) in the pathogenesis of both intrahepatic and extrahepatic inflammation. *Can J Gastroenterol Hepatol.* (2017) 2017:2896809. doi: 10.1155/2017/2896809
21. Hoeffel G, Wang Y, Greter M, See P, Teo P, Malleret B, et al. Adult Langerhans cells derive predominantly from embryonic fetal liver monocytes with a minor contribution of yolk sac-derived macrophages. *J Exp Med.* (2012) 209:1167–81. doi: 10.1084/jem.20120340
22. Jenkins SJ, Ruckerl D, Cook PC, Jones LH, Finkelman FD, van Rooijen N, et al. Local macrophage proliferation, rather than recruitment from the blood, is a signature of TH2 inflammation. *Science* (2011) 332:1284–8. doi: 10.1126/science.1204351
23. Ingersoll MA, Spanbroek R, Lottaz C, Gautier EL, Frankenberger M, Hoffmann R, et al. Comparison of gene expression profiles between human and mouse monocyte subsets. *Blood* (2010) 115:e10-9. doi: 10.1182/blood-2009-07-235028
24. Brown BN, Haschak MJ, Lopresti ST, Stahl EC. Effects of age-related shifts in cellular function and local microenvironment upon the innate immune response to implants. *Semin Immunol.* (2017) 29:24–32. doi: 10.1016/j.smim.2017.05.001
25. Ricard-Blum S, Vallet SD. Fragments generated upon extracellular matrix remodeling: biological regulators and potential drugs. *Matrix Biol.* (2017). doi: 10.1016/j.matbio.2017.11.005 [Epub ahead of print].
26. Mills CD, Kincaid K, Alt JM, Heilman MJ, Hill AM. M-1/M-2 macrophages and the Th1/Th2 paradigm. *J Immunol.* (2000) 164:6166–73. doi: 10.4049/jimmunol.164.12.6166

27. Murray PJ, Allen JE, Biswas SK, Fisher EA, Gilroy DW, Goerdt S, et al. Macrophage activation and polarization: nomenclature and experimental guidelines. *Immunity* (2014) 41:14–20. doi: 10.1016/j.immuni.2014.06.008
28. Martinez FO, Gordon S. The M1 and M2 paradigm of macrophage activation: time for reassessment. *F1000Prime Rep.* (2014) 6:13. doi: 10.12703/P6-13
29. Kapetanovic R, Bokil NJ, Sweet MJ. Innate immune perturbations, accumulating DAMPs and inflammasome dysregulation: a ticking time bomb in ageing. *Ageing Res Rev.* (2015) 24(Pt A):40–53.
30. Latz E, Xiao TS, Stutz A. Activation and regulation of the inflammasomes. *Nat Rev Immunol.* (2013) 13:397–411. doi: 10.1038/nri3452
31. Schroder K, Tschopp J. The inflammasomes. *Cell* (2010) 140:821–32. doi: 10.1016/j.cell.2010.01.040
32. Sutterwala FS, Haasken S, Cassel SL. Mechanism of NLRP3 inflammasome activation. *Ann N Y Acad Sci.* (2014) 1319:82–95. doi: 10.1111/nyas.12458
33. Winkler S, Rosen-Wolff A. Caspase-1: an integral regulator of innate immunity. *Semin Immunopathol.* (2015) 37:419–27. doi: 10.1007/s00281-015-0494-4
34. Novak ML, Koh TJ. Macrophage phenotypes during tissue repair. *J Leukoc Biol.* (2013) 93:875–81. doi: 10.1189/jlb.1012512
35. Sica A, Erreni M, Allavena P, Porta C. Macrophage polarization in pathology. *Cell Mol Life Sci.* (2015) 72:4111–26. doi: 10.1007/s00018-015-1995-y
36. Liu Y, Cao X. The origin and function of tumor-associated macrophages. *Cell Mol Immunol.* (2015) 12:1–4. doi: 10.1038/cmi.2014.83
37. Mass E, Ballesteros I, Farlik M, Halbritter F, Gunther P, Crozet L, et al. Specification of tissue-resident macrophages during organogenesis. *Science* (2016) 353:6304. doi: 10.1126/science.aaf4238
38. Hoeffel G, Chen J, Lavin Y, Low D, Almeida FF, See P, et al. C-Myb(+) erythro-myeloid progenitor-derived fetal monocytes give rise to adult tissue-resident macrophages. *Immunity* (2015) 42:665–78. doi: 10.1016/j.immuni.2015.03.011
39. Movita D, Kreefft K, Biesta P, van Oudenaren A, Leenen PJ, Janssen HL, et al. Kupffer cells express a unique combination of phenotypic and functional characteristics compared with splenic and peritoneal macrophages. *J Leukocyte Biol.* (2012) 92:723–33. doi: 10.1189/jlb.1111566
40. Kinoshita M, Uchida T, Sato A, Nakashima M, Nakashima H, Shono S, et al. Characterization of two F4/80-positive Kupffer cell subsets by their function and phenotype in mice. *J Hepatol.* (2010) 53:903–10. doi: 10.1016/j.jhep.2010.04.037
41. Helmy KY, Katschke KJ, Jr., Gorgani NN, Kljavin NM, Elliott JM, Diehl L, et al. CRIg: a macrophage complement receptor required for phagocytosis of circulating pathogens. *Cell* (2006) 124:915–27. doi: 10.1016/j.cell.2005.12.039
42. Zeng Z, Surewaard BG, Wong CH, Geoghegan JA, Jenne CN, Kubes P. CRIg functions as a macrophage pattern recognition receptor to directly bind and capture blood-borne gram-positive bacteria. *Cell Host Microbe* (2016) 20:99–106. doi: 10.1016/j.chom.2016.06.002
43. Janeway CA Jr. The immune system evolved to discriminate infectious nonself from noninfectious self. *Immunol Today* (1992) 13:11–6. doi: 10.1016/0167-5699(92)90198-G
44. Takeuchi O, Akira S. Pattern recognition receptors and inflammation. *Cell* (2010) 140:805–20. doi: 10.1016/j.cell.2010.01.022
45. Kubes P, Mehal WZ. Sterile inflammation in the liver. *Gastroenterology* (2012) 143:1158–72. doi: 10.1053/j.gastro.2012.09.008
46. Knolle P, Schlaak J, Uhrig A, Kempf P, Meyer zum Buschenfelde KH, Gerken G. Human Kupffer cells secrete IL-10 in response to lipopolysaccharide (LPS) challenge. *J Hepatol.* (1995) 22:226–9. doi: 10.1016/0168-8278(95)80433-1
47. Ju C, Tacke F. Hepatic macrophages in homeostasis and liver diseases: from pathogenesis to novel therapeutic strategies. *Cell Mol Immunol.* (2016) 13:316–27. doi: 10.1038/cmi.2015.104
48. Ginhoux F, Greter M, Leboeuf M, Nandi S, See P, Gokhan S, et al. Fate mapping analysis reveals that adult microglia derive from primitive macrophages. *Science* (2010) 330:841–5. doi: 10.1126/science.1194637
49. Holt MP, Cheng L, Ju C. Identification and characterization of infiltrating macrophages in acetaminophen-induced liver injury. *J Leukoc Biol.* (2008) 84:1410–21. doi: 10.1189/jlb.0308173
50. Klein I, Cornejo JC, Polakos NK, John B, Wuensch SA, Topham DJ, et al. Kupffer cell heterogeneity: functional properties of bone marrow derived and sessile hepatic macrophages. *Blood* (2007) 110:4077–85. doi: 10.1182/blood-2007-02-073841
51. Dal-Secco D, Wang J, Zeng Z, Kolaczkowska E, Wong CH, Petri B, et al. A dynamic spectrum of monocytes arising from the *in situ* reprogramming of CCR2+ monocytes at a site of sterile injury. *J Exp Med.* (2015) 212:447–56. doi: 10.1084/jem.20141539
52. Mossanen JC, Krenkel O, Ergen C, Govaere O, Liepelt A, Puengel T, et al. Chemokine (C-C motif) receptor 2-positive monocytes aggravate the early phase of acetaminophen-induced acute liver injury. *Hepatology* (2016) 64:1667–82. doi: 10.1002/hep.28682
53. Zhang X, Han J, Man K, Li X, Du J, Chu ES, et al. CXC chemokine receptor 3 promotes steatohepatitis in mice through mediating inflammatory cytokines, macrophages and autophagy. *J Hepatol.* (2016) 64:160–70. doi: 10.1016/j.jhep.2015.09.005
54. Heymann F, Hammerich L, Storch D, Bartneck M, Huss S, Russeler V, et al. Hepatic macrophage migration and differentiation critical for liver fibrosis is mediated by the chemokine receptor C-C motif chemokine receptor 8 in mice. *Hepatology* (2012) 55:898–909. doi: 10.1002/hep.24764
55. Seki E, De Minicis S, Gwak GY, Kluwe J, Inokuchi S, Bursill CA, et al. CCR1 and CCR5 promote hepatic fibrosis in mice. *J Clin Invest.* (2009) 119:1858–70. doi: 10.1172/JCI37444
56. Swirski FK, Nahrendorf M, Etzrodt M, Wildgruber M, Cortez-Retamozo V, Panizzi P, et al. Identification of splenic reservoir monocytes and their deployment to inflammatory sites. *Science* (2009) 325:612–6. doi: 10.1126/science.1175202
57. Wang J, Kubes P. A reservoir of mature cavity macrophages that can rapidly invade visceral organs to affect tissue repair. *Cell* (2016) 165:668–78. doi: 10.1016/j.cell.2016.03.009
58. Sato A, Nakashima H, Nakashima M, Ikarashi M, Nishiyama K, Kinoshita M, et al. Involvement of the TNF and FasL produced by CD11b Kupffer cells/macrophages in CCl4-induced acute hepatic injury. *PLoS ONE* (2014) 9:e92515. doi: 10.1371/journal.pone.0092515
59. Nakashima H, Ogawa Y, Shono S, Kinoshita M, Nakashima M, Sato A, et al. Activation of CD11b+ Kupffer cells/macrophages as a common cause for exacerbation of TNF/Fas-ligand-dependent hepatitis in hypercholesterolemic mice. *PLoS ONE* (2013) 8:e49339. doi: 10.1371/journal.pone.0049339
60. Kinoshita M, Miyazaki H, Nakashima H, Nakashima M, Nishikawa M, Ishikiriyama T, et al. *In vivo* lipopolysaccharide tolerance recruits CD11b+ macrophages to the liver with enhanced bactericidal activity and low tumor necrosis factor-releasing capability, resulting in drastic resistance to lethal septicemia. *J Innate Immun.* (2017) 9:493–510. doi: 10.1159/000475931
61. Nakashima H, Nakashima M, Kinoshita M, Ikarashi M, Miyazaki H, Hanaka H, et al. Activation and increase of radio-sensitive CD11b+ recruited Kupffer cells/macrophages in diet-induced steatohepatitis in FGF5 deficient mice. *Sci Rep.* (2016) 6:34466. doi: 10.1038/srep34466
62. Nishiyama K, Nakashima H, Ikarashi M, Kinoshita M, Nakashima M, Aosasa S, et al. Mouse CD11b+kupffer cells recruited from bone marrow accelerate liver regeneration after partial hepatectomy. *PLoS ONE* (2015) 10:e0136774. doi: 10.1371/journal.pone.0136774
63. Theurl I, Hilgendorf I, Nairz M, Tymoszuk P, Haschka D, Asshoff M, et al. On-demand erythrocyte disposal and iron recycling requires transient macrophages in the liver. *Nat Med.* (2016) 22:945–51. doi: 10.1038/nm.4146
64. Scott CL, Zheng F, De Baetselier P, Martens L, Saeys Y, De Prijck S, et al. Bone marrow-derived monocytes give rise to self-renewing and fully differentiated Kupffer cells. *Nat Commun.* (2016) 7:10321. doi: 10.1038/ncomms10321
65. Kingham TP, Chaudhry UI, Plitas G, Katz SC, Raab J, DeMatteo RP. Murine liver plasmacytoid dendritic cells become potent immunostimulatory cells after Flt-3 ligand expansion. *Hepatology* (2007) 45:445–54. doi: 10.1002/hep.21457
66. Kim IH, Kisseleva T, Brenner DA. Aging and liver disease. *Curr Opin Gastroenterol.* (2015) 31:184–91. doi: 10.1097/MOG.0000000000000176
67. Salminen A, Kaarniranta K, Kauppinen A. Inflammaging: disturbed interplay between autophagy and inflammasomes. *Aging (Albany NY)* (2012) 4:166–75. doi: 10.18632/aging.100444
68. Zeeh J, Platt D. The aging liver. *Gerontology* (2002) 48:121–7. doi: 10.1159/000052829

69. McLean AJ, Cogger VC, Chong GC, Warren A, Markus AM, Dahlstrom JE, et al. Age-related pseudocapillarization of the human liver. *J Pathol.* (2003) 200:112–7. doi: 10.1002/path.1328
70. Tietz NW, Shuey DF, Wekstein DR. Laboratory values in fit aging individuals–sexagenarians through centenarians. *Clin Chem.* (1992) 38:1167–85.
71. Wakabayashi H, Nishiyama Y, Ushiyama T, Maeba T, Maeta H. Evaluation of the effect of age on functioning hepatocyte mass and liver blood flow using liver scintigraphy in preoperative estimations for surgical patients: comparison with CT volumetry. *J Surg Res.* (2002) 106:246–53. doi: 10.1006/jsre.2002.6462
72. Sastre J, Pallardo FV, Pla R, Pellin A, Juan G, O'Connor JE, et al. Aging of the liver: age-associated mitochondrial damage in intact hepatocytes. *Hepatology* (1996) 24:1199–205. doi: 10.1002/hep.510240536
73. Hohn A, Grune T. Lipofuscin: formation, effects and role of macroautophagy. *Redox Biol.* (2013) 1:140–4. doi: 10.1016/j.redox.2013.01.006
74. Poulose N, Raju R. Aging and injury: alterations in cellular energetics and organ function. *Aging Dis.* (2014) 5:101–8. doi: 10.14336/AD.2014.0500101
75. American Geriatrics Society Beers Criteria Update Expert P. American geriatrics society updated beers criteria for potentially inappropriate medication use in older adults. *J Am Geriatr Soc.* (2012) 60:616–31. doi: 10.1111/j.1532-5415.2012.03923.x
76. Wang GL, Salisbury E, Shi X, Timchenko L, Medrano EE, Timchenko NA. HDAC1 cooperates with C/EBPalpha in the inhibition of liver proliferation in old mice. *J Biol Chem.* (2008) 283:26169–78. doi: 10.1074/jbc.M803544200
77. Aravinthan AD, Alexander GJM. Senescence in chronic liver disease: Is the future in aging? *J Hepatol.* (2016) 65:825–34. doi: 10.1016/j.jhep.2016.05.030
78. Ben-Porath I, Weinberg RA. The signals and pathways activating cellular senescence. *Int J Biochem Cell Biol.* (2005) 37:961-76. doi: 10.1016/j.biocel.2004.10.013
79. Campisi J. Replicative senescence: an old lives' tale? *Cell* (1996) 84:497–500. doi: 10.1016/S0092-8674(00)81023-5
80. Coppe JP, Patil CK, Rodier F, Sun Y, Munoz DP, Goldstein J, et al. Senescence-associated secretory phenotypes reveal cell-nonautonomous functions of oncogenic RAS and the p53 tumor suppressor. *PLoS Biol.* (2008) 6:2853–68. doi: 10.1371/journal.pbio.0060301
81. Aravinthan A, Challis B, Shannon N, Hoare M, Heaney J, Alexander GJ. Selective insulin resistance in hepatocyte senescence. *Exp Cell Res.* (2015) 331:38–45. doi: 10.1016/j.yexcr.2014.09.025
82. Verma S, Tachtatzis P, Penrhyn-Lowe S, Scarpini C, Jurk D, Von Zglinicki T, et al. Sustained telomere length in hepatocytes and cholangiocytes with increasing age in normal liver. *Hepatology* (2012) 56:1510–20. doi: 10.1002/hep.25787
83. Hilmer SN, Cogger VC, Le Couteur DG. Basal activity of Kupffer cells increases with old age. *J Gerontol A Biol Sci Med Sci.* (2007) 62:973–8. doi: 10.1093/gerona/62.9.973
84. Singh P, Coskun ZZ, Goode C, Dean A, Thompson-Snipes L, Darlington G. Lymphoid neogenesis and immune infiltration in aged liver. *Hepatology* (2008) 47:1680–90. doi: 10.1002/hep.22224
85. Maeso-Diaz R, Ortega-Ribera M, Fernandez-Iglesias A, Hide D, Munoz L, Hessheimer AJ, et al. Effects of aging on liver microcirculatory function and sinusoidal phenotype. *Aging Cell* (2018) 8:e12829. doi: 10.1111/acel.12829
86. Stranks AJ, Hansen AL, Panse I, Mortensen M, Ferguson DJ, Puleston DJ, et al. Autophagy Controls acquisition of aging features in macrophages. *J Innate Immun.* (2015) 7:375–91. doi: 10.1159/000370112
87. Rubinsztein DC, Marino G, Kroemer G. Autophagy and aging. *Cell* (2011) 146:682–95. doi: 10.1016/j.cell.2011.07.030
88. Khalil H, Tazi M, Caution K, Ahmed A, Kanneganti A, Assani K, et al. Aging is associated with hypermethylation of autophagy genes in macrophages. *Epigenetics* (2016) 11:381–8. doi: 10.1080/15592294.2016.1144007
89. Trepanowski JF, Canale RE, Marshall KE, Kabir MM, Bloomer RJ. Impact of caloric and dietary restriction regimens on markers of health and longevity in humans and animals: a summary of available findings. *Nutr J.* (2011) 10:107. doi: 10.1186/1475-2891-10-107
90. Linehan E, Dombrowski Y, Snoddy R, Fallon PG, Kissenpfennig A, Fitzgerald DC. Aging impairs peritoneal but not bone marrow-derived macrophage phagocytosis. *Aging Cell* (2014) 13:699–708. doi: 10.1111/acel.12223
91. Wong CK, Smith CA, Sakamoto K, Kaminski N, Koff JL, Goldstein DR. Aging impairs alveolar macrophage phagocytosis and increases influenza-induced mortality in mice. *J Immunol.* (2017) 199:1060–8. doi: 10.4049/jimmunol.1700397
92. Brouwer A, Knook DL. The reticuloendothelial system and aging: a review. *Mech Ageing Dev.* (1983) 21:205–28. doi: 10.1016/0047-6374(83)90042-8
93. Puzianowska-Kuznicka M, Owczarz M, Wieczorowska-Tobis K, Nadrowski P, Chudek J, Slusarczyk P, et al. Interleukin-6 and C-reactive protein, successful aging, and mortality: the PolSenior study. *Immun Ageing.* (2016) 13:21. doi: 10.1186/s12979-016-0076-x
94. Dimitrijevic M, Stanojevic S, Kustrimovic N, Mitic K, Vujic V, Aleksic I, et al. The influence of aging and estradiol to progesterone ratio on rat macrophage phenotypic profile and NO and TNF-alpha production. *Exp Gerontol.* (2013) 48:1243–54. doi: 10.1016/j.exger.2013.07.001
95. Cecilio CA, Costa EH, Simioni PU, Gabriel DL, Tamashiro WM. Aging alters the production of iNOS, arginase and cytokines in murine macrophages. *Braz J Med Biol Res.* (2011) 44:671–81. doi: 10.1590/S0100-879X2011007500067
96. Suchy D, Labuzek K, Buldak L, Szkudlapski D, Okopien B. Comparison of chosen activation markers of human monocytes/macrophages isolated from the peripheral blood of young and elderly volunteers. *Pharmacol Rep.* (2014) 66:759–65. doi: 10.1016/j.pharep.2014.04.008
97. Hefendehl JK, Neher JJ, Suhs RB, Kohsaka S, Skodras A, Jucker M. Homeostatic and injury-induced microglia behavior in the aging brain. *Aging Cell* (2014) 13:60–9. doi: 10.1111/acel.12149
98. von Leden RE, Khayrullina G, Moritz KE, Byrnes KR. Age exacerbates microglial activation, oxidative stress, inflammatory and NOX2 gene expression, and delays functional recovery in a middle-aged rodent model of spinal cord injury. *J Neuroinflammation* (2017) 14:161. doi: 10.1186/s12974-017-0933-3
99. Cho SH, Chen JA, Sayed F, Ward ME, Gao F, Nguyen TA, et al. SIRT1 deficiency in microglia contributes to cognitive decline in aging and neurodegeneration via epigenetic regulation of IL-1beta. *J Neurosci.* (2015) 35:807–18. doi: 10.1523/JNEUROSCI.2939-14.2015
100. Malm T, Koistinaho M, Muona A, Magga J, Koistinaho J. The role and therapeutic potential of monocytic cells in Alzheimer's disease. *Glia* (2010) 58:889–900. doi: 10.1002/glia.20973
101. Pinto AR, Godwin JW, Chandran A, Hersey L, Ilinykh A, Debuque R, et al. Age-related changes in tissue macrophages precede cardiac functional impairment. *Aging* (2014) 6:399–413. doi: 10.18632/aging.100669
102. Epelman S, Lavine KJ, Beaudin AE, Sojka DK, Carrero JA, Calderon B, et al. Embryonic and adult-derived resident cardiac macrophages are maintained through distinct mechanisms at steady state and during inflammation. *Immunity* (2014) 40:91–104. doi: 10.1016/j.immuni.2013.11.019
103. Lavine KJ, Epelman S, Uchida K, Weber KJ, Nichols CG, Schilling JD, et al. Distinct macrophage lineages contribute to disparate patterns of cardiac recovery and remodeling in the neonatal and adult heart. *Proc Natl. Acad. Sci USA* (2014) 111:16029–34. doi: 10.1073/pnas.1406508111
104. Stahl EC, Brown BN. Cell therapy strategies to combat immunosenescence. *Organogenesis* (2015) 11:159–72. doi: 10.1080/15476278.2015.11 20046
105. Goronzy JJ, Fang F, Cavanagh MM, Qi Q, Weyand CM. Naive T cell maintenance and function in human aging. *J Immunol.* (2015) 194:4073–80. doi: 10.4049/jimmunol.1500046
106. Onyema OO, Njemini R, Forti LN, Bautmans I, Aerts JL, De Waele M, et al. Aging-associated subpopulations of human CD8+T-lymphocytes identified by their CD28 and CD57 phenotypes. *Arch Gerontol Geriat.* (2015) 61:494–502. doi: 10.1016/j.archger.2015.08.007
107. van der Geest KSM, Abdulahad WH, Tete SM, Lorencetti PG, Horst G, Bos NA, et al. Aging disturbs the balance between effector and regulatory CD4+T cells. *Exp Gerontol.* (2014) 60:190–6. doi: 10.1016/j.exger.2014.11.005
108. Garg SK, Delaney C, Shi H, Yung R. Changes in adipose tissue macrophages and T cells during aging. *Crit Rev Immunol.* (2014) 34:1–14. doi: 10.1615/CritRevImmunol.2013006833
109. Urs S, Smith C, Campbell B, Saxton AM, Taylor J, Zhang B, et al. Gene expression profiling in human preadipocytes and adipocytes by microarray analysis. *J Nutr.* (2004) 134:762–70. doi: 10.1093/jn/134.4.762

110. Tchkonia T, Morbeck DE, Von Zglinicki T, Van Deursen J, Lustgarten J, Scrable H, et al. Fat tissue, aging, and cellular senescence. *Aging Cell* (2010) 9:667–84. doi: 10.1111/j.1474-9726.2010.00608.x
111. Duewell P, Kono H, Rayner KJ, Sirois CM, Vladimer G, Bauernfeind FG, et al. NLRP3 inflammasomes are required for atherogenesis and activated by cholesterol crystals. *Nature* (2010) 464:1357–61. doi: 10.1038/nature08938
112. Wang K, Yao Y, Zhu X, Zhang K, Zhou F, Zhu L. Amyloid beta induces NLRP3 inflammasome activation in retinal pigment epithelial cells via NADPH oxidase- and mitochondria-dependent ROS production. *J Biochem Mol Toxicol.* (2017) 31. [Epub ahead of print].
113. Murphy N, Grehan B, Lynch MA. Glial uptake of amyloid beta induces NLRP3 inflammasome formation via cathepsin-dependent degradation of NLRP10. *Neuromolecular Med.* (2014) 16:205–15. doi: 10.1007/s12017-013-8274-6
114. Jin C, Frayssinet P, Pelker R, Cwirka D, Hu B, Vignery A, et al. NLRP3 inflammasome plays a critical role in the pathogenesis of hydroxyapatite-associated arthropathy. *Proc Natl Acad Sci USA* (2011) 108:14867–72. doi: 10.1073/pnas.1111101108
115. Chen CJ, Shi Y, Hearn A, Fitzgerald K, Golenbock D, Reed G, et al. MyD88-dependent IL-1 receptor signaling is essential for gouty inflammation stimulated by monosodium urate crystals. *J Clin Investigat.* (2006) 116:2262–71. doi: 10.1172/JCI28075
116. Mariathasan S, Weiss DS, Newton K, McBride J, O'Rourke K, Roose-Girma M, et al. Cryopyrin activates the inflammasome in response to toxins and ATP. *Nature* (2006) 440:228–32. doi: 10.1038/nature04515
117. Cichoz-Lach H, Michalak A. Oxidative stress as a crucial factor in liver diseases. *World J Gastroenterol.* (2014) 20:8082–91. doi: 10.3748/wjg.v20.i25.8082
118. Abais JM, Xia M, Zhang Y, Boini KM, Li PL. Redox regulation of NLRP3 inflammasomes: ROS as trigger or effector? *Antioxid Redox Signal.* (2015) 22:1111–29. doi: 10.1089/ars.2014.5994
119. Thevaranjan N, Puchta A, Schulz C, Naidoo A, Szamosi JC, Verschoor CP, et al. Age-associated microbial dysbiosis promotes intestinal permeability, systemic inflammation, and macrophage dysfunction. *Cell Host Microbe* (2017) 21:455-66 e4.
120. Cohen-Naftaly M, Friedman SL. Current status of novel antifibrotic therapies in patients with chronic liver disease. *Therap Adv Gastroenterol.* (2011) 4:391–417. doi: 10.1177/1756283X11413002
121. Iwaisako K, Brenner DA, Kisseleva T. What's new in liver fibrosis? The origin of myofibroblasts in liver fibrosis. *J Gastroenterol Hepatol.* (2012) 27(Suppl. 2):65–8. doi: 10.1111/j.1440-1746.2011.07002.x
122. Poynard T, Ratziu V, Charlotte F, Goodman Z, McHutchison J, Albrecht J. Rates and risk factors of liver fibrosis progression in patients with chronic hepatitis c. *J Hepatol.* (2001) 34:730–9. doi: 10.1016/S0168-8278(00)00097-0
123. Mahrouf-Yorgov M, Collin de l'Hortet A, Cosson C, Slama A, Abdoun E, Guidotti JE, et al. Increased susceptibility to liver fibrosis with age is correlated with an altered inflammatory response. *Rejuvenation Res.* (2011) 14:353–63. doi: 10.1089/rej.2010.1146
124. Zimmermann HW, Seidler S, Nattermann J, Gassler N, Hellerbrand C, Zernecke A, et al. Functional contribution of elevated circulating and hepatic non-classical CD14CD16 monocytes to inflammation and human liver fibrosis. *PLoS ONE* (2010) 5:e11049. doi: 10.1371/journal.pone.0011049
125. Liaskou E, Zimmermann HW, Li KK, Oo YH, Suresh S, Stamataki Z, et al. Monocyte subsets in human liver disease show distinct phenotypic and functional characteristics. *Hepatology* (2013) 57:385–98. doi: 10.1002/hep.26016
126. Marra F, DeFranco R, Grappone C, Milani S, Pastacaldi S, Pinzani M, et al. Increased expression of monocyte chemotactic protein-1 during active hepatic fibrogenesis: correlation with monocyte infiltration. *Am J Pathol.* (1998) 152:423–30.
127. Alzaid F, Lagadec F, Albuquerque M, Ballaire R, Orliaguet L, Hainault I, et al. IRF5 governs liver macrophage activation that promotes hepatic fibrosis in mice and humans. *JCI Insight.* (2016) 1:e88689. doi: 10.1172/jci.insight.88689
128. Blazer DG, Wu LT. The epidemiology of at-risk and binge drinking among middle-aged and elderly community adults: National Survey on Drug Use and Health. *Am J Psychiatry* (2009) 166:1162–9. doi: 10.1176/appi.ajp.2009.09010016
129. Kim IH, Xu J, Liu X, Koyama Y, Ma HY, Diggle K, et al. Aging increases the susceptibility of hepatic inflammation, liver fibrosis and aging in response to high-fat diet in mice. *Age (Dordr).* (2016) 38:291–302. doi: 10.1007/s11357-016-9938-6
130. Meier P, Seitz HK. Age, alcohol metabolism and liver disease. Current Opinion in Clinical *Nutr Metab Care* (2008) 11:21-6. doi: 10.1097/MCO.0b013e3282f30564
131. Tacke F. Targeting hepatic macrophages to treat liver diseases. *J Hepatol.* (2017) 66:1300–12. doi: 10.1016/j.jhep.2017.02.026
132. Wang M, You Q, Lor K, Chen F, Gao B, Ju C. Chronic alcohol ingestion modulates hepatic macrophage populations and functions in mice. *J Leukoc Biol.* (2014) 96:657–65. doi: 10.1189/jlb.6A0114-004RR
133. Seitz HK, Stickel F. Risk factors and mechanisms of hepatocarcinogenesis with special emphasis on alcohol and oxidative stress. *Biol Chem.* (2006) 387:349–60. doi: 10.1515/BC.2006.047
134. Tapia-Abellan A, Martinez-Esparza M, Ruiz-Alcaraz AJ, Hernandez-Caselles T, Martinez-Pascual C, Miras-Lopez M, et al. The peritoneal macrophage inflammatory profile in cirrhosis depends on the alcoholic or hepatitis C viral etiology and is related to ERK phosphorylation. *BMC Immunol.* (2012) 13:42. doi: 10.1186/1471-2172-13-42
135. Hartmann P, Chen WC, Schnabl B. The intestinal microbiome and the leaky gut as therapeutic targets in alcoholic liver disease. *Front Physiol.* (2012) 3:402. doi: 10.3389/fphys.2012.00402
136. Mikolasevic I, Filipec-Kanizaj T, Mijic M, Jakopcic I, Milic S, Hrstic I, et al. Nonalcoholic fatty liver disease and liver transplantation - Where do we stand? *World J Gastroenterol.* (2018) 24:1491–506. doi: 10.3748/wjg.v24.i14.1491
137. Wong RJ, Aguilar M, Cheung R, Perumpail RB, Harrison SA, Younossi ZM, et al. Nonalcoholic steatohepatitis is the second leading etiology of liver disease among adults awaiting liver transplantation in the United States. *Gastroenterology* (2015) 148:547–55. doi: 10.1053/j.gastro.2014.11.039
138. Younossi ZM, Koenig AB, Abdelatif D, Fazel Y, Henry L, Wymer M. Global epidemiology of nonalcoholic fatty liver disease-Meta-analytic assessment of prevalence, incidence, and outcomes. *Hepatology* (2016) 64:73–84. doi: 10.1002/hep.28431
139. Barzilai N, Huffman DM, Muzumdar RH, Bartke A. The critical role of metabolic pathways in aging. *Diabetes* (2012) 61:1315–22. doi: 10.2337/db11-1300
140. Koehler EM, Schouten JN, Hansen BE, van Rooij FJ, Hofman A, Stricker BH, et al. Prevalence and risk factors of non-alcoholic fatty liver disease in the elderly: results from the Rotterdam study. *J Hepatol.* (2012) 57:1305–11. doi: 10.1016/j.jhep.2012.07.028
141. Frith J, Day CP, Henderson E, Burt AD, Newton JL. Non-alcoholic fatty liver disease in older people. *Gerontology* (2009) 55:607–13. doi: 10.1159/000235677
142. Noureddin M, Yates KP, Vaughn IA, Neuschwander-Tetri BA, Sanyal AJ, McCullough A, et al. Clinical and histological determinants of nonalcoholic steatohepatitis and advanced fibrosis in elderly patients. *Hepatology* (2013) 58:1644–54. doi: 10.1002/hep.26465
143. Ogrodnik M, Miwa S, Tchkonia T, Tiniakos D, Wilson CL, Lahat A, et al. Cellular senescence drives age-dependent hepatic steatosis. *Nat Commun.* (2017) 8:15691. doi: 10.1038/ncomms15691
144. Mohamad M, Mitchell SJ, Wu LE, White MY, Cordwell SJ, Mach J, et al. Ultrastructure of the liver microcirculation influences hepatic and systemic insulin activity and provides a mechanism for age-related insulin resistance. *Aging Cell* (2016) 15:706–15. doi: 10.1111/acel.12481
145. Gonzalez-Rodriguez A, Mayoral R, Agra N, Valdecantos MP, Pardo V, Miquilena-Colina ME, et al. Impaired autophagic flux is associated with increased endoplasmic reticulum stress during the development of NAFLD. *Cell Death Dis.* (2014) 5:e1179. doi: 10.1038/cddis.2014.162
146. Duval C, Thissen U, Keshtkar S, Accart B, Stienstra R, Boekschoten MV, et al. Adipose tissue dysfunction signals progression of hepatic steatosis towards nonalcoholic steatohepatitis in C57BL/6 mice. *Diabetes* (2010) 59:3181–91. doi: 10.2337/db10-0224
147. Kumar A, Sharma A, Duseja A, Das A, Dhiman RK, Chawla YK, et al. Patients with nonalcoholic fatty liver disease (NAFLD) have higher oxidative stress in comparison to chronic viral hepatitis. *J Clin Exp Hepatol.* (2013) 3:12–8. doi: 10.1016/j.jceh.2012.10.009

148. Fontana L, Zhao E, Amir M, Dong H, Tanaka K, Czaja MJ. Aging promotes the development of diet-induced murine steatohepatitis but not steatosis. *Hepatology* (2013) 57:995–1004. doi: 10.1002/hep.26099
149. Wan J, Benkdane M, Teixeira-Clerc F, Bonnafous S, Louvet A, Lafdil F, et al. M2 Kupffer cells promote M1 Kupffer cell apoptosis: a protective mechanism against alcoholic and nonalcoholic fatty liver disease. *Hepatology* (2014) 59:130–42. doi: 10.1002/hep.26607
150. Reid DT, Reyes JL, McDonald BA, Vo T, Reimer RA, Eksteen B. Kupffer cells undergo fundamental changes during the development of experimental nash and are critical in initiating liver damage and inflammation. *PLoS ONE* (2016) 11:e0159524. doi: 10.1371/journal.pone.0159524
151. Kazankov K, Moller HJ, Lange A, Birkebaek NH, Holland-Fischer P, Solvig J, et al. The macrophage activation marker sCD163 is associated with changes in NAFLD and metabolic profile during lifestyle intervention in obese children. *Pediatr Obes.* (2015) 10:226–33. doi: 10.1111/ijpo.252
152. Shah K, Stufflebam A, Hilton TN, Sinacore DR, Klein S, Villareal DT. Diet and exercise interventions reduce intrahepatic fat content and improve insulin sensitivity in obese older adults. *Obesity (Silver Spring)* (2009) 17:2162–8. doi: 10.1038/oby.2009.126
153. Villareal DT, Chode S, Parimi N, Sinacore DR, Hilton T, Armamento-Villareal R, et al. Weight loss, exercise, or both and physical function in obese older adults. *N Engl J Med.* (2011) 364:1218–29. doi: 10.1056/NEJMoa1008234
154. Friedman S, Sanyal A, Goodman Z, Lefebvre E, Gottwald M, Fischer L, et al. Efficacy and safety study of cenicriviroc for the treatment of non-alcoholic steatohepatitis in adult subjects with liver fibrosis: CENTAUR Phase 2b study design. *Contemp Clin Trials* (2016) 47:356–65. doi: 10.1016/j.cct.2016.02.012
155. Friedman SL, Ratziu V, Harrison SA, Abdelmalek MF, Aithal GP, Caballeria J, et al. A randomized, placebo-controlled trial of cenicriviroc for treatment of nonalcoholic steatohepatitis with fibrosis. *Hepatology* (2018) 67:1754–67. doi: 10.1002/hep.29477
156. Åberg F, Isoniemi H, Höckerstedt K. Long-term results of liver transplantation. *Scand J Surg.* (2011) 100:14–21. doi: 10.1177/145749691110000104
157. Randall HB, Cao S, deVera ME. Transplantation in elderly patients. *Arch Surg.* (2003) 138:1089–92. doi: 10.1001/archsurg.138.10.1089
158. Adani GL, Baccarani U, Lorenzin D, Rossetto A, Nicolini D, Vecchi A, et al. Elderly versus young liver transplant recipients: patient and graft survival. *Transplant Proc.* (2009) 41:1293–4. doi: 10.1016/j.transproceed.2009.03.080
159. Yeung OW, Lo CM, Ling CC, Qi X, Geng W, Li CX, et al. Alternatively activated (M2) macrophages promote tumour growth and invasiveness in hepatocellular carcinoma. *J Hepatol.* (2015) 62:607–16. doi: 10.1016/j.jhep.2014.10.029
160. Tapper EB, Parikh ND. Mortality due to cirrhosis and liver cancer in the United States, 1999-2016: observational study. *BMJ* (2018) 362:k2817. doi: 10.1136/bmj.k2817

11

Contribution of Macrophage Efferocytosis to Liver Homeostasis and Disease

*Andrea Kristina Horst, Gisa Tiegs and Linda Diehl**

Institute for Experimental Immunology and Hepatology, University Medical Center Hamburg-Eppendorf, Hamburg, Germany

***Correspondence:**
Linda Diehl
li.diehl@uke.de

The clearance of apoptotic cells is pivotal for both maintaining tissue homeostasis and returning to homeostasis after tissue injury as part of the regenerative resolution response. The liver is known for its capacity to remove aged and damaged cells from the circulation and can serve as a graveyard for effector T cells. In particular Kupffer cells are active phagocytic cells, but during hepatic inflammatory responses incoming neutrophils and monocytes may contribute to pro-inflammatory damage. To stimulate resolution of such inflammation, myeloid cell function can change, via sensing of environmental changes in the inflammatory milieu. Also, the removal of apoptotic cells via efferocytosis and the signaling pathways that are activated in macrophages/phagocytes upon their engulfment of apoptotic cells are important for a return to tissue homeostasis. Here, we will discuss, how efferocytosis mechanisms in hepatic macrophages/phagocytes may regulate tissue homeostasis and be involved in tissue regeneration in liver disease.

Keywords: liver injury, macrophage, efferocytosis, inflammation, resolution, apoptosis, phagocytosis, cytokines

INTRODUCTION

Under homeostatic conditions, new cells are produced and old cells die constantly within in the body. These aged and damaged cells need to be efficiently removed from the surroundings without inducing inflammation or tissue damage, which is achieved by a process called *efferocytosis*. Here, dying/dead cells are specifically recognized by phagocytes and subsequently engulfed. Inefficient removal of apoptotic cells is associated with the development of (auto) immune-mediated diseases (1–3) highlighting the importance of efferocytosis for homeostasis within the immune system. The liver has long been recognized as a major system for removal of aging/dying/activated cells. Under homeostatic conditions, aging erythrocytes and neutrophils, but also effector $CD8^+$ T cells can be eliminated in the liver (4–7). This is mostly attributed to the activity of the organ-resident macrophages in the liver, the Kupffer cells. However, also during liver disease, both in experimental models as well as in patients, large amounts of dying cells are generated directly due to liver injury and/or following inflammatory responses. Various forms of insults leading to liver damage, such as infections, toxins or inflammation, often leads to rapid death of intrahepatic cell populations (mostly hepatocytes), making the efficient removal of such damaged cells extremely important to prevent unwarranted tissue damage and excessive inflammatory responses and support the restitution of tissue integrity. As the liver is known for its extreme and rapid capacity for regeneration upon liver injury, such as after the experimental procedure of partial hepatectomy, it must harbor efficient mechanisms and pathways to deal with large amounts of dying cells. Although cell death may occur through different mechanisms, such as apoptosis, necrosis or necroptosis (8), in this review we will focus on the role of mechanisms related to the efferocytic clearance of apoptotic cells in the context of liver immune tolerance and liver disease. Most hepatic cell types, including hepatocytes, hepatic stellate cells and liver sinusoidal endothelial cells have been reported to be able to take up apoptotic cells in some way (9, 10). However, the most important hepatic efferocytes are thought to be Kupffer cells together with other myeloid phagocytic cells, like neutrophils and monocytes, which are attracted into the liver after injury for the removal of apoptotic cells. Here, we will discuss the mechanisms and pathways involved in the process of efferocytosis in general, the role for these pathways in hepatic myeloid cells (tissue resident and migrating) and their relevance for both the induction and resolution of liver disease.

FINDING, SENSING, AND CLEARING APOPTOTIC CELLS

The process of efferocytosis is essential for the clearance of apoptotic cells dying from physiological and pathological causes without arousing inflammation. Soluble "find me" signals are released during the onset of apoptosis to attract the phagocytically active myeloid subsets. The most well-known "find me" signals are lyso-phosphatidyl choline (LPC), sphingosine-1-phosphate (S1P), fractalkine (CX_3CL1), and the nucleotides ATP and UTP. LPC is generated via the caspase-3-dependent activation of the inflammatory phospholipase A2 (iPLA2), which hydrolyses phosphatidyl choline (PC) from the cell membrane (11, 12). LPC then functions as an attractant for macrophages via the ligation of the G-protein coupled receptor G2A (13). Additionally, during apoptosis, the activity of sphingosine kinase leads to the caspase-3 dependent generation of S1P from sphingosine. Binding of S1P to sphingosine 1 phosphate receptors (S1PR1-5), expressed on macrophages and other phagocytes, leads to their attraction toward the apoptotic cells (11). Furthermore, membrane-bound or soluble CX_3CL1 from either micro-vesicles of apoptotic cells (12), or cleaved by caspase-3 activity, acts as an attractant for restorative $CX3CR1^+$ phagocytes. Finally, the release of the nucleotides ATP and UTP that function as extracellular alarmins, attract phagocytes via signaling through purinergic P2Y receptors and secretion via pannexin-1 channels.

The main recognition of apoptotic cells by phagocytes occurs via caspase-dependent expulsion of phosphatidyl serine (PS) onto the outer leaflet of the plasma membrane. This characteristic "eat-me" signal can be recognized directly via PS binding receptors on macrophages or indirectly by "bridging molecules" that bind to PS on the one hand and to their cognate receptors on the other hand to trigger engulfment of apoptotic cells. Most prominent are the bridging molecules milk fat globule epidermal growth factor VIII (MFG-E8; also lactadherin), and the vitamin K-dependent proteins growth arrest specific 6 (Gas6) and protein S (11, 14). Macrophages and dendritic cells can secrete MFG-E8, which then interacts with PS and can be recognized via the integrins $\alpha v\beta 3$ or $\alpha v\beta 5$. Both Gas6 and Protein S act as bridging molecules for the TAM receptor family, consisting of Tyro3, Axl, and MerTK (15). These interactions induce efficient clearance of apoptotic cells. Similarly, the binding of the complement factor C1q as an opsonin to PS serves as a bridging molecule for recognition by the scavenger receptor class F member 1 (SCARF1) (16) on phagocytes and endothelial cells, but may also as part of a protein complex containing calreticulin be involved in the initiation of efferocytosis (17). Recently, soluble CD93 was identified to act as an efferocytic opsonin by bridging PS on apoptotic cells with the complement receptor integrin $\alpha x\beta 2$ (CD11c/CD18) (18). Experimentally, the detection of efferocytosis by phagocytes is most often probed with fluorescently labeled apoptotic cells, like dexamethasone-treated thymocytes or neutrophils that die via apoptosis upon *in vitro* culture. Ingestion of such apoptotic cells by phagocytes is then analyzed by microscopy or flow cytometry.

PS receptors are not ubiquitously expressed but are rather tissue and/or cell type-specific: For instance, the T cell immunoglobulin and mucin-domain-containing molecule (Tim) family of receptors act as PS receptors. In particular, Tim3 and Tim4 are expressed on phagocytes, such as macrophages and dendritic cells (DC) (11). Although Tim4 can bind directly to PS, actual clearance of apoptotic cells via phagocytosis requires its cooperation with other receptors, such as MerTK and/or integrin $\beta 1$ (19, 20). The receptors stabilin-1 and-2 both recognize PS on apoptotic cells for engulfment and are expressed by macrophages, but are most prominently known for their role in the capture and elimination of PS-exposed damaged and/or aged erythrocytes by LSEC (9). Besides the uptake of aged erythrocytes by the asialo-glycoprotein receptors (ASGPR) by hepatocytes, this is the only liver cell-specific mechanism for efferocytosis described so far (10).

Like Tim4, stabilin-2 also requires cofactors/receptors [engulfment adapter phospho-tyrosine binding domain-containing protein 1 (GULP1) and thymosin4] for the initiation of engulfment (12). Additionally, some members of the CD300 family of type I transmembrane proteins (CD300a, CD300f, and CD300b) are capable of recognizing phosphatidyl-serine (PS) and -ethanolamine (PE), which are both exposed on the outer leaflet of the plasma membrane early during apoptosis (21–24). Knock-down or knock-out of CD300b and CD300f, respectively, results in impaired efferocytosis by macrophages (23, 24). Also, binding of the receptor for advanced glycation end products (RAGE) to PS increases the potential of macrophages to take up apoptotic cells (25). Contrary, secretion of the pro-inflammatory high mobility group box 1 (HMGB1) during inflammation interferes with RAGE-mediated efferocytosis by binding to PS (26). Similarly, secreted soluble RAGE itself can also inhibit efferocytosis by binding to and masking exposed PS for recognition by other PS receptors. Additional receptors, such as the scavenger receptors SR-A1 and SR-B1 and CD36 (27–29), are also implicated to play a role in (oxidized) PS recognition during efferocytosis, but their definite role has not been determined so far.

Not only do apoptotic cells signal phagocytes in various ways to enhance efferocytosis, healthy viable non-apoptotic cells express surface molecules that prevent efferocytosis. The transmembrane CD47 molecule constitutes such a "don't eat-me" signal via interaction with the ITIM-containing receptor Signal regulatory protein 1 alpha (SIRP1α; CD172a). This leads to the inhibition of actin cytoskeleton rearrangements necessary for phagocytosis (30). Recently, also the sialoglycoprotein CD24 (heat stable antigen) was shown to inhibit phagocytosis via interacting with and signaling via Sialic acid-binding Ig like lectin 10 (Siglec-10) on macrophages (31). In addition to the regulation of apoptotic cell clearance via "find-me," "eat-me," and "don't eat-me" signals for the phagocytotic activity of macrophages cross talk between these signaling pathways can modulate the efferocytosis process. For instance, signaling via the "find-me" receptors S1PR, CX_3CR1 and "eat-me" receptor SCARF1 can enhance the release of the bridging molecules Gas6 and/or MFG-E8, but also upregulate their receptors, e.g., MerTK (11). This feed forward loop further enhances the capability of phagocytes after the engulfment of apoptotic cells has already been initiated.

MODULATION OF PHAGOCYTE FUNCTION DUE TO EFFEROCYTOSIS

The process of efferocytosis and the subsequent signaling events are critical for the upkeep of homeostasis and even more important for the return to tissue homeostasis after tissue damage due to inflammation and/or disease [reviewed in (32) and (33)]. Cellular signaling and metabolic adaptation initiated by efferocytosis enables the return to tissue homeostasis by anti-inflammatory reprogramming of the formerly pro-inflammatory leukocytes: Signaling via the CX_3CR1 receptor, recognizing CX_3CL1 released from apoptotic cells, induces pro-survival signals and expression/generation of antioxidant factors. Signaling via S1PR invokes an anti-inflammatory gene expression program, including reduction of pro-inflammatory Interleukin (IL)-12 and tumor necrosis factor alpha (TNFα) whilst promoting production of anti-inflammatory mediators such as IL-10, vascular endothelial growth factor (VEGF) and prostaglandin E2 (PGE_2) (32). Indeed, after efferocytosis, macrophages can produce several anti-inflammatory and pro-resolving lipid mediators that promote macrophage conversion toward phenotypes associated with resolution of inflammation (34). Also, the ATP released from apoptotic cells can be converted to adenosine by sequentially acting nucleotidases, and subsequent signaling through adenosine receptors suppresses production of proinflammatory mediators and chemokines (35).

In addition to the modulation of cellular signaling, efferocytosis leads to the accumulation of high amounts of cellular material in phagocytes that needs to be processed and digested. The metabolic adaptation to this high ingestion of cargo leads to the activation of several lipid sensing nuclear receptors, such as liver X receptor (LXR) and members of the peroxisome proliferator-activated receptor (PPAR) family (33, 36). The activation of these pathways in macrophages promotes anti-inflammatory reprogramming and can reinforce their efferocytic capacity by upregulation of phagocytic receptors, like MerTK, and inducing the synthesis of precursors for pro-resolving lipid mediators (33, 37). The uptake of apoptotic material is also closely linked to a non-canonical rubicon-dependent autophagy pathway, called light chain (LC)3-associated phagocytosis (LAP) (38, 39). Specific signaling via the TAM receptor Axl induces autophagy, which is not only involved in the physical clearance of apoptotic material, but also prevents NOD, LRR-, and pyrin-domain containing 3 (NLRP3) inflammasome activation and concomitantly reduces IL-1β and IL-18 production (40). Similarly, Tim4-mediated apoptotic cell engulfment connects to LAP after recognition of PS on apoptotic cells (41) and incomplete cargo digestion via defective LAP is associated with development of autoinflammation (42).

Classical activation or polarization of macrophages into M1 (pro-inflammatory, mostly induced by LPS/IFNγ) vs. M2 (alternative or anti-inflammatory, induced by the cytokines IL-4/IL-13) shows that also the cytokine/chemokine microenvironment in which phagocytes encounter apoptotic cells can modulate their cognate response. Classically, Th2 cells are major sources for the cytokines IL-4 and IL-13, and the simultaneous recognition of apoptotic cells (neutrophils) and IL-4/IL-13 stimulation of macrophages is necessary for the induction of an anti-inflammatory, pro-resolving tissue repair gene signature (43). Congruently, expulsion of the helminth *N. Brasiliensis* was unsuccessful in mice lacking the TAM receptors Axl and MerTK even though the capacity to produce IL-4 and IL-13 was not affected (43). IL-13 production is also essential for the induction of efferocytosis in macrophages by regulatory T cells (Treg) during resolution of a zymosan-induced model of peritonitis (44). Treg-derived IL-13 promotes autocrine IL-10 induction in macrophages leading to Vav1-Rac1-dependent phagosome formation thus promoting their capacity to phagocytose apoptotic cells (44). Although anti-inflammatory mediators, like IL-13 and IL-10, can augment efferocytosis in macrophages, not all pro-inflammatory signals reduce efferocytosis. For instance, both interferon (IFN)α, which is produced as a result of signaling via toll-like receptor (TLR)3, or direct TLR3 signaling using Poly:IC down regulates MerTK expression (as do LPS and IFNγ), but at the same time induces Axl expression in human macrophages, which may facilitate efferocytosis during viral infections (45). Signaling via the TLR-dependent upregulated TAM receptors may then interfere with TLR signaling via the induction of suppressor of cytokine signaling proteins (SOCS) 1 and 3, thus scaling down the proinflammatory response induced by the initial TLR signals (46).

RELEVANCE FOR EFFEROCYTOSIS MECHANISMS IN PHAGOCYTES IN THE LIVER

Macrophage populations in adult tissues arise from different origins. Several tissue-resident macrophage populations, like Langerhans cells, microglia and Kupffer cells, are seeded in distinct waves during embryogenesis and are self-sustaining without input from the bone marrow during adulthood (47). The bone marrow also contributes to the myeloid/macrophage cell pool found in different tissues under homeostatic conditions and include $Ly6C^+$ monocyte derived cells and dendritic cells. In particular in the liver, mas cytometry combined with gene expression analysis (48), shows that within the non-B, non-T CD45$^+$ population the most abundant myeloid cells are dendritic cells, Kupffer cells and Ly6C$^+$ monocytes (48). Distinct but small populations of plasmacytoid DC, neutrophils and basophils are also present. F4/80$^+$MHCII$^+$CD11b$^+$ positive Kupffer cells comprise two populations additionally expressing CD11c or CD206, CD317 (plasmacytoid dendritic cell antigen-1, PCDA-1) and CD1d, pointing to a possible functional difference. Within Ly6C$^+$ infiltrating monocytes, an F4/80 positive and F4/80 negative population are present. By intravital microscopy, the expression of F4/80 and/or CX_3CR1, which is not expressed on Kupffer cells under homeostasis (49), shows that F4/80$^+$ cells are exclusively to be found intravascularly (which may include both F4/80$^+$ Kupffer cells and F4/80 expressing monocytes) and CX_3CR1^+ cells extravascularly in the parenchyma, suggesting that in addition to gene signatures another level of functionality is established via localization. Other markers that are used to distinguish tissue-resident Kupffer cells from recruited monocytes/neutrophils include the C-type lectin receptor Clec4f and the V-set and immunoglobulin domain-containing 4 (Vsig4) (50, 51). Interestingly, also the PS-receptor Tim4 is used for identification of liver resident Kupffer cells, indicating that these cells are set for efferocytosis under homeostatic conditions (50, 51). Thus, when studying the contribution of myeloid subsets to different liver diseases and/or injuries, the definition and identification of these different highly plastic myeloid subsets is challenging. Moreover, due to the large influx of pro-inflammatory myeloid subsets [neutrophils and inflammatory monocytes, but possibly also eosinophils (52)] the composition of the myeloid compartment at any given time during inflammatory liver disease can vary dynamically. We will focus on how local and recruited phagocytes are involved in the safeguarding of and return to immunological homeostasis in the liver and how their capacity for efferocytosis plays a role in the pathogenesis and resolution of liver diseases. Due to the highly divergent etiologies of liver disease, being either infectious, toxic or nutritional in origin, and depending on whether liver (immunological) function is being compromised acutely or in a chronic fashion, it is very well-possible that similar mechanisms controlling macrophage efferocytic function may have unexpected opposite effects.

First reports that intrahepatic phagocytes are capable of recognizing PS to trigger phagocytosis relate to the elimination of aged/damage erythrocytes from the circulation (4). The PS receptors Stabilin-1 and -2 expressed on LSEC are important for erythrocyte sequestration in this process (9). However, the removal of erythrocytes is blocked by clodronate-containing liposomes, indicating that Kupffer cells mediate actual phagocytosis. Also, aged erythrocytes that are taken up by Ly6C$^+$ monocytes elsewhere in the circulation are carried to the liver as cargo to recover the iron from hemoglobin (53). Kupffer cells can express several receptors involved in PS recognition, such as MerTK (54) and Tim4 (53), or phagocytic receptors thought to assist in the uptake of PS exposed apoptotic cells like CD36 and scavenger receptors (55). The relevance for recognition of apoptotic cells and its downstream signaling events for potential treatment options in inflammatory diseases of the liver can be taken from experiments using apoptotic cells to treat inflammation and damage in D-galactosamine (D-GalN)/LPS induced liver damage (56). Here, adoptively transferred UV-irradiated splenocytes that are taken up by Kupffer cells prevent mortality in the D-GalN/LPS model, induces expression of IL-4, IL-10, and transforming growth factor beta (TGFβ) and suppresses expression of TNFα, IL-6, and IL-1β (56). Moreover, in a more controlled fashion liposomes expressing phosphatidyl serine may mimic apoptotic cell effects on phagocyte function in immune cells and hepatic disease (57, 58).

INVOLVEMENT OF THE EFFEROCYTOSIS MACHINERY IN LIVER DISEASE

Contribution of Efferocytosis Inducing Signals From Soluble Mediators Released by Apoptotic Cells

Early in the process of apoptosis, soluble mediators, such as ATP and UTP, act as damage-associated molecular patterns (DAMP) and "find-me" signals for efferocytes. In the liver, extracellular nucleotides trigger dichotomous responses; on the one hand, release of nucleotides by apoptotic cells after tissue injury initiates inflammation, and on the other hand, activation of non-parenchymal, liver-resident, and infiltrating efferocytes is a prerequisite for the activation of phagocytosis and the clearance of dead cells. Kupffer cells can detect and respond to the soluble mediator ATP released by apoptotic cells via expression of several P2Y receptors (59) and increase IL-6 production in response. Interestingly, however, Kupffer cells themselves also release ATP in response to LPS, which in an autocrine fashion promotes pro-inflammatory IL-6 release $PY2_{13}$-dependently (59). Thus, attraction to apoptotic cells via ATP may lead to pro-inflammatory cytokine release by Kupffer cells. *In vivo* the recognition of and response to ATP in liver disease is more complex. After partial hepatectomy, both Kupffer cells and hepatocytes release ATP, which is important for the regenerative response in hepatocytes via direct signaling through the $P2Y_2$ receptor (60), indicating that ATP release may have pro-inflammatory effects but at the same time may be indispensable for the initiation of hepatocyte proliferation necessary for liver regeneration. Depending on the longevity of ATP release and the expression of different purinergic receptors capable of recognizing ATP, the outcome of ATP release can be modulated. For instance, in the model of partial hepatectomy ATP release peaks within 15 min (59). In other models, where ATP is likely released over a prolonged time period, effects on intrahepatic phagocytes and disease progression may be different. In acetaminophen (APAP)-mediated liver injury, ATP (and also NAD) signaling via the purinergic $P2X_7$ receptor mediates hepatotoxicity to a large extent as $P2X_7$-deficient mice, and the use of selective $P2X_7$ antagonists decreases APAP-dependent liver toxicity (61). Although direct ATP signaling induces proinflammatory signaling, such as IL-1β and IL-6 production by Kupffer cells (59, 61), ATP released during liver injury and inflammation *in vivo* can be further modulated to attenuate liver inflammation. The cell surface ectonucleotidase CD39 counteracts proinflammatory effects of ATP release by catalyzing the hydrolysis of ATP/ADP to AMP, which can then be further metabolized to adenosine that can results in A_{2A} receptor stimulation. In APAP liver injury, in both a caecal ligation and puncture (CLP) liver dysfunction model and a chemically induced biliary fibrosis model (by 3,5-diethoxycarbonyl-1,4-dihydrocollidine (DCC)-feeding), CD39-deficiency exacerbates disease (61–63). In DCC-dependent biliary fibrosis, CD39 deficiency in myeloid cells, via LysM-Cre-mediated excision of the CD39 gene, was sufficient for exacerbation of disease (63). As ATP signaling via the $P2X_7$ receptor not only induces a proinflammatory phenotype in macrophages but also increases CD39 expression and CD39 activity in macrophages (62), this represents a mechanism to induce an anti-inflammatory pro-resolving response after initial pro-inflammatory signaling in macrophages during inflammation and injury in the liver.

The release of LPC from apoptotic cells and it signaling via the G-protein coupled receptor G2A (13) can function as a "find-me" signal for efferocytes. Additionally, LPC signaling via the G2A receptor may also enhance phagocytic activity by promoting phagosome maturation (64, 65) and induce an anti-inflammatory (M2-like) mRNA expression profile [arginase 1 (Arg1), chitinase-like 3 (Chil3), CD206] and cytokine/mediator production (IL-10, PGE_2) (66). Preventing G2A signaling in CLP leads to higher mortality. However, inhibition Kupffer cell activity by gadolinium chloride treatment prevents this higher mortality in $G2A^{-/-}$ mice (67), indicating that G2A signaling in Kupffer cells reduces mortality in this model. Unexpectedly, G2A deficiency leads to overproduction of not only pro-inflammatory IL-6 and TNFα but also anti-inflammatory IL-10 by Kupffer cells. In CLP, the increased production of IL-10 by $G2A^{-/-}$ Kupffer cells is pivotal for the lack of bacterial clearance (and higher mortality) as this is reversed by either Kupffer cell depletion or IL-10 blockade (67).

The involvement of S1P as an efferocytic "find-me" signal regulating myeloid cells in liver disease has not been studied extensively. S1P is a major factor regulating immune cell migration to and from bone marrow and lymphoid organs and can signal through five S1PR. Reduced S1P serum levels in patients with liver cirrhosis and hepatocellular carcinoma (HCC) are associated with worse outcome and HBV co-infection (68, 69). However, in the experimental model of bile duct ligation, specific inhibition of $S1PR_{2/3}$ diminishes liver injury and fibrosis due to the inhibition of monocyte migration from the bone marrow into the liver (70). Similarly, treatment with the S1P antagonist FTY in mice fed a NASH diet also prevents infiltration of inflammatory monocytes and reduces liver inflammation and injury (71). The disparity between low serum S1P in patients being a predictor for higher mortality and a decreased inflammatory liver injury due to inhibition of S1P signaling in experimental models, may be the result of different timing (prevention and onset in experimental settings vs. end-stage disease in patients) but may also have to with comorbidities in patients. For instance, hyperglycemia, associated with type II diabetes, directly affects intrahepatic myeloid cell function. In mice treated with the pancreatic β cell toxin streptozotocin, that induces hyperglycemia, Kupffer cells produce more IL-6 and TNFα and less IL-10 in response to APAP-mediated injury compared to normoglycaemic animals (72). In these hyperglycemic mice, an imbalance between AMPK and Akt signaling leads to enhanced reactive oxygen species (ROS) production promoting an M1 type instead of M2 type gene signature in Kupffer cells. Hyperglycemia also increases intrahepatic S1P and S1PR3 levels both in patients and experimental animals (73). Targeting ROS production with *N*-acetyl cysteine (72) or treatment with a S1PR3 antagonist (73) both reduces the proinflammatory polarization of Kupffer cells and is associated with less inflammatory liver damage, which suggests that the combination of these treatments might bring additional advantage to counteract pro-inflammatory skewing of intrahepatic macrophages due to hyperglycemia.

The CX_3CR1 chemokine receptor is widely used to identify different populations of myeloid cells with the help of GFP-reporter mice (74). In the non-inflamed murine liver, CX_3CR1 expression identifies a myeloid cell population residing outside of the hepatic sinusoids, whereas $F4/80^+$ Kupffer cells are to be found intravascularly (48). Interestingly, single cell sequencing of healthy human hepatic immune cells did not reveal a similar division based on CX_3CR1 expression, but rather identified two populations of $CD68^+$ myeloid cells according to the expression of the macrophage receptor with collagenous structure (MARCO) receptor, with $MARCO^{pos}$ cells transcriptionally resembling murine Kupffer cells and $MARCO^{neg}$ having a rather inflammatory gene signature (75). It cannot, however, be excluded that CX_3CR1 may play a role in human intrahepatic inflammatory responses, as human peripheral blood monocytes express high levels of CX_3CR1 also in patients with liver disease (76). Although in the murine liver, CX_3CR1 positive cells are present under homeostatic conditions, it is widely accepted that during inflammatory responses, the up-regulation of CX_3CR1 on macrophages signifies their change from largely pro-inflammatory toward an anti-inflammatory, wound healing type of cell. Their anti-inflammatory properties could be enhanced by recognition of CX_3CL1 that is released by apoptotic cells. The change of $CCR2^{high}CX_3CR1^{low}$ inflammatory monocytes locally into $CCR2^{low}CX_3CR1^{high}$ macrophages in a sterile liver injury model leads to optimal repair and is dependent on local production of IL-4 and IL-10 (77). However, in liver disease, also endothelial-related expression of CX_3CL1 may attract $CD16^+$ monocytes CX_3CR1-dependently into areas with active inflammation (78) to dampen inflammation and promote resolution of injury. Fittingly, CX_3CR1-deficient mice develop greater liver fibrosis in both chronic CCl_4 and bile duct ligation models due to development of high amounts of TNFα- and NO-producing macrophages (79). Additionally, in the absence of CX_3CR1 signaling, the pro-inflammatory circle is perpetuated, as expression of the anti-apoptotic B cell lymphoma associated oncogene 2 protein (Bcl-2) is not induced in CX_3CR1-deficient macrophages.

Relevance of Indirect Phosphatidyl Serine Recognizing Receptors for Efferocytosis in the Liver

Recognition of apoptotic cells is mediated by binding to phosphatidyl serine exposed on the outer leaflet cell membrane. PS receptors either engage directly with PS (e.g., Tim family,

CD300 molecules, stabilins) or via bridging molecules that bind to PS (Gas6, Protein S and MGF-E8) that can then be recognized by certain integrins or receptors of the TAM family. Although Protein S is abundant in the circulation, Gas6 expression is more restricted. In acute CCl_4-mediated liver injury, Gas6 expression is induced in liver macrophages, indicating a role for detection of apoptotic cells via Gas6 and TAM receptors in this model. However, Gas6-deficiency does not change acute liver damage after CCl_4, but in the regenerative phase after CCl_4 induced liver injury, hepatocyte proliferation is stunted, and a reduction in Kupffer cell numbers and infiltrating monocytes are observed, with concomitant reduction of pro-inflammatory cytokine production (80). Mechanistically, Gas6 can signal via Axl, which is also induced in the liver after acute CCl_4 damage, and leads to autophagy induction, inhibition of NLRP3 inflammasome activation and subsequent reduction in IL-1β and IL-18 secretion, which is required to reinstall homeostasis (40).

The TAM (Tyro3-Axl-MerTK) family of receptor tyrosine kinases connects the recognition and removal of apoptotic cells to the induction of anti-inflammatory signaling in macrophages. General features of TAM-induced signaling include enhancement of phagocytosis, reduction of Type I IFN induced inflammation, inhibition of NLRP3 inflammasome activation via induction of autophagy and the promotion of anti-inflammatory cytokine production (34). The importance for these receptors in liver immune homeostasis becomes apparent in animals lacking all three TAM receptors. These mice develop an auto-immune hepatitis like disease, with high ALT, auto-antibodies and large immune cell infiltrates (81), which is dependent on bone-marrow derived cells. Individual TAM receptors can also modulate inflammatory response in the liver. In patients with acute liver failure MerTK-expressing macrophages expand, and migrate to the necrotic areas in the liver. Fittingly, in MerTK-deficient mice acute liver failure (ALF) due to APAP administration is aggravated and associated with a reduced number of hepatic macrophages and increased MPO^+ neutrophils (54). This suggests that MerTK may be involved in the removal of apoptotic neutrophils in the course of ALF. By increasing the amounts of MerTK-expressing macrophages, through *in vivo* application of secretory leukocyte protease inhibitor (SLPI), the amount of MPO^+TUNEL^+ neutrophils after APAP administration are reduced and this may constitute a therapeutic approach in acute liver failure after accidental or deliberate paracetamol intoxication (54). However, in patients with decompensated cirrhosis and acute-on-chronic liver failure (ACLF) the opposite may hold true. In ACLF patients, high susceptibility to infections and accompanying monocyte dysfunction correlates with disease severity (82). Here, MerTK expressing monocytes and macrophages are highly increased and are associated with decreased TNFα and IL-6 production. Interestingly, the treatment of $MerTK^+$ monocytes with a MerTK inhibitor increased proinflammatory cytokine production (82). Thus, either inhibiting or promoting expansion of MerTK expressing myeloid cells may be used to prevent immune paralysis in ACLF patients or enhance the clearance of necrotic material and apoptotic neutrophils in ALF patients, respectively.

Other non-TAM PS receptors may influence liver disease as well. The integrins αvβ3 and αvβ5, which recognize apoptotic cells via binding to the bridging molecule MFG-E8, can contribute to limiting fibrosis and the inhibition of proinflammatory mediator production in the chronic liver inflammation models of bile duct ligation and thioacetamine (TAA)-induced fibrosis (83). As the infiltration of macrophages with or without Cilengitide® (an αvβ3 and αvβ5 inhibitor mimicking the RDG-peptide ligand for integrins) treatment remains the same in these models, it is not clear whether or not the effects of αvβ3 and αvβ5 inhibition targets efferocytosis mechanisms in macrophages.

Relevance of Receptors Directly Recognizing Phosphatidyl Serine by Hepatic Macrophages for Liver Disease

The receptor stabilin-1 is well-known for mediating phosphatidyl serine-dependent removal of aged erythrocytes in the liver (9). In chronic CCl_4 liver injury the absence of stabilin-1 aggravates fibrosis and delays resolution after termination of CCl_4 administration. Furthermore, the phenotypic switch of pro-inflammatory macrophages to the pro-resolving $Ly6C^{low}$ macrophage is impaired in stabilin-1-deficient mice (84). Interestingly, stabilin-1 expression in non-injured animals is restricted to endothelial cells, but in inflamed/injured livers an $F4/80^+$stablilin-1^+ macrophage population can be detected (84). In addition to stabilin-1 binding to PS to promote efferocytosis, fibrosis development can additionally be prevented via stabilin-1. Pro-fibrogenic chemokine production can be inhibited via binding of malondialdehyde (MDA)-LDL, generated from lipid peroxidation, to stabilin-1. Furthermore, during resolution of liver injury the absence of stabilin-1 prevents the change to $Ly6C^{low}$ macrophages, which are thought to be pro-resolving macrophages (84). Besides stabilin-1, Tim4 can also bind directly to PS. Tim4 is over-expressed in hepatic macrophages of mice fed both a high fat diet (HFD) and methionine-choline deficient (MCD) diet (85) and its absence leads to increased inflammation and severe steatosis. Tim4 strongly binds to PS, but does not induce efferocytosis independently; it collaborates with TAM receptors to elicit efferocytosis (19, 86). Strikingly, signal transduction via the Tim4 cytoplasmic domain upon PS binding induces activation of AMPKα via LKB1, which is critical to initiate autophagy (85). What is more, the levels of Tim4 expression determine the degree of inhibition of NLRP3 protein complex expression. Tim4 deficiency, therefore, leads to high levels of IL-1β and IL-18 and proinflammatory damage in both NASH diets (85).

Phagocytosis and Autophagy of Apoptotic Cells and Its Relevance for Liver Disease

The sensing and physical uptake of apoptotic cells by macrophages can enhance phagocytosis. The cargo that is taken up needs to be digested and processed appropriately and several intermediates that are generated during this process may have signaling functions to modulate macrophage function toward a pro-resolving phenotype. For instance, the TAM-receptors and also the Tim4 receptor connect the uptake of apoptotic cells to autophagy, which in its turn prevents inflammasome activation and ultimately the production of pro-inflammatory IL-1β and IL-18. This means that macrophages that are incapable of properly digesting their apoptotic cargo may display aberrant inflammatory functions or phagocytosis. For instance, macrophages that can engulf apoptotic cells but are defective in processing their apoptotic cargo, due to the lack of LC3 interacting glycoprotein non-metastatic melanoma protein B (Gpnmb) expression (87) are neither capable to increase pSTAT3-dependent IL-6 transcription and IL-10 release nor sustain efficient efferocytosis by increasing phagocytosis. Addition of exogenous IL-6 and IL-10 increased phagocytosis in Gpnmb-deficient macrophages, indicating that secondary cytokine production is an important mechanism induced by proper cargo digestion to regulate phagocyte function. Indeed, *in vivo* absence of Gpnmb reduces the amount of $Ly6C^{low}$ restorative macrophages in acute APAP-mediated damage and also in chronic CCl_4 induced fibrosis (87) which can be reversed by treatment with IL-6. Different secondary signaling events that influence macrophage efferocytosis and anti-inflammatory function may also depend on the appropriate digestion of apoptotic material. Chemical inhibition of the lysosomal acid lipase (LIPA) reduces cholesterol hydrolysis in macrophages, and leads to mitochondrial stress and pro-inflammatory NLRP3 and caspase-1 activation. Furthermore, anti-inflammatory LXR activation is reduced due to the limited production of oxysterols from cholesterol (88). *In vivo,* the inhibition of LIPA activity reduces efferocytosis of both stressed erythrocytes and apoptotic lymphocytes. Also, under conditions of hypercholesterolemia, in which efferocytosis is constrained (89), additional LIPA inhibition exacerbated this effect and this consequently leads to increased liver inflammation. Interestingly, LIPA inhibition does not only increases the production of *iNos* and *Il1b* mRNA, it is accompanied by an almost complete reduction of *Mertk, Axl,* and *Gas6* mRNA expression (88). The efferocytic uptake of apoptotic cells connects to autophagy, which is achieved via a process called LC3-complex associated phagocytosis (LAP) (38). This non-canonical autophagy pathway requires a so-called class III PI3K complex that comprises the core proteins Beclin1, UV radiation resistance-associated gene protein (UVRAG), and RUN domain containing, Beclin1-interacting protein (Rubicon) (90). During LAP, rubicon localizes to the single membrane LAPosome, which is decorated with LC3-II, and promotes PI(3)P production necessary to recruit downstream autophagic machinery, including the ubiquitin-conjugating enzymes autophagy related proteins ATG5, 7 and 12 (38, 90). As a results, alterations in LAP lead to stalled degradation of apoptotic cells, which is observed in autoimmune disorders such as systemic lupus erythematosus (SLE) (42). Furthermore, LAP that is active during efferocytosis instructs phagocytes to secrete the anti-inflammatory cytokines TGFβ and IL-10, and conversely to repress secretion of the pro-inflammatory cytokines IL-1β, IL-12, and TNFα (37, 91, 92).

In HFD livers, Kupffer cells show defective LC3-I and LC3-II induction after LPS treatment, which leads to overproduction of TNFα. This phenotypically overlaps with ATG7-deficiency in Kupffer cells, which leads to defective induction of autophagy and provokes increased TNFα release (93). Furthermore, ATG5-deficiency restricted to myeloid cells leads to higher inflammatory responses in liver injury models (CCl_4, D-GalN/LPS) (94, 95). The lack of ATG5 expression results most prominently in NLRP3 and caspase-1 dependent IL-1β production, which promotes hepatic stellate cells to synthesize fibrotic factors and augments infiltration of $Ly6C^{high}$ inflammatory monocytes and MPO^+ neutrophils (94). Interestingly, the application of an IL-1R antagonist almost completely reverses injury and inflammatory phenotype due to ATG5 deficiency in mice, and offers a promising potential therapeutic approach in the prevention of liver fibrosis and limitation of acute toxic liver injury (94, 95). Thus, the way in which apoptotic cells are processed and digested in macrophages determines the signaling cascades that impose immunologically quiet anti-inflammatory responses on the liver and could be exploited to protect from liver inflammatory diseases.

Interactions Between Phagocytes Can Affect Efferocytosis Efficiency in the Liver

In infections and inflammatory diseases, neutrophilic granulocytes are first responders and infiltrate into the inflamed injured tissue. Pro-inflammatory cytokine release, protease release and the formation of extracellular nuclear traps (NETs) during the process of NETosis are deployed by neutrophils to combat the infection/injury (96, 97). Neutrophils die partially after NETosis or spontaneously via apoptosis and are cleared by tissue-resident or infiltrating macrophages via efferocytosis and the ordered clearance of apoptotic neutrophils by hepatic macrophages is essential for resolution of liver injury. Expectedly, CCR2-antibody depletion of pro-inflammatory $Ly6C^{high}$ monocytes during acute APAP injury increases the numbers of infiltrating neutrophils. However, these neutrophils are functionally changed and produce less ROS due to decreased NADPH2 expression and seem more long-lived as they upregulate pro survival factors (98). Reversely, changes in neutrophil activity may also influence efferocytic activity in macrophages. Mediators released by neutrophils during NETosis, may promote inflammatory signaling in macrophages but can also directly corrupt recognition of apoptotic cells by phagocytes: HMGB1, for example, can either bind to the PS-recognizing the RAGE receptor or directly binds to PS which interferes with recognition by other PS-binding proteins (26). Alcoholic liver disease (ALD) patients have elevated blood serum levels of HMGB1, which is secreted by neutrophils during NETosis. Interestingly, alcohol can directly increase NETosis by neutrophils (99) and thus in ALD patients the consumption of alcohol may directly affect pro- and anti-inflammatory pathways via HMGB1 in a dichotomous way: first, HMGB1 may act as a damage-associated molecular pattern protein (DAMP) that initiates pro-inflammatory TLR and NLRP3 signaling whilst simultaneously preventing efferocytosis via obscuring PS recognition. Furthermore,

TABLE 1 | Efferocytosis mechanisms in liver disease.

Molecules directly or indirectly involved in efferocytosis	Cell-associated or soluble	Model of gastrointestinal disease, function in the liver, and/or function in efferocytosis	References
IMMUNE RECEPTORS			
Vsig4	KC	Homeostasis	(51)
Tim4	KC	Homeostasis; in HFD and MCD, Tim4 deficiency: increase in inflammation and steatosis	(50, 53, 85)
Tim3	Liver mph	Hepatocellular carcinoma	(114)
SCAVENGER RECEPTORS			
Stabilin-1	LSEC, F4/80$^+$ stabilin1$^+$ mph	Removal of aged erythrocytes; CCl4; absence of Stabilin 1 aggravates fibrosis, delays in resolution	(9, 84)
Stabilin-2	LSEC	Removal of aged erythrocytes	(9)
CD36	KC, other phagocytes		(55)
PURINERGIC G-PROTEIN COUPLED RECEPTORS RECEPTORS			
P2Y receptors, P2Y13	KC	Expression in response to extracellular ATP, attraction of apoptotic cells, partial hepatectomy	(59)
P2Y2	HC	Partial hepatectomy, ATP release, and attraction of apoptotic cells	(60)
P2X7	KC	APAP, ATP release and attraction of apoptotic cells	(61)
G-PROTEIN COUPLED RECEPTORS AND LIGANDS			
G2A	KC	Enhancing phagosome maturation, CLP (cecal ligation and puncture)	(66, 67)
S1PR2/3		Bile duct ligation	(70)
S1P antagonist		NASH, S1P antagonist reduces monocyte infiltration, and reduces inflammation and injury	(71)
S1PR serum levels	Soluble, serum	Reduction of serum levels S1P, worse outcome in human liver cirrhosis, HCC, HBV	
S1P and S1PR3	Intrahepatic levels	Ischemia/reperfusion, hyperglycemia mice, and humans	(73)
S1PR3 antagonist		Reduction of inflammatory KC polarization	(73)
CHEMOKINE RECEPTORS AND LIGANDS			
Potenital: CX3CR1	KC, mph	recognition of CX3CL1 released by apoptotic cells, sterile liver injury	(77)
CX3CL1	LSEC	Potential attraction of CX3CR1 monocytes into areas of inflammation	(78)
CX3CR1		absence in deficient mice: greater liver fibrosis,CCl4 and BDL	(79)
TAM FAMILY RECEPTORS AND LIGANDS			
Gas6, Axl	Liver mph	CCl4, induction of Gas6/Axl expression, induction of autophagy, inhibition NLRP3 inflammasome	(80)
MertTK, Axl, Tyro3		MerTK$^{-/-}$, Axl$^{-/-}$ Tyro3$^{-/-}$ mice, development of auto-immune hepatitis like disease, autoantibodies, immune cell infiltrates	(81)
MerTK	KC	MerTK deficient mice, ALF after APAP	(54)
MerTK		Human ACLF, decompensated cirrhosis, increase in MerTK expressing myeloid cells, immune paralysis, Hepatocellular carcinoma	(82, 107)
INTEGRINS			
avb3 and avb5		binding to MFG-E8, BDL, TAA-induced fibrosis	(83)
INTRACELLULAR MOLECULES			
Gpnmb	mph	Lack of Gpnmb impairs cytokine release and sustaining efferocytosis; in APAP, CCl4: reduction of restorative macrophages	(87)
Lysosomal acid lipase		Reduction Mertk, Axl, Gas6 expression, reduction of LXR activation, reduction of efferocytosis; in hypercholesteremia, increase in liver inflammation	(88, 89)
LC3-I and LC3-II deficiency	KC	HFD induces deficiency in LC3-I and LC3-II, overproduction of inflammatory cytokines	(93)

(Continued)

TABLE 1 | Continued

Molecules directly or indirectly involved in efferocytosis	Cell-associated or soluble	Model of gastrointestinal disease, function in the liver, and/or function in efferocytosis	References
ATG7	KC	ATG7-deficiency in KC, increased release of inflammatory cytokines, defective autophagy	(93)
ATG5	Myeloid cells	Myeloid-restricted ATG5-deletion, hyperinfammation in CCl4/D-GalN/LPS, Hepatocellular carcinoma	(94, 95, 117)
HMGB1		PS or RAGE binding, impairs efferocytosis in ALD	(99)
miR-223	Neutrophils	CCl4, LPS-mediated liver injury: miR-223-releasing neutrophils promote generation of resolving macrophages; miR-223 downregulated in human NASH	(100, 102)
OTHER			
CD47	Non-phagocytes	Hepatocellular carcinoma	(118, 119)

neutrophils can act as anti-inflammatory modulators that support the formation of pro-resolving macrophages via the release of micro-vesicles carrying microRNAs (100). MicroRNA-223, which inhibits NLRP3 inflammasome activation (101), is highly expressed by neutrophils. As such, miR-223-deficient mice are highly susceptible to liver inflammation in response to low-dose LPS injection or CCl_4-mediated liver injury. During the resolution phase of inflammation after 1 week of CCl_4 treatment or during the resolving phase after MCD diet feeding, depletion of $Ly6G^+$ neutrophils impairs spontaneous resolution of liver injury and leads to the prevalence of pro-inflammatory $Ly6C^{high}$ monocytes (100). Due to the lack of neutrophils that release miR-223 to be taken up by macrophages, NLPR3 inflammasome protein expression is exacerbated and liver inflammation persists, as pro-inflammatory macrophages cannot be converted into the $CD163^{pos}$ anti-inflammatory, resolving type. Strikingly, this phenotype can be reversed by application of a miR-223 mimetic or the infusion of miR-223-compentent neutrophils. (100). In line with these observations, miR-223 is amongst the most prominent down regulated microRNAs in NASH patients (100, 102).

Involvement of Efferocytosis Mechanisms in Liver Cancer

The tumor microenvironment (TME) is rich in immune cells of which macrophages and other myeloid cells are the most abundant (103, 104) and the presence of high amounts of CD68 and CD163 positive tumor-associated macrophages is associated with poor prognosis in a number of human cancers (105), including hepatocellular carcinoma (HCC) (106). The presence of tumor-associated macrophages (TAM) is also associated with the expression of efferocytosis receptors like MerTK, and the uptake of apoptotic tumor cells may promote further anti-inflammatory, tumor promoting polarization of TAMs (107). In hepatocellular carcinoma, molecules involved in efferocytosis are clinically relevant. The presence of soluble Axl in the serum of patients, for instance, is used as a biomarker for liver cirrhosis and HCC development (108, 109) and receptor tyrosine kinase inhibitors that can inhibit Axl function are currently being tested in therapeutic settings (110). However, here it is not clear whether Axl function in tumor-associated macrophages plays a role, as hepatocellular cancer cells themselves overexpress Axl, which provides survival advantages via activation of downstream signal transduction promoting epithelial to mesenchymal transition (EMT) (111). Similarly, overexpression of the bridging molecule Gas6 also promotes HCC metastasis via direct signaling through the Axl receptor in carcinoma cells (112). Contrary to this, several studies in preclinical cancer models have provided evidence that efferocytosis, mostly, but not exclusively, dependent on the TAM receptor MerTK is involved in promoting tumor progression, and several Axl, Tyro3, and MerTK targeting small molecular inhibitors are being tested in clinical trials (113). Tim3 expression on TAMs also correlates negatively with HCC patient survival, most likely via the promotion of pro-inflammatory IL-6 production by Tim3 expressing macrophages (114), which is thought to be essential for the development of hepatocellular carcinoma (115). Although the process of efferocytosis is associated with the development of an M2-like pro-resolving anti-inflammatory phenotype in tumor associated macrophages, which supports tumor progression, and oppositely the induction of pro-inflammatory M1-like macrophages promotes anti-tumor immunity (116), boosting the pro-inflammatory milieu in the absence of efferocytosis may contrarily promote tumorigenesis in the preneoplastic stage of carcinogenesis in the liver (117). Lastly, tumors may also evade immunosurveillance, by preventing recognition for efferocytosis. The "don't eat me" ligand CD47 is highly overexpressed in HCC samples and preventing interaction with SIRP1α by blocking anti-CD47 antibodies augments macrophage efferocytosis of HCC cells *in vitro* and diminishes HCC tumor growth in *in vivo* xenograft models (118, 119).

CONCLUSION

The removal of dead cells poses a challenge to the maintenance of tolerance and the return to tissue integrity after inflammation or injury. Also in the liver, the maintenance of and return to immune homeostasis relies on functional efferocytosis (as summarized in **Table 1**), as demonstrated by the development of hepatic autoimmune disease in TAM receptor deficient mice. It has not been elucidated whether specific efferocytosis mechanisms exist in the liver. As during liver disease the most abundant cells involved in efferocytosis are infiltrating myeloid cells, general efferocytosis mechanisms known to be operative in macrophages have been investigated and found to play a role. However, under homeostatic conditions the most abundant myeloid cells in the liver are Kupffer cells. Due to their different ontogeny and expression of specific phagocytic receptors, such as the PS-receptor Tim4, complement receptor Vsig4 and the C-type lectin Clec4f, Kupffer cells may well-utilize additional pathways for efferocytosis under homeostasis. In liver disease, the use of global and cell specific knock-out mouse models for molecules involved in various aspects of efferocytosis has shown that efferocytosis mechanisms are heavily deployed in virtually all settings and stages of disease. The absence of functional efferocytosis in these genetic models can on the one hand lead to exacerbation of liver inflammation and injury or on the other hand to a lack and/or delay of resolution of inflammation and a insufficient return to tissue integrity. These opposite effects can be partly explained by the type of liver injury/inflammatory response (e.g., due to toxins or diet induced), but also by the length of the disease course and the timing of interference with efferocytosis. For instance, the inhibition of sufficient pro-inflammatory signaling can lead to defects in resolution, due to the fact that already early inflammatory responses set the stage for the induction of anti-inflammatory, pro-resolving pathways. The following inefficient induction of efferocytosis mechanisms impairs the clearance of damaged and apoptotic cells and subsequent loss of tissue homeostasis. In different etiologies of liver disease, it will be essential to understand the tempo-spatial contribution of pro- and anti-inflammatory and efferocytosis mechanisms in order to utilize these for treatment and prevention strategies in liver disease.

AUTHOR CONTRIBUTIONS

AH, GT, and LD contributed to analysis of publications, drafting of the manuscript, and critical revision of the content.

REFERENCES

1. Wium M, Paccez JD, Zerbini LF. The dual role of TAM receptors in autoimmune diseases and cancer: an overview. *Cells.* (2018) 7:166. doi: 10.3390/cells7100166
2. Bäck M, Yurdagul A, Tabas I, Öörni K, Kovanen PT. Inflammation and its resolution in atherosclerosis: mediators and therapeutic opportunities. *Nat Rev Cardiol.* (2019) 16:389–406. doi: 10.1038/s41569-019-0169-2
3. Grabiec AM, Hussell T. The role of airway macrophages in apoptotic cell clearance following acute and chronic lung inflammation. *Semin Immunopathol.* (2016) 38:409–23. doi: 10.1007/s00281-016-0555-3
4. Terpstra V, van Berkel TJ. Scavenger receptors on liver Kupffer cells mediate the *in vivo* uptake of oxidatively damaged red blood cells in mice. *Blood.* (2000) 95:2157–63. doi: 10.1182/blood.V95.6.2157
5. Shi J, Fujieda H, Kokubo Y, Wake K. Apoptosis of neutrophils and their elimination by Kupffer cells in rat liver. *Hepatology.* (1996) 24:1256–63. doi: 10.1002/hep.510240545
6. Shi J, Gilbert GE, Kokubo Y, Ohashi T. Role of the liver in regulating numbers of circulating neutrophils. *Blood.* (2001) 98:1226–30. doi: 10.1182/blood.V98.4.1226
7. Crispe IN, Dao T, Klugewitz K, Mehal WZ, Metz DP. The liver as a site of T-cell apoptosis: graveyard, or killing field? *Immunol Rev.* (2000) 174:47–62. doi: 10.1034/j.1600-0528.2002.017412.x
8. Tang D, Kang R, Berghe TV, Vandenabeele P, Kroemer G. The molecular machinery of regulated cell death. *Cell Res.* (2019) 29:347–64. doi: 10.1038/s41422-019-0164-5
9. Lee S-J, Park S-Y, Jung M-Y, Bae SM, Kim I-S. Mechanism for phosphatidylserine-dependent erythrophagocytosis in mouse liver. *Blood.* (2011) 117:5215–23. doi: 10.1182/blood-2010-10-313239
10. Davies SP, Reynolds GM, Stamataki Z. Clearance of apoptotic cells by tissue epithelia: a putative role for hepatocytes in liver efferocytosis. *Front Immunol.* (2018) 9:44. doi: 10.3389/fimmu.2018.00044
11. Park S-Y, Kim I-S. Engulfment signals and the phagocytic machinery for apoptotic cell clearance. *Exp Mol Med.* (2017) 49:e331. doi: 10.1038/emm.2017.52
12. Medina CB, Ravichandran KS. Do not let death do us part: "find-me" signals in communication between dying cells and the phagocytes. *Cell Death Differ.* (2016) 23:979–89. doi: 10.1038/cdd.2016.13
13. Kabarowski JH. G2A and LPC: regulatory functions in immunity. *Prostaglandins Other Lipid Mediat.* (2009) 89:73–81. doi: 10.1016/j.prostaglandins.2009.04.007
14. Bellido-Martín L, de Frutos PG. Vitamin K-dependent actions of Gas6. *Vitam Horm.* (2008) 78:185–209. doi: 10.1016/S0083-6729(07)00009-X
15. Rothlin CV, Lemke G. TAM receptor signaling and autoimmune disease. *Curr Opin Immunol.* (2010) 22:740–6. doi: 10.1016/j.coi.2010.10.001
16. Ramirez-Ortiz ZG, Pendergraft WF, Prasad A, Byrne MH, Iram T, Blanchette CJ, et al. The scavenger receptor SCARF1 mediates the clearance of apoptotic cells and prevents autoimmunity. *Nat Immunol.* (2013) 14:917–26. doi: 10.1038/ni.2670
17. Païdassi H, Tacnet-Delorme P, Verneret M, Gaboriaud C, Houen G, Duus K, et al. Investigations on the C1q-calreticulin-phosphatidylserine interactions yield new insights into apoptotic cell recognition. *J Mol Biol.* (2011) 408:277–90. doi: 10.1016/j.jmb.2011.02.029
18. Blackburn JWD, Lau DHC, Liu EY, Ellins J, Vrieze AM, Pawlak EN, et al. Soluble CD93 is an apoptotic cell opsonin recognized by α xβ 2. *Eur J Immunol.* (2019) 49:600–10. doi: 10.1002/eji.201847801
19. Nishi C, Yanagihashi Y, Segawa K, Nagata S. MERTK tyrosine kinase receptor together with TIM4 phosphatidylserine receptor mediates distinct signal transduction pathways for efferocytosis and cell proliferation. *J Biol Chem.* (2019) 294:7221–30. doi: 10.1074/jbc.RA118.006628
20. Flannagan RS, Canton J, Furuya W, Glogauer M, Grinstein S. The phosphatidylserine receptor TIM4 utilizes integrins as coreceptors to effect phagocytosis. *Mol Biol Cell.* (2014) 25:1511–22. doi: 10.1091/mbc.e13-04-0212
21. Borrego F. The CD300 molecules: an emerging family of regulators of the immune system. *Blood.* (2013) 121:1951–60. doi: 10.1182/blood-2012-09-435057
22. Nakahashi-Oda C, Tahara-Hanaoka S, Honda S-I, Shibuya K, Shibuya A. Identification of phosphatidylserine as a ligand for the CD300a immunoreceptor. *Biochem Biophys Res Commun.* (2012) 417:646–50. doi: 10.1016/j.bbrc.2011.12.025
23. Tian L, Choi S-C, Murakami Y, Allen J, Morse HC, Qi C-F, et al. p85α recruitment by the CD300f phosphatidylserine receptor mediates apoptotic cell clearance required for autoimmunity suppression. *Nat Comms.* (2014) 5:3146. doi: 10.1038/ncomms4146
24. Murakami Y, Tian L, Voss OH, Margulies DH, Krzewski K, Coligan JE. CD300b regulates the phagocytosis of apoptotic cells via phosphatidylserine recognition. *Cell Death Differ.* (2014) 21:1746–57. doi: 10.1038/cdd.2014.86
25. Friggeri A, Banerjee S, Biswas S, de Freitas A, Liu G, Bierhaus A, et al. Participation of the receptor for advanced glycation end products in efferocytosis. *J Immunol.* (2011) 186:6191–8. doi: 10.4049/jimmunol.1004134
26. Davis K, Banerjee S, Friggeri A, Bell C, Abraham E, Zerfaoui M. Poly(ADP-ribosyl)ation of high mobility group box 1 (HMGB1) protein enhances inhibition of efferocytosis. *Mol Med.* (2012) 18:359–69. doi: 10.2119/molmed.2011.00203
27. Zhang Z, Jiang Y, Zhou Z, Huang J, Chen S, Zhou W, et al. Scavenger receptor A1 attenuates aortic dissection via promoting efferocytosis in macrophages.

Biochem Pharmacol. (2019) 168:392–403. doi: 10.1016/j.bcp.2019.07.027
28. Tao H, Yancey PG, Babaev VR, Blakemore JL, Zhang Y, Ding L, et al. Macrophage SR-BI mediates efferocytosis via Src/PI3K/Rac1 signaling and reduces atherosclerotic lesion necrosis. *J Lipid Res.* (2015) 56:1449–60. doi: 10.1194/jlr.M056689
29. Driscoll WS, Vaisar T, Tang J, Wilson CL, Raines EW. Macrophage ADAM17 deficiency augments CD36-dependent apoptotic cell uptake and the linked anti-inflammatory phenotype. *Circ Res.* (2013) 113:52–61. doi: 10.1161/CIRCRESAHA.112.300683
30. Matozaki T, Murata Y, Okazawa H, Ohnishi H. Functions and molecular mechanisms of the CD47-SIRPalpha signalling pathway. *Trends Cell Biol.* (2009) 19:72–80. doi: 10.1016/j.tcb.2008.12.001
31. Barkal AA, Brewer RE, Markovic M, Kowarsky M, Barkal SA, Zaro BW, et al. CD24 signalling through macrophage Siglec-10 is a target for cancer immunotherapy. *Nature.* (2019) 572:392–6. doi: 10.1038/s41586-019-1456-0
32. Elliott MR, Koster KM, Murphy PS. Efferocytosis signaling in the regulation of macrophage inflammatory responses. *J Immunol.* (2017) 198:1387–94. doi: 10.4049/jimmunol.1601520
33. Szondy Z, Sarang Z, Kiss B, Garabuczi É, Köröskényi K. Anti-inflammatory mechanisms triggered by apoptotic cells during their clearance. *Front Immunol.* (2017) 8:909. doi: 10.3389/fimmu.2017.00909
34. Lee C-H, Chun T. Anti-inflammatory role of TAM family of receptor tyrosine kinases via modulating macrophage function. *Mol Cells.* (2019) 42:1–7. doi: 10.14348/molcells.2018.0419
35. Haskó G, Pacher P. Regulation of macrophage function by adenosine. *Arterioscler Thromb Vasc Biol.* (2012) 32:865–9. doi: 10.1161/ATVBAHA.111.226852
36. Röszer T. Transcriptional control of apoptotic cell clearance by macrophage nuclear receptors. *Apoptosis.* (2017) 22:284–94. doi: 10.1007/s10495-016-1310-x
37. A-Gonzalez N, Bensinger SJ, Hong C, Beceiro S, Bradley MN, Zelcer N, et al. Apoptotic cells promote their own clearance and immune tolerance through activation of the nuclear receptor LXR. *Immunity.* (2009) 31:245–8. doi: 10.1016/j.immuni.2009.06.018
38. Heckmann BL, Boada-Romero E, Cunha LD, Magne J, Green DR. LC3-associated phagocytosis and inflammation. *J Mol Biol.* (2017) 429:3561–76. doi: 10.1016/j.jmb.2017.08.012
39. Wong SW, Sil P, Martinez J. Rubicon: LC3-associated phagocytosis and beyond. *FEBS J.* (2017) 285:1379–88. doi: 10.1111/febs.14354
40. Han J, Bae J, Choi C-Y, Choi S-P, Kang H-S, Jo E-K, et al. Autophagy induced by AXL receptor tyrosine kinase alleviates acute liver injury via inhibition of NLRP3 inflammasome activation in mice. *Autophagy.* (2016) 12:2326–43. doi: 10.1080/15548627.2016.1235124
41. Martinez J, Almendinger J, Oberst A, Ness R, Dillon CP, Fitzgerald P, et al. Microtubule-associated protein 1 light chain 3 alpha. (LC3)-associated phagocytosis is required for the efficient clearance of dead cells. *Proc Natl Acad Sci USA.* (2011) 108:17396–401. doi: 10.1073/pnas.1113421108
42. Martinez J, Cunha LD, Park S, Yang M, Lu Q, Orchard R, et al. Non-canonical autophagy inhibits the autoinflammatory, lupus-like response to dying cells. *Nature.* (2016) 533:115–9. doi: 10.1038/nature17950
43. Bosurgi L, Cao YG, Cabeza-Cabrerizo M, Tucci A, Hughes LD, Kong Y, et al. Macrophage function in tissue repair and remodeling requires IL-4 or IL-13 with apoptotic cells. *Science.* (2017) 356:1072–6. doi: 10.1126/science.aai8132
44. Proto JD, Doran AC, Gusarova G, Yurdagul A, Sozen E, Subramanian M, et al. Regulatory T cells promote macrophage efferocytosis during inflammation resolution. *Immunity.* (2018) 49:666–77.e6. doi: 10.1016/j.immuni.2018.07.015
45. Grabiec AM, Goenka A, Fife ME, Fujimori T, Hussell T. Axl and MerTK receptor tyrosine kinases maintain human macrophage efferocytic capacity in the presence of viral triggers. *Eur J Immunol.* (2018) 48:855–60. doi: 10.1002/eji.201747283
46. Rothlin CV, Carrera-Silva EA, Bosurgi L, Ghosh S. TAM receptor signaling in immune homeostasis. *Annu Rev Immunol.* (2015) 33:355–91. doi: 10.1146/annurev-immunol-032414-112103
47. Ginhoux F, Guilliams M. Tissue-resident macrophage ontogeny and homeostasis. *Immunity.* (2016) 44:439–49. doi: 10.1016/j.immuni.2016.02.024
48. David BA, Rezende RM, Antunes MM, Santos MM, Freitas Lopes MA, Diniz AB, et al. Combination of mass cytometry and imaging analysis reveals origin, location, and functional repopulation of liver myeloid cells in mice. *Gastroenterology.* (2016) 151:1176–91. doi: 10.1053/j.gastro.2016.08.024
49. Yona S, Kim K-W, Wolf Y, Mildner A, Varol D, Breker M, et al. Fate mapping reveals origins and dynamics of monocytes and tissue macrophages under homeostasis. *Immunity.* (2013) 38:79–91. doi: 10.1016/j.immuni.2012.12.001
50. Devisscher L, Scott CL, Lefere S, Raevens S, Bogaerts E, Paridaens A, et al. Non-alcoholic steatohepatitis induces transient changes within the liver macrophage pool. *Cell Immunol.* (2017) 322:74–83. doi: 10.1016/j.cellimm.2017.10.006
51. van der Tuin SJL, Li Z, Berbée JFP, Verkouter I, Ringnalda LE, Neele AE, et al. Lipopolysaccharide lowers cholesteryl ester transfer protein by activating $F4/80^{+}Clec4f^{+}Vsig4^{+}Ly6C^{-}$ kupffer cell subsets. *J Am Heart Assoc.* (2018) 7:395. doi: 10.1161/JAHA.117.008105
52. Goh YPS, Henderson NC, Heredia JE, Red Eagle A, Odegaard JI, Lehwald N, et al. Eosinophils secrete IL-4 to facilitate liver regeneration. *Proc Natl Acad Sci USA.* (2013) 110:9914–9. doi: 10.1073/pnas.1304046110
53. Theurl I, Hilgendorf I, Nairz M, Tymoszuk P, Haschka D, Asshoff M, et al. On-demand erythrocyte disposal and iron recycling requires transient macrophages in the liver. *Nat Med.* (2016) 22:945–51. doi: 10.1038/nm.4146
54. Triantafyllou E, Pop OT, Possamai LA, Wilhelm A, Liaskou E, Singanayagam A, et al. MerTK expressing hepatic macrophages promote the resolution of inflammation in acute liver failure. *Gut.* (2018) 67:333–47. doi: 10.1136/gutjnl-2016-313615
55. Trahtemberg U, Mevorach D. Apoptotic cells induced signaling for immune homeostasis in macrophages and dendritic cells. *Front Immunol.* (2017) 8:1356. doi: 10.3389/fimmu.2017.01356
56. Zhang M, Xu S, Han Y, Cao X. Apoptotic cells attenuate fulminant hepatitis by priming Kupffer cells to produce interleukin-10 through membrane-bound TGF-β. *Hepatology.* (2010) 53:306–16. doi: 10.1002/hep.24029
57. Rodriguez-Fernandez S, Pujol-Autonell I, Brianso F, Perna-Barrull D, Cano-Sarabia M, Garcia-Jimeno S, et al. Phosphatidylserine-liposomes promote tolerogenic features on dendritic cells in human type 1 diabetes by apoptotic mimicry. *Front Immunol.* (2018) 9:253. doi: 10.3389/fimmu.2018.00253
58. Yousefi-Manesh H, Shirooie S, Partoazar A, Nikoui V, Estakhri MRA, Bakhtiarian A. Hepatoprotective effects of phosphatidylserine liposomes on carbon tetrachloride-induced hepatotoxicity in rats. *J Cell Biochem.* (2019) 120:11853–8. doi: 10.1002/jcb.28464
59. Ishimaru M, Yusuke N, Tsukimoto M, Harada H, Takenouchi T, Kitani H, et al. Purinergic signaling via P2Y receptors up-mediates IL-6 production by liver macrophages/Kupffer cells. *J Toxicol Sci.* (2014) 39:413–23. doi: 10.2131/jts.39.413
60. Gonzales E, Julien B, Serrière-Lanneau V, Nicou A, Doignon I, Lagoudakis L, et al. ATP release after partial hepatectomy regulates liver regeneration in the rat. *J Hepatol.* (2010) 52:54–62. doi: 10.1016/j.jhep.2009.10.005
61. Hoque R, Sohail MA, Salhanick S, Malik AF, Ghani A, Robson SC, et al. P2X7 receptor-mediated purinergic signaling promotes liver injury in acetaminophen hepatotoxicity in mice. *AJP.* (2012) 302:G1171–9. doi: 10.1152/ajpgi.00352.2011
62. Savio LEB, de Andrade Mello P, Figliuolo VR, de Avelar Almeida TF, Santana PT, Oliveira SDS, et al. CD39 limits P2X7 receptor inflammatory signaling and attenuates sepsis-induced liver injury. *J Hepatol.* (2017) 67:716–26. doi: 10.1016/j.jhep.2017.05.021
63. Rothweiler S, Feldbrügge L, Jiang ZG, Csizmadia E, Longhi MS, Vaid K, et al. Selective deletion of ENTPD1/CD39 in macrophages exacerbates biliary fibrosis in a mouse model of sclerosing cholangitis. *Purinergic Signal.* (2019) 15:375–85. doi: 10.1007/s11302-019-09664-3
64. Frasch SC, Fernandez-Boyanapalli RF, Berry KZ, Leslie CC, Bonventre JV, Murphy RC, et al. Signaling via macrophage G2A enhances efferocytosis of dying neutrophils by augmentation of Rac activity. *J Biol Chem.* (2011) 286:12108–22. doi: 10.1074/jbc.M110.181800
65. Lee H-J, Ko H-J, Song D-K, Jung Y-J. Lysophosphatidylcholine promotes phagosome maturation and regulates inflammatory mediator production through the protein kinase A-phosphatidylinositol 3 kinase-p38 mitogen-activated protein kinase signaling pathway during *Mycobacterium tuberculosis* infection in mouse macrophages. *Front Immunol.* (2018) 9:920. doi: 10.3389/fimmu.2018.00920

66. Assunção LS, Magalhães KG, Carneiro AB, Molinaro R, Almeida PE, Atella GC, et al. Schistosomal-derived lysophosphatidylcholine triggers M2 polarization of macrophages through PPARγ dependent mechanisms. *Biochim Biophys Acta Mol Cell Biol Lipids.* (2017) 1862:246–54. doi: 10.1016/j.bbalip.2016.11.006
67. Li H-M, Jang JH, Jung J-S, Shin J, Park CO, Kim Y-J, et al. G2A protects mice against sepsis by modulating kupffer cell activation: cooperativity with adenosine receptor 2b. *J Immunol.* (2019) 202:527–38. doi: 10.4049/jimmunol.1700783
68. Becker S, Kinny-Köster B, Bartels M, Scholz M, Seehofer D, Berg T, et al. Low sphingosine-1-phosphate plasma levels are predictive for increased mortality in patients with liver cirrhosis. *PLoS ONE.* (2017) 12:e0174424. doi: 10.1371/journal.pone.0174424
69. Dong H, Xiao J, Zhu R, Liu B, Dong M, Luo D, et al. Serum sphingosine 1-phosphate in hepatocellular carcinoma patients is related to HBV infection. *J BUON.* (2018) 23:1711–6.
70. Yang L, Han Z, Tian L, Mai P, Zhang Y, Wang L, et al. Sphingosine 1-phosphate receptor 2 and 3 mediate bone marrow-derived monocyte/macrophage motility in cholestatic liver injury in mice. *Sci Rep.* (2015) 5:13423. doi: 10.1038/srep13423
71. Mauer AS, Hirsova P, Maiers JL, Shah VH, Malhi H. Inhibition of sphingosine 1-phosphate signaling ameliorates murine non-alcoholic steatohepatitis. *AJP: Gastrointest Liver Physiol.* (2017) 312:G300–13. doi: 10.1152/ajpgi.00222.2016
72. Wang Q, Wei S, Zhou H, Shen G, Gan X, Zhou S, et al. Hyperglycemia exacerbates acetaminophen-induced acute liver injury by promoting liver-resident macrophage proinflammatory response via AMPK/PI3K/AKT-mediated oxidative stress. *Cell Death Discov.* (2019) 5:119–12. doi: 10.1038/s41420-019-0198-y
73. Hu Y, Yang C, Shen G, Yang S, Cheng X, Cheng F, et al. Hyperglycemia-triggered sphingosine-1-phosphate and sphingosine-1-phosphate receptor 3 signaling worsens liver ischemia/reperfusion injury by regulating M1/M2 polarization. *Liver Transpl.* (2019) 25:1074–90. doi: 10.1002/lt.25470
74. Jung S, Aliberti J, Graemmel P, Sunshine MJ, Kreutzberg GW, Sher A, et al. Analysis of fractalkine receptor CX(3)CR1 function by targeted deletion and green fluorescent protein reporter gene insertion. *Mol Cell Biol.* (2000) 20:4106–14. doi: 10.1128/MCB.20.11.4106-4114.2000
75. MacParland SA, Liu JC, Ma X-Z, Innes BT, Bartczak AM, Gage BK, et al. Single cell RNA sequencing of human liver reveals distinct intrahepatic macrophage populations. *Nat Comms.* (2018) 9:4383–21. doi: 10.1038/s41467-018-06318-7
76. Gadd VL, Patel PJ, Jose S, Horsfall L, Powell EE, Irvine KM. Altered peripheral blood monocyte phenotype and function in chronic liver disease: implications for hepatic recruitment and systemic inflammation. *PLoS ONE.* (2016) 11:e0157771. doi: 10.1371/journal.pone.0157771
77. Dal-Secco D, Wang J, Zeng Z, Kolaczkowska E, Wong CHY, Petri B, et al. A dynamic spectrum of monocytes arising from the in situ reprogramming of CCR2^{+} monocytes at a site of sterile injury. *J Exp Med.* (2015) 212:447–56. doi: 10.1084/jem.20141539
78. Aspinall AI, Curbishley SM, Lalor PF, Weston CJ, Blahova M, Liaskou E, et al. CX_3CR1 and vascular adhesion protein-1-dependent recruitment of CD16^{+} monocytes across human liver sinusoidal endothelium. *Hepatology.* (2010) 51:2030–9. doi: 10.1002/hep.23591
79. Karlmark KR, Zimmermann HW, Roderburg C, Gassler N, Wasmuth HE, Luedde T, et al. The fractalkine receptor CX3CR1 protects against liver fibrosis by controlling differentiation and survival of infiltrating hepatic monocytes. *Hepatology.* (2010) 52:1769–82. doi: 10.1002/hep.23894
80. Lafdil F, Chobert M-N, Deveaux V, Zafrani E-S, Mavier P, Nakano T, et al. Growth arrest-specific protein 6 deficiency impairs liver tissue repair after acute toxic hepatitis in mice. *J Hepatol.* (2009) 51:55–66. doi: 10.1016/j.jhep.2009.02.030
81. Qi N, Liu P, Zhang Y, Wu H, Chen Y, Han D. Development of a spontaneous liver disease resembling autoimmune hepatitis in mice lacking tyro3, axl and mer receptor tyrosine kinases. *PLoS ONE.* (2013) 8:e66604. doi: 10.1371/journal.pone.0066604
82. Bernsmeier C, Pop OT, Singanayagam A, Triantafyllou E, Patel VC, Weston CJ, et al. Patients with acute-on-chronic liver failure have increased numbers of regulatory immune cells expressing the receptor tyrosine kinase MERTK. *Gastroenterology.* (2015) 148:603–15.e14. doi: 10.1053/j.gastro.2014.11.045
83. Patsenker E, Popov Y, Stickel F, Schneider V, Ledermann M, Sägesser H, et al. Pharmacological inhibition of integrin alphavbeta3 aggravates experimental liver fibrosis and suppresses hepatic angiogenesis. *Hepatology.* (2009) 50:1501–11. doi: 10.1002/hep.23144
84. Rantakari P, Patten DA, Valtonen J, Karikoski M, Gerke H, Dawes H, et al. Stabilin-1 expression defines a subset of macrophages that mediate tissue homeostasis and prevent fibrosis in chronic liver injury. *Proc Natl Acad Sci USA.* (2016) 113:9298–303. doi: 10.1073/pnas.1604780113
85. Liu W, Bai F, Wang H, Liang Y, Du X, Liu C, et al. Tim-4 inhibits NLRP3 inflammasome via the LKB1/AMPKα pathway in macrophages. *J Immunol.* (2019) 203:990–1000. doi: 10.4049/jimmunol.1900117
86. Nishi C, Toda S, Segawa K, Nagata S. Tim4- and MerTK-mediated engulfment of apoptotic cells by mouse resident peritoneal macrophages. *Mol Cell Biol.* (2014) 34:1512–20. doi: 10.1128/MCB.01394-13
87. Campana L, Starkey Lewis PJ, Pellicoro A, Aucott RL, Man J, O'Duibhir E, et al. The STAT3-IL-10-IL-6 pathway is a novel regulator of macrophage efferocytosis and phenotypic conversion in sterile liver injury. *J Immunol.* (2018) 200:1169–87. doi: 10.4049/jimmunol.1701247
88. Viaud M, Ivanov S, Vujic N, Duta-Mare M, Aira L-E, Barouillet T, et al. Lysosomal cholesterol hydrolysis couples efferocytosis to anti-inflammatory oxysterol production. *Circ Res.* (2018) 122:1369–84. doi: 10.1161/CIRCRESAHA.117.312333
89. Tall AR, Yvan-Charvet L. Cholesterol, inflammation and innate immunity. *Nat Rev Immunol.* (2015) 15:104–16. doi: 10.1038/nri3793
90. Green DR, Oguin TH, Martinez J. The clearance of dying cells: table for two. *Cell Death Differ.* (2016) 23:915–26. doi: 10.1038/cdd.2015.172
91. Fadok VA, Bratton DL, Guthrie L, Henson PM. Differential effects of apoptotic versus lysed cells on macrophage production of cytokines: role of proteases. *J Immunol.* (2001) 166:6847–54. doi: 10.4049/jimmunol.166.11.6847
92. Fadok VA, Bratton DL, Konowal A, Freed PW, Westcott JY, Henson PM. Macrophages that have ingested apoptotic cells *in vitro* inhibit proinflammatory cytokine production through autocrine/paracrine mechanisms involving TGF-beta, PGE2, and PAF. *J Clin Invest.* (1998) 101:890–8. doi: 10.1172/JCI1112
93. Fukada H, Yamashina S, Izumi K, Komatsu M, Tanaka K, Ikejima K, et al. Suppression of autophagy sensitizes Kupffer cells to endotoxin. *Hepatol Res.* (2012) 42:1112–8. doi: 10.1111/j.1872-034X.2012.01024.x
94. Lodder J, Denaës T, Chobert M-N, Wan J, El-Benna J, Pawlotsky J-M, et al. Macrophage autophagy protects against liver fibrosis in mice. *Autophagy.* (2015) 11:1280–92. doi: 10.1080/15548627.2015.1058473
95. Ilyas G, Zhao E, Liu K, Lin Y, Tesfa L, Tanaka KE, et al. Macrophage autophagy limits acute toxic liver injury in mice through down regulation of interleukin-1β. *J Hepatol.* (2016) 64:118–27. doi: 10.1016/j.jhep.2015.08.019
96. Kolaczkowska E, Kubes P. Neutrophil recruitment and function in health and inflammation. *Nat Rev Immunol.* (2013) 13:159–75. doi: 10.1038/nri3399
97. Vanden Berghe T, Linkermann A, Jouan-Lanhouet S, Walczak H, Vandenabeele P. Regulated necrosis: the expanding network of non-apoptotic cell death pathways. *Nat Rev Mol Cell Biol.* (2014) 15:135–47. doi: 10.1038/nrm3737
98. Graubardt N, Vugman M, Mouhadeb O, Caliari G, Pasmanik-Chor M, Reuveni D, et al. Ly6Chi monocytes and their macrophage descendants regulate neutrophil function and clearance in acetaminophen-induced liver injury. *Front Immunol.* (2017) 8:626. doi: 10.3389/fimmu.2017.00626
99. Bukong TN, Cho Y, Iracheta-Vellve A, Saha B, Lowe P, Adejumo A, et al. Abnormal neutrophil traps and impaired efferocytosis contribute to liver injury and sepsis severity after binge alcohol use. *J Hepatol.* (2018) 69:1145–54. doi: 10.1016/j.jhep.2018.07.005
100. Calvente CJ, Tameda M, Johnson CD, Del Pilar H, Lin YC, Adronikou N, et al. Neutrophils contribute to spontaneous resolution of liver inflammation and fibrosis via microRNA-223. *J Clin Invest.* (2019) 130:187. doi: 10.1172/JCI122258
101. Bauernfeind F, Rieger A, Schildberg FA, Knolle PA, Schmid-Burgk JL, Hornung V. NLRP3 inflammasome activity is negatively controlled by miR-223. *J Immunol.* (2012) 189:4175–81. doi: 10.4049/jimmunol.1201516
102. Cheung O, Puri P, Eicken C, Contos MJ, Mirshahi F, Maher JW, et al.

Non-alcoholic steatohepatitis is associated with altered hepatic MicroRNA expression. *Hepatology.* (2008) 48:1810–20. doi: 10.1002/hep.22569

103. Biswas SK, Allavena P, Mantovani A. Tumor-associated macrophages: functional diversity, clinical significance, and open questions. *Semin Immunopathol.* (2013) 35:585–600. doi: 10.1007/s00281-013-0367-7
104. Gabrilovich DI, Ostrand-Rosenberg S, Bronte V. Coordinated regulation of myeloid cells by tumours. *Nat Rev Immunol.* (2012) 12:253–68. doi: 10.1038/nri3175
105. Engblom C, Pfirschke C, Pittet MJ. The role of myeloid cells in cancer therapies. *Nat Rev Cancer.* (2016) 16:447–62. doi: 10.1038/nrc.2016.54
106. Wu K, Kryczek I, Chen L, Zou W, Welling TH. Kupffer cell suppression of $CD8^{+}$ T cells in human hepatocellular carcinoma is mediated by B7-H1/programmed death-1 interactions. *Cancer Res.* (2009) 69:8067–75. doi: 10.1158/0008-5472.CAN-09-0901
107. Akalu YT, Rothlin CV, Ghosh S. TAM receptor tyrosine kinases as emerging targets of innate immune checkpoint blockade for cancer therapy. *Immunol Rev.* (2017) 276:165–77. doi: 10.1111/imr.12522
108. Dengler M, Staufer K, Huber H, Stauber R, Bantel H, Weiss KH, et al. Soluble Axl is an accurate biomarker of cirrhosis and hepatocellular carcinoma development: results from a large scale multicenter analysis. *Oncotarget.* (2017) 8:46234–48. doi: 10.18632/oncotarget.17598
109. Staufer K, Dengler M, Huber H, Marculescu R, Stauber R, Lackner C, et al. The non-invasive serum biomarker soluble Axl accurately detects advanced liver fibrosis and cirrhosis. *Cell Death Dis.* (2017) 8:e3135. doi: 10.1038/cddis.2017.554
110. Personeni N, Rimassa L, Pressiani T, Smiroldo V, Santoro A. Cabozantinib for the treatment of hepatocellular carcinoma. *Expert Rev Anticancer Ther.* (2019) 19:847–55. doi: 10.1080/14737140.2019.1674141
111. Pinato DJ, Brown MW, Trousil S, Aboagye EO, Beaumont J, Zhang H, et al. Integrated analysis of multiple receptor tyrosine kinases identifies Axl as a therapeutic target and mediator of resistance to sorafenib in hepatocellular carcinoma. *Br J Cancer.* (2019) 120:512–21. doi: 10.1038/s41416-018-0373-6
112. Lee H-J, Jeng Y-M, Chen Y-L, Chung L, Yuan R-H. Gas6/Axl pathway promotes tumor invasion through the transcriptional activation of Slug in hepatocellular carcinoma. *Carcinogenesis.* (2014) 35:769–75. doi: 10.1093/carcin/bgt372
113. Myers KV, Amend SR, Pienta KJ. Targeting Tyro3, Axl and MerTK (TAM receptors): implications for macrophages in the tumor microenvironment. *Mol Cancer.* (2019) 18:94–14. doi: 10.1186/s12943-019-1022-2
114. Yan W, Liu X, Ma H, Zhang H, Song X, Gao L, et al. Tim-3 fosters HCC development by enhancing TGF-β-mediated alternative activation of macrophages. *Gut.* (2015) 64:1593–604. doi: 10.1136/gutjnl-2014-307671
115. Bergmann J, Müller M, Baumann N, Reichert M, Heneweer C, Bolik J, et al. IL-6 trans-signaling is essential for the development of hepatocellular carcinoma in mice. *Hepatology.* (2017) 65:89–103. doi: 10.1002/hep.28874
116. Capece D, Fischietti M, Verzella D, Gaggiano A, Cicciarelli G, Tessitore A, et al. The inflammatory microenvironment in hepatocellular carcinoma: a pivotal role for tumor-associated macrophages. *BioMed Res Int.* (2013) 2013:187204–15. doi: 10.1155/2013/187204
117. Sun K, Xu L, Jing Y, Han Z, Chen X, Cai C, et al. Autophagy-deficient Kupffer cells promote tumorigenesis by enhancing mtROS-NF-κB-IL1α/β-dependent inflammation and fibrosis during the preneoplastic stage of hepatocarcinogenesis. *Cancer Lett.* (2017) 388:198–207. doi: 10.1016/j.canlet.2016.12.004
118. Lo J, Lau EYT, So FTY, Lu P, Chan VSF, Cheung VCH, et al. Anti-CD47 antibody suppresses tumour growth and augments the effect of chemotherapy treatment in hepatocellular carcinoma. *Liver Int.* (2016) 36:737–45. doi: 10.1111/liv.12963
119. Xiao Z, Chung H, Banan B, Manning PT, Ott KC, Lin S, et al. Antibody mediated therapy targeting CD47 inhibits tumor progression of hepatocellular carcinoma. *Cancer Lett.* (2015) 360:302–9. doi: 10.1016/j.canlet.2015.02.036

12

Review of Defective NADPH Oxidase Activity and Myeloperoxidase Release in Neutrophils from Patients with Cirrhosis

Richard Moreau [1,2,3,4*], *Axel Périanin* [1,2,4] *and Vicente Arroyo* [5]

[1] *Inserm, U1149, Centre de Recherche sur l'Inflammation, Paris, France,* [2] *UMRS1149, Université Paris Diderot-Paris 7, Paris, France,* [3] *Département Hospitalo-Universitaire UNITY, Service d'Hépatologie, Hôpital Beaujon, Assistance Publique-Hôpitaux de Paris, Clichy, France,* [4] *Centre National de la Recherche Scientifique (CNRS), Paris, France,* [5] *EF Clif, EASL-CLIF Consortium and Grifols Chair, Barcelona, Spain*

Correspondence:
Richard Moreau
richard.moreau@inserm.fr

Patients with decompensated cirrhosis are highly susceptible to develop bacterial infections and these can trigger multiorgan failure associated with high in-hospital mortality. Neutrophils from patients with decompensated cirrhosis exhibit marked alterations that may explain the susceptibility of these patients to develop bacterial infections. These neutrophil alterations include marked defects in intracellular signaling pathways involving serine/threonine kinases such as protein kinase B (AKT), p38-mitogen-activated protein kinase (MAPK), and the MAP kinases1/2; activation of the NADPH oxidase complex; myeloperoxidase (MPO) release; and bactericidal activity of neutrophils stimulated by the bacterial peptide formyl-Methionine-Leucine-Phenylalanine (fMLF). Impaired activity of the NADPH oxidase 2 (NOX2) complex is also related to reduced levels of expression of its major components through post-transcriptional mechanisms. In addition, the catalytic NOX2 component gp91^{phox} is subject to degradation by elastase highly present in patients' plasma. A defect in the protein kinase B (AKT) and p38 MAPK-mediated signaling pathways may explain the decrease in phosphorylation of p47^{phox} (an important component of the NADPH oxidase complex) and MPO release, in response to neutrophil stimulation by fMLF. Most of these alterations are reversible *ex vivo* with TLR7/8 agonists (CL097, R848), raising the possibility that these agonists might be used in the future to restore neutrophil antibacterial functions in patients with cirrhosis.

Keywords: liver disease, infection, neutrophil dysfunction, granule exocytosis, serine-threonine protein kinases

INTRODUCTION

The natural history of cirrhosis, the most common chronic liver disease, is characterized by episodes of acute decompensation (e.g., development of ascites, gastrointestinal hemorrhage, or hepatic encephalopathy) (1). Patients with acutely decompensated cirrhosis are usually admitted to the hospital (1). Of these, 70% have traditional acute decompensation do not exhibit any organ dysfunctions or failures and have a 28-day mortality rate of <5%. The 30% remaining patients have acute-on-chronic liver failure (ACLF) which is defined by the presence of organ failures and a 28-day mortality rate ranging from 20 to 80% or more, depending on the number of failing organs (1). Patients with cirrhosis are highly susceptible to develop acute bacterial infection, which is the most common trigger of traditional acute decompensation and ACLF (1, 2). Studies have shown that neutrophils from patients with cirrhosis exhibit *ex vivo* defective adenine dinucleotide phosphate (NADPH) oxidase 2 (NOX2) (3–5) and of myeloperoxidase (MPO) exocytosis (4), which both may contribute to the susceptibility to infection in patients with cirrhosis. Before summarizing our knowledge about the defective neutrophil functions in cirrhosis, it is important to have some general information on NADPH oxidase activity and MPO release in neutrophils.

NADPH OXIDASE ACTIVATION AND MPO RELEASE IN NEUTROPHILS FROM THE GENERAL POPULATION

Almost 90% of granulocytes in peripheral blood are composed of neutrophils which represent the first line of cellular defense against bacterial infections and play an important role in innate immunity and inflammation. Circulating neutrophils are the first to arrive at a site of infection, and they stay for only a short time (the first 24 h), most of them undergoing cell death in the inflamed tissue as a consequence of their antibacterial effector functions (6). Phagocytosis of bacteria at the infection site activates neutrophil functions, such as the release of proteases, bactericidal peptides and reactive oxygen species (ROS) (7, 8). ROS production is initiated by the generation of superoxide anion ($O_2^{-\cdot}$) by the NADPH oxidase. In the phagosomes, $O_2^{-\cdot}$ reacts with protons to form hydrogen peroxide (H_2O_2), which is used by myeloperoxidase (MPO, an azurophilic [or primary] granule lumen protein) to produce the highly bactericidal ROS, hypochlorous acid. The rapid increase in oxygen and glucose consumption, together with ROS overproduction during neutrophil NADPH oxidase activation, is known as "respiratory burst" (RB). NADPH oxidase is a multicomponent protein (see below); an inherited defect in the expression of one of these components results in a rare disease called chronic granulomatous disease, which is characterized by a defect in ROS production in phagocytes and an increased susceptibility to recurrent bacterial and fungal infections (7). On the other hand, excessive neutrophil ROS production can cause tissue damage (7, 8). The importance of effective MPO release is highlighted by the findings in *MPO*-knockout mice of increased prevalence of infections, prolonged inflammation, and shorter survival (9, 10).

NADPH Oxidase Activity

In its active state the NADPH oxidase is a multiprotein complex comprising the catalytic core flavocytochrome b_{558} heterodimer consisting in two associated transmembrane proteins, gp91^{phox} (i.e., cytochrome b-245 heavy chain, commonly called NOX2) and p22^{phox} (i.e., cytochrome b-245 light chain), and four proteins recruited from the cytosol, including p67^{phox} (i.e., neutrophil cytosol factor 2), p47^{phox} (i.e., neutrophil cytosol factor 1), p40^{phox} (i.e., neutrophil cytosol factor 4), and Rac2 (7). The oxidase is fully activated when cytosolic and membrane proteins are assembled into a complex, which makes gp91^{phox} able to use cytosolic NADPH to produce $O_2^{-\cdot}$ (7, 8, 11).

Different molecules can activate neutrophil NADPH oxidase including the bacterial peptide formyl-Met-Leu-Phe (fMLF), the complement fragment C5a, opsonized bacteria, opsonized zymosan and chemical agents such as calcium ionophores and the protein kinase C (PKC) activator, phorbol-myristate acetate (PMA) [reviewed in (11)]. FMLF, engages the surface formyl peptide receptor fPR1, a G-protein-coupled receptor, to activate several intracellular phospholipases, protein tyrosine kinases, serine/threonine kinases, including PKC isoforms, protein kinases B and B beta (hereafter called AKT1and AKT2, respectively), mammalian target of rapamycin (mTOR), and mitogen-activated protein kinases (MAPK), which include p38-MAPK and MAPK 1 (hereafter called ERK2) and MAPK 3 (hereafter called ERK1) (**Figure 1A**). Serine/threonine kinases phosphorylate the components of the NADPH oxidase (**Figure 1A**) at sites which are detailed in **Table 1** and contribute to the assembly of the complex and $O_2^{-\cdot}$ production. Of note, it has recently been shown that during the first hour of their *ex vivo* fMLF stimulation of neutrophils from healthy subjects, these cells release the protease elastase (contained in azurophil granules and specific [or secondary] granules) in the extracellular milieu to induce degradation of transmembrane gp91^{phox} (5). This degradation is followed by that of p22^{phox}, which is an elastase-independent process, and might be a consequence of gp91^{phox} degradation that would render p22^{phox} unstable and degradable by intracellular proteases (5). The two cytosolic components of the NADPH oxidase complex, p47^{phox} and p40^{phox} are not affected by fMLF-induced elastase release (5).

MPO Release

In freshly isolated neutrophils from healthy subjects, fMLF also induces MPO exocytosis from primary granules (4, 12), which is an important part of the oxygen-dependent antibacterial arsenal (8, 12). Other toxic mediators stored in these primary granules are also released such as elastase and defensins. Stimulation of neutrophils triggers also the degranulation of two other cytosolic compartments, secondary and tertiary granules which contain common mediators (gelatinase, lysozyme, and ß2-microglobuline) and specific mediators, i.e., lactoferrin and acetyltransferase, respectively. The membrane of secondary and tertiary granules contains high amounts of gp91^{phox} (NOX2) and the fMLF receptor fPR1. Thus, during the process of MPO release by neutrophils stimulated with bacteria or bacterial peptides, the fusion of granular membranes to plasma membrane and phagosomes bring new pools of NOX2 and fPR1, which contribute to increase ROS production and bacterial killing. Experiments using selective pharmacological antagonists for phosphorylation of AKT, p38-MAPK and ERK1/2 showed that phosphorylation of AKT, p38-MAPK, but not that of ERK1/2, was involved in MPO exocytosis (4). Moreover, these pharmacological experiments have shown that p38-MAPK

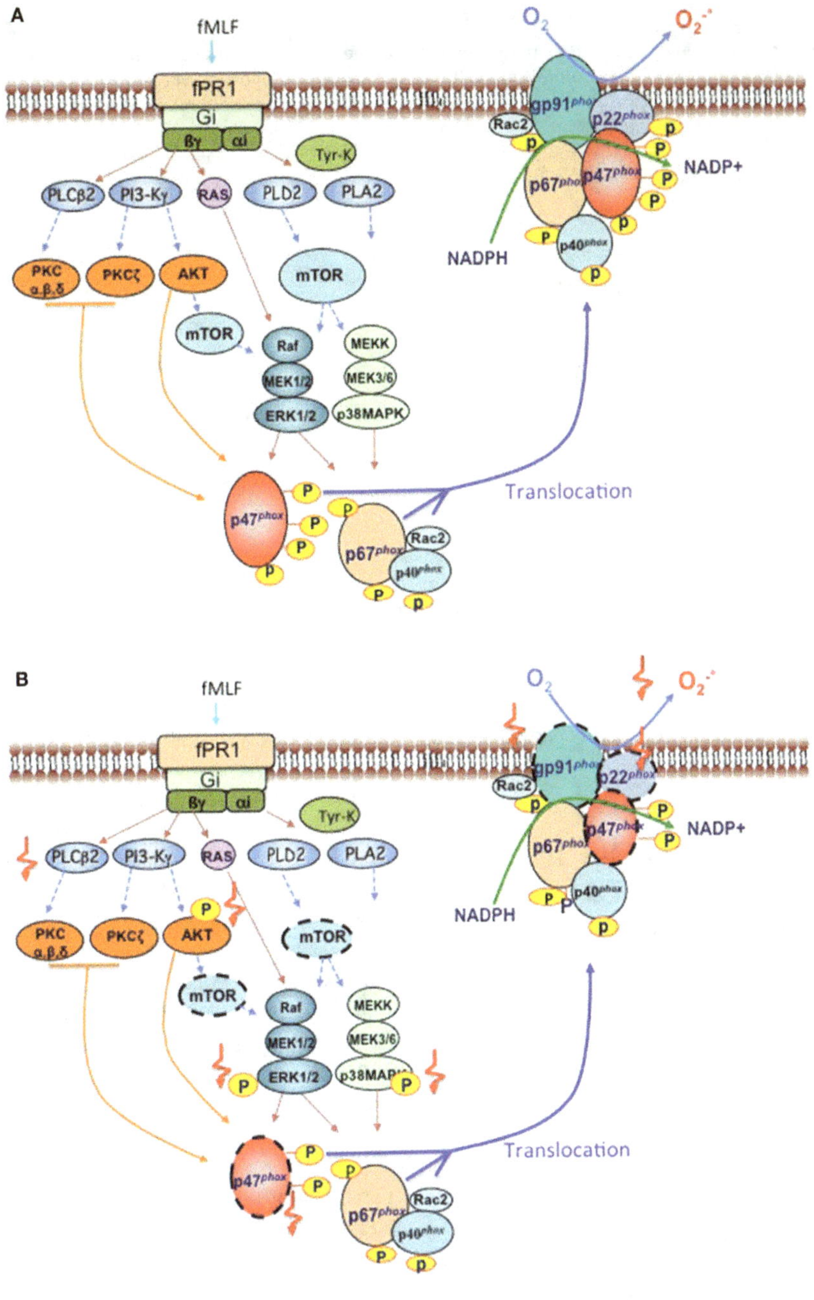

FIGURE 1 | Signaling pathways involved in phosphorylation and activation of the NADPH oxidase induced by bacterial peptides in human neutrophils from respectively "healthy subjects" and "cirrhotic patients". **(A)** Healthy subjects. The binding of the bacterial formylated peptide fMet-leu-Phe (fMLF) to its Gi-protein-coupled receptor fPR1, triggers the activation of various major early signaling effectors such as phospholipase C (PLCß2), Phospholipase D (PLD2), Phospholipase A (PLA2), Phosphatidylinositol-4,5-bisphosphate 3-kinase (PI3-Kγ), tyrosine kinases, and the small G-protein Ras. Second messengers produced by phospholipases stimulate various protein kinases, such as protein kinase C (PKC) isoforms, protein kinase B (AKT1/2), mammalian target of rapamycin (mTOR), which in turn activates two major families of mitogen-activated protein kinases (MAPKs), including ERK1/2 and p38-MAPK. PKCs and MAPKs phosphorylate cytosolic components of the NADPH oxidase (p47^{phox}, p67^{phox}, p40^{phox}) which allows their translocation to the plasma membrane, together with the small G protein Rac2, to activate a cytochrome b, constituted with the gp91^{phox} (also known as NOX2) and its partner p22^{phox}. The activated NOX2 reduces oxygen to superoxide ($O_2^{\cdot -}$) at the expense of NADPH. **(B)** Patients with cirrhosis. Two types of deficiencies have been identified in neutrophils of cirrhotic patients stimulated *in vitro* by bacterial peptides; those which decrease the activation/phosphorylation of signaling effectors such as AKT, MAP-Kinase ERK1/2, and p38-MAP kinase, p47^{phox}; and PLCβ2 activity (indicated by) and those which decrease the expression of protein effectors (indicated by a dashed outline, --------) especially for mTOR, gp91^{phox}, p22^{phox}, and p47^{phox}. These alterations lead to a deficient production of superoxide anion by gp91^{phox}.

TABLE 1 | The different components of the NADPH complex, their site(s) of phosphorylation, phosphorylating serine/threonine kinases, and effects of phosphorylation on the NADPH complex (7, 8, 11).

Gene symbol	Usual name of the protein subunit	Recommended name of the protein subunit	Site(s) of protein phosphorylation: serine/threonine kinase(s) involved	Effects of phosphorylation on the NADPH complex
CYBB	gp91^{phox} (also known as NOX2)	Cytochrome b-245 heavy chain	Ser486: Protein kinase C (PKC) isoforms	Phosphorylation promotes the catalytic activity and assembly of the NADPH oxidase complex
CYBA	p22^{phox}	Cytochrome b-245 light chain	Thr147: Conventional PKC	Phosphorylation promotes NADPH oxidase complex assembly and activation.
NCF1	p47^{phox}	Neutrophil cytosol factor 1	Between Ser303 and Ser379: PKC isoforms Ser304, Ser328: AKT Ser345: p38-MAPK, ERK1/2	Required for complex assembly and activation
NCF4	p40^{phox}	Neutrophil cytosol factor 4	Thr154 and Ser315: PKC	Phosphorylation at Thr154 is required for NADPH oxidase complex assembly and activation at the phagosome
NCF2	p67^{phox}	Neutrophil cytosol factor 2	Thr233: p38-MAPK, ERK1/2, PKC	Unknown

is activated downstream to AKT through mechanisms that remain elusive.

DEFECTIVE RESPONSE TO FMLF IN NEUTROPHILS FROM PATIENTS WITH DECOMPENSATED CIRRHOSIS

Freshly isolated blood neutrophils from patients with decompensated alcoholic cirrhosis stimulated *ex vivo* with fMLF exhibit a marked defect in $O_2^{-\cdot}$ production (i.e., decreased NADPH oxidase activity), RB, and MPO exocytosis, and accordingly reduced bactericidal activity (3–5). These results confirm PN dysfunctions reported by other groups also showing impaired phagocytic activities (13–22). However, in some studies, basal ROS production by patient neutrophils was increased, despite defective bactericidal activity, which suggests a primed and or pre-activated state of patient neutrophils (17–19, 23, 24). We confirmed this paradoxical situation with some of our cirrhotic patients. However, the increased basal ROS production remained low which questions about its relevancy in antibacterial activity, in contrast to the high and rapid production of ROS induced by fMLF which leads to bacterial killing (4, 5). Because patients' neutrophils have decreased baseline protein expression of gp91^{phox}, p22^{phox}, and p47^{phox} (5), these decreased expressions likely contribute to defective fMLF-induced NADPH oxidase activation in these cells (summarized in the **Figure 1B**). The finding that here is no simultaneous decrease in the baseline mRNA levels of *CYBB* (encoding gp91^{phox}, or NOX2), *CYBA* (encoding p22^{phox}), and *NCF1* (encoding p47^{phox}) in patients' neutrophils (5), suggests that decreased expression of the corresponding proteins is related to posttranscriptional mechanisms. Abnormally high plasma levels of elastase are found in patients with decompensated cirrhosis (25). Neutrophils from healthy subjects exposed to plasma from patients or purified elastase, but not neutrophils exposed to plasma from healthy subjects, exhibit a decrease in gp91^{phox} expression which can be prevented by the neutrophil elastase inhibitor, NEI) (5). These findings, together the finding that elastase released by fMLF-stimulated neutrophils from healthy subjects causes gp91^{phox} degradation (see above), suggest that high plasma elastase levels in patients may explain that their neutrophils have low baseline expression of neutrophil gp91^{phox} and p22^{phox}. Since increased extracellular elastase levels do not affect p47^{phox} expression in neutrophils from healthy subjects (see above), high plasma elastase levels cannot explain decreased baseline expression of p47^{phox} in neutrophils from patients with decompensated cirrhosis. The mTOR protein complex 1 (known as mTORC1) promotes protein synthesis by regulating translation of several mRNAs into proteins (26) including gp91^{phox} (5). Because neutrophils from patients with decompensated cirrhosis exhibit decreased mTOR protein (5), this has been suggested to result in reduced translation of *NCF1* into p47^{phox} in these cells as well-translation of gp91^{phox} (5).

In addition to these alterations in protein expression of the NADPH oxidase complex, defects in signaling pathways have been shown in neutrophils from patients with decompensated alcoholic cirrhosis. Following fMLF stimulation, neutrophils from patients have decreased phosphorylation (i.e., activation) of AKTs, p38-MAPK, and ERK1/2 with no changes in the expression levels of corresponding unphosphorylated proteins and in the expression of the formyl peptide receptor [(3, 4), **Figure 1B**]. Together these findings suggest the existence of an important defect in signaling pathway, somewhere between the surface receptor and effector proteins. Alterations in the G proteins which are coupled to the formyl peptide receptor have been suggested to exist in neutrophils from patients with cirrhosis based on the impaired phospholipase C (PLC) activity in response to fMLF and fluoride, a G protein activator (16).

Neutrophil dysfunctions associated with cirrhosis are caused by intrinsic cellular alterations because they persist after cell washing (13). Neutrophils from healthy subjects exhibit decreased fMLF-induced MPO exocytosis when they are cultured with plasma from patients but not with plasma from healthy subjects (4), which reveals the presence of cell-permeant inhibitors in patients' plasma. Neutrophil dysfunctions have been shown to be reversible after removal of endotoxins (i.e., lipolysaccharide) from patients' plasma (17).

The defect in signaling pathways in patients' neutrophils may have several functional consequences. Decreased phosphorylation of AKT and p38-MAPK is associated with a defect in MPO exocytosis in patients' neutrophils (4) indicating a decrease in exocytosis of primary granules. In addition, activated AKT and p38-MAPK both phosphorylate a main component of NADPH oxidase, $p47^{phox}$, at Ser304/Ser328 and Ser 345, respectively (**Table 1**). Therefore, defective activation of AKT and p38-MAPK may contribute to the defect in NADPH oxidase activity in patients' neutrophils. Finally, the defect in ERK1/2 phosphorylation may contribute to decrease NADPH oxidase activity, because ERK1/2 activation accounts for 30% of ROS production by fMLF-stimulated neutrophils from healthy subjects (4). Unlike ROS production, the MPO exocytosis induced by fMLF does not appear to be regulated by ERK1/2 (4, 27), but via the p38 MAPK, AKT (4), and PLC/calcium signaling pathways (12). These later are impaired in neutrophils from cirrhotic patients with may contribute to the defective MPO release (4, 16).

Interestingly, the defects in $O_2^{-\cdot}$ production, MPO release, decreased phosphorylation of AKT, p38 MAPK, and bactericidal activity in patients' neutrophils can be reversed *ex vivo* by treatment of patients' neutrophils with toll-like receptor 7/8 (TLR7/8) agonists (4, 5). This treatment also stimulates a rapid *CYBB* transcription and translation into $gp91^{phox}$ which is inhibited by rapamycin, indicating a mTOR-dependent process. These findings suggest that TLR7/8 agonists might be used in the future to restore neutrophil functions in patients with decompensated alcoholic cirrhosis. In support to this assumption, the TLR7/8 agonist R848 (Resiquimod) was recently shown to restore the impaired production of ROS in whole blood of cirrhotic rats and improve the survival of cirrhotic rats infected by bacteria (28). In this murine model of cirrhosis treated with R848, both neutrophils and mononuclear leukocytes (monocytes and lymphocytes) were modified as indicated by a decreased amount of these cells in the blood of ~40–50%, although modifications of their immune function remain not known.

In patients with decompensated cirrhosis, various defects have also been described in peripheral blood mononuclear cells (PBMCs), notably an impaired expression of genes induced by interferon type 1 (29), a decrease in antigenic presentation by lymphocytes and monocycte/dentritic cells and a decrease in lymphocyte proliferation (30). The effects of TLR7/8 agonists on these adaptive immunity cells in the context of cirrhosis are not known.

However, *in vitro* models, TLR7/8 agonists are particularly effective in inducing robust immune responses (31) including TNFα production in monocytes, IL12 production in human adult and newborn monocytes, INFα production in the dentridic cells, and the activation of T-regulatory cells. Because of their potent immunostimulatory properties, the TLR7/8 agonists are used in non-clinical and clinical studies as vaccine adjuvants (32). TLR 7/8 agonists are also evaluated for a variety of indications in clinical studies and animal models to treat various viral infections and skin cancer (31).

AREAS OF FUTURE RESEARCH

Studies should be performed in patients with cirrhosis to address several questions including the mechanisms for acquired defective signaling pathways in response to fMLF. In particular, the role of LPS should be investigated because it has been shown to be present in the plasma of patients with cirrhosis who did not have ongoing infection by Gram-negative bacteria (33) and because LPS may have effects on neutrophil ROS production (5). In addition, the responses to other potential stimuli for neutrophil activation should investigated in patients' neutrophils.

The phenomenon of neutrophil extracellular traps (NETs, which are mainly composed of DNA that is released from neutrophils upon pathogen encounter) has been considered an alternative to other nonlytic (apoptosis) or lytic (pyroptosis, necroptosis) cell death and called NETosis (6). NETs can entrap bacteria, fungi, and even viruses and contribute to antimicrobial defense. NETosis relies on the presence of the major neutrophil serine protease elastase, MPO and active NADPH oxidase (8). Therefore, NETosis would not be expected to occur in neutrophils from patients with cirrhosis which have defect in NADPH oxidase and in MPO exocytosis. Because defective NETosis might contribute to the fact that patients' neutrophils have decreased ability to kill bacteria, NETosis should be investigated in these cells.

It will be also important to investigate, in patients with cirrhosis, the phenotype of circulating neutrophils according to the severity of the disease identifying cell-surface markers and transcriptome profile, and investigating their ability to leave circulation toward tissues.

Finally, the efficacy and safety of TLR7/8 agonists should be further investigated *in vivo* preclinical experiments performed in mouse models of chronic liver disease.

CONCLUSIONS

Neutrophils from patients with decompensated cirrhosis exhibit marked alterations that may explain the susceptibility of these patients to develop bacterial infections. These neutrophil alterations include marked defects in fMLF-induced activity of the NADPH oxidase complex, MPO release, and bactericidal activity. Decreased activity of the NADPH oxidase complex is related to reduced levels of expression of its major components through post-transcriptional mechanisms. A defect in the AKT/p38 MAPK signaling pathway may explain the decrease in phosphorylation of $p47^{phox}$ (an important component of the NADPH oxidase complex) and MPO release, in response to fMLF stimulation. Most of these alterations are reversible *ex vivo* with TLR7/8 agonists.

AUTHOR CONTRIBUTIONS

RM and AP wrote the manuscript. AP and VA provided critical revision of the manuscript for important intellectual content. AP drew the figures.

REFERENCES

1. Moreau R, Jalan R, Gines P, Pavesi M, Angeli P, Cordoba J, et al. Acute-on-chronic liver failure is a distinct syndrome that develops in patients with acute decompensation of cirrhosis. *Gastroenterology.* (2013) 60:1426–37. doi: 10.1053/j.gastro.2013.02.042
2. Moreau R, Elkrief L, Bureau C, Perarnau JM, Thévenot T, Saliba F, et al. Effects of long-term norfloxacin therapy in patients with advanced cirrhosis. *Gastroenterology.* (2018) 155:1816–27. doi: 10.1053/j.gastro.2018.08.026
3. Rolas L, Makhezer N, Hadjoudj S, El-Benna J, Djerdjouri B, Elkrief L, et al. Inhibition of mammalian target of rapamycin aggravates the respiratory burst defect of neutrophils from decompensated patients with cirrhosis. *Hepatology.* (2013) 57:1163–71. doi: 10.1002/hep.26109
4. Boussif A, Rolas L, Weiss E, Bouriche H, Moreau R, Périanin A. Impaired intracellular signaling, myeloperoxidase release and bactericidal activity of neutrophils from patients with alcoholic cirrhosis. *J Hepatol.* (2016) 64:1041–8. doi: 10.1016/j.jhep.2015.12.005
5. Rolas L, Boussif A, Weiss E, Lettéron P, Haddad O, El-Benna J, et al. NADPH oxidase depletion in neutrophils from patients with cirrhosis and restoration via toll-like receptor 7/8 activation. *Gut.* (2018) 67:1505–16. doi: 10.1136/gutjnl-2016-313443
6. Manz MG, Boettcher S. Emergency granulopoiesis. *Nat Rev Immunol.* (2014) 14:302–14. doi: 10.1038/nri3660
7. Babior BM. NADPH oxidase: an update. *Blood.* (1999) 93:1464–76.
8. Nauseef WM, Borregaard N. Neutrophils at work. *Nat Immunol.* (2014) 15:602–11. doi: 10.1038/ni.2921
9. Aratani Y, Kura F, Watanabe H, Akagawa H, Takano Y, Suzuki K, et al. *In vivo* role of myeloperoxidase for the host defense. *Jpn J Infect Dis.* (2004) 57:S15.
10. El Kebir D, József L, Pan W, Filep JG. Myeloperoxidase delays neutrophil apoptosis through CD11b/CD18 integrins and prolongs inflammation. *Circ Res.* (2008) 103:352–9. doi: 10.1161/01.RES.0000326772.76822.7a
11. Belambri SA, Rolas L, Raad H, Hurtado-Nedelec M, Dang PM, El-Benna J. NADPH oxidase activation in neutrophils: role of the phosphorylation of its subunits. *Eur J Clin Invest.* (2018) 48(Suppl. 2):e12951. doi: 10.1111/eci.12951
12. Lacy P. Mechanisms of degranulation of neutrophils. *Allergy Asthma Clin Immunol.* (2006) 2:98–108. doi: 10.1186/1710-1492-2-3-98
13. Feliu E, Gougerot MA, Hakim J, Cramer E, Auclair C, Rueff B, et al. Blood polymorphonuclear dysfunction in patients with alcoholic cirrhosis. *Eur J Clin Invest.* (1977) 7:571–7.
14. Rajkovic IA, Williams R. Abnormalities of neutrophil phagocytosis, intracellular killing and metabolic activity in alcoholic cirrhosis and hepatitis. *Hepatology.* (1986) 6:252–62.
15. Lebrun L, Pelletier G, Briantais MJ, Galanaud P, Etienne JP. Impaired functions of normal peripheral polymorphonuclear leukocytes in cirrhotic ascitic fluid. *J Hepatol.* (1992) 16:98–101.
16. Garfia C, García-Ruiz I, Solís-Herruzo JA. Deficient phospholipase C activity in blood of polymorphonuclear neutrophils from patients with liver cirrhosis. *J Hepatol.* (2004) 40:749–56. doi: 10.1016/j.jhep.2004.01.004
17. Mookerjee RP, Stadlbauer V, Lidder S, Wright GA, Hodges SJ, Davies NA, et al. Neutrophil dysfunction in alcoholic hepatitis superimposed on cirrhosis is reversible and predicts the outcome. *Hepatology.* (2007) 46:831–40. doi: 10.1002/hep.21737
18. Shawcross Dl, Shabbir SS, Taylor NJ, Hughes RD. Ammonia and the neutrophil in the pathogenesis of hepatic encephalopathy in cirrhosis. *Hepatology.* (2010) 51:1062–9. doi: 10.1002/hep.23367
19. Bruns T, Peter J, Hagel S, Herrmann A, Stallmach A. The augmented neutrophil respiratory burst in response to *Escherichia coli* is reduced in liver cirrhosis during infection. *Clin Exp Immunol.* (2011) 164:346–56. doi: 10.1111/j.1365-2249.2011.04373.x
20. Tritto G, Bechlis Z, Stadlbauer V, Davies N, Francés R, Shah N, et al. Evidence of neutrophil functional defect despite inflammation in stable cirrhosis. *Hepatology.* (2011) 55:574–81. doi: 10.1016/j.jhep.2010.11.034
21. Engelmann C, Becker C, Boldt A, Herta T, Boehlig A, Splith K, et al. Ascites neutrophil function is significantly impaired in patients with decompensated cirrhosis but can be restored by autologous plasma incubation. *Sci Rep.* (2016) 6:37926. doi: 10.1038/srep37926
22. Khanam A, Trehanpati N, Riese P, Rastogi A, Guzman CA, Sarin SK. Blockade of neutrophil's chemokine receptors CXCR1/2 abrogate liver damage in acute-on-chronic liver failure. *Front Immunol.* (2017) 8:464. doi: 10.3389/fimmu.2017.00464
23. Taylor NJ, Manakkat Vijay GK, Abeles RD, Auzinger G, Bernal W, Ma Y, et al. Patients with cirrhosis are susceptible. The severity of circulating neutrophil dysfunction in patients with cirrhosis is associated with 90-day and 1-year mortality. *Aliment Pharmacol Ther.* (2014) 40:705–15. doi: 10.1111/apt.12886
24. Tranah TH, Vijay GK, Ryan JM, Abeles RD, Middleton PK, Shawcross DL. Dysfunctional neutrophil effector organelle mobilization and microbicidal protein release in alcohol-related cirrhosis. *Am J Physiol Gastrointest Liver Physiol.* (2017) 313:G203–1. doi: 10.1152/ajpgi.00112.2016
25. Stanley AJ, MacGregor IR, Dillon JF, Bouchier IA, Hayes PC. Neutrophil activation in chronic liver disease. *Eur J Gastroenterol Hepatol.* (1996) 8:135–8.
26. Saxton RA, Sabatini DM. mTOR signaling in growth, metabolism, and disease. *Cell.* (2017) 168:960–76. doi: 10.1016/j.cell.2017.02.004
27. Mócsai A, Jakus Z, Vántus T, Berton G, Lowell CA, Ligeti E. Kinase pathways in chemoattractant-induced degranulation of neutrophils: the role of p38-mitogen-activated protein kinase activated by Src family kinases. *J Immunol.* (2000) 164:4321–31. doi: 10.4049/jimmunol.164.8.4321
28. Périanin A, Rolas L. *Methods and Pharmaceutical Compositions for The Treatment of Bacterial Infections in Patients Suffering From Cirrhosis.* US patent BIO15052-US-PCT (2019) N° 10, 201,536. Munich: European Patent Office.
29. Weiss E, Rautou PE, Fasseu M, Giabicani M, de Chambrun M, Wan J, et al. Type I interferon signaling in systemic immune cells from patients with alcoholic cirrhosis and its association with outcome. *J Hepatol.* (2017) 66:930–41. doi: 10.1016/j.jhep.2016.12.008
30. Gustot T, Fernandez J, Szabo G, Albillos A, Louvet A, Jalan R, et al. Sepsis in alcohol-related liver disease. *J Hepatol.* (2017) 67:1031–50. doi: 10.1016/j.jhep.2017.06.013
31. Philbin VJ, Levy O. Immunostimulatory activity of Toll-like receptor 8 agonists towards human leucocytes: basic mechanisms and translational opportunities. *Biochem Soc Trans.* (2007) 35:1485–91. doi: 10.1042/BST0351485

32. Vasilakos JP, Tomai MA. The use of Toll-like receptor 7/8 agonists as vaccine adjuvants. *Expert Rev Vaccines.* (2013) 12:809–19. doi: 10.1586/14760584.2013.811208

33. Arroyo V, Moreau R, Kamath PS, Jalan R, Ginès P, Nevens F, et al. Acute-on-chronic liver failure in cirrhosis. *Nat Rev Dis Primers.* (2016) 2:16041. doi: 10.1038/nrdp.2016.41

13

Macrophage Function in the Pathogenesis of Non-Alcoholic Fatty Liver Disease: The Mac Attack

Jarren R. Oates [1,2,3], Melanie C. McKell [1,3,4], Maria E. Moreno-Fernandez [1,2], Michelle S. M. A. Damen [1,2], George S. Deepe Jr. [5], Joseph E. Qualls [1,3,4] and Senad Divanovic [1,2,3,6]*

[1] Department of Pediatrics, University of Cincinnati College of Medicine, Cincinnati, OH, United States, [2] Division of Immunobiology, Cincinnati Children's Hospital Medical Center and the University of Cincinnati College of Medicine, Cincinnati, OH, United States, [3] Immunology Graduate Program, Cincinnati Children's Hospital Medical Center and the University of Cincinnati College of Medicine, Cincinnati, OH, United States, [4] Division of Infectious Diseases, Cincinnati Children's Hospital Medical Center and the University of Cincinnati College of Medicine, Cincinnati, OH, United States, [5] Department of Medicine, University of Cincinnati College of Medicine, Cincinnati, OH, United States, [6] Center for Inflammation and Tolerance, Cincinnati Children's Hospital Medical Center, Cincinnati, OH, United States

***Correspondence:**
Senad Divanovic
senad.divanovic@cchmc.org

Obesity is a prevalent predisposing factor to non-alcoholic fatty liver disease (NAFLD), the most common chronic liver disease in the developed world. NAFLD spectrum of disease involves progression from steatosis (NAFL), to steatohepatitis (NASH), cirrhosis and hepatocellular carcinoma (HCC). Despite clinical and public health significance, current FDA approved therapies for NAFLD are lacking in part due to insufficient understanding of pathogenic mechanisms driving disease progression. The etiology of NAFLD is multifactorial. The induction of both systemic and tissue inflammation consequential of skewed immune cell metabolic state, polarization, tissue recruitment, and activation are central to NAFLD progression. Here, we review the current understanding of the above stated cellular and molecular processes that govern macrophage contribution to NAFLD pathogenesis and how adipose tissue and liver crosstalk modulates macrophage function. Notably, the manipulation of such events may lead to the development of new therapies for NAFLD.

Keywords: macrophage, metabolism, NAFLD, inflammation, cytokines

INTRODUCTION

The unabated obesity pandemic is directly linked with the incidence of non-alcoholic fatty liver disease (NAFLD). NAFLD afflicts ~35% of obese individuals worldwide (1, 2). Current epidemiological estimates suggest that NAFLD will soon surpass chronic hepatitis C infection as the leading cause of liver transplantation. Given the lack of effective therapies for NAFLD, costs of care and management of associated symptoms come with a considerable economic burden (3).

NAFLD spectrum of disease progresses from non-alcoholic fatty liver (NAFL) or hepatic steatosis, to non-alcoholic steatohepatitis (NASH), to cirrhosis and hepatocellular carcinoma (HCC). Steatosis is characterized by increased macrovesicular and microvesicular lipid droplet accumulation that occurs in more than 5% of hepatocytes (1, 2, 4). Approximately 25% of individuals afflicted with NAFL progress to NASH (1). NASH is characterized by hepatocellular ballooning, in part due to increased immune cell infiltration, activation, and proinflammatory cytokine production (4–6). These mechanisms coupled with others such as adipokine production and activation of endoplasmic reticulum stress and reactive oxygen species (ROS) promote hepatic fibrosis and progression to cirrhosis and HCC (7, 8).

The contribution of various immune cells in hepatic inflammation and the mechanisms that govern their migration to the liver, polarization, and inflammatory capabilities, in NAFLD progression represent an intense area of investigation. Here, we specifically focus on the contribution of macrophages to NAFLD pathogenesis. We review the landscape of underlying mechanisms that regulate macrophage effector functions and macrophage interplay with other immune cells/tissues/organs which collectively contribute to NAFLD progression.

CURRENT KNOWLEDGE AND DISCUSSION

Immune Responses in NAFLD

Dysregulated immune responsiveness is central to the development and progression of NAFLD (9, 10). In obesity, both liver resident (e.g., Kupffer cells, [KC], hepatic stellate cells, [HSC], hepatocytes) and infiltrating immune cells (e.g., neutrophils, dendritic cells [DC], natural killer [NK] cells, NKT cells, blood monocytes, T cells, B cells, and macrophages) contribute to NAFLD development and progression via systemic and tissue inflammatory mediator production (e.g., interleukin [IL]-17A, IL-6, tumor necrosis factor [TNF], IL-1β) (5, 11). Obesity-associated intestinal permeability and augmented circulating levels of inflammatory ligands (e.g., lipopolysaccharide [LPS]) (12) via activation of pattern recognition receptors (PRRs) on hematopoietic and non-hematopoietic cells activate multiple proinflammatory cascades that in unison promote liver injury (13). The contribution of PRRs to NAFLD progression has been reviewed in detail elsewhere (14, 15). PRR signaling in macrophages, also contributes to activation of adaptive immune responses, with macrophage-T cell interplay having a particularly important role in NAFLD progression (16). In this setting, activated, liver infiltrating T cells produce proinflammatory cytokines and amplify macrophage polarization and activation to in turn propagate overall hepatic inflammation, hepatocellular damage and hepatocyte release of damage associated molecular patterns (DAMPs). Cumulatively these processes fuel and support a chronic inflammatory state in the liver that is a hallmark of NAFLD progression. Due to the extent of various immune processes in NAFLD, here we selectively focus on the role of macrophage-mediated inflammation and their contribution to NAFLD pathology. The contribution of other immune cells (e.g., T cells, neutrophils, DC, NK cells, and NKT cells) and cytokines in NAFLD has been discussed elsewhere (14, 17, 18).

Macrophage Recruitment to the Liver

Liver infiltration by inflammatory monocytes/macrophages is associated with NAFLD progression (19). Increased release of free fatty acid (FFA) by white adipose tissue (WAT) augments triglyceride synthesis and storage in hepatocytes and induces hepatocyte release of inflammatory mediators including proinflammatory cytokines and macrophage recruiting chemokines (e.g., CCL2, CXCL10) (20, 21). In addition to hepatocytes, HSCs, myofibroblast and macrophages themselves can also produce various chemokines (e.g., CCL2, CCL3, CCL4, CCL5, CCL8, and CXCL10) to fuel increased macrophage recruitment (22).

The contribution of hepatic macrophage recruitment to NAFLD pathogenesis is supported in part by increased systemic and hepatic chemokine levels in NAFLD progression in humans (23). One of the most widely explored pathways of recruiting inflammatory and fibrogenic monocytes to the injured liver is the CCR2/CCL2 axis (24). Pharmacological inhibition of CCR2 and genetic deletion of CCL2 reduced liver steatosis in obese mice (25–27). Additionally, use of CCR1-, CCR2-, CCR5-, and CCR8-deficient mice or pharmacological inhibition of these axes reduced hepatic macrophage infiltration, hepatic fibrosis, and hepatocellular damage in experimental models of chronic liver injury (28–32). Recent evidence also suggests that CXCR3-deficient mice are protected from macrophage infiltration and hepatocellular damage in obesity (33, 34). Further, CXCL10-deficient mice exhibit reduced NAFL (34). Despite its promising effects in animal models, targeting of the CCR2 axis in human NALFD using Cenicriviroc (CVC) did not impact hepatic lobular inflammation and only mildly improved fibrosis and decreased circulating levels of sCD14 (a marker of monocyte activation) (35). Characterization of the intrahepatic immune cells will be required to elucidate the effects of CVC on immune cells, monocyte and macrophage recruitment and fibrogenesis. The results of such could give insight to observed difference of effects of CVC on NAFLD progression between murine models and humans.

Like chemokines, inflammatory cytokines can also alter macrophage activation and tissue recruitment in NAFLD. For example, the IL-17A axis impacts macrophage recruitment in the liver (36), while IL-17RA depletion on macrophages ameliorates NAFLD severity (37). However, as IL-17A can also activate liver parenchymal cells to modulate macrophage recruitment. Thus, detailed studies focused on the role of IL-17 family members, their cognate receptors and cell specific expression in NAFLD pathogenesis are needed. The overall role of the IL-17 axis in NAFLD pathogenesis has been reviewed in detail elsewhere (18).

Macrophage Subsets

KCs reside in the anatomical areas that receive venous blood from the gut including hepatic sinusoids, hepatic lymph nodes and portal tract (38). Approximately 80% of the liver blood supply comes from the gut via the portal vein (39). As such, KCs act as key sentinels of the gut-liver interface. Under homeostatic conditions, PRR signaling instructs KCs to govern liver immunity by maintaining tolerance to harmless immunogens and cellular debris while in parallel enabling them to mount a response against pathogenic invaders via phagocytosis, cytokine production and antigen presentation. Collectively, the adaptation to latter events is central to preventing dissemination of microbes into peripheral circulation (5, 39, 40). In obesity, increased intestinal permeability, trafficking of bacteria into the gut lumen and LPS sensing (2, 40, 41) fuel KC activation and alter their function (42). In this context, activated KCs favor inflammatory responses that contribute to NAFLD pathogenesis (13). *In vitro* treatment of KCs with FFAs (e.g., palmitate) promotes activation and secretion of inflammatory cytokines (e.g., IL-6, TNF, IL-1β) (43) while KC depletion *in vivo* protects from obesity-driven hepatic steatosis (13).

Common bone marrow myeloid progenitors give rise to granulocyte-macrophage progenitors (GMP) from which monocytes are derived. Upon egression from the bone marrow, and following hepatic inflammatory insult, circulating monocytes traffic to the liver. Once in the liver, in response to cytokines and various pathogen associated molecular patterns (PAMPs)/DAMPs, monocytes activate unique transcriptional profiles and differentiate into macrophages. In response to IFNγ or PRR signaling, recruited monocytes differentiate into "classically" activated macrophages that produce proinflammatory cytokines (e.g., IL-6, TNF, IL-1β, IL-12), drive liver recruitment of various immune cells and enhance the overall hepatic inflammation (5, 13, 44). Conversely, in response to either IL-4 or IL-13, tissue recruited monocytes differentiate into "alternatively" activated macrophages that produce anti-inflammatory and wound healing mediators (e.g., IL-8, MCP-1, IL-10) (38, 45, 46). The overall balance of "classically" and "alternatively" activated macrophages in the liver regulates hepatic inflammation, liver scarring and fibrosis. Targeting of inflammatory signaling pathways in macrophages via deletion of JNK, IKKβ, or Toll-like receptor (TLR) 4 is sufficient to reduce hepatic steatosis and inflammation (47–49). A brief summary of the above discussed processes is depicted in **Figure 1**.

Macrophages and Proinflammatory Cytokine Production

Macrophage produced cytokines (e.g., IL-6, TNF, IL-1β) can directly target hepatocytes and promote steatosis, inflammation and hepatocellular damage (5). Systemic increase of these proinflammatory cytokines positively correlates with hepatocellular damage in humans and is recapitulated in NAFLD experimental mouse models (50, 51).

IL-6 is a multifunctional cytokine that regulates immune responses, acute phase reactions, hematopoiesis, and plays key roles in inflammation, host defense and tissue injury (52, 53). IL-6 stimulates hepatic lipogenesis (54), and is associated with obesity (55), impaired insulin signaling (56, 57), and altered insulin sensitivity by activating key steps in the insulin signaling pathway (58). IL-6 is also a biomarker of insulin resistance and cardiovascular diseases risk (50, 59, 60). In humans with NASH, there is a positive correlation between IL-6 expression in hepatocytes and the severity of NAFLD (61). IL-6-deficient mice display a milder NAFLD severity and antibody mediated IL-6 receptor (IL-6R) neutralization improved liver damage in mice fed methionine choline deficient (MCD) diet, despite enhanced steatosis (51, 62).

TNF stimulates hepatic fatty acid synthesis (FAS), increases serum triglyceride (TG) levels (63), stimulates very low density lipoprotein (VLDL) production from liver and contributes to impaired insulin signaling (64, 65). TNF also activates harmful proatherogenic pathways via the reduction of high-density lipoprotein (HDL)-cholesterol, elevated expression of cholesterogenic genes, accompanied by an increase in potentially harmful precholesterol metabolites, and suppression of cholesterol elimination (66). Thus, it is not surprising that TNF sensing by hepatocytes promotes hepatocyte cell death and hepatocyte proliferation (67), and as such directly contributes to NAFLD pathogenesis (68). Further, deletion of TNF in experimental mouse models of NAFLD correlates with decreased steatosis, fibrosis and improved glucose tolerance (69).

IL-1β promotes liver steatosis, inflammation and fibrosis via activation of the IL-1 receptor (IL-1R) signaling (70). IL-1β stimulates TG and cholesterol accumulation in hepatocytes and as such contributes to the development of hepatic steatosis (71). Mechanistically, IL-1β also promotes liver inflammation by inducing IL-6 production, upregulating ICAM-1 and neutrophil infiltration and accrual in the liver (72). IL-1R-deficient mice are protected from liver fibrosis (73). Hepatocyte-specific deletion of IL-1R attenuates liver injury in a model of acute liver disease (74). Whether similar effects are observed in animal models of NAFLD have not been examined. Further, IL-1R activates Myd88 signaling similar to TLRs (75). Thus, the role of IL-1R signaling in NAFLD warrants further investigation. In addition, blockade of IL-1 signaling with anakinra improved glycemic control in patients with T2D (76), suggesting the importance of inflammatory mediators in liver disease pathogenesis.

Macrophages and ROS Production

Reactive oxygen species (ROS) production, a central antimicrobial effector function of macrophages, can be induced in part via macrophage sensing of proinflammatory cytokines. Macrophages generate ROS via numerous mechanisms including ER stress, mitochondrial damage and activation of nicotinamide adenine dinucleotide phosphate (NADPH) oxidases (NOXs). NOX2, also known as the phagocytic nicotinamide adenine dinucleotide phosphate NADPH oxidase, is constitutively associated with p22phox at the plasma membrane. PRR signaling in KCs and infiltrating macrophages causes complexing of NOX2 with other proteins (p67, P40, Rac GTPases) to generate superoxide, drive proinflammatory cytokine production (e.g., IL-6, TNF, IL-1β, transforming growth factor-β [TGFβ]) and promote hepatic steatosis, hepatocellular damage and fibrosis (43, 77, 78). NOX2-deficient mice display reduced macrophage-associated proinflammatory cytokine production, hepatic steatosis and fibrosis, and overall NAFLD severity in obesity (43, 79, 80). However, the underlying mechanisms regulating macrophage ROS production in NAFLD are not fully understood. Thus, in depth interrogation of the interplay between inflammatory cytokines and NADPH components on macrophage ROS production in NAFLD progression is needed.

Macrophage Cellular Metabolism

Metabolic pathways regulate immune cell function and inflammation (81, 82). Obesity alters cellular metabolism (83). In fact, both obesity-associated and inflammation-driven derangements in cellular metabolism are implicated in NAFLD

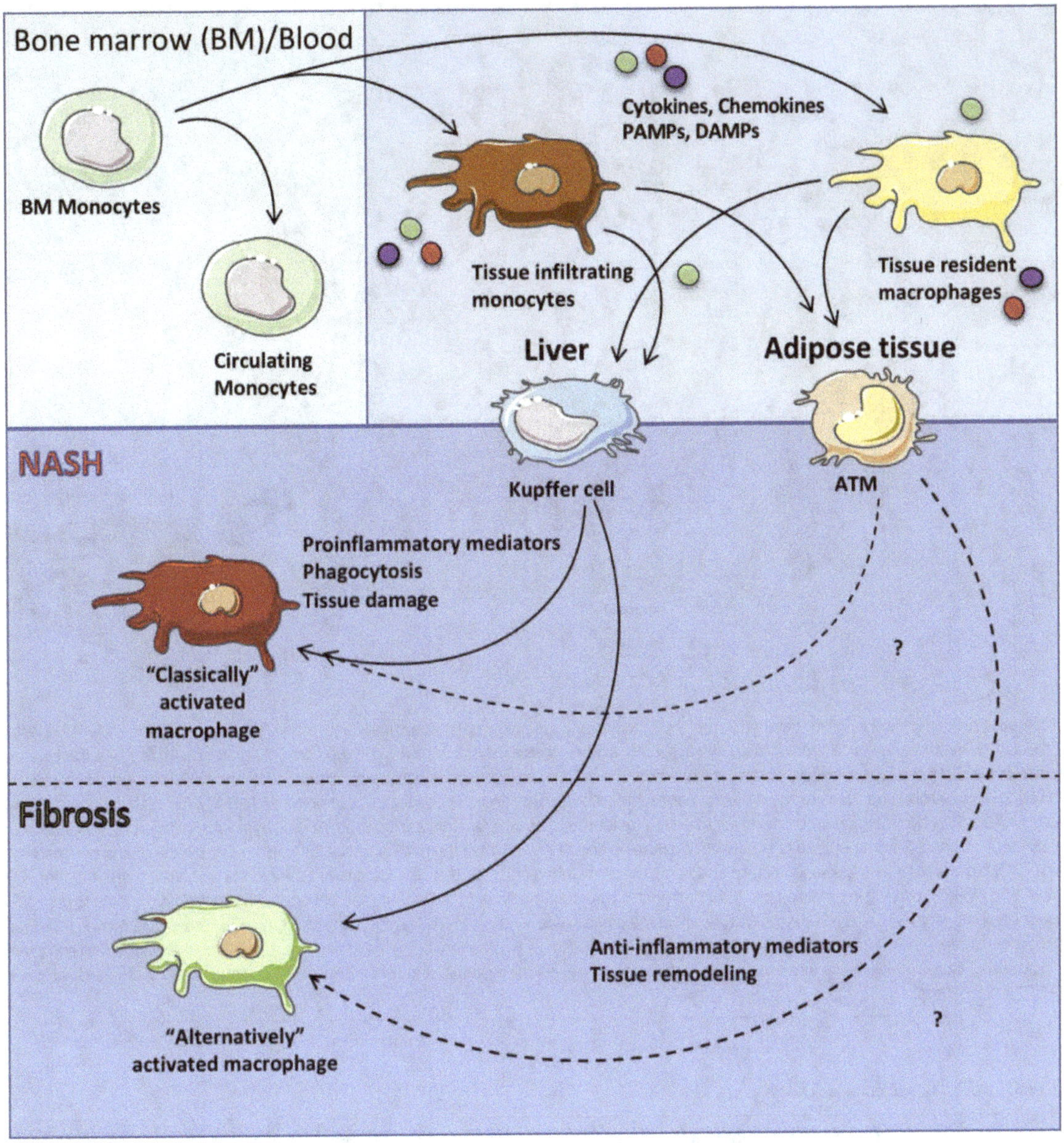

FIGURE 1 | Macrophage subsets in health and disease. Circulating monocytes originating from the bone marrow are recruited to specific tissues and differentiate into tissue resident macrophages. In the context of systemic inflammation, circulating monocytes as well as tissue resident macrophages are activated by sensing of proinflammatory mediators (i.e., IL-6, TNF, IL-1β), chemokines and ROS or anti-inflammatory mediators (i.e., IL-10) leading to "classically" or "alternatively" activated tissue macrophages, respectively which then contribute to tissue pathology.

progression (84–86). The full discovery of specific metabolic pathways and genes detrimental to NAFLD pathogenesis however remains an intense area of investigation. Macrophage-driven inflammation and resolution of inflammation are intricately linked to various metabolic pathways and several clinical phenotypes (i.e., insulin resistance, hyperlipidemia, etc.) (86, 87). Here we review metabolic pathways that contribute to macrophage-intrinsic inflammation and resolution in NAFLD. A brief summary of these processes is depicted in **Figure 2** and **Table 1**.

Glycolysis

Macrophage reliance on glycolysis to meet energetic demands has been demonstrated in several murine models of "classical" macrophage activation (88). Upon stimulation with cytokines or activation of PRR signaling, macrophages acquire a proinflammatory phenotype that correlates with robust upregulation of glycolytic pathways including hypoxia inducing factor alpha (HIF1α) (88). Activation of HIF1α induces transcription of hypoxic genes (e.g., glucose transporters, glycolytic genes) and IL-1β production by macrophages.

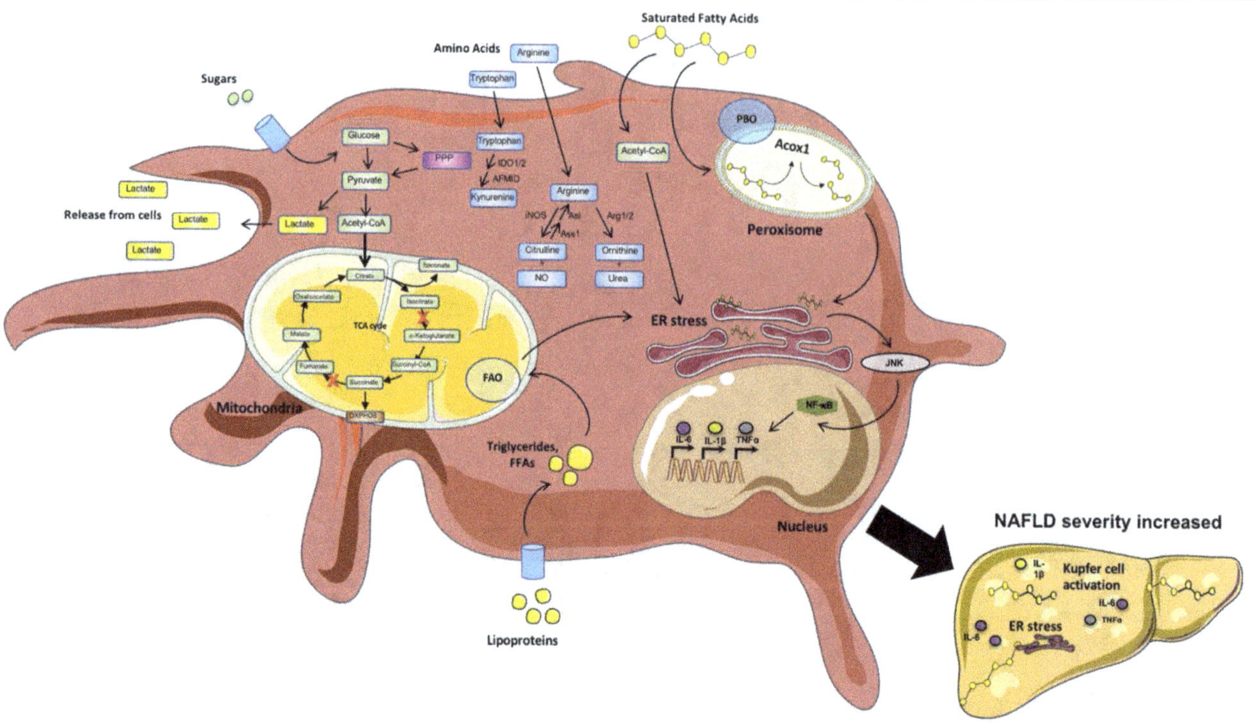

FIGURE 2 | Metabolic processes within inflammatory macrophages. Macrophages are highly metabolically active cells. Their metabolic identity is impacted by inflammatory mediators. In contrast, specific metabolic pathways (Fatty acid synthesis [FAS], Glycolysis, Amino acid [AA] metabolism) regulate the type of mediators produced by these cells. During a proinflammatory state, inflammatory mediators (e.g., sugars, lipoproteins, saturated fatty acids [SFAs], cytokines [IL6, TNF]) trigger "classical" activation of circulating and tissue resident macrophages (e.g., Kupfer cells and adipose tissue macrophages [ATMs]). Circulating sugars are taken up and processed via glycolysis/TCA cycle. In addition, several intermediate metabolites, as well as amino acids L-arginine, L-tryptophan and glutamine, can impact macrophage effector functions. Sensing/uptake of excessive lipoproteins and SFAs activates the mitochondrial fatty acid oxidation (FAO) and peroxisomal fatty acid beta-oxidation (PBO) pathways to breakdown long chain and very long chain fatty acids, respectively. Excessive activation of these pathways triggers ER stress and signaling via JNK and NF-kB, resulting in amplified production of proinflammatory mediators. "Classical" macrophage activation shifts the cells toward preferential utilization of glycolytic pathways with altered enzyme activity within the tricarboxylic acid cycle (TCA) cycle generating more lactate and fast energy production in the form of ATP to generate inflammatory mediators (e.g., IL-6, TNF, IL1). Metabolism of tryptophan (L-TRP) and arginine (L-ARG) by macrophages regulates key immunologic processes. Cumulatively, these inflammatory mechanisms fuel the overall systemic and tissue inflammation, hepatocyte death, and fibrosis in turn amplifying NAFLD pathogenesis.

TABLE 1 | Metabolic function in macrophage subsets.

Pathway	"Classically" activated macrophage	"Alternatively" activated macrophage
Reactive oxygen species	Increased ROS production through mitochondrial ROS and NADPH oxidase	Mitochondrial ROS and NADPH oxidase activity minimal
Glycolysis	High aerobic glycolysis resulting in lactate production	Low glycolytic rate resulting in acetyl-coA production
Pentose phosphate pathway	Increased pentose phosphate pathway	Decreased pentose phosphate pathway
Tricarboxylic Acid Cycle	Fractured TCA cycle, broken at Idh and Sdh	Functional TCA cycle fed by acetyl-coA from beta-oxidation and glycolysis
Electron transport chain	Dysfunctional electron transport chain, resulting in mitochondrial ROS production	Functional electron transport chain resulting in ATP production
Fatty acid	Fatty acid synthesis from fractured TCA	Fatty acid beta-oxidation from lipoproteins
L-Tryptophan catabolism	L-Tryptophan catabolism by IDO results in suppression of aberrant inflammation	L-Tryptophan catabolism not induced
L-Arginine metabolism*	L-Arginine metabolism by iNOS resulting in nitric oxide production	L-Arginine metabolism by arginase resulting in L-ornithine and downstream metabolites

*ATP, adenosine triphosphate; Idh, isocitrate dehydrogenase; IDO, indoleamine-2,3-dioxygenase; iNOS, inducible nitric oxide synthase; NADPH, nicotinamide adenine dinucleotide phosphate; ROS, reactive oxygen species; Sdh, succinate dehydrogenase; TCA, tricarboxylic acid. Unless noted, references are in main text. *Arginase 1 (Arg1) expression occurs along with iNOS in macrophages during intracellular infection, and is not sufficient on its own to define alternative activation.*

Preferential skewing toward glycolysis favors proinflammatory macrophage effector functions as administration of the glucose analog, 2-deoxyglucose (2-DG), decreases macrophage inflammatory polarization, cytokine production and phagocytosis (88). Mice fed MCD diet and patients with NASH display increased hepatic macrophage HIF1α expression and exacerbated hepatic steatosis and inflammation (89). However, given the functional relevance of HIF1α to macrophage-mediated inflammation, additional studies are warranted to determine the impact of macrophage-intrinsic HIF1α in inflammation and NAFLD progression.

Pentose Phosphate Pathway

Pentose phosphate pathway (PPP) branches off glycolysis at glucose-6-phosphate, the second step in glycolysis. Through a series of dehydration and decarboxylation reactions, glucose-6-phosphate is converted to ribulose-5-phosphate. Macrophages upregulate the PPP in response to LPS, which yields two NADPH (used as cofactors for NOXs) and in turn promote inflammation and cellular damage (90–92). Additionally, the PPP is necessary for limiting the dissemination of various pathogens (93). In contrast, macrophages also use the PPP to resolve inflammation and ROS, as PPP results in glutathione reduction and subsequently maintains proper redox balance, limiting the consequences of extraneous ROS activity (94, 95). During hypercholesterolemia, cholesterol inhibits LPS-mediated PPP activity in inflammatory macrophages, leading to a foamy macrophage phenotype (96). Further, adipocytes are known to use NADPH metabolism to regulate lipid metabolism, and dysregulation of enzymes involved in the production of NADPH contributes to obesity and obesity-related pathology (97, 98). Despite the role of PPP in modulating inflammation, the contribution of this metabolic pathway to macrophage-intrinsic inflammation in the context of NAFLD is underdefined and requires in-depth examination.

Tricarboxylic Acid Cycle

Acetyl CoA, generated following glycolysis or beta-oxidation, enters the tricarboxylic acid (TCA) cycle, resulting in H_2O, CO_2, NADH and $FADH_2$ generation. The latter two are utilized in the electron transport chain (ETC) to produce ATP. Despite the high energy yield of the TCA cycle, the process is time consuming and requires oxygen. In the context of a rapid inflammatory response, the TCA is downregulated and fractured in macrophages. Specifically, inflammatory macrophages reduce isocitrate dehydrogenase (Idh) and succinate dehydrogenase (Sdh) activity (90, 91). This results in decreased α-ketoglutarate formation but increased production of itaconate - a key anti-microbial metabolite. Accumulation of succinate in macrophages can inhibit the HIF1α-suppressing molecules prolyl hydroxylases (PHDs), allowing HIF1α to drive IL-1β and other inflammatory processes (90). Sdh is complex II of the ETC, which donates two electrons from $FADH_2$ to produce the electron gradient that drives ATP synthesis. During LPS stimulation, the breakdown of Sdh feeds electrons through complex I, known as reverse electron transport, resulting in mitochondrial ROS production (99). The contribution of Idh and Sdh to NAFLD has not been investigated. However, it can be hypothesized that the hepatic inflammatory environment in NAFLD would drive the breakdown of the TCA cycle, as seen in LPS stimulated macrophages. Hence, additional studies are needed to formally address these postulates.

Fatty Acid Synthesis (FAS)

Excessive hepatocellular uptake of glucose is diverted to FAS pathways where glucose is converted into TGs and secreted to adipose tissue (AT) as VLDL (100). Under pathological conditions, *de novo* FAS by the liver is a primary cause of excessive hepatic steatosis (100). In contrast to glucose, insulin reduces AT lipolysis via suppression of hormone-sensitive lipase (HSL), thus regulating the circulation of FFAs in the periphery (100, 101). However, obesity-and NAFLD-associated insulin resistance limits HSL suppression, leading to increased AT lipolysis and FFA deposition in the liver (102). FAS is essential for immune cell proliferation in response to inflammatory insult. Macrophages upregulate FAS when undergoing "classical" activation. Monocyte treatment with macrophage colony stimulating factor promotes "classical" activation and expression of sterol regulatory element binding transcription protein 1c (SREBP1c), FAS target genes and increases lipid synthesis (103). Inhibition of SREBP1c reduces macrophage inflammatory capacity (104). Increased FAS drives KC inflammasome activation via nucleotide-binding oligomerization (NOD)-like receptor 3 (NLR3) signaling (103, 105). In fact, increased inflammasome activation has been observed in both murine experimental models and human NAFLD (105–107). Inflammasomes, reviewed elsewhere (105), are multiprotein complexes containing nucleotide-binding oligomerization domains NLRs. KCs are a key source of IL-1β and caspase 1, a critical NLR3 component that regulates downstream proinflammatory signaling (e.g., pro-IL-1β, pro-IL-18, ASC), and are elevated in livers from NASH patients (105, 108, 109). However, given the complexity of inflammasome signaling the underlying mechanism unique to macrophage inflammasome-driven inflammation in NAFLD, these processes warrant further examination. Additional studies are also needed to determine if targeted inhibition of FAS pathways in macrophages is sufficient to reverse inflammasome activation and subsequently improve NAFLD pathology.

Beta-Oxidation

Beta-oxidation of fatty acids (FA) is central for ensuring cellular and tissue energetic demands by breakdown and conversion of lipids into ATP. Under homeostatic conditions, fat storage and lipolysis are regulated in part by beta-oxidation. Members of the nuclear hormone receptor superfamily known as peroxisome proliferator activated receptors (PPARα, PPARβ, and PPARγ) are transcriptional modulators of beta-oxidation. PPARα, which is primarily expressed in the liver, has several endogenous ligands (e.g., FA, eicosanoids and other complex lipids) and acts as a master regulator for FA beta-oxidation (110, 111). Given the importance of hepatic steatosis in NAFLD and the relevance of beta-oxidation in immune responses, below we discuss the contribution of both mitochondrial and peroxisomal beta-oxidation to macrophage inflammation.

Mitochondrial beta-oxidation

Mitochondrial-beta oxidation breaks down short ($<C_8$), medium (C_8-C_{14}) and long chain FA (C_{14}-C_{20}) (85). Long chain FA, which are a major component of the standard diet, are shuttled into the mitochondria via carnitine shuttles (carnitine palmitoyltransferase I) by linking with coenzyme A (acyl-CoA) (85, 112). Once acylcarnitine exchanges the carnitine molecule with CoA via exchange with carnitine palmitoyltransferase II the acyl-CoA proceeds into the beta-oxidation cycle. At the inner membrane the enzymatic activity of very long chain acyl-CoA dehydrogenase (VCLAD), shortens long chain acyl-CoAs. Shortened fatty acyl-CoAs are further oxidized by a trifunctional protein complex consisting of: Enoyl-CoA hydratase, 3-hydroxyacyl CoA dehydrogenase, and 3 ketoacyl CoA thiolase. Impaired beta-oxidation in macrophages prevents the degradation of lipids leading to the FA overload and rupture and release of toxic lipid species (85). Although, the traditional view is that FA beta-oxidation is essential for polarization of "alternatively" activated macrophages, recent evidence suggest that inhibition of this pathway may in fact promote a "classical" macrophage phenotype. Etomoxir driven inhibition of beta-oxidation or knockdown of CPT-1 results in reduced fatty acid oxidation (FAO) but increased proinflammatory signaling, cytokine production, ER stress and ROS levels (113–115). Thus, additional studies are needed to formally determine how mitochondrial FAO impacts macrophage inflammation and NAFLD progression.

Peroxisomal beta oxidation

Oxidation of very long chain fatty acids (VLCFAs) ($C>_{21}$) is exclusive to the peroxisome due to the selective presence of very long chain acyl-CoA synthetase (85). Aside from VLCFAs, long chain dicarboxylic acid, eicosanoids, and bile acid precursors are also oxidized within the peroxisomes. Compared to mitochondria, 3 enzymes Acyl-CoA oxidase 1 (Acox1), enoyl CoA hydratase/L-3-hydroxyacyl CoA dehydrogenase bifunctional protein and 3-ketoacyl CoA thiolase regulate peroxisomal beta-oxidation (85). Whole body *Acox1* null mice and $Acox1^{Lampe1}$ mice, which features a point mutation rendering the *Acox1* gene inactive, spontaneously develop steatosis and steatohepatitis (85, 116). $Acox1^{Lampe1}$ mice also exhibit increased systemic inflammation both at baseline and after LPS challenge *in vivo*, increased hepatic expression of macrophage recruiting chemokines and macrophage infiltration into the liver following short term high fat diet (HFD) feeding. HFD feeding combined with secondary LPS insult *in vivo* further exacerbates liver pathologies in $Acox1^{Lampe1}$ mice (86). Together, these data suggest that peroxisomal beta-oxidation regulates macrophage-intrinsic inflammation and NAFLD pathogenesis. However, the underlying processes by which peroxisomal beta-oxidation regulates macrophage function and inflammation remain understudied. Similarly, the contribution of peroxisomal beta-oxidation to inflammatory potential of other immune cells and their contribution to NAFLD progression remains poorly understood.

Amino Acid Metabolism

Amino acids (AA) are critical precursors for several metabolic pathways. For example, glutamine and aspartate are necessary for purine and pyrimidine synthesis as well as feeding the TCA cycle via α-ketoglutarate production. Valine and leucine fuel the synthesis of branched chain FA. Direct metabolism of tryptophan (L-TRP) and arginine (L-ARG) by macrophages and other myeloid cells regulate key immunologic processes. For this reason, below we focus on how metabolism of tryptophan and arginine within macrophages modulates their inflammatory potential.

Tryptophan

In macrophages, L-TRP metabolism is tightly regulated by two isoforms of the enzyme indoleamine 2,3-dioxygenase (IDO1 and IDO2). IDO is the rate limiting enzyme that converts L-TRP into N-formylkynurenine (117). Early reports focused on L-TRP depletion as the central mechanism of immune modulation, yet more recent literature deemphasizes L-TRP depletion and reports kynurenine production as the key regulator of immune responses (117, 118). The downstream products of kynurenine modulate immune responses to infection, cancer, and autoimmune diseases (117, 119, 120). IDO activity is induced in macrophages following IFNγ, LPS, or TNF stimulation and can be further enhanced with IL-1β co-stimulation (121–125). Several studies have begun to address the contribution of IDO-mediated L-TRP metabolism during NAFLD. Kynurenine is increased in the serum of obese subjects, and IDO1 is upregulated in the liver and WAT in obesity (126). IDO-deficient mice displayed elevated liver fibrosis, increased hepatic macrophage infiltration, and higher concentrations of IL-1β, IL-6, and IFNγ in obesity. However, these mice are protected from HFD-driven weight gain, hepatic steatosis, and oxidative stress (127). Interestingly, mice lacking IDO1 expression in macrophages and neutrophils exhibited normal weight gain and insulin sensitivity in obesity (128). Mice with an intact bone-marrow derived immune system, but lacking IDO1 in all other tissues, displayed a similar protection from HFD-induced metabolic disease as the mice with global IDO1 deletion. In sum, these data suggest that IDO contributes to multiple aspects of NAFLD progression and that non-hematopoietic IDO activity may play a key role in regulating NAFLD pathogenesis. Follow-up studies are needed however to dissect the contribution of IDO activity during the full spectrum of NAFLD pathogenesis and to evaluate IDO activity within radiation-resistant tissue macrophages.

L-TRP supplementation has been explored in multiple studies. Mice fed a high fructose diet exhibit reduced liver weight and hepatic lipid accumulation when supplemented with L-TRP (129). Clinical studies examining patients with hepatic steatosis or NASH found supplementation, twice daily, with L-TRP for 14 months result in decreased plasma LDL, TG, and gamma gluthamylo transpeptidase levels with a correlative decrease in plasma IL-1β, IL-6, and TNF (130, 131). Key studies, however, are needed to identify where supplemental L-TRP and its downstream metabolites accumulate, and whether L-TRP is available for IDO activity within the diseased liver. Considering the availability of conditional IDO1 knockout mice (128), it is now feasible to separate the contribution of IDO activity by macrophages as well as other immune and non-immune cell types during the initiation and progression of NAFLD. These, studies would help determine how IDO modulates immune responses and NAFLD pathogenesis.

Arginine

Historically, macrophage polarization was characterized in part by the ability to metabolize L-ARG. "Classically" activated macrophages upregulate inducible nitric oxide synthase (iNOS) which converts L-ARG to L-citrulline and anti-microbial nitric oxide (NO). In contrast, "alternatively" activated macrophages upregulate arginase 1 (Argl) to metabolize L-ARG into ornithine and urea (132, 133). It is now appreciated that Argl and iNOS expression can occur within similarly stimulated macrophages, adding to the complexity of defining "classical" and "alternative" macrophage activation profiles (134–136). Regardless, macrophage L-ARG metabolism has been documented to restrict intrinsic and extrinsic immune cell function. Blocking arginase activity or eliminating Argl within macrophages allows for increased L-arginine availability for NO production and anti-microbial activity but can also be associated with unrestricted lymphocyte activity and increased tissue pathology (132, 136–141). Thus, understanding how L-ARG metabolism is regulated during altered inflammatory and metabolic states, including NAFLD, is of considerable interest.

Limited studies have focused on the contribution of enzymes involved in the breakdown of L-ARG in NAFLD. Mammals possess two arginase isoforms (Argl, Arg2) that are differentially expressed within tissues. The importance of macrophage Argl in NAFLD has not been addressed. The role of Arg2 in NAFLD, despite published studies, remains undefined. Opposing findings employing Arg2-deficient mice have shown that Arg2-deficiency results in development of spontaneous hepatic steatosis and increased liver injury (142) or promotes decreased NAFLD severity in obesity (143). Although NO contributes to NAFLD, additional studies are needed to determine the critical source of NO as NO inhibitors have various specificities and differ in their ability to regulate disease severity (144). L-ARG supplementation has also been shown to reduce NAFLD severity (145). As such, studies determining the contribution not only of L-ARG utilization, but also of L-ARG synthesis during NAFLD are warranted. The necessity of L-ARG synthesis within macrophages has recently been described during infection, suggesting extracellular L-ARG is not available in sufficient concentrations to drive effective macrophage function (135, 146, 147). Accounting for the considerable influx of inflammatory macrophages in NAFLD, future studies aimed at addressing macrophage-specific modulation of L-ARG metabolism with existing molecular tools (e.g., $Argl^{flox}$, Asl^{flox}, Nos2-deficient) (148–150) will be necessary to dissect how various macrophage populations manipulate the liver microenvironment and NAFLD progression.

Macrophages and Trace Metals

Trace metals including iron, zinc and copper are essential for many cellular functions and for optimal adaptive and innate immune responses (151). Among these three metals, iron and copper exert an important influence on the genesis of NAFLD (152–155). Adults, but not children, with NAFLD manifest increased circulating concentrations of ferritin; however, both age groups exhibit increased transferrin saturation (153, 154). Excess iron accrual in the liver, specifically KCs (156) is associated with elevated amounts of hepcidin, which blocks iron egress mediated by ferroportin. Hepcidin binds to ferroportin and enhances its degradation. The accumulation of iron promotes "classically" activated macrophage polarization and production of proinflammatory cytokines that enhance the inflammatory response (157, 158). Excessive iron accumulation in both KCs and hepatocytes is associated with NAFLD (152). Inflammatory mediators, induced by lipid overload, drive increased hepcidin and decreased iron export from KCs and hepatocytes, in turn exacerbating NAFLD severity. Although copper is connected to iron homeostasis, the former metal is diminished in patients with NAFLD. Copper deficiency is associated with a decrease in ceruloplasmin ferroxidase which promotes iron release (152, 159). Aside from the effects of copper on iron regulation, the paucity of copper would reduce generation of copper/zinc superoxide dismutases that scavenge ROS and subsequently impairing the cellular defenses to ROS-mediated damage. Despite the knowledge of low zinc concentrations in chronic liver disease and damage (160) the role of zinc in NAFLD has not been investigated. How zinc deficiency augments liver damage is not well defined. Experiments determining the necessity of superoxide dismutases to combat excess ROS would provide valuable insight but have yet to be performed.

Adipose Tissue/Adipocytes and NAFLD

The traditional perspective of AT was that of a simplistic fat storing/releasing organ playing a role in energy homeostasis (161). It is now well-appreciated that AT is a highly metabolic, active and plastic organ comprised of various types of cells (e.g., adipocytes, progenitor stem cells within the stromal vascular fraction, endothelial cells, fibroblasts, and immune cells) (162, 163). The AT regulates the accommodation of excess energy through storage of circulating dietary lipids and *de novo* lipogenesis. In the case of nutrient shortage, lipolysis controls/regulates the release of hydrolyzed TGs as glycerol and FFAs to provide energy to surrounding tissues (164–166). Obesity-associated changes in AT robustly modify AT function including production of hormones, cytokines and adipokines. Which cells within AT tissue contribute to such changes and how the low-grade systemic and AT inflammatory state in obesity/metabolic disease impacts AT function is poorly understood.

Adipose tissue macrophages (ATMs) are believed to play a major role in regulating AT inflammation. In general, healthy AT, is believed to contain a balance between "alternatively" and "classically" activated ATMs. In contrast, the unhealthy/inflammatory AT, houses an increased number of "classically" activated ATMs. "Classically" activated ATMs produce an array of proinflammatory mediators (e.g., IL-6, TNF, IL-1β, IFNγ) that further amplify AT inflammation and promote additional macrophage and other immune cell recruitment and activation. Cumulatively, such events, in obesity, fuel a chronic low-grade inflammation within the AT (167, 168). In addition to the enhanced release of soluble mediators, AT inflammation drives expression of integrin α4 on macrophages and vascular cell adhesion molecule 1 (VCAM-1) on adipocytes allowing for AT macrophage accrual (43). The inhibition of integrin α4 reduces ATM retention and AT inflammation. Notably, individuals with NAFLD exhibit high expression of VCAM-1 in AT underlining the importance of this cell-cell interaction pathways (169).

Adipocytes play a pivotal role in metabolic disease by promoting chronic inflammation via release of FFAs in response to increased circulating levels of TNF. These FFAs translocate to the liver and skeletal muscle propagating inflammation and insulin resistance (170, 171). Mechanistically, TNF inhibits PPARγ (172) and CCAAT/enhancer binding protein (C/EBPα) in adipocytes that is needed for the expression of adipocyte-specific GLUT4 and insulin receptor (IR) to maintain insulin sensitivity (173, 174). This suggests that like ATMs, adipocytes themselves play an important role in maintaining AT metabolic processes. Recent studies demonstrate that adipocytes, like immune cells, exhibit immune-like potential (175, 176). Specifically, adipocytes express various innate immune receptors including RIG-I-like receptors (RLR), NLRs, and nucleotide oligomerization domains (NODs) (177, 178). NOD-1 signaling suppresses adipocyte differentiation and contributes to induction of the NF-kB (177, 179). Adipocyte sensing of various PAMPs leads to production of multiple inflammatory mediators (e.g., cytokines, chemokines, adipokines) (180). In obesity, the main mechanisms associated with unlocking adipocyte-intrinsic inflammation are: (a) obesity-associated endotoxemia and (b) AT hypoxic micro-environment which leads to ER stress, inflammatory cytokine production, cell death, release of lipid content and debris and induction of the inflammatory mediators (181). Adipocyte production of inflammatory mediators is potentially sensed by ATMs and leads to their activation (161, 168, 180, 182). Adiponectin, an adipokine, exerts either

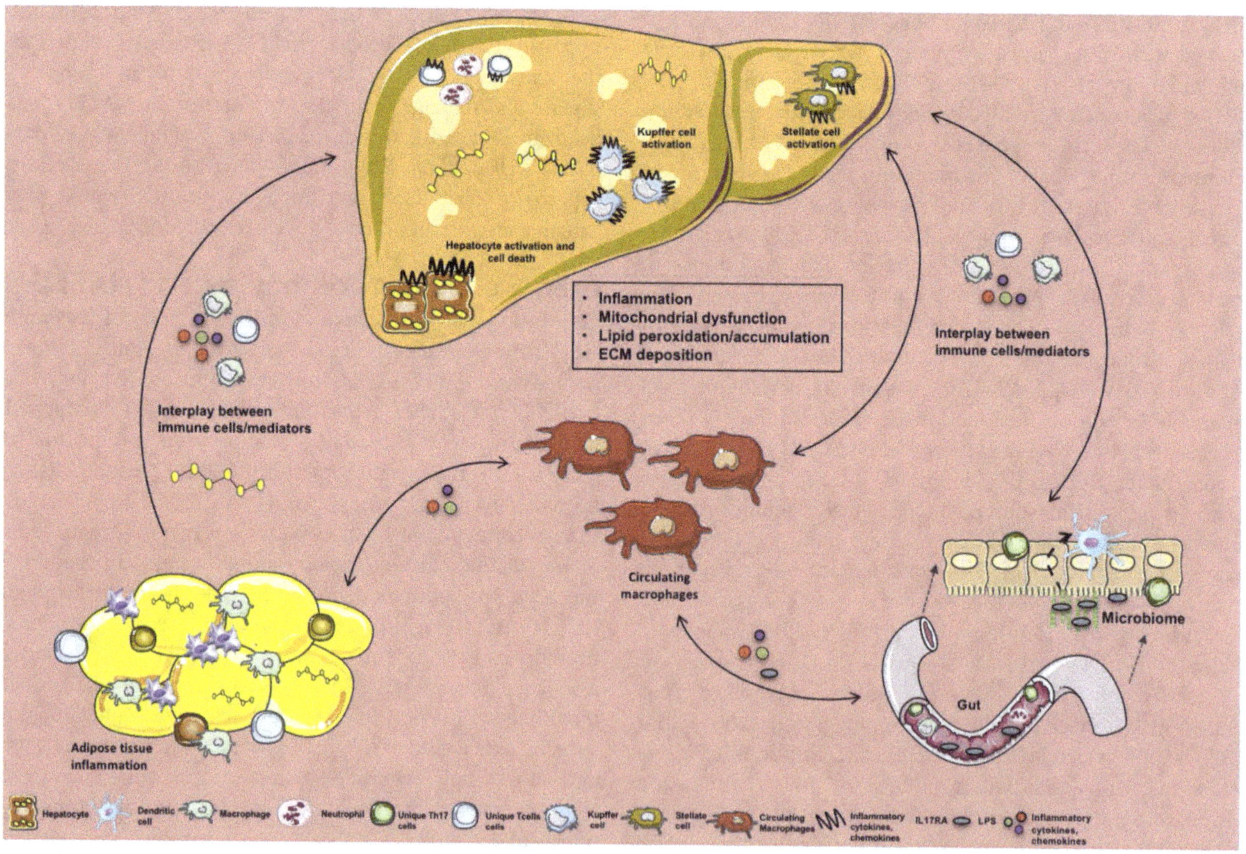

FIGURE 3 | Crosstalk between tissue-specific inflammation and macrophage function in NAFLD. Schematic overview of the crosstalk between various organs, their specific immune cells and inflammatory mediators during NAFLD. Obesity-associated low-grade, chronic inflammation and altered gut microbiome impacts immune cell crosstalk between the gut, circulating monocytes/macrophages, and the liver. In addition, obesity-associated adipocyte expansion promotes hypoxia leading to adipose tissue (AT) inflammation, activation of adipose tissue macropahes (ATMs) and fuels infiltration of various immune cells and inflammatory mediator production (e.g., FFAs, ROS, cytokines, chemokines) to be sensed by circulating macrophages and hepatocytes. Collectively these processes alter hepatocellular lipid metabolism, contributing to steatosis and proinflammatory cytokine (IL-17, TNF, IFNγ, IL-6) and chemokine production (CCL2, CXCL9, CXCL10). Moreover, this inflammatory state activates hepatic stellate cells (HSCs) and Kupffer cells (KCs) in turn contributing to extracellular matrix deposition (collagen fibers) and progression to fibrosis.

anti- or pro-inflammatory effects on macrophages. It inhibits macrophage functions (e.g., phagocytosis, cytokine production) and induces proliferation of "alternatively" activated macrophage in AT (183–185). Conversely, adiponectin also induces pro-inflammatory signaling cascades through NF-kB activation and upregulation of pro-inflammatory cytokines (e.g., TNF-α, IL-6, and IL-8) (186, 187). However, detailed analysis of specific adipocyte mediators and adipokines relevant to altered ATMs polarization and activation is needed. Similarly, whether obesity-activated adipocytes or ATMs directly play a role in NAFLD pathogenesis is not fully understood and should be further investigated. A brief summary of the above discussed processes is depicted in **Figure 3**.

Therapies

Ultimately, the improvement of experimental models to more closely recapitulate human NAFLD would be ideal for the discovery and development of therapies targeting various metabolic pathways in macrophages. Diet and lifestyle changes help in reversing NAFLD progression. Thus, it is not surprising that several pharmacological drugs that target metabolic and inflammatory and molecular mechanisms important in NAFLD progression are currently being examined (188). Hepatic lipid accumulation is an initial driver of NAFLD pathogenesis (9 84). Intuitively, use of therapeutic drugs that target lipid metabolism is actively pursued. Glitazones, which are a class of insulin-sensitizing drugs, are effective in regulating lipid metabolism. They increase FAS and FA uptake by adipocytes, thus increasing lipid loading in AT instead of ectopic organs (e.g., liver and muscle) (189, 190). However, due to their association with increased risks of heart failure the use of glitazones as a treatment option has not been pursued in the clinic (191, 192). Sodium glucose co-transporter 2 (SGLT2) inhibitors have also proven efficacious in regulating NAFLD-associated dyslipidemia by inhibiting hepatic expression of lipogenic genes (e.g., sterol regulatory-element binding protein 1-c, fatty acid synthase, acetyl-CoA carboxylase 1, and sterol CoA desaturase), hepatic macrophage infiltration and expression of inflammatory cytokine production (190, 193, 194). However, underlying mechanisms that govern this process remains an area of investigation. Upregulation of oxidative stress, inflammation and apoptosis pathways are associated with NAFLD pathogenesis. NASH patients display increased hepatic activation of apoptosis signal-regulating kinase 1 (Ask1). Activation of Ask1 by TNF causes oxidative and ER stress, and induction of p38 and JNK signaling (188, 190, 195). Ask1 inhibition reduced hepatic steatosis, inflammation and fibrosis (196, 197). However, given that phenotypical outcomes of Ask1 inhibition in mice are not often recapitulated in humans, more effective "humanized" mouse models are needed (198, 199). Further, the effects of Ask1 inhibition on macrophage inflammation in NAFLD pathogenesis remains underdefined. Limiting the detrimental effects of obesity-associated microbiome alteration and subsequent systemic endotoxemia which contribute to NAFLD pathogenesis is another active area of investigation for drug development. Excessive PRR activation and inflammation resulting in liver injury is characteristic of NAFLD. JKB-121, a TLR4 antagonist, prevents LPS induced inflammatory liver injury in MCD diet models of NAFLD. However, given that obesity modulates the expression of multiple TLRs, more studies are needed to determine the impact of ablation of other TLRs in NAFLD pathogenesis. In addition, there are several other therapeutic approaches regarding use of ACC inhibitors, fructose inhibitors and obetocholic acid inhibitors (188, 190) for the treatment of NAFLD. In sum, several potential avenues for NAFLD therapies are being pursued. Specifically, there is a need for studies to allow for HFD-driven induction of hepatic fibrosis (41), eliminate gender bias by employing a more "human"-like disease state (e.g., thermoneutrality) (200), CCL4 experimental models of fibrosis (201) use of various murine strains/genotypes to mimic genetic diversity as well as expansion of such findings into non-human primate models of NAFLD (198). Use of such wide ranging experimental models would be beneficial in the development of therapeutic targets that may prove more effective in the clinic. Thus, in sum, given the interplay between metabolism and inflammation, additional therapies targeting macrophage polarization, chemo-attracting, inflammatory and metabolic pathways are needed—something that may be achieved by improving experimental modeling of disease.

CONCLUSION

Overall, this review highlights the inflammatory processes associated with macrophage polarization, tissue recruitment and inflammation and the role of such processes in NAFLD. We also extensively discuss how cellular metabolic pathways may contribute to macrophage-driven inflammation. Given the metabolic changes in obesity and inflammation the potential benefits to be gained from understanding the interplay between various metabolic and inflammatory pathways in macrophages are immense. Further elucidation of the crosstalk between macrophages and other tissues/immune cells similarly remains an exciting area of exploration. However, subsequent to the detailed interrogation of the afore discussed cellular and molecular processes in NAFLD, validation of such processes in multiple experimental models of NAFLD will be required.

AUTHOR CONTRIBUTIONS

JO, MM, MM-F, MD, GD, JQ, and SD wrote the manuscript. All authors have reviewed the manuscript and approve the final version.

ACKNOWLEDGMENTS

We thank Jessica R. Doll for the careful review of the manuscript.

REFERENCES

1. Perumpail BJ, Khan MA, Yoo ER, Cholankeril G, Kim D, Ahmed A. Clinical epidemiology and disease burden of nonalcoholic fatty liver disease. *World J Gastroenterol.* (2017) 23:8263–76. doi: 10.3748/wjg.v23.i47.8263
2. Fabbrini E, Sullivan S, Klein S. Obesity and nonalcoholic fatty liver disease: biochemical, metabolic, and clinical implications. *Hepatology.* (2010) 51:679–89. doi: 10.1002/hep.23280
3. Younossi ZM, Blissett D, Blissett R, Henry L, Stepanova M, Younossi Y, et al. The economic and clinical burden of nonalcoholic fatty liver disease in the United States and Europe. *Hepatology.* (2016) 64:1577–86. doi: 10.1002/hep.28785
4. Hardy T, Oakley F, Anstee QM, Day CP. Nonalcoholic Fatty Liver Disease: Pathogenesis and Disease Spectrum. *Annu Rev Pathol.* (2016) 11:451–96. doi: 10.1146/annurev-pathol-012615-044224
5. Arrese M, Cabrera D, Kalergis AM, Feldstein AE. Innate immunity and inflammation in NAFLD/NASH. *Dig Dis Sci.* (2016) 61:1294–303. doi: 10.1007/s10620-016-4049-x
6. Cha JY, Kim DH, Chun KH. The role of hepatic macrophages in nonalcoholic fatty liver disease and nonalcoholic steatohepatitis. *Lab Anim Res.* (2018) 34:133–9. doi: 10.5625/lar.2018.34.4.133
7. Kwon H, Pessin JE. Adipokines mediate inflammation and insulin resistance. *Front Endocrinol.* (2013) 4:71. doi: 10.3389/fendo.2013.00071
8. Huang J, Viswakarma N, Yu S, Jia Y, Bai L, Vluggens A, et al. Progressive endoplasmic reticulum stress contributes to hepatocarcinogenesis in fatty acyl-CoA oxidase 1-deficient mice. *Am J Pathol.* (2011) 179:703–13. doi: 10.1016/j.ajpath.2011.04.030
9. Cobbina E, Akhlaghi F. Non-alcoholic fatty liver disease (NAFLD) - pathogenesis, classification, and effect on drug metabolizing enzymes and transporters. *Drug Metab Rev.* (2017) 49:197–211. doi: 10.1080/03602532.2017.1293683
10. Giles DA, Moreno-Fernandez ME, Stankiewicz TE, Cappelletti M, Huppert SS, Iwakura Y, et al. Regulation of Inflammation by IL-17A and IL-17F Modulates Non-Alcoholic Fatty Liver Disease Pathogenesis. *PLoS ONE.* (2016) 11:e0149783. doi: 10.1371/journal.pone.0 149783
11. Rosso C, Kazankov K, Younes R, Esmaili S, Marietti M, Sacco M, et al. Crosstalk between adipose tissue insulin resistance and liver macrophages in non-alcoholic fatty liver disease. *J Hepatol.* (2019) 71:1012–21. doi: 10.1016/j.jhep.2019.06.031
12. Cani PD, Amar J, Iglesias MA, Poggi M, Knauf C, Bastelica D, et al. Metabolic endotoxemia initiates obesity and insulin resistance. *Diabetes.* (2007) 56:1761–72. doi: 10.2337/db06-1491
13. Grunhut J, Wang W, Aykut B, Gakhal I, Torres-Hernandez A, Miller G. Macrophages in nonalcoholic steatohepatitis: friend or foe? *Eur Med J Hepatol.* (2018) 6:100–9.
14. Wree A, Broderick L, Canbay A, Hoffman HM, Feldstein AE. From NAFLD to NASH to cirrhosis-new insights into disease mechanisms. *Nat Rev Gastroenterol Hepatol.* (2013) 10:627–36. doi: 10.1038/nrgastro.2013.149
15. Miura K, Ohnishi H. Role of gut microbiota and Toll-like receptors in nonalcoholic fatty liver disease. *World J Gastroenterol.* (2014) 20:7381–91. doi: 10.3748/wjg.v20.i23.7381
16. Phan AT, Goldrath AW, Glass CK. Metabolic and epigenetic coordination of T cell and macrophage immunity. *Immunity.* (2017) 46:714–29. doi: 10.1016/j.immuni.2017.04.016
17. Braunersreuther V, Viviani GL, Mach F, Montecucco F. Role of cytokines and chemokines in non-alcoholic fatty liver disease. *World J Gastroenterol.* (2012) 18:727–35. doi: 10.3748/wjg.v18.i8.727
18. Giles DA, Moreno-Fernandez ME, Divanovic S. IL-17 Axis driven inflammation in non-alcoholic fatty liver disease progression. *Curr Drug Targets.* (2015) 16:1315–23. doi: 10.2174/1389450116666150531153627
19. Karlmark KR, Weiskirchen R, Zimmermann HW, Gassler N, Ginhoux F, Weber C, et al. Hepatic recruitment of the inflammatory Gr1+ monocyte subset upon liver injury promotes hepatic fibrosis. *Hepatology.* (2009) 50:261–74. doi: 10.1002/hep.22950
20. Wasmuth HE, Tacke F, Trautwein C. Chemokines in liver inflammation and fibrosis. *Semin Liver Dis.* (2010) 30:215–25. doi: 10.1055/s-0030-1255351
21. Obstfeld AE, Sugaru E, Thearle M, Francisco AM, Gayet C, Ginsberg HN, et al. C-C chemokine receptor 2 (CCR2) regulates the hepatic recruitment of myeloid cells that promote obesity-induced hepatic steatosis. *Diabetes.* (2010) 59:916–25. doi: 10.2337/db09-1403
22. Holt AP, Haughton EL, Lalor PF, Filer A, Buckley CD, Adams DH. Liver myofibroblasts regulate infiltration and positioning of lymphocytes in human liver. *Gastroenterology.* (2009) 136:705–14. doi: 10.1053/j.gastro.2008.10.020
23. Kazankov K, Jorgensen SMD, Thomsen KL, Moller HJ, Vilstrup H, George J, et al. The role of macrophages in nonalcoholic fatty liver disease and nonalcoholic steatohepatitis. *Nat Rev Gastroenterol Hepatol.* (2019) 16:145–59. doi: 10.1038/s41575-018-0082-x
24. Mak A, Uetrecht J. Involvement of CCL2/CCR2 macrophage recruitment in amodiaquine-induced liver injury. *J Immunotoxicol.* (2019) 2019:1–6. doi: 10.1080/1547691X.2018.1516014
25. Kanda H, Tateya S, Tamori Y, Kotani K, Hiasa K, Kitazawa R, et al. MCP-1 contributes to macrophage infiltration into adipose tissue, insulin resistance, and hepatic steatosis in obesity. *J Clin Invest.* (2006) 116:1494–505. doi: 10.1172/JCI26498
26. Weisberg SP, Hunter D, Huber R, Lemieux J, Slaymaker S, Vaddi K, et al. CCR2 modulates inflammatory and metabolic effects of high-fat feeding. *J Clin Invest.* (2006) 116:115–24. doi: 10.1172/JCI24335
27. Tamura Y, Sugimoto M, Murayama T, Minami M, Nishikaze Y, Ariyasu H, et al. C-C chemokine receptor 2 inhibitor improves diet-induced development of insulin resistance and hepatic steatosis in mice. *J Atheroscler Thromb.* (2010) 17:219–28. doi: 10.5551/jat.3368
28. Seki E, De Minicis S, Gwak GY, Kluwe J, Inokuchi S, Bursill CA, et al. CCR1 and CCR5 promote hepatic fibrosis in mice. *J Clin Invest.* (2009) 119:1858–70. doi: 10.1172/JCI37444
29. Berres ML, Koenen RR, Rueland A, Zaldivar MM, Heinrichs D, Sahin H, et al. Antagonism of the chemokine Ccl5 ameliorates experimental liver fibrosis in mice. *J Clin Invest.* (2010) 120:4129–40. doi: 10.1172/JCI41732
30. Miura K, Yang L, van Rooijen N, Ohnishi H, Seki E. Hepatic recruitment of macrophages promotes nonalcoholic steatohepatitis through CCR2. *Am J Physiol Gastrointest Liver Physiol.* (2012) 302:G1310–21. doi: 10.1152/ajpgi.00365.2011
31. Heymann F, Hammerich L, Storch D, Bartneck M, Huss S, Russeler V, et al. Hepatic macrophage migration and differentiation critical for liver fibrosis is mediated by the chemokine receptor C-C motif chemokine receptor 8 in mice. *Hepatology.* (2012) 55:898–909. doi: 10.1002/hep.24764
32. Baeck C, Wei X, Bartneck M, Fech V, Heymann F, Gassler N, et al. Pharmacological inhibition of the chemokine C-C motif chemokine ligand 2 (monocyte chemoattractant protein 1) accelerates liver fibrosis regression by suppressing Ly-6C(+) macrophage infiltration in mice. *Hepatology.* (2014) 59:1060–72. doi: 10.1002/hep.26783
33. Zhang X, Han J, Man K, Li X, Du J, Chu ES, et al. CXC chemokine receptor 3 promotes steatohepatitis in mice through mediating inflammatory cytokines, macrophages and autophagy. *J Hepatol.* (2016) 64:160–70. doi: 10.1016/j.jhep.2015.09.005
34. Tomita K, Freeman BL, Bronk SF, LeBrasseur NK, White TA, Hirsova P, et al. CXCL10-Mediates Macrophage, but not Other Innate Immune Cells-Associated Inflammation in Murine Nonalcoholic Steatohepatitis. *Sci Rep.* (2016) 6:28786. doi: 10.1038/srep28786
35. Friedman SL, Ratziu V, Harrison SA, Abdelmalek MF, Aithal GP, Caballeria J, et al. A randomized, placebo-controlled trial of cenicriviroc for treatment of nonalcoholic steatohepatitis with fibrosis. *Hepatology.* (2018) 67:1754–67. doi: 10.1002/hep.29477
36. Harley IT, Stankiewicz TE, Giles DA, Softic S, Flick LM, Cappelletti M, et al. IL-17 signaling accelerates the progression of nonalcoholic fatty liver disease in mice. *Hepatology.* (2014) 59:1830–9. doi: 10.1002/hep.26746
37. Gomes AL, Teijeiro A, Buren S, Tummala KS, Yilmaz M, Waisman A, et al. Metabolic inflammation-associated IL-17A causes non-alcoholic steatohepatitis and hepatocellular carcinoma. *Cancer Cell.* (2016) 30:161–75. doi: 10.1016/j.ccell.2016.05.020
38. Baffy G. Kupffer cells in non-alcoholic fatty liver disease: the emerging view. *J Hepatol.* (2009) 51:212–23. doi: 10.1016/j.jhep.2009.03.008
39. Robinson MW, Harmon C, O'Farrelly C. Liver immunology and its role in inflammation and homeostasis. *Cell Mol Immunol.* (2016) 13:267–76. doi: 10.1038/cmi.2016.3

40. Takeuchi O, Akira S. Pattern recognition receptors and inflammation. *Cell.* (2010) 140:805–20. doi: 10.1016/j.cell.2010.01.022
41. Kohli R, Kirby M, Xanthakos SA, Softic S, Feldstein AE, Saxena V, et al. High-fructose, medium chain trans fat diet induces liver fibrosis and elevates plasma coenzyme Q9 in a novel murine model of obesity and nonalcoholic steatohepatitis. *Hepatology.* (2010) 52:934–44. doi: 10.1002/hep.23797
42. Mayoral Monibas R, Johnson AM, Osborn O, Traves PG, Mahata SK. Distinct hepatic macrophage populations in lean and obese mice. *Front Endocrinol (Lausanne).* (2016) 7:152. doi: 10.3389/fendo.2016.00152
43. Kim SY, Jeong JM, Kim SJ, Seo W, Kim MH, Choi WM, et al. Pro-inflammatory hepatic macrophages generate ROS through NADPH oxidase 2 via endocytosis of monomeric TLR4-MD2 complex. *Nat Commun.* (2017) 8:2247. doi: 10.1038/s41467-017-02325-2
44. Classen A, Lloberas J, Celada A. Macrophage activation: classical versus alternative. *Methods Mol Biol.* (2009) 531:29–43. doi: 10.1007/978-1-59745-396-7_3
45. Kang K, Reilly SM, Karabacak V, Gangl MR, Fitzgerald K, Hatano B, et al. Adipocyte-derived Th2 cytokines and myeloid PPARdelta regulate macrophage polarization and insulin sensitivity. *Cell Metab.* (2008) 7:485–95. doi: 10.1016/j.cmet.2008.04.002
46. Gordon S. Alternative activation of macrophages. *Nat Rev Immunol.* (2003) 3:23–35. doi: 10.1038/nri978
47. Saberi M, Woods NB, de Luca C, Schenk S, Lu JC, Bandyopadhyay G, et al. Hematopoietic cell-specific deletion of toll-like receptor 4 ameliorates hepatic and adipose tissue insulin resistance in high-fat-fed mice. *Cell Metab.* (2009) 10:419–29. doi: 10.1016/j.cmet.2009.09.006
48. Solinas G, Vilcu C, Neels JG, Bandyopadhyay GK, Luo JL, Naugler W, et al. JNK1 in hematopoietically derived cells contributes to diet-induced inflammation and insulin resistance without affecting obesity. *Cell Metab.* (2007) 6:386–97. doi: 10.1016/j.cmet.2007.09.011
49. Arkan MC, Hevener AL, Greten FR, Maeda S, Li ZW, Long JM, et al. IKK-beta links inflammation to obesity-induced insulin resistance. *Nat Med.* (2005) 11:191–8. doi: 10.1038/nm1185
50. Cai D, Yuan M, Frantz DF, Melendez PA, Hansen L, Lee J, et al. Local and systemic insulin resistance resulting from hepatic activation of IKK-beta and NF-kappaB. *Nat Med.* (2005) 11:183–90. doi: 10.1038/nm1166
51. Mas E, Danjoux M, Garcia V, Carpentier S, Segui B, Levade T. IL-6 deficiency attenuates murine diet-induced non-alcoholic steatohepatitis. *PLoS ONE.* (2009) 4:e7929. doi: 10.1371/journal.pone.0007929
52. Papanicolaou DA, Wilder RL, Manolagas SC, Chrousos GP. The pathophysiologic roles of interleukin-6 in human disease. *Ann Intern Med.* (1998) 128:127–37. doi: 10.7326/0003-4819-128-2-199801150-00009
53. Ray A, Tatter SB, Santhanam U, Helfgott DC, May LT, Sehgal PB. Regulation of expression of interleukin-6. Molecular and clinical studies. *Ann N Y Acad Sci.* (1989) 557:353–61; discussion 61–2. doi: 10.1111/j.1749-6632.1989.tb24028.x
54. Brass EP, Vetter WH. Interleukin-6, but not tumour necrosis factor-alpha, increases lipogenesis in rat hepatocyte primary cultures. *Biochem J.* (1994) 301 (Pt 1):193–7. doi: 10.1042/bj3010193
55. Fernandez-Real JM, Lopez-Bermejo A, Ricart W. Cross-talk between iron metabolism and diabetes. *Diabetes.* (2002) 51:2348–54. doi: 10.2337/diabetes.51.8.2348
56. Wellen KE, Hotamisligil GS. Obesity-induced inflammatory changes in adipose tissue. *J Clin Invest.* (2003) 112:1785–8. doi: 10.1172/JCI20514
57. Senn JJ, Klover PJ, Nowak IA, Mooney RA. Interleukin-6 induces cellular insulin resistance in hepatocytes. *Diabetes.* (2002) 51:3391–9. doi: 10.2337/diabetes.51.12.3391
58. Bastard JP, Maachi M, Lagathu C, Kim MJ, Caron M, Vidal H, et al. Recent advances in the relationship between obesity, inflammation, and insulin resistance. *Eur Cytokine Netw.* (2006) 17:4–12.
59. Kugelmas M, Hill DB, Vivian B, Marsano L, McClain CJ. Cytokines and NASH: a pilot study of the effects of lifestyle modification and vitamin E. *Hepatology.* (2003) 38:413–9. doi: 10.1053/jhep.2003.50316
60. Haukeland JW, Damas JK, Konopski Z, Loberg EM, Haaland T, Goverud I, et al. Systemic inflammation in nonalcoholic fatty liver disease is characterized by elevated levels of CCL2. *J Hepatol.* (2006) 44:1167–74. doi: 10.1016/j.jhep.2006.02.011
61. Wieckowska A, Feldstein AE. Diagnosis of nonalcoholic fatty liver disease: invasive versus noninvasive. *Semin Liver Dis.* (2008) 28:386–95. doi: 10.1055/s-0028-1091983
62. Yamaguchi K, Itoh Y, Yokomizo C, Nishimura T, Niimi T, Fujii H, et al. Blockade of interleukin-6 signaling enhances hepatic steatosis but improves liver injury in methionine choline-deficient diet-fed mice. *Lab Invest.* (2010) 90:1169–78. doi: 10.1038/labinvest.2010.75
63. Harris HW, Grunfeld C, Feingold KR, Rapp JH. Human very low density lipoproteins and chylomicrons can protect against endotoxin-induced death in mice. *J Clin Invest.* (1990) 86:696–702. doi: 10.1172/JCI114765
64. Grunfeld C, Pang M, Doerrler W, Shigenaga JK, Jensen P, Feingold KR. Lipids, lipoproteins, triglyceride clearance, and cytokines in human immunodeficiency virus infection and the acquired immunodeficiency syndrome. *J Clin Endocrinol Metab.* (1992) 74:1045–52. doi: 10.1210/jcem.74.5.1373735
65. Borst SE. The role of TNF-alpha in insulin resistance. *Endocrine.* (2004) 23(2–3):177–82. doi: 10.1385/ENDO:23:2-3:177
66. Fon Tacer K, Kuzman D, Seliskar M, Pompon D, Rozman D. TNF-alpha interferes with lipid homeostasis and activates acute and proatherogenic processes. *Physiol Genomics.* (2007) 31:216–27. doi: 10.1152/physiolgenomics.00264.2006
67. Wullaert A, van Loo G, Heyninck K, Beyaert R. Hepatic tumor necrosis factor signaling and nuclear factor-kappaB: effects on liver homeostasis and beyond. *Endocr Rev.* (2007) 28:365–86. doi: 10.1210/er.2006-0031
68. Tomita K, Tamiya G, Ando S, Ohsumi K, Chiyo T, Mizutani A, et al. Tumour necrosis factor alpha signalling through activation of Kupffer cells plays an essential role in liver fibrosis of non-alcoholic steatohepatitis in mice. *Gut.* (2006) 55:415–24. doi: 10.1136/gut.2005.071118
69. Kakino S, Ohki T, Nakayama H, Yuan X, Otabe S, Hashinaga T, et al. Pivotal role of TNF-alpha in the development and progression of nonalcoholic fatty liver disease in a murine model. *Horm Metab Res.* (2018) 50:80–7. doi: 10.1055/s-0043-118666
70. Tan Q, Hu J, Yu X, Guan W, Lu H, Yu Y, et al. The role of IL-1 family members and kupffer cells in liver regeneration. *Biomed Res Int.* (2016) 2016:6495793. doi: 10.1155/2016/6495793
71. Negrin KA, Roth Flach RJ, DiStefano MT, Matevossian A, Friedline RH, Jung D, et al. IL-1 signaling in obesity-induced hepatic lipogenesis and steatosis. *PLoS ONE.* (2014) 9:e107265. doi: 10.1371/journal.pone.0107265
72. Garlanda C, Dinarello CA, Mantovani A. The interleukin-1 family: back to the future. *Immunity.* (2013) 39:1003–18. doi: 10.1016/j.immuni.2013.11.010
73. Meier RPH, Meyer J, Montanari E, Lacotte S, Balaphas A, Muller YD, et al. Interleukin-1 receptor antagonist modulates liver inflammation and fibrosis in mice in a model-dependent manner. *Int J Mol Sci.* (2019) 20:E1295. doi: 10.3390/ijms20061295
74. Gehrke N, Hovelmeyer N, Waisman A, Straub BK, Weinmann-Menke J, Worns MA, et al. Hepatocyte-specific deletion of IL1-RI attenuates liver injury by blocking IL-1 driven autoinflammation. *J Hepatol.* (2018) 68:986–95. doi: 10.1016/j.jhep.2018.01.008
75. Janssens S, Beyaert R. A universal role for MyD88 in TLR/IL-1R-mediated signaling. *Trends Biochem Sci.* (2002) 27:474–82. doi: 10.1016/S0968-0004(02)02145-X
76. Larsen CM, Faulenbach M, Vaag A, Volund A, Ehses JA, Seifert B, et al. Interleukin-1-receptor antagonist in type 2 diabetes mellitus. *N Engl J Med.* (2007) 356:1517–26. doi: 10.1056/NEJMoa065213
77. Gomez R, Villalvilla A, Largo R, Gualillo O, Herrero-Beaumont G. TLR4 signalling in osteoarthritis–finding targets for candidate DMOADs. *Nat Rev Rheumatol.* (2015) 11:159–70. doi: 10.1038/nrrheum.2014.209
78. Day CP, James OF. Steatohepatitis: a tale of two "hits"? *Gastroenterology.* (1998) 114:842–5. doi: 10.1016/S0016-5085(98)70599-2
79. Crosas-Molist E, Fabregat I. Role of NADPH oxidases in the redox biology of liver fibrosis. *Redox Biol.* (2015) 6:106–11. doi: 10.1016/j.redox.2015.07.005
80. Mukherjee R, Moreno-Fernandez ME, Giles DA, Cappelletti M, Stankiewicz TE, Chan CC, et al. Nicotinamide adenine dinucleotide phosphate (reduced) oxidase 2 modulates inflammatory vigor during nonalcoholic fatty liver disease progression in mice. *Hepatol Commun.* (2018) 2:546–60. doi: 10.1002/hep4.1162
81. Chapman NM, Shrestha S, Chi H. Metabolism in immune cell differentiation and function. *Adv Exp Med Biol.* (2017) 1011:1–85. doi: 10.1007/978-94-024-1170-6_1

82. Krzywinska E, Stockmann C. Hypoxia, metabolism and immune cell function. *Biomedicines.* (2018) 6:E56. doi: 10.3390/biomedicines6020056
83. Cirulli ET, Guo L, Leon Swisher C, Shah N, Huang L, Napier LA, et al. Profound perturbation of the metabolome in obesity is associated with health risk. *Cell Metab.* (2019) 29:488–500 e2. doi: 10.1016/j.cmet.2018.09.022
84. Reddy JK, Rao MS. Lipid metabolism and liver inflammation. II. Fatty liver disease and fatty acid oxidation. *Am J Physiol Gastrointest Liver Physiol.* (2006) 290:G852–8. doi: 10.1152/ajpgi.00521.2005
85. Reddy JK, Hashimoto T. Peroxisomal beta-oxidation and peroxisome proliferator-activated receptor alpha: an adaptive metabolic system. *Annu Rev Nutr.* (2001) 21:193–230. doi: 10.1146/annurev.nutr.21.1.193
86. Moreno-Fernandez ME, Giles DA, Stankiewicz TE, Sheridan R, Karns R, Cappelletti M, et al. Peroxisomal beta-oxidation regulates whole body metabolism, inflammatory vigor, and pathogenesis of nonalcoholic fatty liver disease. *JCI Insight.* (2018) 3:93626. doi: 10.1172/jci.insight.93626
87. Olefsky JM, Glass CK. Macrophages, inflammation, and insulin resistance. *Annu Rev Physiol.* (2010) 72:219–46. doi: 10.1146/annurev-physiol-021909-135846
88. Diskin C, Palsson-McDermott EM. Metabolic modulation in macrophage effector function. *Front Immunol.* (2018) 9:270. doi: 10.3389/fimmu.2018.00270
89. Wang X, de Carvalho Ribeiro M, Iracheta-Vellve A, Lowe P, Ambade A, Satishchandran A, et al. Macrophage-specific hypoxia-inducible factor-1alpha contributes to impaired autophagic flux in nonalcoholic steatohepatitis. *Hepatology.* (2019) 69:545–63. doi: 10.1002/hep.30215
90. Tannahill GM, Curtis AM, Adamik J, Palsson-McDermott EM, McGettrick AF, Goel G, et al. Succinate is an inflammatory signal that induces IL-1beta through HIF-1alpha. *Nature.* (2013) 496:238–42. doi: 10.1038/nature11986
91. Jha AK, Huang SC, Sergushichev A, Lampropoulou V, Ivanova Y, Loginicheva E, et al. Network integration of parallel metabolic and transcriptional data reveals metabolic modules that regulate macrophage polarization. *Immunity.* (2015) 42:419–30. doi: 10.1016/j.immuni.2015.02.005
92. Haschemi A, Kosma P, Gille L, Evans CR, Burant CF, Starkl P, et al. The sedoheptulose kinase CARKL directs macrophage polarization through control of glucose metabolism. *Cell Metab.* (2012) 15:813–26. doi: 10.1016/j.cmet.2012.04.023
93. Koo SJ, Szczesny B, Wan X, Putluri N, Garg NJ. Pentose phosphate shunt modulates reactive oxygen species and nitric oxide production controlling trypanosoma cruzi in macrophages. *Front Immunol.* (2018) 9:202. doi: 10.3389/fimmu.2018.00202
94. Pollak N, Dolle C, Ziegler M. The power to reduce: pyridine nucleotides–small molecules with a multitude of functions. *Biochem J.* (2007) 402:205–18. doi: 10.1042/BJ20061638
95. Ray PD, Huang BW, Tsuji Y. Reactive oxygen species (ROS) homeostasis and redox regulation in cellular signaling. *Cell Signal.* (2012) 24:981–90. doi: 10.1016/j.cellsig.2012.01.008
96. Baardman J, Verberk SGS, Prange KHM, van Weeghel M, van der Velden S, Ryan DG, et al. A Defective pentose phosphate pathway reduces inflammatory macrophage responses during hypercholesterolemia. *Cell Rep.* (2018) 25:2044–52 e5. doi: 10.1016/j.celrep.2018.10.092
97. Koh HJ, Lee SM, Son BG, Lee SH, Ryoo ZY, Chang KT, et al. Cytosolic NADP+-dependent isocitrate dehydrogenase plays a key role in lipid metabolism. *J Biol Chem.* (2004) 279:39968–74. doi: 10.1074/jbc.M402260200
98. Al-Dwairi A, Pabona JM, Simmen RC, Simmen FA. Cytosolic malic enzyme 1 (ME1) mediates high fat diet-induced adiposity, endocrine profile, and gastrointestinal tract proliferation-associated biomarkers in male mice. *PLoS ONE.* (2012) 7:e46716. doi: 10.1371/journal.pone.0046716
99. Chouchani ET, Pell VR, Gaude E, Aksentijevic D, Sundier SY, Robb EL, et al. Ischaemic accumulation of succinate controls reperfusion injury through mitochondrial ROS. *Nature.* (2014) 515:431–5. doi: 10.1038/nature13909
100. Postic C, Girard J. Contribution of *de novo* fatty acid synthesis to hepatic steatosis and insulin resistance: lessons from genetically engineered mice. *J Clin Invest.* (2008) 118:829–38. doi: 10.1172/JCI34275
101. Carmen GY, Victor SM. Signalling mechanisms regulating lipolysis. *Cell Signal.* (2006) 18:401–8. doi: 10.1016/j.cellsig.2005.08.009
102. Lewis GF, Carpentier A, Adeli K, Giacca A. Disordered fat storage and mobilization in the pathogenesis of insulin resistance and type 2 diabetes. *Endocr Rev.* (2002) 23:201–29. doi: 10.1210/edrv.23.2.0461
103. O'Neill LA, Kishton RJ, Rathmell J. A guide to immunometabolism for immunologists. *Nat Rev Immunol.* (2016) 16:553–65. doi: 10.1038/nri.2016.70
104. Ecker J, Liebisch G, Englmaier M, Grandl M, Robenek H, Schmitz G. Induction of fatty acid synthesis is a key requirement for phagocytic differentiation of human monocytes. *Proc Natl Acad Sci USA.* (2010) 107:7817–22. doi: 10.1073/pnas.0912059107
105. Wu X, Dong L, Lin X, Li J. Relevance of the NLRP3 Inflammasome in the pathogenesis of chronic liver disease. *Front Immunol.* (2017) 8:1728. doi: 10.3389/fimmu.2017.01728
106. Csak T, Ganz M, Pespisa J, Kodys K, Dolganiuc A, Szabo G. Fatty acid and endotoxin activate inflammasomes in mouse hepatocytes that release danger signals to stimulate immune cells. *Hepatology.* (2011) 54:133–44. doi: 10.1002/hep.24341
107. Wree A, McGeough MD, Pena CA, Schlattjan M, Li H, Inzaugarat ME, et al. NLRP3 inflammasome activation is required for fibrosis development in NAFLD. *J Mol Med.* (2014) 92:1069–82. doi: 10.1007/s00109-014-1170-1
108. Dixon LJ, Berk M, Thapaliya S, Papouchado BG, Feldstein AE. Caspase-1-mediated regulation of fibrogenesis in diet-induced steatohepatitis. *Lab Invest.* (2012) 92:713–23. doi: 10.1038/labinvest.2012.45
109. Miura K, Kodama Y, Inokuchi S, Schnabl B, Aoyama T, Ohnishi H, et al. Toll-like receptor 9 promotes steatohepatitis by induction of interleukin-1beta in mice. *Gastroenterology.* (2010) 139:323–34 e7. doi: 10.1053/j.gastro.2010.03.052
110. Wahli W, Michalik L. PPARs at the crossroads of lipid signaling and inflammation. *Trends Endocrinol Metab.* (2012) 23:351–63. doi: 10.1016/j.tem.2012.05.001
111. Yu K, Bayona W, Kallen CB, Harding HP, Ravera CP, McMahon G, et al. Differential activation of peroxisome proliferator-activated receptors by eicosanoids. *J Biol Chem.* (1995) 270:23975–83. doi: 10.1074/jbc.270.41.23975
112. Bjorndal B, Alteras EK, Lindquist C, Svardal A, Skorve J, Berge RK. Associations between fatty acid oxidation, hepatic mitochondrial function, and plasma acylcarnitine levels in mice. *Nutr Metab.* (2018) 15:10. doi: 10.1186/s12986-018-0241-7
113. Namgaladze D, Lips S, Leiker TJ, Murphy RC, Ekroos K, Ferreiros N, et al. Inhibition of macrophage fatty acid beta-oxidation exacerbates palmitate-induced inflammatory and endoplasmic reticulum stress responses. *Diabetologia.* (2014) 57:1067–77. doi: 10.1007/s00125-014-3173-4
114. O'Connor RS, Guo L, Ghassemi S, Snyder NW, Worth AJ, Weng L, et al. The CPT1a inhibitor, etomoxir induces severe oxidative stress at commonly used concentrations. *Sci Rep.* (2018) 8:6289. doi: 10.1038/s41598-018-24676-6
115. Pike LS, Smift AL, Croteau NJ, Ferrick DA, Wu M. Inhibition of fatty acid oxidation by etomoxir impairs NADPH production and increases reactive oxygen species resulting in ATP depletion and cell death in human glioblastoma cells. *Biochim Biophys Acta.* (2011) 1807:726–34. doi: 10.1016/j.bbabio.2010.10.022
116. Sheridan R, Lampe K, Shanmukhappa SK, Putnam P, Keddache M, Divanovic S, et al. Lampe1: an ENU-germline mutation causing spontaneous hepatosteatosis identified through targeted exon-enrichment and next-generation sequencing. *PLoS ONE.* (2011) 6:e21979. doi: 10.1371/journal.pone.0021979
117. Moffett JR, Namboodiri MA. Tryptophan and the immune response. *Immunol Cell Biol.* (2003) 81:247–65. doi: 10.1046/j.1440-1711.2003.t01-1-01177.x
118. Badawy AA, Namboodiri AM, Moffett JR. The end of the road for the tryptophan depletion concept in pregnancy and infection. *Clin Sci.* (2016) 130:1327–33. doi: 10.1042/CS20160153
119. McGaha TL, Huang L, Lemos H, Metz R, Mautino M, Prendergast GC, et al. Amino acid catabolism: a pivotal regulator of innate and adaptive immunity. *Immunol Rev.* (2012) 249:135–57. doi: 10.1111/j.1600-065X.2012.01149.x
120. Grohmann U, Bronte V. Control of immune response by amino acid metabolism. *Immunol Rev.* (2010) 236:243–64. doi: 10.1111/j.1600-065X.2010.00915.x

121. Hissong BD, Byrne GI, Padilla ML, Carlin JM. Upregulation of interferon-induced indoleamine 2,3-dioxygenase in human macrophage cultures by lipopolysaccharide, muramyl tripeptide, and interleukin-1. *Cell Immunol.* (1995) 160:264–9. doi: 10.1016/0008-8749(95)80037-J
122. Hu B, Hissong BD, Carlin JM. Interleukin-1 enhances indoleamine 2,3-dioxygenase activity by increasing specific mRNA expression in human mononuclear phagocytes. *J Interferon Cytokine Res.* (1995) 15:617–24. doi: 10.1089/jir.1995.15.617
123. Hissong BD, Carlin JM. Potentiation of interferon-induced indoleamine 2,3-dioxygenase mRNA in human mononuclear phagocytes by lipopolysaccharide and interleukin-1. *J Interferon Cytokine Res.* (1997) 17:387–93. doi: 10.1089/jir.1997.17.387
124. Carlin JM, Borden EC, Sondel PM, Byrne GI. Interferon-induced indoleamine 2,3-dioxygenase activity in human mononuclear phagocytes. *J Leukoc Biol.* (1989) 45:29–34. doi: 10.1002/jlb.45.1.29
125. Currier AR, Ziegler MH, Riley MM, Babcock TA, Telbis VP, Carlin JM. Tumor necrosis factor-alpha and lipopolysaccharide enhance interferon-induced antichlamydial indoleamine dioxygenase activity independently. *J Interferon Cytokine Res.* (2000) 20:369–76. doi: 10.1089/107999000312306
126. Wolowczuk I, Hennart B, Leloire A, Bessede A, Soichot M, Taront S, et al. Tryptophan metabolism activation by indoleamine 2,3-dioxygenase in adipose tissue of obese women: an attempt to maintain immune homeostasis and vascular tone. *Am J Physiol Regul Integr Comp Physiol.* (2012) 303:R135–43. doi: 10.1152/ajpregu.00373.2011
127. Nagano J, Shimizu M, Hara T, Shirakami Y, Kochi T, Nakamura N, et al. Effects of indoleamine 2,3-dioxygenase deficiency on high-fat diet-induced hepatic inflammation. *PLoS ONE.* (2013) 8:e73404. doi: 10.1371/journal.pone.0073404
128. Laurans L, Venteclef N, Haddad Y, Chajadine M, Alzaid F, Metghalchi S, et al. Genetic deficiency of indoleamine 2,3-dioxygenase promotes gut microbiota-mediated metabolic health. *Nat Med.* (2018) 24:1113–20. doi: 10.1038/s41591-018-0060-4
129. Ritze Y, Bardos G, Hubert A, Bohle M, Bischoff SC. Effect of tryptophan supplementation on diet-induced non-alcoholic fatty liver disease in mice. *Br J Nutr.* (2014) 112:1–7. doi: 10.1017/S0007114514000440
130. Cichoz-Lach H, Celinski K, Konturek PC, Konturek SJ, Slomka M. The effects of L-tryptophan and melatonin on selected biochemical parameters in patients with steatohepatitis. *J Physiol Pharmacol.* (2010) 61:577–80.
131. Celinski K, Konturek PC, Slomka M, Cichoz-Lach H, Brzozowski T, Konturek SJ, et al. Effects of treatment with melatonin and tryptophan on liver enzymes, parameters of fat metabolism and plasma levels of cytokines in patients with non-alcoholic fatty liver disease—14 months follow up. *J Physiol Pharmacol.* (2014) 65:75–82.
132. Munder M, Eichmann K, Modolell M. Alternative metabolic states in murine macrophages reflected by the nitric oxide synthase/arginase balance: competitive regulation by CD4+ T cells correlates with Th1/Th2 phenotype. *J Immunol.* (1998) 160:5347–54.
133. Shearer JD, Richards JR, Mills CD, Caldwell MD. Differential regulation of macrophage arginine metabolism: a proposed role in wound healing. *Am J Physiol.* (1997) 272:E181–90. doi: 10.1152/ajpendo.1997.272.2.E181
134. Mattila JT, Ojo OO, Kepka-Lenhart D, Marino S, Kim JH, Eum SY, et al. Microenvironments in tuberculous granulomas are delineated by distinct populations of macrophage subsets and expression of nitric oxide synthase and arginase isoforms. *J Immunol.* (2013) 191:773–84. doi: 10.4049/jimmunol.1300113
135. Qualls JE, Subramanian C, Rafi W, Smith AM, Balouzian L, DeFreitas AA, et al. Sustained generation of nitric oxide and control of mycobacterial infection requires argininosuccinate synthase 1. *Cell Host Microbe.* (2012) 12:313–23. doi: 10.1016/j.chom.2012.07.012
136. Murray PJ, Allen JE, Biswas SK, Fisher EA, Gilroy DW, Goerdt S, et al. Macrophage activation and polarization: nomenclature and experimental guidelines. *Immunity.* (2014) 41:14–20. doi: 10.1016/j.immuni.2014.06.008
137. Modolell M, Corraliza IM, Link F, Soler G, Eichmann K. Reciprocal regulation of the nitric oxide synthase/arginase balance in mouse bone marrow-derived macrophages by TH1 and TH2 cytokines. *Eur J Immunol.* (1995) 25:1101–4. doi: 10.1002/eji.1830250436
138. Munder M, Eichmann K, Moran JM, Centeno F, Soler G, Modolell M. Th1/Th2-regulated expression of arginase isoforms in murine macrophages and dendritic cells. *J Immunol.* (1999) 163:3771–7.
139. Rutschman R, Lang R, Hesse M, Ihle JN, Wynn TA, Murray PJ. Cutting edge: Stat6-dependent substrate depletion regulates nitric oxide production. *J Immunol.* (2001) 166:2173–7. doi: 10.4049/jimmunol.166.4.2173
140. Barron L, Smith AM, El Kasmi KC, Qualls JE, Huang X, Cheever A, et al. Role of arginase 1 from myeloid cells in th2-dominated lung inflammation. *PLoS ONE.* (2013) 8:e61961. doi: 10.1371/journal.pone.0061961
141. Duque-Correa MA, Kuhl AA, Rodriguez PC, Zedler U, Schommer-Leitner S, Rao M, et al. Macrophage arginase-1 controls bacterial growth and pathology in hypoxic tuberculosis granulomas. *Proc Natl Acad Sci USA.* (2014) 111:E4024–32. doi: 10.1073/pnas.1408839111
142. Navarro LA, Wree A, Povero D, Berk MP, Eguchi A, Ghosh S, et al. Arginase 2 deficiency results in spontaneous steatohepatitis: a novel link between innate immune activation and hepatic *de novo* lipogenesis. *J Hepatol.* (2015) 62:412–20. doi: 10.1016/j.jhep.2014.09.015
143. Liu C, Rajapakse AG, Riedo E, Fellay B, Bernhard MC, Montani JP, et al. Targeting arginase-II protects mice from high-fat-diet-induced hepatic steatosis through suppression of macrophage inflammation. *Sci Rep.* (2016) 6:20405. doi: 10.1038/srep20405
144. Pasarin M, La Mura V, Gracia-Sancho J, Garcia-Caldero H, Rodriguez-Vilarrupla A, Garcia-Pagan JC, et al. Sinusoidal endothelial dysfunction precedes inflammation and fibrosis in a model of NAFLD. *PLoS ONE.* (2012) 7:e32785. doi: 10.1371/journal.pone.0032785
145. Sellmann C, Degen C, Jin CJ, Nier A, Engstler AJ, Hasan Alkhatib D, et al. Oral arginine supplementation protects female mice from the onset of non-alcoholic steatohepatitis. *Amino Acids.* (2017) 49:1215–25. doi: 10.1007/s00726-017-2423-4
146. Rapovy SM, Zhao J, Bricker RL, Schmidt SM, Setchell KD, Qualls JE. Differential Requirements for L-Citrulline and L-Arginine during antimycobacterial macrophage activity. *J Immunol.* (2015) 195:3293–300. doi: 10.4049/jimmunol.1500800
147. Lange SM, McKell MC, Schmidt SM, Zhao J, Crowther RR, Green LC, et al. L-arginine synthesis from l-citrulline in myeloid cells drives host defense against mycobacteria *in vivo*. *J Immunol.* (2019) 202:1747–54. doi: 10.4049/jimmunol.1801569
148. Erez A, Nagamani SC, Shchelochkov OA, Premkumar MH, Campeau PM, Chen Y, et al. Requirement of argininosuccinate lyase for systemic nitric oxide production. *Nat Med.* (2011) 17:1619–26. doi: 10.1038/nm.2544
149. MacMicking JD, Nathan C, Hom G, Chartrain N, Fletcher DS, Trumbauer M, et al. Altered responses to bacterial infection and endotoxic shock in mice lacking inducible nitric oxide synthase. *Cell.* (1995) 81:641–50. doi: 10.1016/0092-8674(95)90085-3
150. El Kasmi KC, Qualls JE, Pesce JT, Smith AM, Thompson RW, Henao-Tamayo M, et al. Toll-like receptor-induced arginase 1 in macrophages thwarts effective immunity against intracellular pathogens. *Nat Immunol.* (2008) 9:1399–406. doi: 10.1038/ni.1671
151. Failla ML. Trace elements and host defense: recent advances and continuing challenges. *J Nutr.* (2003) 133(5 Suppl 1):1443S–7S. doi: 10.1093/jn/133.5.1443S
152. Aigner E, Theurl I, Haufe H, Seifert M, Hohla F, Scharinger L, et al. Copper availability contributes to iron perturbations in human nonalcoholic fatty liver disease. *Gastroenterology.* (2008) 135:680–8. doi: 10.1053/j.gastro.2008.04.007
153. Aigner E, Weiss G, Datz C. Dysregulation of iron and copper homeostasis in nonalcoholic fatty liver. *World J Hepatol.* (2015) 7:177–88. doi: 10.4254/wjh.v7.i2.177
154. Feldman A, Aigner E, Weghuber D, Paulmichl K. The Potential role of iron and copper in pediatric obesity and nonalcoholic fatty liver disease. *Biomed Res Int.* (2015) 2015:287401. doi: 10.1155/2015/287401
155. Tarantino G, Porcu C, Arciello M, Andreozzi P, Balsano C. Prediction of carotid intima-media thickness in obese patients with low prevalence of comorbidities by serum copper bioavailability. *J Gastroenterol Hepatol.* (2018) 33:1511–7. doi: 10.1111/jgh.14104
156. Turlin B, Mendler MH, Moirand R, Guyader D, Guillygomarc'h A, Deugnier Y. Histologic features of the liver in insulin resistance-associated iron overload. A study of 139 patients. *Am J Clin Pathol.* (2001) 116:263–70. doi: 10.1309/WWNE-KW2C-4KTW-PTJ5
157. Handa P, Thomas S, Morgan-Stevenson V, Maliken BD, Gochanour E, Boukhar S, et al. Iron alters macrophage polarization status and leads

to steatohepatitis and fibrogenesis. *J Leukoc Biol.* (2019) 105:1015–26. doi: 10.1002/JLB.3A0318-108R

158. Handa P, Vemulakonda AL, Maliken BD, Morgan-Stevenson V, Nelson JE, Dhillon BK, et al. Differences in hepatic expression of iron, inflammation and stress-related genes in patients with nonalcoholic steatohepatitis. *Ann Hepatol.* (2017) 16:77–85. doi: 10.5604/16652681.1226818
159. Sharp P. The molecular basis of copper and iron interactions. *Proc Nutr Soc.* (2004) 63:563–9. doi: 10.1079/PNS2004386
160. Himoto T, Masaki T. Associations between zinc deficiency and metabolic abnormalities in patients with chronic liver disease. *Nutrients.* (2018) 10:88. doi: 10.3390/nu10010088
161. Trayhurn P. Hypoxia and adipose tissue function and dysfunction in obesity. *Physiol Rev.* (2013) 93:1–21. doi: 10.1152/physrev.00017.2012
162. Ghaben AL, Scherer PE. Adipogenesis and metabolic health. *Nat Rev Mol Cell Biol.* (2019) 20:242–58. doi: 10.1038/s41580-018-0093-z
163. Sarantopoulos CN, Banyard DA, Ziegler ME, Sun B, Shaterian A, Widgerow AD. Elucidating the preadipocyte and its role in adipocyte formation: a comprehensive review. *Stem Cell Rev Rep.* (2018) 14:27–42. doi: 10.1007/s12015-017-9774-9
164. Langin D, Dicker A, Tavernier G, Hoffstedt J, Mairal A, Ryden M, et al. Adipocyte lipases and defect of lipolysis in human obesity. *Diabetes.* (2005) 54:3190–7. doi: 10.2337/diabetes.54.11.3190
165. Ebbert JO, Jensen MD. Fat depots, free fatty acids, and dyslipidemia. *Nutrients.* (2013) 5:498–508. doi: 10.3390/nu5020498
166. Frayn KN. Adipose tissue as a buffer for daily lipid flux. *Diabetologia.* (2002) 45:1201–10. doi: 10.1007/s00125-002-0873-y
167. Kamada Y, Takehara T, Hayashi N. Adipocytokines and liver disease. *J Gastroenterol.* (2008) 43:811–22. doi: 10.1007/s00535-008-2213-6
168. O'Rourke RW, White AE, Metcalf MD, Olivas AS, Mitra P, Larison WG, et al. Hypoxia-induced inflammatory cytokine secretion in human adipose tissue stromovascular cells. *Diabetologia.* (2011) 54:1480–90. doi: 10.1007/s00125-011-2103-y
169. Lefere S, Van de Velde F, Devisscher L, Bekaert M, Raevens S, Verhelst X, et al. Serum vascular cell adhesion molecule-1 predicts significant liver fibrosis in non-alcoholic fatty liver disease. *Int J Obes.* (2017) 41:1207–13. doi: 10.1038/ijo.2017.102
170. van Herpen NA, Schrauwen-Hinderling VB. Lipid accumulation in non-adipose tissue and lipotoxicity. *Physiol Behav.* (2008) 94:231–41. doi: 10.1016/j.physbeh.2007.11.049
171. Ranjit S, Boutet E, Gandhi P, Prot M, Tamori Y, Chawla A, et al. Regulation of fat specific protein 27 by isoproterenol and TNF-alpha to control lipolysis in murine adipocytes. *J Lipid Res.* (2011) 52:221–36. doi: 10.1194/jlr.M008771
172. Sung CK, She H, Xiong S, Tsukamoto H. Tumor necrosis factor-alpha inhibits peroxisome proliferator-activated receptor gamma activity at a posttranslational level in hepatic stellate cells. *Am J Physiol Gastrointest Liver Physiol.* (2004) 286:G722–9. doi: 10.1152/ajpgi.00411.2003
173. Stephens JM, Lee J, Pilch PF. Tumor necrosis factor-alpha-induced insulin resistance in 3T3-L1 adipocytes is accompanied by a loss of insulin receptor substrate-1 and GLUT4 expression without a loss of insulin receptor-mediated signal transduction. *J Biol Chem.* (1997) 272:971–6. doi: 10.1074/jbc.272.2.971
174. Ruan H, Hacohen N, Golub TR, Van Parijs L, Lodish HF. Tumor necrosis factor-alpha suppresses adipocyte-specific genes and activates expression of preadipocyte genes in 3T3-L1 adipocytes: nuclear factor-kappaB activation by TNF-alpha is obligatory. *Diabetes.* (2002) 51:1319–36. doi: 10.2337/diabetes.51.5.1319
175. Tilg H, Moschen AR. Adipocytokines: mediators linking adipose tissue, inflammation and immunity. *Nat Rev Immunol.* (2006) 6:772–83. doi: 10.1038/nri1937
176. Chan CC, Damen M, Alarcon PC, Sanchez-Gurmaches J, Divanovic S. Inflammation and immunity: from an adipocyte's perspective. *J Interferon Cytokine Res.* (2019) 39:459–71. doi: 10.1089/jir.2019.0014
177. Zhou YJ, Zhou H, Li Y, Song YL. NOD1 activation induces innate immune responses and insulin resistance in human adipocytes. *Diabetes Metab.* (2012) 38:538–43. doi: 10.1016/j.diabet.2012.08.001
178. Ballak DB, van Diepen JA, Moschen AR, Jansen HJ, Hijmans A, Groenhof GJ, et al. IL-37 protects against obesity-induced inflammation and insulin resistance. *Nat Commun.* (2014) 5:4711. doi: 10.1038/ncomms5711
179. Zhou YJ, Liu C, Li CL, Song YL, Tang YS, Zhou H, et al. Increased NOD1, but not NOD2, activity in subcutaneous adipose tissue from patients with metabolic syndrome. *Obesity.* (2015) 23:1394–400. doi: 10.1002/oby.21113
180. Kopp A, Buechler C, Neumeier M, Weigert J, Aslanidis C, Scholmerich J, et al. Innate immunity and adipocyte function: ligand-specific activation of multiple Toll-like receptors modulates cytokine, adipokine, and chemokine secretion in adipocytes. *Obesity.* (2009) 17:648–56. doi: 10.1038/oby.2008.607
181. Marra F, Svegliati-Baroni G. Lipotoxicity and the gut-liver axis in NASH pathogenesis. *J Hepatol.* (2018) 68:280–95. doi: 10.1016/j.jhep.2017.11.014
182. Frasca D, Diaz A, Romero M, Thaller S, Blomberg BB. Secretion of autoimmune antibodies in the human subcutaneous adipose tissue. *PLoS ONE.* (2018) 13:e0197472. doi: 10.1371/journal.pone.0197472
183. Yokota T, Oritani K, Takahashi I, Ishikawa J, Matsuyama A, Ouchi N, et al. Adiponectin, a new member of the family of soluble defense collagens, negatively regulates the growth of myelomonocytic progenitors and the functions of macrophages. *Blood.* (2000) 96:1723–32. doi: 10.1182/blood.V96.5.1723
184. Hui X, Gu P, Zhang J, Nie T, Pan Y, Wu D, et al. Adiponectin enhances cold-induced browning of subcutaneous adipose tissue via promoting M2 macrophage proliferation. *Cell Metab.* (2015) 22:279–90. doi: 10.1016/j.cmet.2015.06.004
185. Luo Y, Liu M. Adiponectin: a versatile player of innate immunity. *J Mol Cell Biol.* (2016) 8:120–8. doi: 10.1093/jmcb/mjw012
186. Lappas M, Yee K, Permezel M, Rice GE. Release and regulation of leptin, resistin and adiponectin from human placenta, fetal membranes, and maternal adipose tissue and skeletal muscle from normal and gestational diabetes mellitus-complicated pregnancies. *J Endocrinol.* (2005) 186:457–65. doi: 10.1677/joe.1.06227
187. Tsatsanis C, Zacharioudaki V, Androulidaki A, Dermitzaki E, Charalampopoulos I, Minas V, et al. Peripheral factors in the metabolic syndrome: the pivotal role of adiponectin. *Ann N Y Acad Sci.* (2006) 1083:185–95. doi: 10.1196/annals.1367.013
188. Sumida Y, Yoneda M. Current and future pharmacological therapies for NAFLD/NASH. *J Gastroenterol.* (2018) 53:362–76. doi: 10.1007/s00535-017-1415-1
189. Munteanu MA, Nagy GA, Mircea PA. Current Management of NAFLD. *Clujul Med.* (2016) 89:19–23. doi: 10.15386/cjmed-539
190. Friedman SL, Neuschwander-Tetri BA, Rinella M, Sanyal AJ. Mechanisms of NAFLD development and therapeutic strategies. *Nat Med.* (2018) 24:908–22. doi: 10.1038/s41591-018-0104-9
191. Wang CH, Weisel RD, Liu PP, Fedak PW, Verma S. Glitazones and heart failure: critical appraisal for the clinician. *Circulation.* (2003) 107:1350–4. doi: 10.1161/01.CIR.0000054675.30348.9A
192. Nesto RW, Bell D, Bonow RO, Fonseca V, Grundy SM, Horton ES, et al. Thiazolidinedione use, fluid retention, and congestive heart failure: a consensus statement from the American Heart Association and American Diabetes Association. *Diabetes Care.* (2004) 27:256–63. doi: 10.2337/diacare.27.1.256
193. Komiya C, Tsuchiya K, Shiba K, Miyachi Y, Furuke S, Shimazu N, et al. Ipragliflozin improves hepatic steatosis in obese mice and liver dysfunction in type 2 diabetic patients irrespective of body weight reduction. *PLoS ONE.* (2016) 11:e0151511. doi: 10.1371/journal.pone.0151511
194. Takase T, Nakamura A, Miyoshi H, Yamamoto C, Atsumi T. Amelioration of fatty liver index in patients with type 2 diabetes on ipragliflozin: an association with glucose-lowering effects. *Endocr J.* (2017) 64:363–7. doi: 10.1507/endocrj.EJ16-0295
195. Brenner C, Galluzzi L, Kepp O, Kroemer G. Decoding cell death signals in liver inflammation. *J Hepatol.* (2013) 59:583–94. doi: 10.1016/j.jhep.2013.03.033
196. Wang PX, Ji YX, Zhang XJ, Zhao LP, Yan ZZ, Zhang P, et al. Targeting CASP8 and FADD-like apoptosis regulator ameliorates nonalcoholic steatohepatitis in mice and nonhuman primates. *Nat Med.* (2017) 23:439–49. doi: 10.1038/nm.4290
197. Yamamoto E, Dong YF, Kataoka K, Yamashita T, Tokutomi Y, Matsuba S, et al. Olmesartan prevents cardiovascular injury and hepatic steatosis in obesity and diabetes, accompanied by apoptosis

signal regulating kinase-1 inhibition. *Hypertension.* (2008) 52:573–80. doi: 10.1161/HYPERTENSIONAHA.108.112292

198. Farrell G, Schattenberg JM, Leclercq I, Yeh MM, Goldin R, Teoh N, et al. Mouse models of nonalcoholic steatohepatitis: toward optimization of their relevance to human nonalcoholic steatohepatitis. *Hepatology.* (2019) 69:2241–57. doi: 10.1002/hep.30333
199. Loomba R, Lawitz E, Mantry PS, Jayakumar S, Caldwell SH, Arnold H, et al. The ASK1 inhibitor selonsertib in patients with nonalcoholic steatohepatitis: a randomized, phase 2 trial. *Hepatology.* (2018) 67:549–59. doi: 10.1002/hep.29514
200. Giles DA, Moreno-Fernandez ME, Stankiewicz TE, Graspeuntner S, Cappelletti M, Wu D, et al. Thermoneutral housing exacerbates nonalcoholic fatty liver disease in mice and allows for sex-independent disease modeling. *Nat Med.* (2017) 23:829–38. doi: 10.1038/nm.4346
201. Yanguas SC, Cogliati B, Willebrords J, Maes M, Colle I, van den Bossche B, et al. Experimental models of liver fibrosis. *Arch Toxicol.* (2016) 90:1025–48. doi: 10.1007/s00204-015-1543-4

14

Compartmentalization of Immune Response and Microbial Translocation in Decompensated Cirrhosis

Camila Alvarez-Silva[1†], *Robert Schierwagen*[2,3†], *Alessandra Pohlmann*[3†], *Fernando Magdaleno*[3], *Frank E. Uschner*[2,3], *Patrick Ryan*[3], *Maria J. G. T. Vehreschild*[4], *Joan Claria*[5], *Eicke Latz*[6,7,8,9], *Benjamin Lelouvier*[10], *Manimozhiyan Arumugam*[1,11*] and *Jonel Trebicka*[2,3,5,11,12*]

[1] Novo Nordisk Foundation Center for Basic Metabolic Research, Faculty of Health and Medical Sciences, University of Copenhagen, Copenhagen, Denmark, [2] Department of Internal Medicine I, Goethe University Clinic Frankfurt, Frankfurt, Germany, [3] Department of Internal Medicine I, University of Bonn, Bonn, Germany, [4] Medical Clinic II, University Center for Infectious Diseases, University Hospital Frankfurt, Frankfurt, Germany, [5] European Foundation for the Study of Chronic Liver Failure, Barcelona, Spain, [6] Institute of Innate Immunity, University of Bonn, Bonn, Germany, [7] Division of Infectious Diseases and Immunology, University of Massachusetts Medical School, Worcester, MA, United States, [8] German Center for Neurodegenerative Diseases (DZNE), Bonn, Germany, [9] Centre for Inflammation Research, Norwegian University of Science and Technology, Trondheim, Norway, [10] Vaiomer, Labège, France, [11] Department of Gastroenterology and Hepatology, Odense University Hospital, Odense, Denmark, [12] Institute for Bioengineering of Catalonia, Barcelona, Spain

***Correspondence:**
Manimozhiyan Arumugam
arumugam@sund.ku.dk
Jonel Trebicka
jonel.trebicka@kgu.de

†These authors share first authorship

Background: Acquired dysfunctional immunity in cirrhosis predisposes patients to frequent bacterial infections, especially spontaneous bacterial peritonitis (SBP), leading to systemic inflammation that is associated with poor outcome. But systemic inflammation can also be found in the absence of a confirmed infection. Detection of bacterial DNA has been investigated as a marker of SBP and as a predictor of prognosis. Data is, however, contradictory. Here we investigated whether levels of IL-6 and IL-8 putatively produced by myeloid cells in ascites are associated with systemic inflammation and whether inflammation depends on the presence of specific bacterial DNA.

Methods and Materials: We enrolled 33 patients with decompensated liver cirrhosis from whom we collected paired samples of blood and ascites. IL-6 and IL-8 were measured in serum samples of all patients using ELISA. In a subset of 10 representative patients, bacterial DNA was extracted from ascites and whole blood, followed by 16S rRNA gene amplicon sequencing.

Results: There were significantly higher levels of IL-6 in ascites fluid compared to blood samples in all patients. Interestingly, IL-6 levels in blood correlated tightly with disease severity and surrogates of systemic inflammation, while IL-6 levels in ascites did not. Moreover, patients with higher blood CRP levels showed greater SBP prevalence compared to patients with lower levels, despite similar positive culture results. Bacterial richness was also significantly higher in ascites compared to the corresponding patient blood. We identified differences in microbial composition and diversity between ascites and blood, but no tight relationship with surrogates of systemic inflammation could be observed.

Discussion: In decompensated cirrhosis, markers of systemic inflammation and microbiota composition seem to be dysregulated in ascites and blood. While a relationship between systemic inflammation and microbiota composition seems to exist in blood, this is not the case for ascites in our hands. These data may suggest compartmentalization of the immune response and interaction of the latter with the microbiota especially in the blood compartment.

Keywords: microbiome, systemic inflammation, myeloid cells, cirrhosis, ascites, cytokines, acute-on-chronic liver failure

INTRODUCTION

Acquired dysfunctional immunity in cirrhosis predisposes patients to frequent bacterial infections contributing to disease progression and may lead to the development of acute-on-chronic liver failure (ACLF) (1). Especially, spontaneous bacterial peritonitis (SBP) is one of the most frequent infections in cirrhosis and therefore a trigger for ACLF (2). Interestingly, SBP is defined by the number of granulocytes in ascites and not by cultural detection of bacteria (3). This is because many patients with SBP show negative bacterial cultivation from ascites, while in many other patients, viable bacteria can be cultivated in the absence of peritonitis, so-called bacterascites (3). Lack of bacterial cultivation in the presence of SBP can be explained by the concept of dormant microbiota, meaning that bacteria can reside inside circulating and resident immune cells but cannot be cultured and hence detected (4).

The source of infection, especially in the case of SBP, is suspected to be bacterial translocation from the gut (2), which is facilitated by impaired intestinal defense and increased intestinal permeability, processes which are correlated with the stage of cirrhosis (5). Not only viable bacteria (1, 6), but also bacterial components broadly termed pathogen-associated molecular patterns (PAMPs) may induce an immune response and aggravate systemic inflammation (2). As a consequence, the presence of circulating bacterial DNA reflects bacterial translocation in cirrhosis. However, the relationship of bacterial DNA with systemic inflammation is still controversially discussed (7, 8). PAMP-associated immune response requires recognition by innate immune cells and is reflected by synthesis and secretion of cytokines. Especially levels of the cytokines IL-6 and IL-8 are closely related to ACLF and clinical outcome (9). At the same time, the antibacterial capacity of myeloid cells and myelopoiesis is impaired during decompensation and ACLF (10, 11). Interestingly, these effects are not only induced by PAMPs (deriving from pathogens), but in general by bacterial-derived molecules, so-called microbe-associated molecular patterns (MAMPs).

Recent data from our group suggest that specific circulating bacteria or MAMPs in blood are associated with myeloid cell dysregulation and systemic inflammation (12). Therefore, a specific microbial DNA may be more crucial than just detecting any bacterial DNA in circulation. In ascites, the detection of bacterial DNA in ascites does not seem to correlate with SBP or clinical signs of infection (13). Therefore, the question remains, whether specific bacteria in ascites lead to myeloid cell activation with subsequent cytokine release and a systemic inflammatory response. To address this question, we investigated whether the representative cytokine (IL-6, IL-8) levels produced by myeloid cells in ascites reflect systemic inflammation. Moreover, we compared the levels of cytokines in paired ascites and blood samples, together with the general bacterial composition and specific species abundances of the microbiota estimated by 16S ribosomal RNA gene sequencing. Our study focused not only on common pathogens but also on the role of MAMPs in activating myeloid cells of the innate immune response. We hypothesize that DNA from specific bacterial species, but not any bacterial DNA, induces an inflammatory response in cirrhotic patients.

MATERIALS AND METHODS

Patient Recruitment and Sample Collection

Ascites and blood were collected in 33 cirrhotic patients scheduled for paracentesis. Paracentesis was performed by international standards (14). The study was performed in accordance with the declaration of Helsinki and approved by the local ethics committee at the University of Bonn (Nr. 121/14). Patients gave their written informed consent.

Microbiological Analysis

Microbiological culture of blood and ascites was performed at the clinical microbiology department at the University of Bonn in accordance with Microbiology Procedures Quality Standards of the German Society for Hygiene and Microbiology (15, 16). Ten milliliters of peripheral whole blood or ascitic fluid were transferred into aerobic, anaerobic and fungal blood culture bottles and incubated for up to 5 days using the Bactex FX blood culture system as described previously (17). SBP was diagnosed based on a leucocyte count in ascites >250/μl (3).

Enzyme-Linked Immunosorbent Assay

Ascites and peripheral blood samples (serum, EDTA-plasma and whole-blood) were collected during paracentesis and stored immediately at −80°C until further use. Enzyme-linked immunosorbent assay for cytokines IL-6 and IL-8 (DY206 and DY208, respectively; R&D Systems Inc., Minneapolis, MN, USA) were performed according to the manufacturer's protocols. All samples were measured in duplicates.

16S Ribosomal RNA Gene Sequencing

For extraction of total DNA, 100 μl of whole blood or ascitic fluid were used. Samples were mechanically lysed two times for 30 s at 20 Hz in a bead beater (TissueLyser, Qiagen, Hilden, Germany) with 0.1 mm glass beads (MoBio, CA, USA). DNA extraction was performed using the NucleoSpin Blood Kit (Macherey-Nagel, Düren, Germany). Quality and quantity of extracted nucleic acids were controlled by gel electrophoresis. 16S rRNA gene V3-V4 hypervariable regions were amplified and quantified by qPCR, and sequenced using MiSeq technology (Illumina, San Diego, CA, USA) as described previously producing 2 × 300 bp paired-end reads (18, 19).

Bioinformatics and Statistical Analysis

Paired-ends reads were processed in DADA2 version 1.6.0 (20) using the following parameters: "trimLeft = 10, truncLen = (260;230), maxN = 0, maxEE = (2,5), minOverlap = 20, maxMismatch = 1, pool=TRUE." The resulting output was an amplicon sequence variant (ASV) table. The ASVs were mapped against SILVA database (21) release 128. Data analysis was performed in R version 3.5, using phyloseq package (22) version 1.24.2. Genus level relative abundances were generated by combining ASVs annotated with the same genus using phyloseq package. The alpha-diversity measures were calculated based on rarefied data at 6,000 reads/sample. Significant differences in alpha-diversity between ascites and blood samples as well as between samples with different inflammation status were determined using *t*-test.

Beta-diversity was calculated using unweighted and weighted UniFrac measures. Effects of different factors on beta-diversity were determined using Adonis Permutational Multivariate Analysis of Variance (PERMANOVA) test from the vegan package (23) version 2.5.2. For differential abundance analysis, we chose a *t*-test based on the evaluation using DAtest package (24) version 2.7.11, which showed that, compared with different statistical tests, *t*-test has the highest area under the curve (AUC = 0.608) while keeping the false discovery rate (FDR) under 0.05.

Statistical analysis of patient characteristics and clinical measures was performed using SPSS version 24 (IBM, Armonk, NY) and Mann–Whitney test for metric variables and Chi-square test for nominal variables. Receiver operator characteristic curve analysis was used to define a cut-off for CRP and divide the cohort into one group with low CRP profile and one group with high CRP profile. *P*-values were adjusted for multiple testing using Benjamini–Hochberg FDR procedure. An FDR-adjusted *P*-value below 0.05 was considered statistically significant.

RESULTS

General Description of the Cohort

General characteristics of the patients are summarized in **Table 1**. The cohort consists of patients with decompensated liver cirrhosis as reflected by the model for end-stage liver disease (MELD) and Child-Pugh (CHILD) scores, which assess severity of liver disease, prognosis and mortality. The median MELD score of 15 represents a value at which patients would benefit from liver transplantation. The median CHILD score of 10 is associated with a 1-year survival below 50%. Seventy-two percent of the patients (24/33) showed ACLF at baseline.

The median C-reactive protein (CRP) level of 48.8 mg/l in the blood were compatible with bacterial infections (upper limit of normal 5 mg/l), together with findings of SBP in 21% of the patients (**Table 1**). CRP performed well to detect SBP using receiver operator characteristic curve analysis (AUC = 0.901, $P \leq 0.001$). In blood cultures, we detected members of the bacterial genera *Enterococcus, Escherichia, Sporosarcina,* and *Staphylococcus* in five patients. Additionally, we detected *Candida* spp. in blood culture of one patient. In ascites, we detected the genera *Enterococcus, Serratia,* and *Staphylococcus* in five patients and *Candida* spp. in one patient. None of the patients presented with cultural evidence of bacteria in both, blood and ascites.

There was also evidence of systemic inflammation with elevated levels of cytokines IL-6 (and IL-8, although not statistically significant), which are mainly produced by myeloid cells. The median levels assessed by ELISA assays were 33.53 and 68.78 pg/ml, respectively (**Table 1**). Reported mean levels in healthy individuals are 1.46 and 12.9 pg/ml, respectively, assessed by the same technique (25, 26). Ascites fluid showed higher median levels of both cytokines, with an almost 20-fold increase of median IL-6 levels in ascites compared to blood from the same patient.

Differences in Patients With Systemic Inflammation

In order to decipher the role of systemic inflammation, we divided the cohort into two groups according to their CRP level. A cut-off of 25 mg/l (sensitivity = 1.0, specificity = 0.54 for detection of SBP) was used to divide the cohort into 12 patients with a low CRP profile and 21 patients with a high CRP profile. Patients with the high CRP profile showed higher MELD, CHILD, and Chronic Liver Failure Consortium (CLIF-C)-ACLF scores (**Table 1**; $P = 0.06$, $P = 0.03$, and $P = 0.002$, respectively). SBP was detected in 50% of the patients (7 out of 14) with the high CRP profile, but in none of 12 patients with the low CRP profile ($P = 0.02$). Therefore, the positive predictive value, the probability for patients with high CRP profile to have SBP, is 35%. In contrast, the negative predictive value, the chance for patients with low CRP profile to not have SBP, is 100%. A high negative predictive value in this regards is extremely important since CRP level may be elevated also in absence of infection. Furthermore, patients with the high CRP profile showed a significant increase in blood granulocyte counts ($P = 0.001$), leucocyte counts ($P = 0.004$), and IL-6 levels ($P = 0.002$). However, there was no difference in ascitic cytokine levels between these two groups (**Table 1**). Similarly, IL-6 levels in blood strongly correlate with MELD, CHILD score, and CLIF-C-ACLF score and surrogate markers of systemic inflammation (leucocytes and CRP). However, blood IL-8 levels only slightly reflected disease stage and did not correlate significantly with markers of inflammation (**Figure 1A**). Even though median cytokine levels were higher in ascites than

TABLE 1 | Patient characteristics.

	Parameters	All ($n = 33$)	Low CRP profile ($n = 12$)	High CRP profile ($n = 21$)	*P*
General characteristics	Sex (male/female)	23/10	8/4	15/6	0.78
	Age, years	57 (33–105)	53.5 (40.0–75.0)	60.0 (33.0–105.0)	0.19
	Etiology of cirrhosis (alcohol/viral/other)	18/8/7	8/4/0	10/4/7	0.08
	MELD	15.71 (3.66–39.65)	13.87 (9.79–38.25)	20.50 (3.66–39.65)	0.06
	CHILD	10 (7–15)	9 (7–13)	10 (7–15)	**0.03**
	ACLF (no/yes)	9/24	5/7	4/17	0.16
	CLIF-C-ACLF	57 (39–84)	44 (39–57)	60 (47–84)	**0.002**
	Esophageal varices (absent/small/large)	14/8/11	6/2/4	8/6/7	0.38
	Hepatic encephalopathy (absent/grade 1/grade 2/grade 3/grade 4)	22/4/3/2/2	11/1/0/0/0	11/3/3/2/2	0.20
	Hepatorenal syndrome (no/yes)	14/19	6/6	8/13	0.51
	Spontaneous bacterial peritonitis (no/yes)	26/7	12/0	14/7	**0.02**
	Blood culture (negative/positive/NA)	12/6/15	4/2/6	8/4/9	1.00
	Ascites culture (negative/positive/NA)	24/6/3	11/1/0	13/5/3	0.19
Laboratory blood	Creatinine [mg/dl]	1.40 (0.57–4.68)	1.30 (0.57–2.59)	1.58 (0.86–4.68)	0.10
	Platelets [10^6/l]	120 (7–685)	108 (38–235)	120 (7–685)	0.84
	INR	1.4 (1.0–5.5)	1.35 (1.00–2.10)	1.40 (1.00–5.50)	0.78
	Bilirubin [mg/dl]	2.08 (0.37–45.21)	1.92 (0.75–45.21)	3.20 (0.37–35.41)	0.81
	GGT [U/l]	152 (26–1,139)	139 (33–585)	181 (26–1,139)	0.76
	ALT [U/l]	32 (8–1,050)	49.5 (17.0–269.0)	30.0 (8.0–1050.0)	0.75
	CRP [mg/l]	48.8 (5.7–205.0)	13.55 (5.70–22.20)	60.20 (27.60–205.00)	**0.000**
	Granulocytes [10^6/l]	100 (10–1,070)	40 (10–170)	230 (10–1,070)	**0.001**
	Leucocytes [10^6/l]	9.81 (3.34–31.18)	7.01 (3.60–22.20)	15.09 (3.34–31.18)	**0.004**
	Monocytes [10^3/l]	1.09 (0.24–12.80)	0.86 (0.24–1.90)	1.13 (0.26–12.80)	0.43
	IL6 [pg/ml]	33.53 (3.63–684.84)	10.97 (3.95–236.71)	83.42 (3.63–684.84)	**0.002**
	IL8 [pg/ml]	68.78 (5.67–752.26)	43.76 (15.54–752.26)	77.84 (7.87–1487.36)	0.46
Laboratory ascites	Protein [g/l]	10 (1–44)	9.5 (4.0–19.0)	10.0 (1.0–44.0)	0.65
	Granulocytes [10^6/l]	48 (2–2,333)	48 (7–250)	48 (2–2,333)	0.97
	Leucocytes [10^3/l]	256 (11–3,031)	467 (52–887)	218 (11–3,031)	0.40
	Lymphocytes/Monocytes [10^3/l]	127 (5–740)	300 (39–740)	127 (5–698)	0.15
	IL6 [pg/ml]	642.67 (7.87–1487.36)	596.15 (109.56–1226.54)	653.58 (7.87–1487.36)	0.45
	IL8 [pg/ml]	83.75 (10.91–988.56)	44.91 (15.17–277.70)	95.55 (10.90–988.56)	0.15

Data are medians and (ranges). The results of Mann–Whitney test for metric variables and Chi-square test for nominal variables comparing patients with low CRP profile to those with high CRP profile are shown with P-value (significantly different comparisons are marked in bold).

in blood (**Figure 1B**), ascitic cytokine levels reflected neither disease severity nor systemic inflammation (**Figures 1A,C**). Therefore, ascites cytokine levels did not seem to be affected by systemic inflammation or by the presence of SBP, which was diagnosed in one third of the patients with the high CRP profile (**Figure 1C**).

The rate of positive blood cultures was identical in patients with the low and high CRP profile. There were three positive blood and three positive ascites cultures in patients with a high CRP against two positive blood and one positive ascites cultures in the patients with lower CRP values.

Characterizing the Microbiome in Ascites and Blood

We selected a subset of 10 representative patients (accounting for etiology and inflammation markers in ascites) from the whole cohort and performed 16S rRNA gene sequencing of ascites and blood to identify differences in microbial composition and diversity between ascites and blood. These 10 patients were also

TABLE 2 | Patient characteristics for the subpopulation in which 16S rRNA gene amplicon sequencing was performed in blood and ascites.

	Parameters	Low CRP profile ($n = 6$)	High CRP profile ($n = 4$)	P
General characteristics	Sex (male/female)	5/1	2/2	0.26
	Age, years	52.5 (40.0–67.0)	56.0 (33–76)	0.76
	Etiology of cirrhosis (alcohol/viral/other)	5/1/0	3/0/1	0.34
	MELD	10.26 (9.79–38.25)	18.72 (11.21–24.16)	0.17
	CHILD	9.0 (8.0–13.0)	9.5 (8.0–10.0)	0.91
	ACLF (no/yes)	4/2	1/3	0.20
	Esophageal varices (absent/small/large)	3/0/3	2/1/1	0.17
	Hepatic encephalopathy (absent/grade 1/grade 2/grade 3/grade 4)	5/1/0/0	3/1/0/0	0.34
	Hepatorenal syndrome (no/yes)	4/2	2/2	0.60
	Spontaneous bacterial peritonitis (no/yes)	6/0	3/1	0.20
	Blood culture (negative/positive/NA)	2/1/3	0/1/3	0.25
	Ascites culture (negative/positive/NA)	6/0/0	3/1/0	0.20
Laboratory blood	Creatinine [mg/dl]	0.98 (0.57–2.59)	2.27 (1.07–4.68)	0.17
	Platelets [10^6/l]	69.5 (38.0–235.0)	191.5 (123.5–237.5)	0.26
	INR	1.35 (1.00–2.10)	1.20 (1.00–1.20)	0.47
	Bilirubin [mg/dl]	2.78 (0.75–45.21)	1.54 (0.73–7.97)	0.61
	GGT [U/l]	226.0 (152.0–585.0)	149.5 (78.0–1139.0)	0.47
	CRP [mg/l]	14.4 (5.7–22.2)	94.6 (27.6–205.0)	**0.01**
	Leucocytes [10^6/l]	5.33 (3.60–9.07)	7.37 (6.59–17.30)	0.07
	Monocytes [10^3/l]	0.57 (0.24–0.87)	1.10 (0.73–1.17)	0.10
	IL6 [pg/ml]	8.32 (3.95–236.71)	81.66 (19.94–97.29)	0.39
	IL8 [pg/ml]	41.80 (15.54–752.26)	66.61 (25.08–192.48)	0.61
Laboratory ascites	Protein [g/l]	8 (5–17)	21 (10–44)	0.11
	Granulocytes [10^6/l]	18.5 (7–250)	24.0 (10.0–117.0)	0.91
	Leucocytes [10^3/l]	130.5 (52.0–824.0)	163.0 (47.0–480.0)	0.61
	Lymphocytes/Monocytes [10^3/l]	120.0 (39.0–740.0)	139.5 (37.0–363.0)	0.61
	IL6 [pg/ml]	757.19 (109.56–1226.54)	529.64 (7.87–816.83)	0.35
	IL8 [pg/ml]	29.93 (17.46–277.70)	116.82 (43.12–224.85)	0.17

Data are medians and (ranges). The results of Mann–Whitney test for metric variables and Chi-square test for nominal variables comparing patients with low CRP profile to those with high CRP profile are shown with P-value (significantly different comparisons are marked in bold).

divided into two groups based on CRP levels ($n = 4$ for high CRP profile and $n = 6$ for low CRP profile, see **Table 2**). Their disease profiles with regard to stage of liver cirrhosis and inflammatory markers in blood were comparable to those of the respective subgroups and also of the whole cohort.

Microbiota compositions at the phylum level were in line with previously reported bacterial compositions of ascites (27) and peripheral blood (12). The most abundant phylum detected in ascites samples was Proteobacteria (mean relative abundance 77.7%), followed by Firmicutes (9.4%), Actinobacteria (7.9%), Bacteroidetes (3.9%), and Gemmatimonadetes (0.6%) (**Figure 2**). The phylum composition was slightly different in the blood samples, with Proteobacteria accounting for 87.4% on average, while Actinobacteria, Firmicutes, and Bacteroidetes accounted for small proportions (5.3, 3.7, and 3.5, respectively; **Figure 2**). We identified 53 bacterial families in ascites and 48 families in blood samples. Among these, we found a set of six core families detected in all samples in both compartments: *Pseudomonadaceae*, *Oxalobacteriaceae*, *Neisseriaceae*, *Enterobacteriaceae*, *Sphingomonadaceae*, and *Moraxellaceae*. These results were in line with previous studies that reported an increase in potentially pathogenic families such as *Enterobacteriaceae* on the gut microbiome of liver patients and as well a high prevalence in ascites samples (28).

We identified 97 bacterial genera from ascites and 89 genera from blood (**Figure S2**). There were no statistical significant differences between the microbiota compositions of ascites and blood samples at phylum level. At genus level, alpha-diversity indices, such as richness (number of observed genera in a sample) and Shannon diversity (richness as well as evenness of genera in a sample), showed that the ascites microbiome was significantly more diverse than the peripheral blood microbiome ($P < 0.01$; **Figure 3A**).

Translocation of the gut microbiota into the circulatory system and into ascites is increasingly recognized as a driver

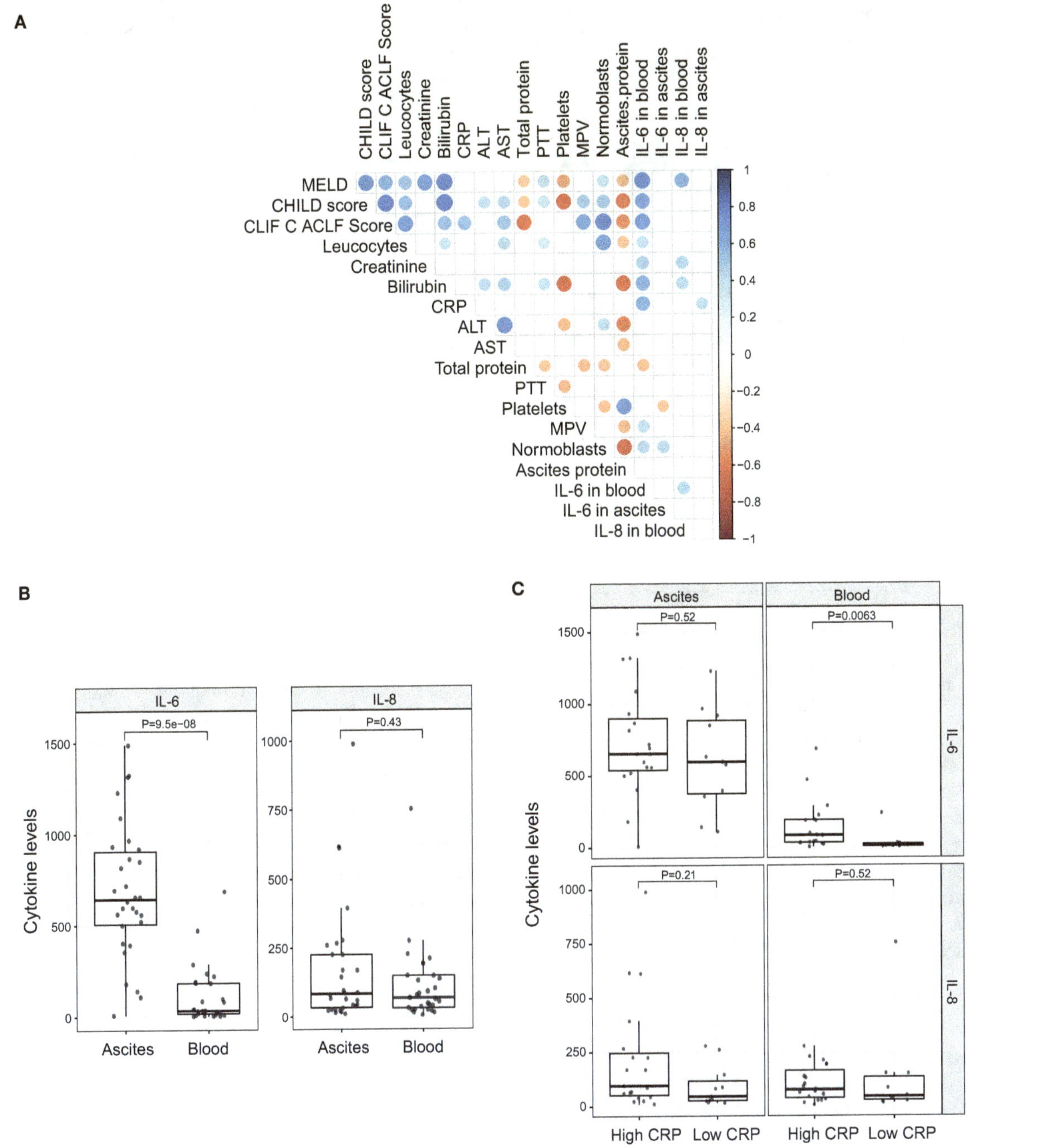

FIGURE 1 | Pro-inflammatory cytokines. **(A)** Correlation of clinical markers for disease progression and systemic inflammation with cytokines IL-6 and IL-8 in blood and ascites. **(B)** Comparison between cytokines levels in ascites and peripheral blood. **(C)** Comparison between cytokines levels in ascites and peripheral blood under different systemic inflammation status (low CRP profile vs. high CRP profile).

of complication in advanced liver disease (27, 29). As we showed above, the levels of pro-inflammatory cytokines (IL-6 and IL-8) were higher in ascites compared to blood, suggesting different drivers of inflammation. To determine the relation of the microbiota with cytokine levels and systemic inflammation, we investigated the differences in the microbiome composition of ascites and blood samples, in patients with low and high CRP levels. CRP levels did not appear to affect microbiota diversity of ascites or blood samples (**Figure 3B**).

Distinct Bacterial Signatures of Ascites and Blood Microbiome

To study the variation in the microbial structure between ascites and peripheral blood samples, we used unweighted

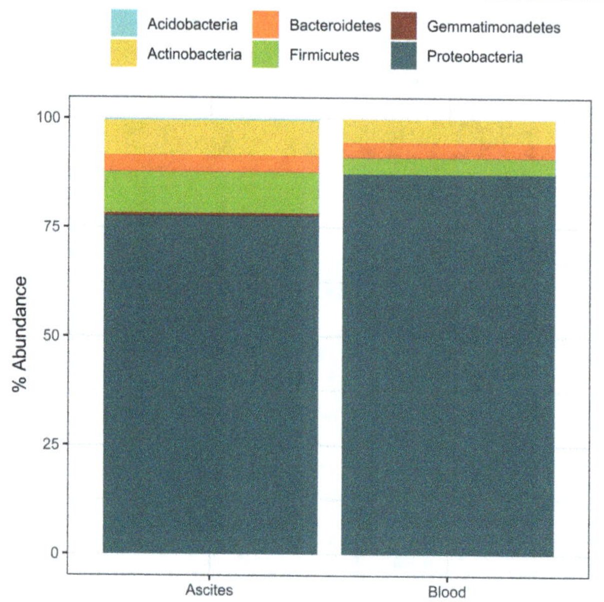

FIGURE 2 | Average microbiome phylum composition in ascites and blood samples (n = 10 each).

and weighted UniFrac metrics (30) as measures of the beta-diversity. Unweighted UniFrac uses a phylogenetic tree taking into account only the phylogenetic affiliation of members to evaluate the community structure and diversity, while weighted UniFrac additionally considers the relative abundance of the members of the community. Both measures clearly separated ascites from blood samples (**Figure 4**). The sampling compartment explained 11% of the variance in beta-diversity when using unweighted UniFrac metric (PERMANOVA test, $P = 0.006$), whereas it explained 21.2% of the variance when using weighted UniFrac metric (PERMANOVA test, $P = 0.001$). Additionally, the first principal coordinate (PC1) of microbiome beta-diversity explained 20.4% of the variance in the samples under unweighted UniFrac metric, whereas it explained 34% of the variance in the samples under weighted UniFrac metric (**Figure 4**).

We then investigated specific bacterial signatures that differentiated ascites from peripheral blood samples. We used DAtest (24) to select the most suitable statistical method to identify differentially abundant bacteria. Compared with other statistical methods evaluated by DAtest, t-test had the highest power to distinguish between two simulated sample groups based on our cohort, while keeping the false discovery rate of simulated differential taxa under 0.05. Therefore, we performed t-tests between the ascites and blood microbiomes using the relative abundances of 99 genera. We found that *Janthinobacterium, Serratia,* and *Rugamonas* were significantly enriched in ascites, while *Escherichia/Shigella* and *Pseudomonas* were enriched in blood (**Figure 5**, **Table 3**). These findings were in concordance with our cultivation results, where *Serratia* was detected in ascites culture and *Escherichia* in peripheral blood.

Since the presence of bacteria in blood is generally associated with systemic inflammation, we investigated whether there were differences in the bacterial composition of patients with systemic inflammation (high CRP levels, n = 4) and patients without systemic inflammation (low CRP levels, n = 6). There was no significant difference between groups, potentially due to limited sample size. We then examined the 5 bacterial genera that were significantly different between ascites and blood samples to determine their relationship with systemic inflammation. Although there were no statistically significant differences between the samples with and without systemic inflammation, *Escherichia/Shigella* and *Janthinobacterium* were more abundant in patients with elevated systemic inflammation, both in ascites and blood samples, while *Pseudomonas* and *Serratia* were increased only in the ascites samples with systemic inflammation (**Figure S1**).

DISCUSSION

The present study demonstrates that the levels of inflammatory cytokines and microbial richness are significantly higher in ascites of patients with decompensated cirrhosis than in their blood compartment. Neither the levels of cytokines nor the overall abundance of bacterial DNA nor microbial richness seemed to be related to the extent of systemic inflammation in these patients.

These findings are particularly striking, since the cell count in circulating blood is several fold higher than in ascites. Still, the levels of inflammatory cytokines were several fold reduced in blood compared to ascites. Moreover, the relationship between the surrogates of systemic inflammation (e.g., leucocyte count, CRP) and severity scores of liver cirrhosis were correlated with the levels of blood cytokines, but no relationship was detected in the same patients in ascites.

A recent study described the role of alcohol consumption for circulating microbiome composition and associated metabolic functions. Even though leucocyte count and endotoxemia increased with the severity of disease in this study, soluble CD14, as a marker for monocyte activation, decreased in severe alcoholic hepatitis underlining the dysregulation of the immune response (31).

Overall, these results may suggest a dysregulation in myeloid cell function in cirrhosis with an excess of cytokine synthesis in ascites. This does, however, not result in at least the two main markers of systemic inflammation investigated here. Although rather descriptive, our study suggests compartmentalization of the immune response in this setting. This compartmental dysregulation may occur as a response to MAMPs, e.g., bacterial DNA.

The reason for this compartmentalization of the immune response remains elusive. Granulocytes, as one of the main producers of cytokines, besides macrophages and monocytes, but crucial for the diagnosis of SBP, were similar or lower in ascites samples than blood samples, although levels of IL-6 and IL-8 were many times higher in ascites. This suggests an external source of these cytokines and inflammation in

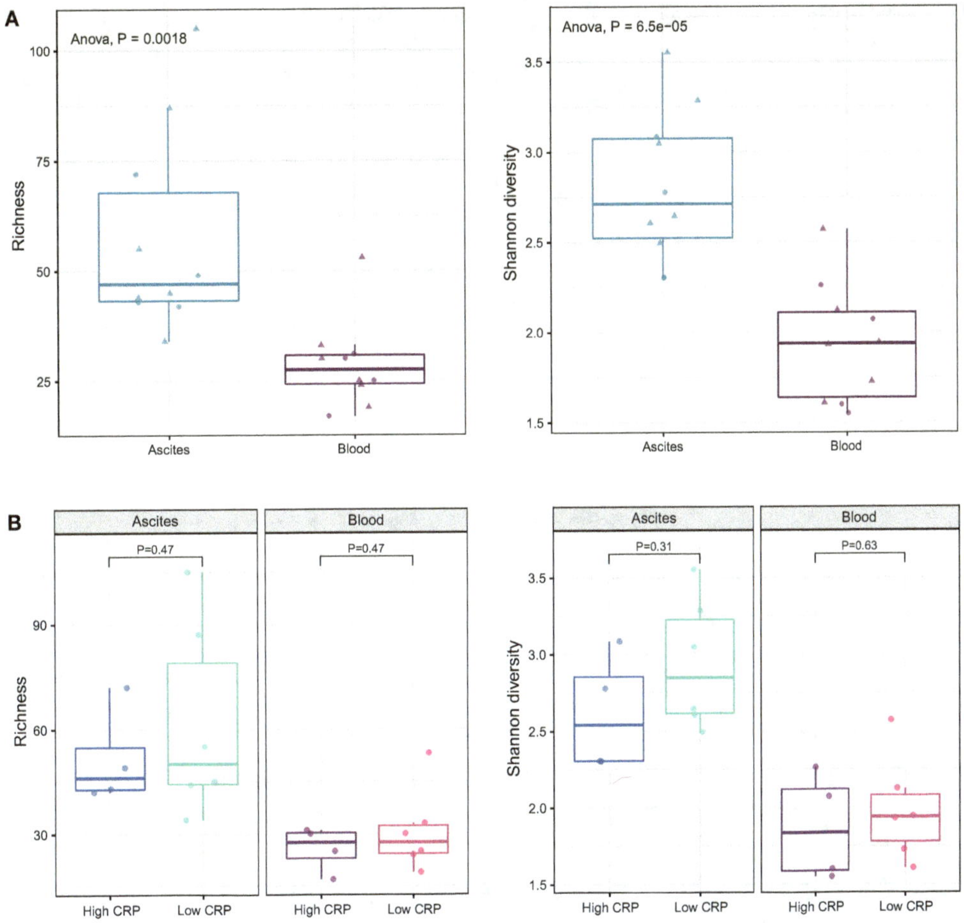

FIGURE 3 | (A) Alpha diversity indices at genus level. Ascites microbiota has higher richness and diversity compared to peripheral blood microbiome. **(B)** Alpha diversity indices under different systemic inflammation status. The inflammation status does not affect the microbial diversity of the ascites or blood samples.

ascites. Bacterial translocation from the gut is suspected to be the primary source of infection in SBP (2). However, bacteria not associated to the gut can also be found in ascites, suggesting other additional sources of infection (27). Bacterial translocation has been associated with impaired immune response and decompensation of liver cirrhosis, but the efforts to elaborate simple biomarkers such as detection and cut-off levels of bacterial DNA have shown discrepant results. Such discrepancies highlight that the relationship of presence or amount of bacterial DNA is not a strong predictor for decompensation and systemic inflammation in these patients, and probably also does not explain compartmentalization of the immune response. However, recent studies show an association of bacterial DNA levels in ascites and survival (32, 33).

Therefore, we have characterized the microbiome of matched ascites and blood samples from patients with decompensated liver cirrhosis. While ascites and blood harbored the same phyla with marginally different proportions, they showed distinct compositions at genus level. Genus alpha-diversity represented by richness and Shannon's diversity was significantly higher in ascites than in blood. Depending on the choice of the beta-diversity measure, 11% (unweighted UniFrac), or 21.2% (weighted UniFrac) of the variance in beta-diversity was dependent on the sampling compartment. These results suggest that the phylogeny of the members as well as their relative abundance have a significant yet cumulative effect in explaining the differences between ascites and blood microbial communities.

Culture-positive organisms *per se* do not seem to trigger systemic inflammation assessed by two representative cytokines (9) in patients with cirrhosis as demonstrated by the blood and ascites culture results in the two sub cohorts stratified by their CRP profile. Therefore, we hypothesize that abundance of specific genera must play a prominent role in the induction of systemic inflammation in cirrhosis. This hypothesis is supported by other studies where specific bacterial species correlate with clinical measures (27, 31).

We also identified five bacterial genera that were significantly different between ascites and blood samples, despite the small cohort size. Some of these genera were also cultivated from additional samples of the respective compartments,

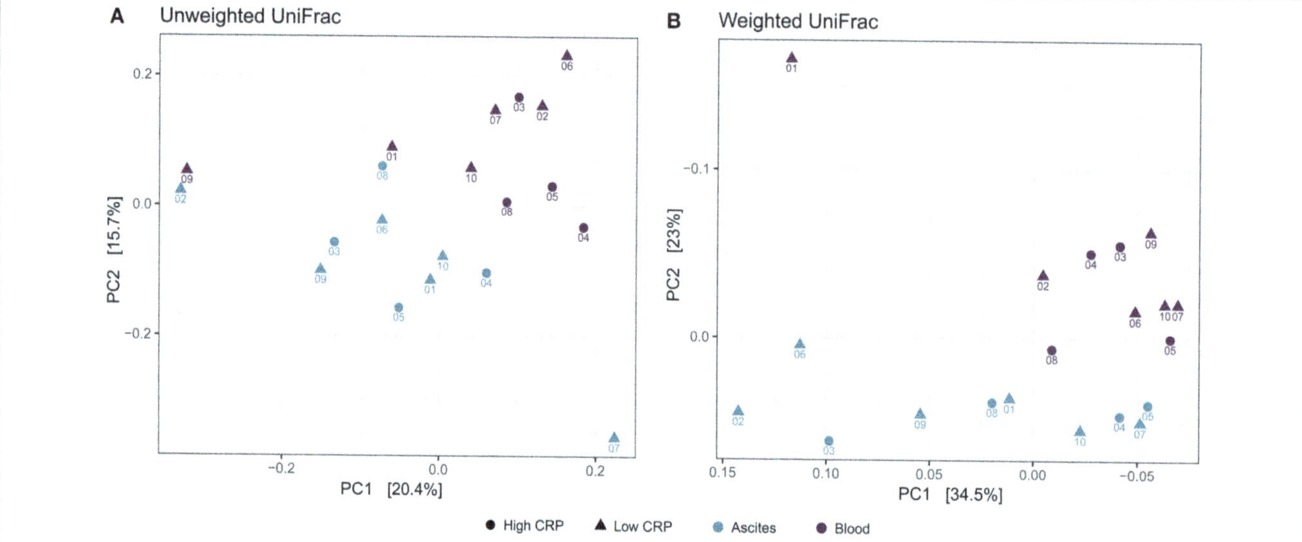

FIGURE 4 | Beta-diversity analysis. Principal coordinate analysis shows clear separation between ascites and peripheral blood samples, but samples do not cluster based on inflammation status. **(A)** Unweighted UniFrac **(B)** Weighted UniFrac.

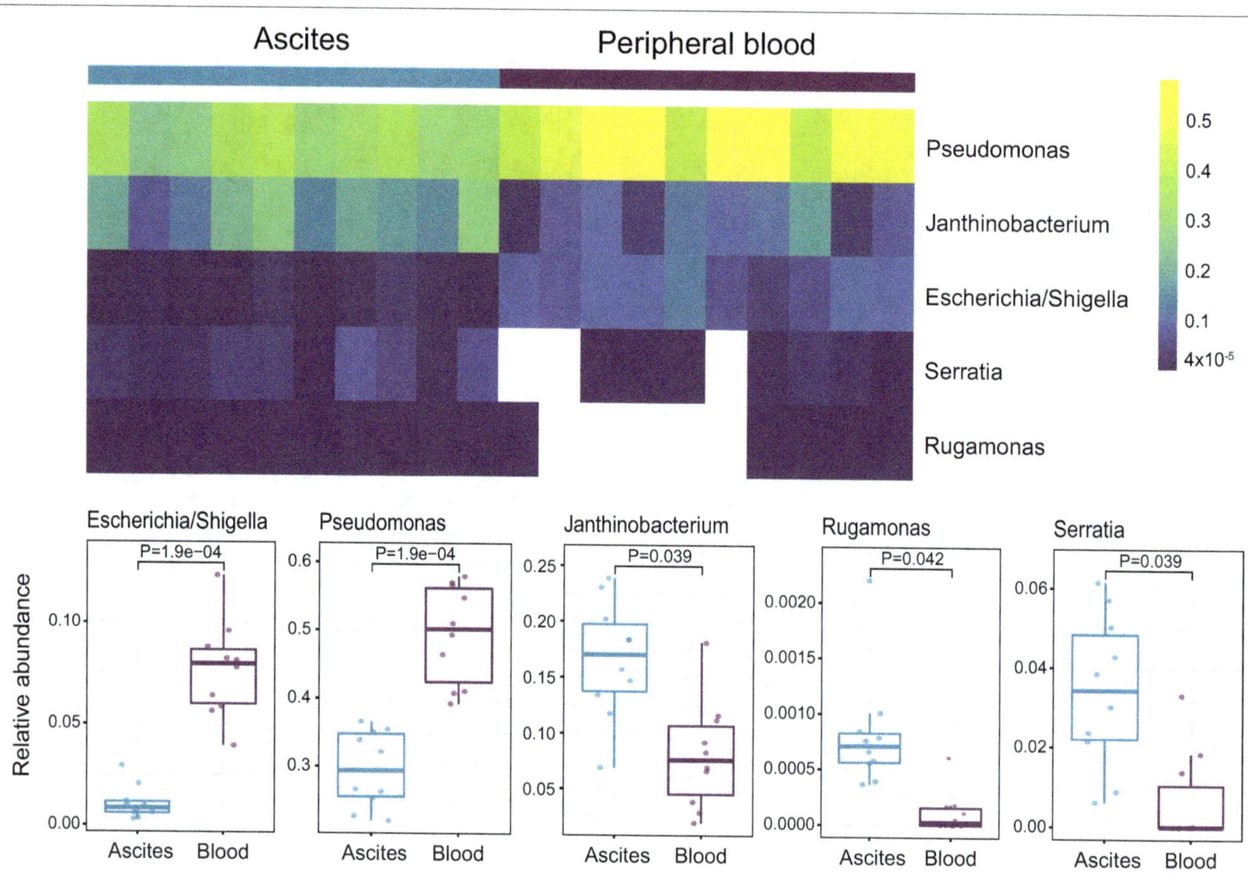

FIGURE 5 | Genera differentially abundant among ascites and blood samples.

TABLE 3 | Differentially abundant genera between ascites and blood.

Kingdom	Phylum	Class	Order	Family	Genus	Padj	Sig.	log2FC	Dir
Bacteria	Proteobacteria	Gammaproteobacteria	Enterobacteriales	Enterobacteriaceae	Escherichia/Shigella	0.00019243	***	2.75	Blood
Bacteria	Proteobacteria	Gammaproteobacteria	Pseudomonadales	Pseudomonadaceae	Pseudomonas	0.00019243	***	0.74	Blood
Bacteria	Proteobacteria	Betaproteobacteria	Burkholderiales	Oxalobacteraceae	Janthinobacterium	0.038589035	*	−1.04	Ascites
Bacteria	Proteobacteria	Gammaproteobacteria	Enterobacteriales	Enterobacteriaceae	Serratia	0.038589035	*	−2.21	Ascites
Bacteria	Proteobacteria	Betaproteobacteria	Burkholderiales	Oxalobacteraceae	Rugamonas	0.041897934	*	−0.71	Ascites

*Padj, adjusted P-value; Sig., significance level; ***P < 0.001, *P < 0.05; Dir, direction of enrichment; log2FC, log2 of fold change.*

confirming the viability of at least some of the bacteria reported in our study. Even though high CRP levels were associated with SBP, we did not see a significant difference in microbiome composition between high and low CRP samples, possibly due to reduced statistical power. However, the genera *Escherichia/Shigella* and *Janthinobacterium* showed higher abundance in blood samples of patients with systemic inflammation. *Escherichia* is already known for its pathogenic capabilities via lipopolysaccharides binding to Toll-like receptor 4, especially in individuals with dysfunctional immune response. *Janthinobacterium*, another Gram-negative bacterium, has not been described in relation to bacteremia previously, but could also induce inflammation via the same mechanism. On the other hand, while relative abundance of *Escherichia* was decreased in ascites samples, *Janthinobacterium* was increased. We speculate that the compartmentalization of immune dysfunction might be the reason behind the different behavior of these two bacteria, both of which are Gram-negative, in the different compartments.

In decompensated cirrhosis, representative markers of systemic inflammation and the microbiota seem to be dysregulated in ascites and blood. While a relationship between systemic inflammation and the microbiota seems to exist in blood, this is not found in ascites. These data may suggest the compartmentalization of the immune response and its interaction with the microbiome is especially important and evident in blood, while in ascites not found in our hands.

AUTHOR CONTRIBUTIONS

CA-S, RS, MA, and JT: conceptualization and methodology. CA-S, RS, AP, MA, and JT: formal analysis. CA-S, RS, AP, FM, FU, and PR: investigation. FM, FU, PR, and EL: resources. BL: data curation. CA-S, RS, EL, BL, JC, MV, MA, and JT: writing—original draft. CA-S, RS, MA, and JT: visualization. MA and JT: supervision.

ACKNOWLEDGMENTS

We thank Gudrun Hack and Silke Bellinghausen for excellent technical assistance. We were supported by grants from the Deutsche Forschungsgemeinschaft (SFB TRR57), Cellex Foundation, and Novo Nordisk Foundation (NNF10CC1016515 and NNF16CC0020896). This study was inspired, but not funded, by European Union's Horizon 2020 research and innovation program's GALAXY study (No 668031). The study was supported by Challenge Grant MicrobLiver grant number NNF15OC0016692 from the Novo Nordisk Foundation. The funders had no influence on study design, data collection and analysis, decision to publish or preparation of the manuscript.

REFERENCES

1. Laleman W, Claria J, Van der Merwe S, Moreau R, Trebicka J. Systemic inflammation and acute-on-chronic liver failure: too much, not enough. *Can J Gastroenterol Hepatol.* (2018) 2018:1027152. doi: 10.1155/2018/1027152
2. Arroyo V, Moreau R, Kamath PS, Jalan R, Ginès P, Nevens F, et al. Acute-on-chronic liver failure in cirrhosis. *Nat Rev Dis Primers* (2016) 2:16041. doi: 10.1038/nrdp.2016.41
3. European Association for the Study of the Liver. Electronic address: easloffice@easloffice.eu, European Association for the Study of the Liver. EASL Clinical Practice Guidelines for the management of patients with decompensated cirrhosis. *J Hepatol.* (2018) 69:406–60. doi: 10.1016/j.jhep.2018.03.024
4. Potgieter M, Bester J, Kell DB, Pretorius E. The dormant blood microbiome in chronic, inflammatory diseases. *FEMS Microbiol Rev.* (2015) 39:567–91. doi: 10.1093/femsre/fuv013
5. Wiest R, Garcia-Tsao G. Bacterial translocation (BT) in cirrhosis. *Hepatology* (2005) 41:422–33. doi: 10.1002/hep.20632
6. Mücke MM, Rumyantseva T, Mücke VT, Schwarzkopf K, Joshi S, Kempf VAJ, et al. Bacterial infection-triggered acute-on-chronic liver failure is associated with increased mortality. *Liver Int.* (2018) 38:645–53. doi: 10.1111/liv.13568
7. Mortensen C, Jensen JS, Hobolth L, Dam-Larsen S, Madsen BS, Andersen O, et al. Association of markers of bacterial translocation with immune activation in decompensated cirrhosis. *Eur J Gastroenterol Hepatol.* (2014) 26:1360–6. doi: 10.1097/MEG.0000000000000217
8. González-Navajas JM, Bellot P, Francés R, Zapater P, Muñoz C, García-Pagán JC, et al. Presence of bacterial-DNA in cirrhosis identifies a subgroup of patients with marked inflammatory response not related to endotoxin. *J Hepatol.* (2008) 48:61–7. doi: 10.1016/j.jhep.2007.08.012
9. Clària J, Stauber RE, Coenraad MJ, Moreau R, Jalan R, Pavesi M, et al. Systemic inflammation in decompensated cirrhosis: characterization and role in acute-on-chronic liver failure. *Hepatology* (2016) 64:1249–64. doi: 10.1002/hep.28740
10. Hackstein C-P, Assmus LM, Welz M, Klein S, Schwandt T, Schultze J, et al. Gut microbial translocation corrupts myeloid cell function to control bacterial infection during liver cirrhosis. *Gut* (2017) 66:507–18. doi: 10.1136/gutjnl-2015-311224
11. Thaiss CA, Zmora N, Levy M, Elinav E. The microbiome and innate immunity. *Nature* (2016) 535:65–74. doi: 10.1038/nature18847
12. Schierwagen R, Alvarez-Silva C, Madsen MSA, Kolbe CC, Meyer C, Thomas D, et al. Circulating microbiome in blood of different circulatory compartments. *Gut* (2018). doi: 10.1136/gutjnl-2018-316227. [Epub ahead of print].
13. Appenrodt B, Lehmann LE, Thyssen L, Gentemann M, Rabe C, Molitor E, et al. Is detection of bacterial DNA in ascitic fluid of

clinical relevance? *Eur J Gastroenterol Hepatol.* (2010) 22:1487–94. doi: 10.1097/MEG.0b013e328340c43a

14. European Association for the Study of the Liver. EASL clinical practice guidelines on the management of ascites, spontaneous bacterial peritonitis, and hepatorenal syndrome in cirrhosis. *J Hepatol.* (2010) 53:397–417. doi: 10.1016/j.jhep.2010.05.004
15. Mauch H. *Mikrobiologisch-Infektiologische Qualitätsstandards: MiQ; Qualitätsstandards in der Mikrobiologisch-Infektiologischen Diagnostik.* Munich: Elsevier (2007).
16. Vehreschild MJGT, Hamprecht A, Peterson L, Schubert S, Häntschel M, Peter S, et al. A multicentre cohort study on colonization and infection with ESBL-producing *Enterobacteriaceae* in high-risk patients with haematological malignancies. *J Antimicrob Chemother.* (2014) 69:3387–92. doi: 10.1093/jac/dku305
17. Lutz P, Goeser F, Kaczmarek DJ, Schlabe S, Nischalke HD, Nattermann J, et al. Relative ascites polymorphonuclear cell count indicates bacterascites and risk of spontaneous bacterial peritonitis. *Dig Dis Sci.* (2017) 62:2558–68. doi: 10.1007/s10620-017-4637-4
18. Lelouvier B, Servant F, Païssé S, Brunet AC, Benyahya S, Serino M, et al. Changes in blood microbiota profiles associated with liver fibrosis in obese patients: a pilot analysis. *Hepatology* (2016) 64:2015–27. doi: 10.1002/hep.28829
19. Païssé S, Valle C, Servant F, Courtney M, Burcelin R, Amar J, et al. Comprehensive description of blood microbiome from healthy donors assessed by 16S targeted metagenomic sequencing. *Transfusion* (2016) 56:1138–47. doi: 10.1111/trf.13477
20. Callahan BJ, McMurdie PJ, Rosen MJ, Han AW, Johnson AJA, Holmes SP. DADA2: High-resolution sample inference from Illumina amplicon data. *Nat Methods* (2016) 13:581–3. doi: 10.1038/nmeth.3869
21. Quast C, Pruesse E, Yilmaz P, Gerken J, Schweer T, Yarza P, et al. The SILVA ribosomal RNA gene database project: improved data processing and web-based tools. *Nucleic Acids Res.* (2013) 41:D590–6. doi: 10.1093/nar/gks1219
22. McMurdie PJ, Holmes S. Phyloseq: an R package for reproducible interactive analysis and graphics of microbiome census data. *PLoS ONE* (2013) 8:e61217. doi: 10.1371/journal.pone.0061217
23. Callahan BJ, Sankaran K, Fukuyama JA, McMurdie PJ, Holmes SP. Bioconductor workflow for microbiome data analysis: from raw reads to community analyses. *F1000Res.* (2016) 5:1492. doi: 10.12688/f1000research.8986.2
24. Russel J, Thorsen J, Brejnrod AD, Bisgaard H, Sorensen SJ, Burmolle M. DAtest: a framework for choosing differential abundance or expression method. *bioRxiv* (2018) 2018:241802. doi: 10.1101/241802
25. Ridker PM, Rifai N, Stampfer MJ, Hennekens CH. Plasma concentration of interleukin-6 and the risk of future myocardial infarction among apparently healthy men. *Circulation* (2000) 101:1767–72. doi: 10.1161/01.CIR.101.15.1767
26. Arican O, Aral M, Sasmaz S, Ciragil P. Serum levels of TNF-α, IFN-γ, IL-6, IL-8, IL-12, IL-17, and IL-18 in patients with active psoriasis and correlation with disease severity. *Mediators Inflamm.* (2005) 2005:273–9. doi: 10.1155/MI.2005.273
27. Rogers GB, van der Gast CJ, Bruce KD, Marsh P, Collins JE, Sutton J, et al. Ascitic microbiota composition is correlated with clinical severity in cirrhosis with portal hypertension. *PLoS ONE* (2013) 8:e74884. doi: 10.1371/journal.pone.0074884
28. Tuomisto S, Pessi T, Collin P, Vuento R, Aittoniemi J, Karhunen PJ. Changes in gut bacterial populations and their translocation into liver and ascites in alcoholic liver cirrhotics. *BMC Gastroenterol.* (2014) 14:40. doi: 10.1186/1471-230X-14-40
29. Zhu L, Baker SS, Gill C, Liu W, Alkhouri R, Baker RD, et al. Characterization of gut microbiomes in nonalcoholic steatohepatitis (NASH) patients: a connection between endogenous alcohol and NASH. *Hepatology* (2013) 57:601–9. doi: 10.1002/hep.26093
30. Lozupone C, Knight R. UniFrac: a new phylogenetic method for comparing microbial communities. *Appl Environ Microbiol.* (2005) 71:8228–35. doi: 10.1128/AEM.71.12.8228-8235.2005
31. Puri P, Liangpunsakul S, Christensen JE, Shah VH, Kamath PS, Gores GJ, et al. The circulating microbiome signature and inferred functional metagenomics in alcoholic hepatitis. *Hepatology* (2018) 67:1284–302. doi: 10.1002/hep.29623
32. Fagan KJ, Rogers GB, Melino M, Arthur DM, Costello M-E, Morrison M, et al. Ascites bacterial burden and immune cell profile are associated with poor clinical outcomes in the absence of overt infection. *PLoS ONE* (2015) 10:e0120642. doi: 10.1371/journal.pone.0120642
33. Engelmann C, Krohn S, Prywerek D, Hartmann J, Herber A, Boehlig A, et al. Detection of molecular bacterascites in decompensated cirrhosis defines a risk with decreased survival. *Eur J Gastroenterol Hepatol.* (2016) 28:1285–92. doi: 10.1097/MEG.0000000000000712

15

PNPLA3—A Potential Therapeutic Target for Personalized Treatment of Chronic Liver Disease

*Xiaocheng Charlie Dong**

Center for Diabetes and Metabolic Diseases, Department of Biochemistry and Molecular Biology, Indiana University School of Medicine, Indianapolis, IN, United States

***Correspondence:**
Xiaocheng Charlie Dong
xcdong@iu.edu

Patatin-like phospholipase domain-containing protein 3 (PNPLA3) is a lipid droplet-associated protein that has been shown to have hydrolase activity toward triglycerides and retinyl esters. The first evidence of PNPLA3 being associated with fatty liver disease was revealed by a genome-wide association study (GWAS) of Hispanic, African American, and European American individuals in the Dallas Heart Study back in 2008. Since then, numerous GWAS reports have shown that PNPLA3 rs738409[G] (148M) variant is associated with hepatic triglyceride accumulation (steatosis), inflammation, fibrosis, cirrhosis, and even hepatocellular carcinoma regardless of etiologies including alcohol- or obesity-related and others. The frequency of PNPLA3(148M) variant ranges from 17% in African Americans, 23% in European Americans, to 49% in Hispanics in the Dallas Heart Study. Due to high prevalence of obesity and alcohol consumption in modern societies, the PNPLA3(148M) gene variant and environment interaction poses a serious concern for public health, especially chronic liver diseases including alcohol-related liver disease (ALD) and nonalcoholic fatty liver disease (NAFLD). Therefore, PNPLA3(148M) variant is a potential therapeutic target for chronic liver disease in the rs738409 allele carriers. Currently, there is no approved drug specifically targeting the PNPLA3(148M) variant yet. With additional mechanistic studies, novel therapeutic strategies are expected to be developed for the treatment of the PNPLA3(148M) variant-associated chronic liver diseases in the near future.

Keywords: PNPLA3, rs738409, nonalcoholic steatohepatitis, alcoholic liver disease, fibrosis, cirrhosis, hepatocellular carcinoma

Alcoholic and non-alcoholic fatty liver diseases (ALD and NAFLD) have become serious public health burdens in the modern societies (1). ALD and NAFLD are chronic liver disorders that begin with hepatic triglyceride accumulation (steatosis) and progress to hepatic inflammation and fibrosis, cirrhosis and even liver cancer (2, 3). The causes of these liver diseases are multifactorial, including genetic, and environmental factors. Excess alcohol consumption, over nutrition, and physical inactivity are significant environmental risk factors (4, 5). It is believed that hepatic steatosis sets a stage for elevated susceptibility to acute and chronic inflammation in the liver. Multiple cytokines and chemokines including transforming growth factor-β (TGF-β) secreted from inflammatory immune cells trigger an activation of hepatic stellate cells (HSCs) and subsequently hepatic fibrogenesis (6).

In addition to those environmental factors, numerous genetic variants have been shown to be associated with ALD and NAFLD, including patatin-like phospholipase domain-containing protein 3 (PNPLA3), transmembrane 6 superfamily member 2 (TM6SF2), glucokinase regulator (GCKR), membrane bound O-acyltransferase domain-containing 7 (MBOAT7), and hydroxysteriod 17-beta dehydrogenase 13 (HSD17B13) (7, 8). TM6SF2 is involved in the VLDL secretion (9–15). The rs58542926 C>T variant of TM6SF2 decreases the VLDL secretion and increases hepatic triglycerides (16–25). GCKR regulates the glucokinase activity in the liver (26). The rs780094 A>G and rs1260326 C>T variants of GCKR lead to the loss of control of hepatic glucose influx and therefore increase hepatic lipogenesis (27–38). MBOAT7 catalyzes the acyl chain remodeling of phosphatidylinositol and decreases free arachidonic acid levels (39, 40). The rs641738 C>T variant of MBOAT7 increases arachidonic acid levels and hepatic inflammation (41–54). HSD17B13 has been shown to have retinol dehydrogenase activity (55). The rs72613567:TA variant of HSD17B13 is associated with increased steatosis and decreased inflammation and fibrosis (56–64). PNPLA3 has drawn a remarkable attention in the liver field since the first genome-wide association study (GWAS) revealed that a single nucleotide polymorphism (SNP) in the human PNPLA3 gene—rs738409[G] (148M) is the only non-synonymous sequence variant significantly associated with hepatic fat content in the Dallas Heart Study cohort (65). Multiple genetic studies have since validated the association of PNPLA3(148M) with a broad spectrum of liver diseases ranging from ALD and NAFLD, non-alcoholic steatohepatitis (NASH), fibrosis, cirrhosis, and hepatocellular carcinoma (HCC) (33, 66–117). However, the underlying pathogenic mechanisms remain elusive. This review aims to briefly summarize the PNPLA3 biology, clinical implications, and therapeutic development strategies.

PNPLA3 GENE FUNCTION

PNPLA3 has multiple names in the literature including adiponutrin (ADPN), calcium-independent phospholipase A2-epsilon (IPLA2epsilon, and chromosome 22 open reading frame 20 (C22orf20). In 2001, PNPLA3 was initially cloned from mouse 3T3 preadipocytes as a feeding-inducible gene, therefore named adiponutrin (118). In 2004, PNPLA3 was rediscovered as IPLA2epsilon by nucleotide sequence similarity search (119). In 2006, human patatin-like phospholipases including adiponutrin were grouped to the PNPLA family (120), which has 9 members (PNPLA1-9). The common feature of the PNPLA family members is the patatin-like phospholipase domain (**Figure 1**).

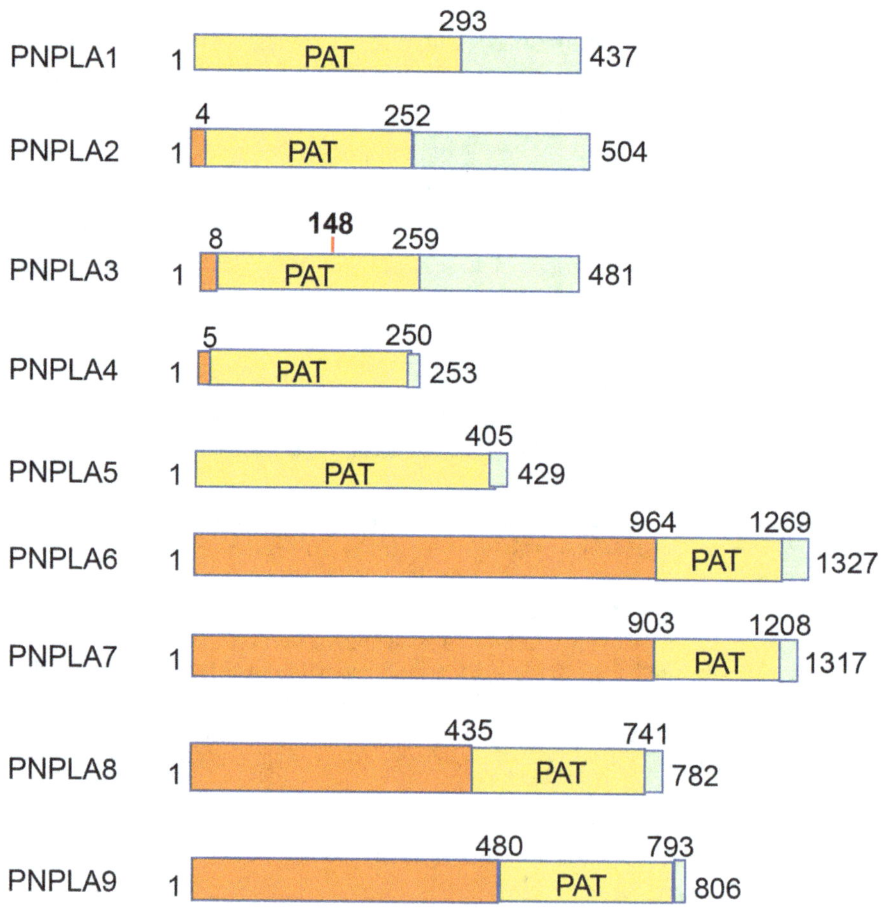

FIGURE 1 | PNPLA family members. Nine PNPLA family members are depicted by the size and localization of the conserved patatin (PAT) domains.

Protein sequence alignments show that the overall sequence conservation is low except a few conserved regions including the glycine-rich region and the aspartate-glycine residues of the catalytic site (120).

PNPLA3 GENE CHARACTERIZATION

Human PNPLA3 gene is localized on chromosome 22 (22q13.31). It has 9 exons that encode a 481-amino acid protein. In contrast, mouse Pnpla3 (384 amino acids) is much smaller than human PNPLA3 protein (**Figure 2**), as both proteins share high homology in the N-terminal half of the amino acid sequences. But the mouse Pnpla3 lacks the middle 17 residues and the C-terminal 75 residues in the human PNPLA3 protein. Therefore, it should be cautioned when implying the mouse Pnpla3 function to human PNPLA3. Another major difference between mouse and human PNPLA3 genes is the tissue-wise gene expression profiles. The human PNPLA3 gene is expressed highly in the liver and moderately in the adipose tissue, brain, kidney, and skin (120, 121); however, the mouse Pnpla3 gene is expressed at very high levels in both white and brown adipose tissues but at low levels in other tissues (118, 122). PNPLA3 is regulated by carbohydrate-response element binding protein (ChREBP) and sterol regulatory element binding protein 1c (SREBP1c) in mouse and human hepatocytes (123–125). Surprisingly, Pnpla3 gene knockout mice have normal levels of plasma and hepatic triglyceride contents and they do not develop fatty liver disease (126, 127). Interestingly, human PNPLA3(148M) transgenic mice develop hepatic steatosis on chow or high-sucrose diet (128). Pnpla3(148M) knockin mice also develop hepatic steatosis on the high-sucrose diet (129, 130) and hepatic inflammation and fibrosis on a NASH diet (131).

PNPLA3 ENZYMATIC ACTIVITIES

PNPLA3 has been shown to possess triacylglycerol lipase and acylglycerol transacylase activities using recombinant human PNPLA3 protein purified from Sf9 insect cells and triolein and mono-olein as substrates, respectively (119). However, when Huang et al. used similar recombinant human PNPLA3 protein from Sf9 cells to analyze lipase and transacylase activities, they only detected the lipase activity against major

```
Human   1    MYDAERGWSLSFAGCGFLGFYHVGATRCLSEHAPHLLRDARMLFGASAGALHCVGVLSGI  60
             MYD ER WSLSFAGCGFLGFYHVGAT CLSE APHLLRDAR  FG SAGALH V  +  +
Mouse   1    MYDPERRWSLSFAGCGFLGFYHVGATLCLSERAPHLLRDARTFFGCSAGALHAVTFVCSL  60

Human   61   PLEQTLQVLSDLVRKARSRNIGIFHPSFNLSKFLRQGLCKCLPANVHQLISGKIGISLTR  120
             PL + +++L DLVRKARSRNIG  HP FN++K +R GL + LP NVHQ+ISGK+ ISLTR
Mouse   61   PLGRIMEILMDLVRKARSRNIGTLHPFFNINKCIRDGLQESLPDNVHQVISGKVHISLTR  120

Human   121  VSDGENVLVSDFRSKDEVVDALVCSCFIPFYSGLIPPSFRGVRYVDGGVSDNVPFIDAKT  180
             VSDGENVLVS+F SKDEVVDALVCSCFIP +SGLIPPSFRG RYVDGGVSDNVP +DAKT
Mouse   121  VSDGENVLVSEFHSKDEVVDALVCSCFIPLFSGLIPPSFRGERYVDGGVSDNVPVLDAKT  180
                                         *

Human   181  TITVSPFYGEYDICPKVKSTNFLHVDITKLSLRLCTGNLYLLSRAFVPPDLKVLGEICLR  240
             TITVSPFYGE+DICPKVKSTNF HV+IT LSLRLCTGNL LL+RA  P D+KV+GE+C +
Mouse   181  TITVSPFYGEHDICPKVKSTNFFHVNITNLSLRLCTGNLQLLTRALFPSDVKVMGELCYQ  240

Human   241  GYLDAFRFLEEKGICNRPQPGLKSSSEGMDPEVAMPSWANMSLDSSPESAALAVRLEGDE  300
             GYLDAFRFLEE GICN PQ  L                 ++SL   +PE+    +L GD+
Mouse   241  GYLDAFRFLEENGICNGPQRSL-----------------SLSL-VAPEACLENGKLVGDK  282

Human   301  LLDHLRLSILPWDESILDTLSPRLATALSEEMKDKGGYMSKICNLLPIRIMSYVMLPCTL  360
                 + +S+   DE+I +TLSP L+TALSE +KD+ GY+SK+CNLLP+RI+SY+MLPC+L
Mouse   283  ----VPVSLCFTDENIWETLSPELSTALSEAIKDREGYLSKVCNLLPVRILSYIMLPCSL  338

Human   361  PVESAIAIVQRLVTWLPDMPDDVLWLQWVTSQVFTRVLMCLLPASR  406 ..........481
             PVESAIA V RLVTWLPD+ DD+ WLQW TSQV  R+ MCLLP++R
Mouse   339  PVESAIAAVHRLVTWLPDIQDDIQWLQWATSQVCARMTMCLLPSTR  384
```

FIGURE 2 | Human and mouse Pnpla3 protein sequence alignments. The protein sequences were aligned using the NCBI BLAST program. The identical residues are in red. The PAT domain is underlined. The 148I residue is marked by asterisk.

glycerolipids including triacylglyceride, diacylglyceride, and monoacylglyceride but not transacylase activity (132). In another study, human PNPLA3 was overexpressed and purified from HEK293 cells and showed to have a lipase activity on 1,2-o-dilauryl-rac-glycerol-3-glutaric acid-(6'-methylresorufin) ester (122). Mutation of the active-site serine within the Ser^{47}-Asp^{166} catalytic dyad motif abolished the lipase activity; however, overexpression of human PNPLA3 in HEK293 cells did not decrease the cellular triglyceride levels (122). The recombinant human PNPLA3(148M) mutant from Sf9 cells was shown to lose the triglyceride hydrolase activity using triolein as substrate (133). Human wildtype PNPLA3 but not the 148M mutant recombinant protein from yeast cells also showed triglyceride hydrolase activity (134). In addition, wildtype recombinant human PNPLA3 protein purified from yeast cells also showed retinyl esterase activity using retinyl-palmitate as substrate whereas the 148M mutant protein had diminished activity (135). Retinoic acids (all-trans) have been shown to activate retinoic acid receptor (RAR) and retinoid X receptor (RXR) and subsequently downregulate fibrotic genes in HSCs (136–138). PNPLA3(148M) mutant causes an decrease in retinol levels and downregulation of RAR/RXR target genes in the LX-2 hepatic stellate cell line (139).

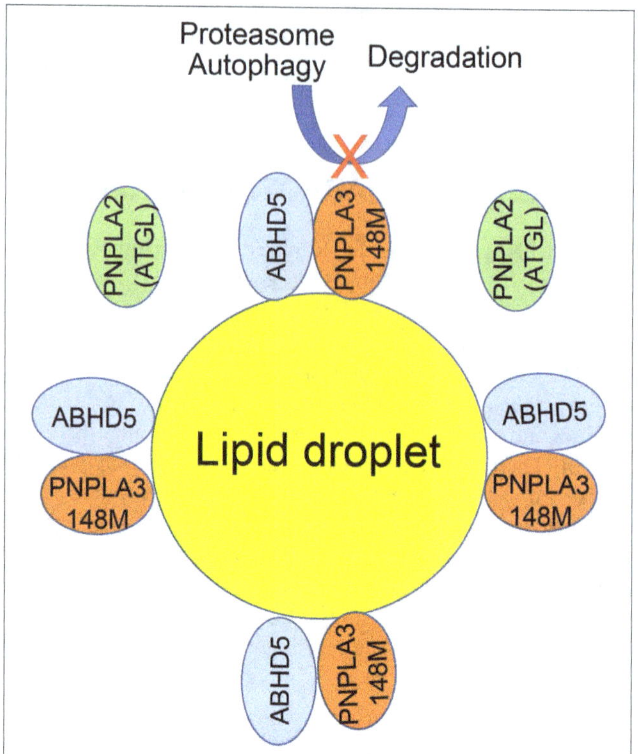

FIGURE 3 | A working model for the PNPLA3 function on lipid droplet. ATGL and ABHD5 normally interact to promote triglyceride breakdown from lipid droplets. The 148M mutation impairs the turnover of PNPLA3 protein by ubiquitin or autophagy mediated degradation. When PNPLA3(148M) variant proteins accumulate on lipid droplets, PNPLA3(148M) competes with ATGL for the interaction with ABHD5. As a result, the ATGL activity is reduced and lipid droplets are accumulated.

PNPLA3 IN LIPID DROPLET HOMEOSTASIS

PNPLA3 is mostly bound to lipid droplets in mammalian cells (133, 140–142), but how this protein functions on lipid droplet remains elusive (**Figure 3**). Several lines of evidence suggest that PNPLA3(148M) abnormally accumulating on lipid droplets links to the impairment of lipid droplet metabolism. Wildtype PNPLA3 turns over according to fasting/feeding cycles; however, the 148M mutant PNPLA3 is resistant to ubiquitin- or autophagy-mediated protein degradation (129, 143, 144). Excess PNPLA3 on the lipid droplets seems to impair the activity of PNPLA2, also called adipose triglyceride lipase (ATGL), likely through competing with the ATGL activator —comparative gene identification 58 (CGI-58) or officially abhydrolase domain containing 5 (ABHD5) (140, 142, 145). Some data suggest that PNPLA3(148M) tends to interact with CGI-58 more strongly than the wildtype counterpart does (145). CGI-58 is also required for the targeting of PNPLA3 to lipid droplet since PNPLA3 cannot localize onto lipid droplet in the CGI-58 knockout liver cells (140).

PNPLA3 IN HEPATIC FIBROSIS

In addition to hepatocytes, human PNPLA3 gene is also abundantly expressed in HSCs (121, 139). PNPLA3 can be induced by TGF-β but not platelet-derived growth factor (PDGF) in human HSCs (146). The same report also shows that overexpression of the wildtype PNPLA3 but not the PNPLA3(148M) mutant reduces the intracellular retinyl esters in HSCs. Interestingly, after incubation with retinol and palmitate, wildtype, but not mutant PNPLA3 decreases the secretion of matrix metallopeptidase 2 (MMP2), tissue inhibitor of metalloproteinase 1 (TIMP1), and TIMP2 from HSCs (146). Another report shows that the PNPLA3 gene expression is induced during the primary human HSC activation and knockdown of PNPLA3 by siRNA attenuates the HSC activation (139). Human HSCs with the PNPLA3(148M) variant have higher expression of inflammatory cytokines and chemokines including granulocyte-macrophage colony-stimulating factor (GM-CSF), chemokine (C-X-C motif) ligand 8 (CXCL8), and TGF-β. Overexpression of the PNPLA3(148M) variant enhances the HSC proliferation and chemotaxis (139). In contrast to the previous report regarding the retinyl palmitate lipase activity of PNPLA3 (135), Bruschi et al. have found that total retinol content and RXR and RAR signaling are both lower in the PNPLA3(148M) mutant HSCs than that in the PNPLA3 wildtype HSCs (139). Further signaling analysis has revealed that c-Jun N-terminal kinase (JNK) is highly activated in the PNPLA3(148M) HSCs. As a consequence, peroxisome proliferator-activated receptor gamma (PPARγ), a key HSC quiescence regulator, is inhibited, whereas activator protein 1 (AP-1), a proinflammatory transcription factor, is activated (139). Collectively, these dysregulations contribute to the fibrogenic phenotype in the PNPLA3(148M) HSCs. The inhibition of

TABLE 1 | Human PNPLA3 genetic association studies in liver diseases.

PNPLA3 SNP	Study population	Associated phenotype and significance	References
rs738409[G]	Hispanics, African Americans, European Americans, $N = 9{,}229$	Positive association with hepatic fat content ($P = 5.9 \times 10^{-10}$), serum ALT ($P = 1.3 \times 10^{-5}$ in Hispanics)	(65)
rs2281135[A], rs738409[G]	Europeans, $N = 12{,}419$	Positive association with ALT ($P = 8.4 \times 10^{-16}$, $P = 3.7 \times 10^{-10}$)	(110)
rs738409[G]	West-Eurasian populations, $N = 23{,}274$	Negative association with total cholesterol ($P = 8.87 \times 10^{-7}$), non-HDL cholesterol ($P = 2.27 \times 10^{-6}$), LDL cholesterol ($P = 7.99 \times 10^{-4}$)	(148)
rs738409[G]	Mestizo (mixed European and Native American ancestry), $N = 1{,}221$	Positive association with ALD (OR = 1.45, $P = 8.4 \times 10^{-4}$) and alcoholic liver cirrhosis (OR = 2.25, $P = 1.7 \times 10^{-10}$)	(89)
rs738409[G]	Caucasian (82.1%), African American (2.3%), Asian (5.4%), American Indian (3.2%), other (7%), $N = 1{,}117$	Positive association with hepatic steatosis (OR = 1.46, $P = 0.03$), portal inflammation (OR = 1.57, $P = 2.5 \times 10^{-4}$), lobular inflammation (OR = 1.84, $P = 0.005$), Mallory-Denk bodies (OR = 1.6, $P = 0.015$), NAFLD activity score ($P = 0.004$), hepatic fibrosis (OR = 1.5, $P = 7.7 \times 10^{-6}$)	(68)
rs738409[G]	Japanese, $N = 831$	Positive association with NAFLD (OR = 1.73, $P = 9.4 \times 10^{-10}$)	(149)
rs738409[G]	German, $N = 1{,}419$	Positive association with alcoholic liver cirrhosis (OR = 2.79, $P = 1.6 \times 10^{-6}$)	(84)
rs738409[G]	Americans and Europeans, $N = 1{,}997$	Positive association with NAFLD (OR = 3.26, $P = 3.6 \times 10^{-43}$)	(83)
rs738409[G]	European Caucasians, $N = 537$	Positive association with chronic hepatitis C related hepatic steatosis (OR = 2.55, $P = 0.034$), fibrosis (OR = 3.13, $P = 0.002$)	(94)
rs738409[G]	German, $N = 899$	Positive association with liver cirrhosis (OR = 1.56, $P = 0.005$)	(150)
rs738409[G]	European Caucasians, $N = 658$	Positive association with liver cirrhosis (OR = 2.08, $P = 0.02$)	(91)
rs738409[G]	Japanese, $N = 1{,}326$	Positive association with NAFLD (OR = 2.05, $P = 6.8 \times 10^{-14}$)	(151)
rs738409[G]	American Caucasians, African Americans, Mexican Americans, $N = 4{,}804$	Positive association with hepatic steatosis and high ALT (OR = 1.36, $P = 0.01$)	(152)
rs738409[G]	American Caucasians, $N = 751$	Positive association with HCC (OR = 3.21, $P = 0.02$)	(153)
rs738409[G]	European Caucasians, $N = 2{,}138$	Positive association with alcoholic liver cirrhosis (OR = 2.19, $P = 1.54 \times 10^{-48}$)	(42)
rs738409[G]	Chinese Han, $N = 768$	Positive association with NAFLD (OR = 1.52, $P = 8.7 \times 10^{-4}$)	(102)
rs738409[G]	Eastern European, $N = 969$	Positive association with liver fibrosis (OR = 1.65, $P = 0.001$), liver cirrhosis (OR = 1.92, $P = 5.57 \times 10^{-7}$)	(154)
rs738409[G]	European Caucasians, $N = 183$	Positive association with alcoholic hepatitis (OR = 1.9, $P = 0.01$)	(155)
rs738409[G]	Korean, $N = 4{,}409$	Positive association with NAFLD (OR = 1.54, $P = 1.74 \times 10^{-15}$)	(156)
rs738409[G]	Chinese Han, $N = 1{,}152$	Positive association with ALD (OR = 1.93, $P = 6.25 \times 10^{-14}$)	(115)
rs738409[G]	Europeans, $N = 5{,}525$	Positive association with HCC (OR = 1.67, $P = 0.005$), HCC in ALD patients (OR = 3.91, $P = 1.14 \times 10^{-9}$), HCC in non-fibrotic patients (OR = 2.19, $P = 0.007$)	(106)
rs738409[G]	American Caucasians, $N = 9{,}677$	Positive association with NAFLD (OR = 1.79, $P = 1.7 \times 10^{-20}$)	(157)
rs4823173[A], rs2896019[G], rs2281135[A]	Mexican Americans, $N = 3{,}757$	Positive association with AST ($P = 3.44 \times 10^{-10}$, $P = 7.29 \times 10^{-9}$, $P = 8.73 \times 10^{-9}$)	(109)

PPARγ in the PNPLA3(148M) HSCs also negatively affects the liver X receptor alpha (LXRα) activity. As a result, cholesterol is accumulated in those mutant HSCs, and this also contributes to the inflammation and fibrogenesis in the PNPLA3(148M) HSCs (147).

PNPLA3 GENE POLYMORPHISM AND CHRONIC LIVER DISEASE

Alcoholic and non-alcoholic liver diseases often begin with simple steatosis and progress to hepatitis, fibrosis/cirrhosis, and even liver cancer. Both environmental and genetic factors contribute to the development of these chronic liver diseases. Among the well documented genes, PNPLA3 has the broad impact on ALD and NAFLD. The involvement of PNPLA3 variant rs738409 (148 M) in the broad spectrum of chronic liver disease has been shown by numerous GWAS (see **Table 1**). In 2008, Romeo et al. identified a strong association between the PNPLA3(148M) variant and hepatic fat concentration in a GWAS on Hispanic, African American, and European American individuals (65). The 148M variant frequencies are concordant with the prevalence of NAFLD in these three ancestry groups, and their allele frequencies are: Hispanics (0.49), European Americans (0.23), and African Americans (0.17). Since then, multiple GWASs have reported a strong association of PNPLA3(148M) variant with both ALD and NAFLD (**Table 1** and **Figure 4**). Several studies have documented a strong association of the 148 M variant with liver cirrhosis (42, 76, 154, 158–160). A number of

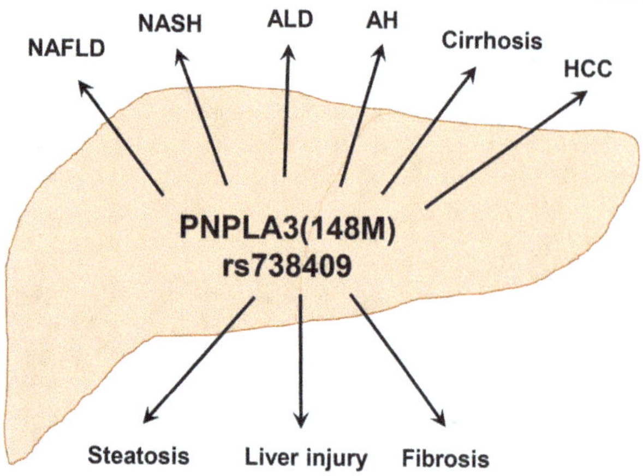

FIGURE 4 | PNPLA3(148M) is associated with a wide-spectrum of chronic liver diseases. Hepatic accumulation of PNPLA3(148M) protein leads to triglyceride accumulation, liver injury, and fibrosis. With different etiologies, this may lead to the development of various liver disorders including NAFLD, NASH, ALD, alcoholic hepatitis (AH), cirrhosis, and HCC.

reports have also shown that the 148M variant is also associated with higher risk for HCC (77, 85, 92, 93, 106, 108, 153, 160–169). In addition, the PNPLA3 variant rs738409 could lead to differential gene regulation via microRNAs. An in silico analysis has identified hsa-miR-769-3p and hsa-miR-516a-3p as potential microRNAs targeting the 3' UTR of the human PNPLA3 mRNA (170). Experimental validations are needed to demonstrate their functional relevance to the PNPLA3(148M) variant.

THERAPEUTIC STRATEGIES FOR TARGETING PNPLA3 FOR PERSONIZED TREATMENT OF CHRONIC LIVER DISEASE

As the PNPLA3(148M) variant is quite prevalent in most populations, especially among Hispanics (65), it is very significant to develop therapeutics targeting this genetic polymorphism. According to the PNPLA3(148M) biology, there are several potential ways of targeting the 148M variant. First, the PNPLA3(148M) variant can be targeted at the RNA levels by small interfering RNA (siRNA), small hairpin RNA (shRNA), or antisense RNA oligonucleotide. A recent report has shown that triantennary N-acetylgalactosamine ($GalNAC_3$) conjugated antisense oligonucleotides (ASO) targeting Pnpla3 in a 148M knockin mouse model significantly reduce hepatic steatosis, inflammation, and fibrosis (131), suggesting the utility of the ASO strategy. In another report, targeting Pnpla3 in the 148M knockin mice by AAV-mediated shRNA has also showed effective reduction of hepatic triglyceride contents (143). For the translational perspective, PNPLA3(148M)-allele-specific RNAi is preferred for human patients in order to avoid affecting the PNPLA3 wildtype allele as we do not fully understand the PNPLA3 biology. With the encouraging phase III clinical trial data on proprotein convertase subtilisin/kexin type 9 (PCSK9) RNAi (171), targeting the PNPLA3(148M) variant by RNAi can be an attractive strategy. Second, PNPLA3 can be targeted at the protein level. Recent data suggested that an accumulation of PNPLA3(148M) on lipid droplets is very critical for the pathogenesis of fatty liver disease (129, 130, 140, 143). Therefore, targeting PNPLA3(148M) for degradation can be a useful strategy. Recently, a proof-of-concept study using proteolysis-targeting chimera (PROTAC)-mediated degradation of Halo-tagged PNPLA3(148M) has shown a significant effect on lowering hepatic triglyceride content (143). The question will be how to degrade endogenous PNPLA3(148M) protein in a variant-specific manner. To date, there are no effective ways to specifically target the PNPLA3(148M) mutant protein. However, targeting PNPLA3 may work from another angle —an interaction between PNPLA3 and CGI-58, as the interaction can be regulated by fatty acids or synthetic CGI-58 ligands (145). Taken together, targeting PNPLA3(148M) has been increasingly appreciated for therapeutic development for multiple chronic liver diseases including ALD and NASH.

In summary, PNPLA3 is an enigmatic protein that has broad implications in metabolic liver diseases from simple steatosis to cirrhosis and liver cancer. Better understanding the biological function of PNPLA3 in lipid droplet metabolism should facilitate the therapeutic development. Targeting the PNPLA3(148M) variant is expected to be an excellent example of the modern personalized medicine.

AUTHOR CONTRIBUTIONS

XD conceived the idea, gathered the data, and wrote the manuscript.

REFERENCES

1. Younossi Z, Tacke F, Arrese M, Sharma BC, Mostafa I, Bugianesi E, et al. Global perspectives on non-alcoholic fatty liver disease and non-alcoholic steatohepatitis. *Hepatology.* (2018) 69:2672–82. doi: 10.1002/hep.30251
2. Friedman SL, Neuschwander-Tetri BA, Rinella M, Sanyal AJ. Mechanisms of NAFLD development and therapeutic strategies. *Nat Med.* (2018) 24:908–22. doi: 10.1038/s41591-018-0104-9
3. Seitz HK, Bataller R, Cortez-Pinto H, Gao B, Gual A, Lackner C, et al. Alcoholic liver disease. *Nat Rev Dis Primers.* (2018) 4:16. doi: 10.1038/s41572-018-0014-7
4. Hydes T, Gilmore W, Sheron N, Gilmore I. Treating alcohol-related liver disease from a public health perspective. *J Hepatol.* (2019) 70:223–36. doi: 10.1016/j.jhep.2018.10.036
5. Stefan N, Haring HU, Cusi K. Non-alcoholic fatty liver disease: causes, diagnosis, cardiometabolic consequences, and treatment strategies. *Lancet Diabetes Endocrinol.* (2019) 7:313–324. doi: 10.1016/S2213-8587(18)30154-2
6. Manne V, Handa P, Kowdley KV. Pathophysiology of nonalcoholic fatty liver disease/nonalcoholic steatohepatitis. *Clin Liver Dis.* (2018) 22:23–37. doi: 10.1016/j.cld.2017.08.007
7. Eslam M, Valenti L, Romeo S. Genetics and epigenetics of NAFLD and NASH: clinical impact. *J Hepatol.* (2018) 68:268–79. doi: 10.1016/j.jhep.2017.09.003
8. Eslam M, George J. Genetic contributions to NAFLD: leveraging shared genetics to uncover systems biology. *Nat Rev Gastroenterol Hepatol.* (2019). doi: 10.1038/s41575-019-0212-0. [Epub ahead of print].

9. Mahdessian H, Taxiarchis A, Popov S, Silveira A, Franco-Cereceda A, Hamsten A, et al. TM6SF2 is a regulator of liver fat metabolism influencing triglyceride secretion and hepatic lipid droplet content. *Proc Natl Acad Sci USA.* (2014) 111:8913–8. doi: 10.1073/pnas.1323785111
10. Fan Y, Lu H, Guo Y, Zhu T, Garcia-Barrio MT, Jiang Z, et al. Hepatic Transmembrane 6 superfamily member 2 regulates cholesterol metabolism in mice. *Gastroenterology.* (2016) 150:1208–18. doi: 10.1053/j.gastro.2016.01.005
11. Smagris E, Gilyard S, BasuRay S, Cohen JC, Hobbs HH. Inactivation of Tm6sf2, a gene defective in fatty liver disease, impairs lipidation but not secretion of very low density lipoproteins. *J Biol Chem.* (2016) 291:10659–76. doi: 10.1074/jbc.M116.719955
12. Ehrhardt N, Doche ME, Chen S, Mao HZ, Walsh MT, Bedoya C, et al. Hepatic Tm6sf2 overexpression affects cellular ApoB-trafficking, plasma lipid levels, hepatic steatosis and atherosclerosis. *Hum Mol Genet.* (2017) 26:2719–31. doi: 10.1093/hmg/ddx159
13. Luukkonen PK, Zhou Y, Nidhina Haridas PA, Dwivedi OP, Hyotylainen T, Ali A, et al. Impaired hepatic lipid synthesis from polyunsaturated fatty acids in TM6SF2 E167K variant carriers with NAFLD. *J Hepatol.* (2017) 67:128–36. doi: 10.1016/j.jhep.2017.02.014
14. Musso G, Cipolla U, Cassader M, Pinach S, Saba F, De Michieli F, et al. TM6SF2 rs58542926 variant affects postprandial lipoprotein metabolism and glucose homeostasis in NAFLD. *J Lipid Res.* (2017) 58:1221–9. doi: 10.1194/jlr.M075028
15. O'Hare EA, Yang R, Yerges-Armstrong LM, Sreenivasan U, McFarland R, Leitch CC, et al. TM6SF2 rs58542926 impacts lipid processing in liver and small intestine. *Hepatology.* (2017) 65:1526–42. doi: 10.1002/hep.29021
16. Kozlitina J, Smagris E, Stender S, Nordestgaard BG, Zhou HH, Tybjaerg-Hansen A, et al. Exome-wide association study identifies a TM6SF2 variant that confers susceptibility to nonalcoholic fatty liver disease. *Nat Genet.* (2014) 46:352–6. doi: 10.1038/ng.2901
17. Milano M, Aghemo A, Mancina RM, Fischer J, Dongiovanni P, De Nicola S, et al. Transmembrane 6 superfamily member 2 gene E167K variant impacts on steatosis and liver damage in chronic hepatitis C patients. *Hepatology.* (2015) 62:111–7. doi: 10.1002/hep.27811
18. Pirola CJ, Sookoian S. The dual and opposite role of the TM6SF2-rs58542926 variant in protecting against cardiovascular disease and conferring risk for nonalcoholic fatty liver: a meta-analysis. *Hepatology.* (2015) 62:1742–56. doi: 10.1002/hep.28142
19. Sookoian S, Castano GO, Scian R, Mallardi P, Fernandez Gianotti T, Burgueno AL, et al. Genetic variation in transmembrane 6 superfamily member 2 and the risk of nonalcoholic fatty liver disease and histological disease severity. *Hepatology.* (2015) 61:515–25. doi: 10.1002/hep.27556
20. Wang X, Liu Z, Peng Z, Liu W. The TM6SF2 rs58542926T allele is significantly associated with non-alcoholic fatty liver disease in Chinese. *J Hepatol.* (2015) 62:1438–9. doi: 10.1016/j.jhep.2015.01.040
21. Eslam M, Mangia A, Berg T, Chan HL, Irving WL, Dore GJ, et al. Diverse impacts of the rs58542926 E167K variant in TM6SF2 on viral and metabolic liver disease phenotypes. *Hepatology.* (2016) 64:34–46. doi: 10.1002/hep.28475
22. Goffredo M, Caprio S, Feldstein AE, D'Adamo E, Shaw MM, Pierpont B, et al. Role of TM6SF2 rs58542926 in the pathogenesis of nonalcoholic pediatric fatty liver disease: a multiethnic study. *Hepatology.* (2016) 63:117–125. doi: 10.1002/hep.28283
23. Grandone A, Cozzolino D, Marzuillo P, Cirillo G, Di Sessa A, Ruggiero L, et al. TM6SF2 Glu167Lys polymorphism is associated with low levels of LDL-cholesterol and increased liver injury in obese children. *Pediatr Obes.* (2016) 11:115–9. doi: 10.1111/ijpo.12032
24. Mancina RM, Sentinelli F, Incani M, Bertoccini L, Russo C, Romeo S, et al. Transmembrane-6 superfamily member 2. (TM6SF2) E167K variant increases susceptibility to hepatic steatosis in obese children. *Dig Liver Dis.* (2016) 48:100–101. doi: 10.1016/j.dld.2015.10.003
25. Viitasalo A, Pihlajamaki J, Paananen J, Atalay M, Lindi V, Lakka TA. Associations of TM6SF2 167K allele with liver enzymes and lipid profile in children: the PANIC Study. *Pediatr Res.* (2016) 79:684–8. doi: 10.1038/pr.2016.3
26. Brown KS, Kalinowski SS, Megill JR, Durham SK, Mookhtiar KA. Glucokinase regulatory protein may interact with glucokinase in the hepatocyte nucleus. *Diabetes.* (1997) 46:179–86. doi: 10.2337/diabetes.46.2.179
27. Lin YC, Chang PF, Chang MH, Ni YH. Genetic variants in GCKR and PNPLA3 confer susceptibility to nonalcoholic fatty liver disease in obese individuals. *Am J Clin Nutr.* (2014) 99:869–74. doi: 10.3945/ajcn.113.079749
28. Tam CH, Ma RC, So WY, Wang Y, Lam VK, Germer S, et al. Interaction effect of genetic polymorphisms in glucokinase. (GCK) and glucokinase regulatory protein. (GCKR) on metabolic traits in healthy Chinese adults and adolescents. *Diabetes.* (2009) 58:765–9. doi: 10.2337/db08-1277
29. Yang Z, Wen J, Tao X, Lu B, Du Y, Wang M, et al. Genetic variation in the GCKR gene is associated with non-alcoholic fatty liver disease in Chinese people. *Mol Biol Rep.* (2011) 38:1145–50. doi: 10.1007/s11033-010-0212-1
30. Zain SM, Mohamed Z, Mohamed R. Common variant in the glucokinase regulatory gene rs780094 and risk of nonalcoholic fatty liver disease: a meta-analysis. *J Gastroenterol Hepatol.* (2015) 30:21–7. doi: 10.1111/jgh.12714
31. Petit JM, Masson D, Guiu B, Rollot F, Duvillard L, Bouillet B, et al. GCKR polymorphism influences liver fat content in patients with type 2 diabetes. *Acta Diabetol.* (2016) 53:237–42. doi: 10.1007/s00592-015-0766-4
32. Santoro N, Caprio S, Pierpont B, Van Name M, Savoye M, Parks EJ. Hepatic *de novo* lipogenesis in obese youth is modulated by a common variant in the GCKR gene. *J Clin Endocrinol Metab.* (2015) 100:E1125–32. doi: 10.1210/jc.2015-1587
33. Santoro N, Feldstein AE, Enoksson E, Pierpont B, Kursawe R, Kim G, et al. The association between hepatic fat content and liver injury in obese children and adolescents: effects of ethnicity, insulin resistance, and common gene variants. *Diabetes Care.* (2013) 36:1353–60. doi: 10.2337/dc12-1791
34. Santoro N, Zhang CK, Zhao H, Pakstis AJ, Kim G, Kursawe R, et al. Variant in the glucokinase regulatory protein. (GCKR) gene is associated with fatty liver in obese children and adolescents. *Hepatology.* (2012) 55:781–9. doi: 10.1002/hep.24806
35. Simons N, Dekker JM, van Greevenbroek MM, Nijpels G, t Hart LM, van der Kallen CJ, et al. A common gene variant in glucokinase regulatory protein interacts with glucose metabolism on diabetic dyslipidemia: the combined CODAM and hoorn studies. *Diabetes Care.* (2016) 39:1811–7. doi: 10.2337/dc16-0153
36. Sliz E, Sebert S, Wurtz P, Kangas AJ, Soininen P, Lehtimaki T, et al. NAFLD risk alleles in PNPLA3, TM6SF2, GCKR and LYPLAL1 show divergent metabolic effects. *Hum Mol Genet.* (2018) 27:2214–23. doi: 10.1093/hmg/ddy124
37. Tan HL, Zain SM, Mohamed R, Rampal S, Chin KF, Basu RC, et al. Association of glucokinase regulatory gene polymorphisms with risk and severity of non-alcoholic fatty liver disease: an interaction study with adiponutrin gene. *J Gastroenterol.* (2014) 49:1056–64. doi: 10.1007/s00535-013-0850-x
38. Trico D, Caprio S, Rosaria Umano G, Pierpont B, Nouws J, Galderisi A, et al. Metabolic features of nonalcoholic fatty liver. (NAFL) in obese adolescents: findings from a multiethnic cohort. *Hepatology.* (2018) 68:1376–90. doi: 10.1002/hep.30035
39. Caddeo A, Jamialahmadi O, Solinas G, Pujia A, Mancina RM, Pingitore P, et al. MBOAT7 is anchored to endomembranes by six transmembrane domains. *J Struct Biol.* (2019) 206:349–60. doi: 10.1016/j.jsb.2019.04.006
40. Lee HC, Inoue T, Sasaki J, Kubo T, Matsuda S, Nakasaki Y, et al. LPIAT1 regulates arachidonic acid content in phosphatidylinositol and is required for cortical lamination in mice. *Mol Biol Cell.* (2012) 23:4689–700. doi: 10.1091/mbc.e12-09-0673
41. Basyte-Bacevice V, Skieceviciene J, Valantiene I, Sumskiene J, Petrenkiene V, Kondrackiene J, et al. TM6SF2 and MBOAT7 gene variants in liver fibrosis and cirrhosis. *Int J Mol Sci.* (2019) 20:1277. doi: 10.3390/ijms20061277
42. Buch S, Stickel F, Trepo E, Way M, Herrmann A, Nischalke HD, et al. A genome-wide association study confirms PNPLA3 and identifies TM6SF2 and MBOAT7 as risk loci for alcohol-related cirrhosis. *Nat Genet.* (2015) 47:1443–8. doi: 10.1038/ng.3417
43. Di Sessa A, Umano GR, Cirillo G, Del Prete A, Iacomino R, Marzuillo P, et al. The membrane-bound O-acyltransferase7 rs641738 variant in pediatric nonalcoholic fatty liver disease. *J Pediatr Gastroenterol Nutr.* (2018) 67:69–74. doi: 10.1097/MPG.0000000000001979
44. Dursun A, Yalnizoglu D, Ozgul RK, Karli Oguz K, Yucel-Yilmaz D. Clinical highlights of a very rare phospholipid remodeling disease due to MBOAT7 gene defect. *Am J Med Genet B Neuropsychiatr Genet.* (2019) 183:3–4. doi: 10.1002/ajmg.b.32762

45. Helsley RN, Varadharajan V, Brown AL, Gromovsky AD, Schugar RC, Ramachandiran I, et al. Obesity-linked suppression of membrane-bound O-acyltransferase 7. (MBOAT7) drives non-alcoholic fatty liver disease. *Elife.* (2019) 8:e49882. doi: 10.7554/eLife.49882
46. Krawczyk M, Rau M, Schattenberg JM, Bantel H, Pathil A, Demir M, et al. Combined effects of the PNPLA3 rs738409, TM6SF2 rs58542926, and MBOAT7 rs641738 variants on NAFLD severity: a multicenter biopsy-based study. *J Lipid Res.* (2017) 58:247–55. doi: 10.1194/jlr.P067454
47. Luukkonen PK, Zhou Y, Hyotylainen T, Leivonen M, Arola J, Orho-Melander M, et al. The MBOAT7 variant rs641738 alters hepatic phosphatidylinositols and increases severity of non-alcoholic fatty liver disease in humans. *J Hepatol.* (2016) 65:1263–5. doi: 10.1016/j.jhep.2016.07.045
48. Mancina RM, Dongiovanni P, Petta S, Pingitore P, Meroni M, Rametta R, et al. The MBOAT7-TMC4 variant rs641738 increases risk of nonalcoholic fatty liver disease in individuals of european descent. *Gastroenterology.* (2016) 150:1219–30.e1216. doi: 10.1053/j.gastro.2016.01.032
49. Thabet K, Asimakopoulos A, Shojaei M, Romero-Gomez M, Mangia A, Irving WL, et al. MBOAT7 rs641738 increases risk of liver inflammation and transition to fibrosis in chronic hepatitis C. *Nat Commun.* (2016) 7:12757. doi: 10.1038/ncomms12757
50. Thabet K, Chan HLY, Petta S, Mangia A, Berg T, Boonstra A, et al. The membrane-bound O-acyltransferase domain-containing 7 variant rs641738 increases inflammation and fibrosis in chronic hepatitis B. *Hepatology.* (2017) 65:1840–50. doi: 10.1002/hep.29064
51. Umano GR, Caprio S, Di Sessa A, Chalasani N, Dykas DJ, Pierpont B, et al. The rs626283 Variant in the MBOAT7 gene is associated with insulin resistance and fatty liver in caucasian obese youth. *Am J Gastroenterol.* (2018) 113:376–83. doi: 10.1038/ajg.2018.1
52. Viitasalo A, Eloranta AM, Atalay M, Romeo S, Pihlajamaki J, Lakka TA. Association of MBOAT7 gene variant with plasma ALT levels in children: the PANIC study. *Pediatr Res.* (2016) 80:651–5. doi: 10.1038/pr.2016.139
53. Xia Y, Huang CX, Li GY, Chen KH, Han L, Tang L, et al. Meta-analysis of the association between MBOAT7 rs641738, TM6SF2 rs58542926 and nonalcoholic fatty liver disease susceptibility. *Clin Res Hepatol Gastroenterol.* (2019) 43:533–41. doi: 10.1016/j.clinre.2019.01.008
54. Yalnizoglu D, Ozgul RK, Oguz KK, Ozer B, Yucel-Yilmaz D, Gurbuz B, et al. Expanding the phenotype of phospholipid remodelling disease due to MBOAT7 gene defect. *J Inherit Metab Dis.* (2019) 42:381–8. doi: 10.1002/jimd.12016
55. Ma Y, Belyaeva OV, Brown PM, Fujita K, Valles K, Karki S, et al. 17-beta hydroxysteroid dehydrogenase 13 is a hepatic retinol dehydrogenase associated with histological features of nonalcoholic fatty liver disease. *Hepatology.* (2019) 69:1504–19. doi: 10.1002/hep.30350
56. About F, Abel L, Cobat A. HCV-associated liver fibrosis and HSD17B13. *N Engl J Med.* (2018) 379:1875–6. doi: 10.1056/NEJMc1804638
57. Abul-Husn NS, Cheng X, Li AH, Xin Y, Schurmann C, Stevis P, et al. A protein-truncating HSD17B13 variant and protection from chronic liver disease. *N Engl J Med.* (2018) 378:1096–106. doi: 10.1056/nejmoa 1712191
58. Basyte-Bacevice V, Skieceviciene J, Valantiene I, Sumskiene J, Petrenkiene V, Kondrackiene J, et al. SERPINA1 and HSD17B13 gene variants in patients with liver fibrosis and cirrhosis. *J Gastrointestin Liver Dis.* (2019) 28:297–302. doi: 10.15403/jgld-168
59. Chen J, Zhuo JY, Yang F, Liu ZK, Zhou L, Xie HY, et al. 17-beta-hydroxysteroid dehydrogenase 13 inhibits the progression and recurrence of hepatocellular carcinoma. *Hepatobil Pancreat Dis Int.* (2018) 17:220–6. doi: 10.1016/j.hbpd.2018.04.006
60. Gellert-Kristensen H, Nordestgaard BG, Tybjaerg-Hansen A, Stender S. High risk of fatty liver disease amplifies the alanine transaminase-lowering effect of a HSD17B13 variant. *Hepatology.* (2019). doi: 10.1002/hep.30799. [Epub ahead of print].
61. Kozlitina J, Stender S, Hobbs HH, Cohen JC. HSD17B13 and chronic liver disease in blacks and hispanics. *N Engl J Med.* (2018) 379:1876–7. doi: 10.1056/NEJMc1804027
62. Pirola CJ, Garaycoechea M, Flichman D, Arrese M, San Martino J, Gazzi C, et al. Splice variant rs72613567 prevents worst histologic outcomes in patients with nonalcoholic fatty liver disease. *J Lipid Res.* (2019) 60:176–85. doi: 10.1194/jlr.P089953
63. Stickel F, Lutz P, Buch S, Nischalke HD, Silva I, Rausch V, et al. Genetic variation in HSD17B13 reduces the risk of developing cirrhosis and hepatocellular carcinoma in alcohol misusers. *Hepatology.* (2019). doi: 10.1002/hep.30996
64. Yang J, Trepo E, Nahon P, Cao Q, Moreno C, Letouze E, et al. A 17-beta-hydroxysteroid dehydrogenase 13 variant protects from hepatocellular carcinoma development in alcoholic liver disease. *Hepatology.* (2019) 70:231–40. doi: 10.1002/hep.30623
65. Romeo S, Kozlitina J, Xing C, Pertsemlidis A, Cox D, Pennacchio LA, et al. Genetic variation in PNPLA3 confers susceptibility to nonalcoholic fatty liver disease. *Nat Genet.* (2008) 40:1461–5. doi: 10.1038/ng.257
66. Romeo S, Sentinelli F, Cambuli VM, Incani M, Congiu T, Matta V, et al. The 148M allele of the PNPLA3 gene is associated with indices of liver damage early in life. *J Hepatol.* (2010) 53:335–8. doi: 10.1016/j.jhep.2010.02.034
67. Romeo S, Sentinelli F, Dash S, Yeo GS, Savage DB, Leonetti F, et al. Morbid obesity exposes the association between PNPLA3 I148M. (rs738409) and indices of hepatic injury in individuals of European descent. *Int J Obes.* (2010) 34:190–4. doi: 10.1038/ijo.2009.216
68. Rotman Y, Koh C, Zmuda JM, Kleiner DE, Liang TJ, Nash CRN. The association of genetic variability in patatin-like phospholipase domain-containing protein 3. (PNPLA3) with histological severity of nonalcoholic fatty liver disease. *Hepatology.* (2010) 52:894–903. doi: 10.1002/hep.23759
69. Salameh H, Hanayneh MA, Masadeh M, Naseemuddin M, Matin T, Erwin A, et al. PNPLA3 as a genetic determinant of risk for and severity of non-alcoholic fatty liver disease spectrum. *J Clin Transl Hepatol.* (2016) 4:175–91. doi: 10.14309/00000434-201510001-02091
70. Salameh H, Raff E, Erwin A, Seth D, Nischalke HD, Falleti E, et al. PNPLA3 gene polymorphism is associated with predisposition to and severity of alcoholic liver disease. *Am J Gastroenterol.* (2015) 110:846–56. doi: 10.1038/ajg.2015.137
71. Santoro N, Kursawe R, D'Adamo E, Dykas DJ, Zhang CK, Bale AE, et al. A common variant in the patatin-like phospholipase 3 gene. (PNPLA3) is associated with fatty liver disease in obese children and adolescents. *Hepatology.* (2010) 52:1281–90. doi: 10.1002/hep.23832
72. Scheiner B, Mandorfer M, Schwabl P, Payer BA, Bucsics T, Bota S, et al. The impact of PNPLA3 rs738409 SNP on liver fibrosis progression, portal hypertension and hepatic steatosis in HIV/HCV coinfection. *PLoS ONE.* (2015) 10:e0143429. doi: 10.1371/journal.pone.0143429
73. Seko Y, Yamaguchi K, Mizuno N, Okuda K, Takemura M, Taketani H, et al. Combination of PNPLA3 and TLL1 polymorphism can predict advanced fibrosis in Japanese patients with nonalcoholic fatty liver disease. *J Gastroenterol.* (2018) 53:438–48. doi: 10.1007/s00535-017-1372-8
74. Shen J, Wong GL, Chan HL, Chan HY, Yeung DK, Chan RS, et al. PNPLA3 gene polymorphism accounts for fatty liver in community subjects without metabolic syndrome. *Aliment Pharmacol Ther.* (2014) 39:532–9. doi: 10.1111/apt.12609
75. Shen J, Wong GL, Chan HL, Chan RS, Chan HY, Chu WC, et al. PNPLA3 gene polymorphism and response to lifestyle modification in patients with nonalcoholic fatty liver disease. *J Gastroenterol Hepatol.* (2015) 30:139–46. doi: 10.1111/jgh. 12656
76. Shen JH, Li YL, Li D, Wang NN, Jing L, Huang YH. The rs738409. (I148M) variant of the PNPLA3 gene and cirrhosis: a meta-analysis. *J Lipid Res.* (2015) 56:167–75. doi: 10.1194/jlr.M048777
77. Singal AG, Manjunath H, Yopp AC, Beg MS, Marrero JA, Gopal P, et al. The effect of PNPLA3 on fibrosis progression and development of hepatocellular carcinoma: a meta-analysis. *Am J Gastroenterol.* (2014) 109:325–34. doi: 10.1038/ajg.2013.476
78. Song G, Xiao C, Wang K, Wang Y, Chen J, Yu Y, et al. Association of patatin-like phospholipase domain-containing protein 3 gene polymorphisms with susceptibility of nonalcoholic fatty liver disease in a Han Chinese population. *Medicine.* (2016) 95:e4569. doi: 10.1097/MD.0000000000004569
79. Sookoian S, Castano GO, Burgueno AL, Gianotti TF, Rosselli MS, Pirola CJ. A nonsynonymous gene variant in the adiponutrin gene is associated with nonalcoholic fatty liver disease severity. *J Lipid Res.* (2009) 50:2111–6. doi: 10.1194/jlr.P900013-JLR200
80. Sookoian S, Castano GO, Pirola CJ. PNPLA3 I148M variant is associated with metabolic stress-response phenotype in patients with nonalcoholic fatty liver disease. *Hepatology.* (2015) 61:1769. doi: 10.1002/hep.27390
81. Sookoian S, Pirola CJ. Meta-analysis of the influence of I148M variant of patatin-like phospholipase domain containing 3 gene. (PNPLA3) on the susceptibility and histological severity of nonalcoholic fatty liver disease.

Hepatology. (2011) 53:1883–94. doi: 10.1002/hep.24283

82. Speliotes EK, Butler JL, Palmer CD, Voight BF, Consortium G, Consortium MI, et al. PNPLA3 variants specifically confer increased risk for histologic nonalcoholic fatty liver disease but not metabolic disease. *Hepatology.* (2010) 52:904–12. doi: 10.1002/hep.23768
83. Speliotes EK, Yerges-Armstrong LM, Wu J, Hernaez R, Kim LJ, Palmer CD, et al. Genome-wide association analysis identifies variants associated with nonalcoholic fatty liver disease that have distinct effects on metabolic traits. *PLoS Genet.* (2011) 7:e1001324. doi: 10.1371/journal.pgen.1001324
84. Stickel F, Buch S, Lau K, Meyer zu Schwabedissen H, Berg T, Ridinger M, et al. Genetic variation in the PNPLA3 gene is associated with alcoholic liver injury in caucasians. *Hepatology.* (2011) 53:86–95. doi: 10.1002/hep.24017
85. Stickel F, Buch S, Nischalke HD, Weiss KH, Gotthardt D, Fischer J, et al. Genetic variants in PNPLA3 and TM6SF2 predispose to the development of hepatocellular carcinoma in individuals with alcohol-related cirrhosis. *Am J Gastroenterol.* (2018) 113:1475–83. doi: 10.1038/s41395-018-0041-8
86. Tai CM, Huang CK, Tu HP, Hwang JC, Yeh ML, Huang CF, et al. Interactions of a PPARGC1A variant and a PNPLA3 variant affect nonalcoholic steatohepatitis in severely obese taiwanese patients. *Medicine.* (2016) 95:e3120. doi: 10.1097/MD.0000000000003120
87. Takeuchi Y, Ikeda F, Moritou Y, Hagihara H, Yasunaka T, Kuwaki K, et al. The impact of patatin-like phospholipase domain-containing protein 3 polymorphism on hepatocellular carcinoma prognosis. *J Gastroenterol.* (2013) 48:405–12. doi: 10.1007/s00535-012-0647-3
88. Tamaki N, Kurosaki M, Higuchi M, Takada H, Nakakuki N, Yasui Y, et al. Genetic polymorphisms of IL28B and PNPLA3 are predictive for HCV related rapid fibrosis progression and identify patients who require urgent antiviral treatment with new regimens. *PLoS ONE.* (2015) 10:e0137351. doi: 10.1371/journal.pone.0137351
89. Tian C, Stokowski RP, Kershenobich D, Ballinger DG, Hinds DA. Variant in PNPLA3 is associated with alcoholic liver disease. *Nat Genet.* (2010) 42:21–3. doi: 10.1038/ng.488
90. Tong J, Guo J, Hu J, Hou S, Zhang Y, Li Q. Correlation between patatin-like phospholipase domain-containing protein 3 gene polymorphisms and liver cirrhosis in a chinese han population with chronic hepatitis B. *Hepat Mon.* (2014) 14:e18943. doi: 10.5812/hepatmon.18943
91. Trepo E, Gustot T, Degre D, Lemmers A, Verset L, Demetter P, et al. Common polymorphism in the PNPLA3/adiponutrin gene confers higher risk of cirrhosis and liver damage in alcoholic liver disease. *J Hepatol.* (2011) 55:906–12. doi: 10.1016/j.jhep.2011.01.028
92. Trepo E, Guyot E, Ganne-Carrie N, Degre D, Gustot T, Franchimont D, et al. PNPLA3. (rs738409 C>G) is a common risk variant associated with hepatocellular carcinoma in alcoholic cirrhosis. *Hepatology.* (2012) 55:1307–8. doi: 10.1002/hep.25518
93. Trepo E, Nahon P, Bontempi G, Valenti L, Falleti E, Nischalke HD, et al. Association between the PNPLA3. (rs738409 C>G) variant and hepatocellular carcinoma: Evidence from a meta-analysis of individual participant data. *Hepatology.* (2014) 59:2170–7. doi: 10.1002/hep.26767
94. Trepo E, Pradat P, Potthoff A, Momozawa Y, Quertinmont E, Gustot T, et al. Impact of patatin-like phospholipase-3. (rs738409 C>G) polymorphism on fibrosis progression and steatosis in chronic hepatitis C. *Hepatology.* (2011) 54:60–9. doi: 10.1002/hep.24350
95. Ueyama M, Nishida N, Korenaga M, Korenaga K, Kumagai E, Yanai H, et al. The impact of PNPLA3 and JAZF1 on hepatocellular carcinoma in non-viral hepatitis patients with type 2 diabetes mellitus. *J Gastroenterol.* (2016) 51:370–9. doi: 10.1007/s00535-015-1116-6
96. Valenti L, Alisi A, Galmozzi E, Bartuli A, Del Menico B, Alterio A, et al. I148M patatin-like phospholipase domain-containing 3 gene variant and severity of pediatric nonalcoholic fatty liver disease. *Hepatology.* (2010) 52:1274–80. doi: 10.1002/hep.23823
97. Valenti L, Al-Serri A, Daly AK, Galmozzi E, Rametta R, Dongiovanni P, et al. Homozygosity for the patatin-like phospholipase-3/adiponutrin I148M polymorphism influences liver fibrosis in patients with nonalcoholic fatty liver disease. *Hepatology.* (2010) 51:1209–17. doi: 10.1002/hep.23622
98. Verrijken A, Beckers S, Francque S, Hilden H, Caron S, Zegers D, et al. A gene variant of PNPLA3, but not of APOC3, is associated with histological parameters of NAFLD in an obese population. *Obesity.* (2013) 21:2138–45. doi: 10.1002/oby.20366
99. Vespasiani-Gentilucci U, Gallo P, Porcari A, Carotti S, Galati G, Piccioni L, et al. The PNPLA3 rs738409 C > G polymorphism is associated with the risk of progression to cirrhosis in NAFLD patients. *Scand J Gastroenterol.* (2016) 51:967–73. doi: 10.3109/00365521.2016.1161066
100. Vigano M, Valenti L, Lampertico P, Facchetti F, Motta BM, D'Ambrosio R, et al. Patatin-like phospholipase domain-containing 3 I148M affects liver steatosis in patients with chronic hepatitis B. *Hepatology.* (2013) 58:1245–52. doi: 10.1002/hep.26445
101. Wang CW, Lin HY, Shin SJ, Yu ML, Lin ZY, Dai CY, et al. The PNPLA3 I148M polymorphism is associated with insulin resistance and nonalcoholic fatty liver disease in a normoglycaemic population. *Liver Int.* (2011) 31:1326–31. doi: 10.1111/j.1478-3231.2011.02526.x
102. Wang X, Liu Z, Wang K, Wang Z, Sun X, Zhong L, et al. Additive effects of the risk alleles of PNPLA3 and TM6SF2 on non-alcoholic fatty liver disease. (NAFLD) in a Chinese population. *Front Genet.* (2016) 7:140. doi: 10.3389/fgene.2016.00140
103. Xia MF, Ling Y, Bian H, Lin HD, Yan HM, Chang XX, et al. I148M variant of PNPLA3 increases the susceptibility to non-alcoholic fatty liver disease caused by obesity and metabolic disorders. *Aliment Pharmacol Ther.* (2016) 43:631–42. doi: 10.1111/apt.13521
104. Xu M, Li Y, Zhang S, Wang X, Shen J, Zhang S. Interaction of TM6SF2 E167K and PNPLA3 I148M variants in NAFLD in northeast China. *Ann Hepatol.* (2019) 18:456–60. doi: 10.1016/j.aohep.2018.10.005
105. Xu R, Tao A, Zhang S, Deng Y, Chen G. Association between patatin-like phospholipase domain containing 3 gene. (PNPLA3) polymorphisms and nonalcoholic fatty liver disease: a HuGE review and meta-analysis. *Sci Rep.* (2015) 5:9284. doi: 10.1038/srep09284
106. Yang J, Trepo E, Nahon P, Cao Q, Moreno C, Letouze E, et al. PNPLA3 and TM6SF2 variants as risk factors of hepatocellular carcinoma across various etiologies and severity of underlying liver diseases. *Int J Cancer.* (2019) 144:533–44. doi: 10.1002/ijc.31910
107. Yasui K, Kawaguchi T, Shima T, Mitsuyoshi H, Seki K, Sendo R, et al. Effect of PNPLA3 rs738409 variant. (I148 M) on hepatic steatosis, necroinflammation, and fibrosis in Japanese patients with chronic hepatitis C. *J Gastroenterol.* (2015) 50:887–93. doi: 10.1007/s00535-014-1018-z
108. Yen YH, Tsai MC, Wu CK, Chang KC, Hung CH, Chiu KW, et al. Association between PNPLA3. (rs738409 C>G) variant and hepatocellular carcinoma in Asian chronic hepatitis C patients: a longitudinal study. *J Formos Med Assoc.* (2018) 117:833–40. doi: 10.1016/j.jfma.2017.10.003
109. Young KA, Palmer ND, Fingerlin TE, Langefeld CD, Norris JM, Wang N, et al. Genome-wide association study identifies loci for liver enzyme concentrations in mexican americans: the GUARDIAN consortium. *Obesity.* (2019) 27:1331–37. doi: 10.1002/oby.22527
110. Yuan X, Waterworth D, Perry JR, Lim N, Song K, Chambers JC, et al. Population-based genome-wide association studies reveal six loci influencing plasma levels of liver enzymes. *Am J Hum Genet.* (2008) 83:520–8. doi: 10.1016/j.ajhg.2008.09.012
111. Zain SM, Mohamed R, Mahadeva S, Cheah PL, Rampal S, Basu RC, et al. A multi-ethnic study of a PNPLA3 gene variant and its association with disease severity in non-alcoholic fatty liver disease. *Hum Genet.* (2012) 131:1145–52. doi: 10.1007/s00439-012-1141-y
112. Zampino R, Coppola N, Cirillo G, Boemio A, Grandone A, Stanzione M, et al. Patatin-like phospholipase domain-containing 3 I148M variant is associated with liver steatosis and fat distribution in chronic hepatitis B. *Dig Dis Sci.* (2015) 60:3005–10. doi: 10.1007/s10620-015-3716-7
113. Zhang S, Wu H, Wu X, Lian W, Wang Y, Zhang X, et al. Association between PNPLA3 rs738409 polymorphisms and risk of hepatocellular carcinoma and its development in patients with cirrhosis: a meta-analysis. *Int J Clin Exp Med.* (2015) 8:6638–49.
114. Zhang Y, Cai W, Song J, Miao L, Zhang B, Xu Q, et al. Association between the PNPLA3 I148M polymorphism and non-alcoholic fatty liver disease in the Uygur and Han ethnic groups of northwestern China. *PLoS ONE.* (2014) 9:e108381. doi: 10.1371/journal.pone.0108381
115. Zhang Y, Guo T, Yang F, Mao Y, Li L, Liu C, et al. Single-nucleotide rs738409 polymorphisms in the PNPLA3 gene are strongly associated with alcoholic liver disease in Han Chinese males. *Hepatol Int.* (2018) 12:429–37. doi: 10.1007/s12072-018-9889-3
116. Liangpunsakul S, Beaudoin JJ, Shah VH, Puri P, Sanyal AJ, Kamath PS,

et al. Interaction between the patatin-like phospholipase domain-containing protein 3 genotype and coffee drinking and the risk for acute alcoholic hepatitis. *Hepatol Commun.* (2018) 2:29–34. doi: 10.1002/hep4.1123
117. Shang L, Mashek DG. The underpinnings of PNPLA3-mediated fatty liver emerge. *Hepatology.* (2019). doi: 10.1002/hep.30888. [Epub ahead of print].
118. Baulande S, Lasnier F, Lucas M, Pairault J. Adiponutrin, a transmembrane protein corresponding to a novel dietary- and obesity-linked mRNA specifically expressed in the adipose lineage. *J Biol Chem.* (2001) 276:33336–44. doi: 10.1074/jbc.M105193200
119. Jenkins CM, Mancuso DJ, Yan W, Sims HF, Gibson B, Gross RW. Identification, cloning, expression, and purification of three novel human calcium-independent phospholipase A2 family members possessing triacylglycerol lipase and acylglycerol transacylase activities. *J Biol Chem.* (2004) 279:48968–75. doi: 10.1074/jbc.M407841200
120. Wilson PA, Gardner SD, Lambie NM, Commans SA, Crowther DJ. Characterization of the human patatin-like phospholipase family. *J Lipid Res.* (2006) 47:1940–9. doi: 10.1194/jlr.M600185-JLR200
121. Huang Y, He S, Li JZ, Seo YK, Osborne TF, Cohen JC, et al. A feed-forward loop amplifies nutritional regulation of PNPLA3. *Proc Natl Acad Sci USA.* (2010) 107:7892–7. doi: 10.1073/pnas.1003585107
122. Lake AC, Sun Y, Li JL, Kim JE, Johnson JW, Li D, et al. Expression, regulation, and triglyceride hydrolase activity of Adiponutrin family members. *J Lipid Res.* (2005) 46:2477–87. doi: 10.1194/jlr.M500290-JLR200
123. Dubuquoy C, Robichon C, Lasnier F, Langlois C, Dugail I, Foufelle F, et al. Distinct regulation of adiponutrin/PNPLA3 gene expression by the transcription factors ChREBP and SREBP1c in mouse and human hepatocytes. *J Hepatol.* (2011) 55:145–53. doi: 10.1016/j.jhep.2010.10.024
124. Liang H, Xu J, Xu F, Liu H, Yuan D, Yuan S, Cai M, et al. The SRE motif in the human PNPLA3 promoter. (-97 to−88 bp) mediates transactivational effects of SREBP-1c. *J Cell Physiol.* (2015) 230:2224–32. doi: 10.1002/jcp.24951
125. Perttila J, Huaman-Samanez C, Caron S, Tanhuanpaa K, Staels B, Yki-Jarvinen H, et al. PNPLA3 is regulated by glucose in human hepatocytes, and its I148M mutant slows down triglyceride hydrolysis. *Am J Physiol Endocrinol Metab.* (2012) 302:E1063–9. doi: 10.1152/ajpendo.00125.2011
126. Basantani MK, Sitnick MT, Cai L, Brenner DS, Gardner NP, Li JZ, et al. Pnpla3/Adiponutrin deficiency in mice does not contribute to fatty liver disease or metabolic syndrome. *J Lipid Res.* (2011) 52:318–29. doi: 10.1194/jlr.M011205
127. Chen W, Chang B, Li L, Chan L. Patatin-like phospholipase domain-containing 3/adiponutrin deficiency in mice is not associated with fatty liver disease. *Hepatology.* (2010) 52:1134–42. doi: 10.1002/hep.23812
128. Li JZ, Huang Y, Karaman R, Ivanova PT, Brown HA, Roddy T, et al. Chronic overexpression of PNPLA3I148M in mouse liver causes hepatic steatosis. *J Clin Invest.* (2012) 122:4130–44. doi: 10.1172/JCI65179
129. BasuRay S, Smagris E, Cohen JC, Hobbs HH. The PNPLA3 variant associated with fatty liver disease. (I148M) accumulates on lipid droplets by evading ubiquitylation. *Hepatology.* (2017) 66:1111–24. doi: 10.1002/hep.29273
130. Smagris E, BasuRay S, Li J, Huang Y, Lai KM, Gromada J, et al. Pnpla3I148M knockin mice accumulate PNPLA3 on lipid droplets and develop hepatic steatosis. *Hepatology.* (2015) 61:108–18. doi: 10.1002/hep.27242
131. Linden D, Ahnmark A, Pingitore P, Ciociola E, Ahlstedt I, Andreasson AC, et al. Pnpla3 silencing with antisense oligonucleotides ameliorates nonalcoholic steatohepatitis and fibrosis in Pnpla3 I148M knock-in mice. *Mol Metab.* (2019) 22:49–61. doi: 10.1016/j.molmet.2019.01.013
132. Huang Y, Cohen JC, Hobbs HH. Expression and characterization of a PNPLA3 protein isoform. (I148M) associated with nonalcoholic fatty liver disease. *J Biol Chem.* (2011) 286:37085–93. doi: 10.1074/jbc.M111.290114
133. He S, McPhaul C, Li JZ, Garuti R, Kinch L, Grishin NV, et al. A sequence variation. (I148M) in PNPLA3 associated with nonalcoholic fatty liver disease disrupts triglyceride hydrolysis. *J Biol Chem.* (2010) 285:6706–15. doi: 10.1074/jbc.M109.064501
134. Pingitore P, Pirazzi C, Mancina RM, Motta BM, Indiveri C, Pujia A, et al. Recombinant PNPLA3 protein shows triglyceride hydrolase activity and its I148M mutation results in loss of function. *Biochim Biophys Acta.* (2014) 1841:574–80. doi: 10.1016/j.bbalip.2013.12.006
135. Pirazzi C, Valenti L, Motta BM, Pingitore P, Hedfalk K, Mancina RM, et al. PNPLA3 has retinyl-palmitate lipase activity in human hepatic stellate cells. *Hum Mol Genet.* (2014) 23:4077–85. doi: 10.1093/hmg/ddu121
136. Hellemans K, Grinko I, Rombouts K, Schuppan D, Geerts A. All-trans and 9-cis retinoic acid alter rat hepatic stellate cell phenotype differentially. *Gut.* (1999) 45:134–42. doi: 10.1136/gut.45.1.134
137. Hellemans K, Verbuyst P, Quartier E, Schuit F, Rombouts K, Chandraratna RA, et al. Differential modulation of rat hepatic stellate phenotype by natural and synthetic retinoids. *Hepatology.* (2004) 39:97–108. doi: 10.1002/hep.20015
138. Wang L, Tankersley LR, Tang M, Potter JJ, Mezey E. Regulation of alpha 2(I) collagen expression in stellate cells by retinoic acid and retinoid X receptors through interactions with their cofactors. *Arch Biochem Biophys.* (2004) 428:92–8. doi: 10.1016/j.abb.2004.05.004
139. Bruschi FV, Claudel T, Tardelli M, Caligiuri A, Stulnig TM, Marra F, et al. The PNPLA3 I148M variant modulates the fibrogenic phenotype of human hepatic stellate cells. *Hepatology.* (2017) 65:1875–90. doi: 10.1002/hep.29041
140. Wang Y, Kory N, BasuRay S, Cohen JC, Hobbs HH. PNPLA3, CGI-58, and inhibition of hepatic triglyceride hydrolysis in mice. *Hepatology.* (2019) 69:2427–41. doi: 10.1002/hep.30583
141. Murugesan S, Goldberg EB, Dou E, Brown WJ. Identification of diverse lipid droplet targeting motifs in the PNPLA family of triglyceride lipases. *PLoS ONE.* (2013) 8:e64950. doi: 10.1371/journal.pone.0064950
142. Chamoun Z, Vacca F, Parton RG, Gruenberg J. PNPLA3/adiponutrin functions in lipid droplet formation. *Biol Cell.* (2013) 105:219–33. doi: 10.1111/boc.201200036
143. BasuRay S, Wang Y, Smagris E, Cohen JC, Hobbs HH. Accumulation of PNPLA3 on lipid droplets is the basis of associated hepatic steatosis. *Proc Natl Acad Sci USA.* (2019) 116:9521–6. doi: 10.1073/pnas.1901974116
144. Negoita F, Blomdahl J, Wasserstrom S, Winberg ME, Osmark P, Larsson S, et al. PNPLA3 variant M148 causes resistance to starvation-mediated lipid droplet autophagy in human hepatocytes. *J Cell Biochem.* (2019) 120:343–56. doi: 10.1002/jcb.27378
145. Yang A, Mottillo EP, Mladenovic-Lucas L, Zhou L, Granneman JG. Dynamic interactions of ABHD5 with PNPLA3 regulate triacylglycerol metabolism in brown adipocytes. *Nat Metab.* (2019) 1:560–9. doi: 10.1038/s42255-019-0066-3
146. Pingitore P, Dongiovanni P, Motta BM, Meroni M, Lepore SM, Mancina RM, et al. PNPLA3 overexpression results in reduction of proteins predisposing to fibrosis. *Hum Mol Genet.* (2016) 25:5212–22. doi: 10.1093/hmg/ddw341
147. Bruschi FV, Claudel T, Tardelli M, Starlinger P, Marra F, Trauner M. PNPLA3 I148M Variant impairs liver X receptor signaling and cholesterol homeostasis in human hepatic stellate cells. *Hepatol Commun.* (2019) 3:1191–204. doi: 10.1002/hep4.1395
148. Kollerits B, Coassin S, Beckmann ND, Teumer A, Kiechl S, Doring A, et al. Genetic evidence for a role of adiponutrin in the metabolism of apolipoprotein B-containing lipoproteins. *Hum Mol Genet.* (2009) 18:4669–76. doi: 10.1093/hmg/ddp424
149. Hotta K, Yoneda M, Hyogo H, Ochi H, Mizusawa S, Ueno T, et al. Association of the rs738409 polymorphism in PNPLA3 with liver damage and the development of nonalcoholic fatty liver disease. *BMC Med Genet.* (2010) 11:172. doi: 10.1186/1471-2350-11-172
150. Krawczyk M, Grunhage F, Zimmer V, Lammert F. Variant adiponutrin. (PNPLA3) represents a common fibrosis risk gene: non-invasive elastography-based study in chronic liver disease. *J Hepatol.* (2011) 55:299–306. doi: 10.1016/j.jhep.2010.10.042
151. Kitamoto T, Kitamoto A, Yoneda M, Hyogo H, Ochi H, Nakamura T, et al. Genome-wide scan revealed that polymorphisms in the PNPLA3, SAMM50, and PARVB genes are associated with development and progression of nonalcoholic fatty liver disease in Japan. *Hum Genet.* (2013) 132:783–92. doi: 10.1007/s00439-013-1294-3
152. Hernaez R, McLean J, Lazo M, Brancati FL, Hirschhorn JN, Borecki IB, et al. Association between variants in or near PNPLA3, GCKR, and PPP1R3B with ultrasound-defined steatosis based on data from the third National Health and Nutrition Examination Survey. *Clin Gastroenterol Hepatol.* (2013) 11:1183–90.e1182. doi: 10.1016/j.cgh.2013.02.011
153. Hassan MM, Kaseb A, Etzel CJ, El-Serag H, Spitz MR, Chang P, et al. Genetic variation in the PNPLA3 gene and hepatocellular carcinoma in USA: risk and prognosis prediction. *Mol Carcinog.* (2013) 52(Suppl 1):E139–47. doi: 10.1002/mc.22057
154. Kupcinskas J, Valantiene I, Varkalaite G, Steponaitiene R, Skieceviciene J, Sumskiene J, et al. PNPLA3 and RNF7 gene variants are associated with the risk of developing liver fibrosis and cirrhosis in an eastern

european population. *J Gastrointestin Liver Dis.* (2017) 26:37–43. doi: 10.15403/jgld.2014.1121.261.pnp
155. Beaudoin JJ, Long N, Liangpunsakul S, Puri P, Kamath PS, Shah V, et al. An exploratory genome-wide analysis of genetic risk for alcoholic hepatitis. *Scand J Gastroenterol.* (2017) 52:1263–9. doi: 10.1080/00365521.2017.1359664
156. Chung GE, Lee Y, Yim JY, Choe EK, Kwak MS, Yang JI, et al. Genetic polymorphisms of PNPLA3 and SAMM50 are associated with nonalcoholic fatty liver disease in a korean population. *Gut Liver.* (2018) 12:316–23. doi: 10.5009/gnl17306
157. Namjou B, Lingren T, Huang Y, Parameswaran S, Cobb BL, Stanaway IB, et al. GWAS and enrichment analyses of non-alcoholic fatty liver disease identify new trait-associated genes and pathways across eMERGE Network. *BMC Med.* (2019) 17:135. doi: 10.1186/s12916-019-1364-z
158. Burza MA, Molinaro A, Attilia ML, Rotondo C, Attilia F, Ceccanti M, et al. PNPLA3 I148M. (rs738409) genetic variant and age at onset of at-risk alcohol consumption are independent risk factors for alcoholic cirrhosis. *Liver Int.* (2014) 34:514–20. doi: 10.1111/liv.12310
159. Chamorro AJ, Torres JL, Miron-Canelo JA, Gonzalez-Sarmiento R, Laso FJ, Marcos M. Systematic review with meta-analysis: the I148M variant of patatin-like phospholipase domain-containing 3 gene. (PNPLA3) is significantly associated with alcoholic liver cirrhosis. *Aliment Pharmacol Ther.* (2014) 40:571–81. doi: 10.1111/apt.12890
160. Falleti E, Fabris C, Cmet S, Cussigh A, Bitetto D, Fontanini E, et al. PNPLA3 rs738409C/G polymorphism in cirrhosis: relationship with the aetiology of liver disease and hepatocellular carcinoma occurrence. *Liver Int.* (2011) 31:1137–43. doi: 10.1111/j.1478-3231.2011.02534.x
161. Burza MA, Pirazzi C, Maglio C, Sjoholm K, Mancina RM, Svensson PA, et al. PNPLA3 I148M. (rs738409) genetic variant is associated with hepatocellular carcinoma in obese individuals. *Dig Liver Dis.* (2012) 44:1037–41. doi: 10.1016/j.dld.2012.05.006
162. Falleti E, Cussigh A, Cmet S, Fabris C, Toniutto P. PNPLA3 rs738409 and TM6SF2 rs58542926 variants increase the risk of hepatocellular carcinoma in alcoholic cirrhosis. *Dig Liver Dis.* (2016) 48:69–75. doi: 10.1016/j.dld.2015.09.009
163. Gao X, Liu W, Yang L, Zhang X, Ma N, Wang L, et al. Association between PNPLA3 gene polymorphisms and risk of hepatitis B virus-related hepatocellular carcinoma in Han population in China:a case-control study. *Scand J Gastroenterol.* (2017) 52:1120–7. doi: 10.1080/00365521.2017.1334088
164. Guyot E, Sutton A, Rufat P, Laguillier C, Mansouri A, Moreau R, et al. PNPLA3 rs738409, hepatocellular carcinoma occurrence and risk model prediction in patients with cirrhosis. *J Hepatol.* (2013) 58:312–8. doi: 10.1016/j.jhep.2012.09.036
165. Huang Z, Guo X, Zhang G, Liang L, Nong B. Correlation between PNPLA3 rs738409 polymorphism and hepatocellular carcinoma: a meta-analysis of 10,330 subjects. *Int J Biol Markers.* (2019) 34:117–22. doi: 10.1177/1724600818812471
166. Li JF, Zheng EQ, Xie M. Association between rs738409 polymorphism in patatin-like phospholipase domain-containing protein 3. (PNPLA3) gene and hepatocellular carcinoma susceptibility: evidence from case-control studies. *Gene.* (2019) 685:143–8. doi: 10.1016/j.gene.2018.11.012
167. Liu YL, Patman GL, Leathart JB, Piguet AC, Burt AD, Dufour JF, et al. Carriage of the PNPLA3 rs738409 C >G polymorphism confers an increased risk of non-alcoholic fatty liver disease associated hepatocellular carcinoma. *J Hepatol.* (2014) 61:75–81. doi: 10.1016/j.jhep.2014.02.030
168. Nischalke HD, Berger C, Luda C, Berg T, Muller T, Grunhage F, et al. The PNPLA3 rs738409 148M/M genotype is a risk factor for liver cancer in alcoholic cirrhosis but shows no or weak association in hepatitis C cirrhosis. *PLoS ONE.* (2011) 6:e27087. doi: 10.1371/journal.pone.0027087
169. Raksayot M, Chuaypen N, Khlaiphuengsin A, Pinjaroen N, Treeprasertsuk S, Poovorawan Y, et al. Independent and additive effects of PNPLA3 and TM6SF2 polymorphisms on the development of non-B, non-C hepatocellular carcinoma. *J Gastroenterol.* (2019) 54:427–36. doi: 10.1007/s00535-018-01533-x
170. Sookoian S, Pirola CJ. PNPLA3, the triacylglycerol synthesis/hydrolysis/storage dilemma, and nonalcoholic fatty liver disease. *World J Gastroenterol.* (2012) 18:6018–26. doi: 10.3748/wjg.v18.i42.6018
171. Mullard A. PCSK9-lowering RNAi contender clears first phase III trial. *Nat Rev Drug Discov.* (2019) 18:737. doi: 10.1038/d41573-019-00153-1

16

Biliary Epithelial Senescence in Liver Disease: There will be SASP

Vik Meadows[1], Leonardo Baiocchi[2], Debjyoti Kundu[1], Keisaku Sato[1], Yessenia Fuentes[3], Chaodong Wu[4], Sanjukta Chakraborty[5], Shannon Glaser[5], Gianfranco Alpini[1,6], Lindsey Kennedy[1,6]† and Heather Francis[1,6]*†*

[1]Hepatology and Gastroenterology, Medicine, Indiana University, Indianapolis, IN, United States, [2]Hepatology Unit, University of Tor Vergata, Rome, Italy, [3]Clinical and Translational Sciences Institute, STEM GEHCS Program, Indiana University School of Medicine, Indianapolis, IN, United States, [4]Department of Nutrition, Texas A&M University, College Station, TX, United States, [5]Department of Medical Physiology, Texas A&M University College of Medicine, Bryan, TX, United States, [6]Richard L. Roudebush VA Medical Center, Indianapolis, IN, United States

***Correspondence:**
Lindsey Kennedy
linkenn@iu.edu
Heather Francis
heafranc@iu.edu

†These authors share senior authorship

Cellular senescence is a pathophysiological phenomenon in which proliferative cells enter cell cycle arrest following DNA damage and other stress signals. Natural, permanent DNA damage can occur after repetitive cell division; however, acute stress or other injuries can push cells into premature senescence and eventually a senescence-associated secretory phenotype (SASP). In recent years, there has been increased evidence for the role of premature senescence in disease progression including diabetes, cardiac diseases, and end-stage liver diseases including cholestasis. Liver size and function change with aging, and presumably with increasing cellular senescence, so it is important to understand the mechanisms by which cellular senescence affects the functional nature of the liver in health and disease. As well, cells in a SASP state secrete a multitude of inflammatory and pro-fibrogenic factors that modulate the microenvironment. Cellular SASP and the associated, secreted factors have been implicated in the progression of liver diseases, such as cholestatic injury that target the biliary epithelial cells (i.e., cholangiocytes) lining the bile ducts. Indeed, cholangiocyte senescence/SASP is proposed to be a driver of disease phenotypes in a variety of liver injuries. Within this review, we will discuss the impact of cholangiocyte senescence and SASP in the pathogenesis of cholestatic disorders.

Keywords: cholestasis, fatty liver, cell cycle arrest, bile duct, aging

INTRODUCTION

Cholangiocytes, which are morphologically heterogenous, polarized cells lining the biliary epithelium (Han et al., 2013; Banales et al., 2019), have high absorptive/secretory functions and play a role in the *1*) modification of canalicular bile, *2*) paracrine communication with portal cells, and *3*) regulation of immune cell infiltration (Nathanson and Boyer, 1991; Chen et al., 2008; Banales et al., 2019). Cholangiocytes are the target of various liver diseases such as fatty liver diseases (non-alcoholic fatty liver disease [NAFLD], non-alcoholic steatohepatitis [NASH]), alcoholic liver disease (ALD) and chronic cholestatic liver diseases including primary biliary cholangitis (PBC), primary sclerosing cholangitis (PSC), biliary atresia, and cholangiocarcinoma. Biliary secretory functions regulate liver inflammation and fibrosis (by both autocrine and paracrine pathways) through secretion of cytokines and other factors which may contribute to liver damage (Kennedy et al., 2021; Kyritsi et al., 2021). Cellular senescence increases in cholangiocytes of PSC patients, likely contributing to disease progression (Tabibian et al., 2014a). Moreover, many factors secreted from cholangiocytes, such as interleukin (IL)-1β, IL-6, monocyte chemoattractant protein (MCP)-1, stem cell factor (SCF), transforming growth factor β1 (TGF-β1), and platelet derived growth factor (PDGF), are components of the senescence-associated secretory phenotype (SASP) (Rao and Jackson, 2016; Lopes-Paciencia et al., 2019; Blokland et al., 2020). Senescence and SASP secretion have gained considerable attention in studies of cholestatic liver disease progression, demonstrating a new role for senescent cholangiocytes in the pathogenesis of liver diseases (Knop et al., 1987; Wu et al., 2016).

CHOLANGIOCYTE CELL CYCLE ARREST AND PROGRESSION

The liver is composed of two main types of epithelial cells: hepatocytes and biliary epithelial cells (i.e., cholangiocytes). In normal conditions, cholangiocytes represent less than 10% of total hepatic cellular mass in humans and 2–3% in rodents (Alpini et al., 1988); however, upon stimulation, they support bile acid (BA)-independent bile flow accounting for approximately 50% of total bile secretion (Kanno et al., 2000). Small and large cholangiocytes line small (<15 μm diameter) and large (≥15 μm diameter) bile ducts, respectively (Cheung et al., 2018). Heterogeneity in size closely relates to the difference in activity and functions of cholangiocytes. Large, cyclic adenosine monophosphate (cAMP)-dependent cholangiocytes represent the mature, hormone-dependent portion of biliary epithelium, while small Ca^{2+}-dependent cholangiocytes are considered a typically quiescent population (Hall et al., 2017; Banales et al., 2019). Specifically, only small cholangiocytes proliferate when stimulated with a specific histamine receptor agonist (HRH1); however, small cholangiocytes can also acquire large cholangiocyte phenotypes after insult such as GABA treatment (Francis et al., 2008; Mancinelli et al., 2013). Secretory and proliferative activities of the cholangiocytes are finely tuned by several hormones, neuropeptides and angiogenic factors (Alvaro et al., 2007; Franchitto et al., 2013). For instance, secretin binding to the cholangiocyte-specific secretin receptor (SR, a G-protein coupled receptor) stimulates bicarbonate enriched choleresis, thereby increasing intracellular cAMP and activating the biliary cAMP/protein kinase A (PKA)-dependent cystic fibrosis transmembrane conductance regulator (CFTR) opening and subsequent anion exchange protein 2 (AE2) activation (Glaser et al., 2009; Mancinelli et al., 2013; Wu et al., 2020). Fluctuations in intracellular levels of cAMP, and its role as a second messenger, are important in the biliary epithelia not only for secretory activities, but also for proliferative processes (Baiocchi et al., 2021). Large cholangiocyte proliferation is tightly regulated by cAMP-dependent PKA/proto-oncogene tyrosine-protein kinase Src (Src)/mitogen activated protein kinase kinase (MEK)/ extracellular signal-regulated protein kinases 1/2 (ERK1/2) signaling axis (Francis et al., 2004). Three proliferative modalities have been identified in experiments in normal and pathological biliary conditions (Alvaro et al., 2000). Type I (typical proliferation) is represented by an inordinate hyperplastic growth of bile ducts and is observed in the cholestatic injury model of bile duct ligation (BDL) in rodents (Alvaro et al., 2007; Glaser et al., 2009). Conversely, Type II (atypical proliferation) spreads outside the portal space, with irregular truncated ducts and is associated with chronic cholestatic diseases or severe injuries (Franchitto et al., 2013). Finally, Type III proliferation is characterized by expansion of the "oval" cells (i.e., hepatic progenitor cells, located in the Canals of Hering) and is characteristic of BDL and 3,5-diethoxycarbonyl-1,4-dihydrocollidine (DDC) diet in rodent models and in human PBC (Olynyk et al., 1998; Carpino et al., 2018; Fragoulis et al., 2019). While each type of proliferative modality is separate, many cholestatic models, such as BDL, may exhibit multiple subtypes during disease progression.

On the opposite side of active eukaryotic cell division and growth stands cell cycle arrest (Toettcher et al., 2009). This molecular process promptly activates during conditions of cellular stress and DNA damage, thus preventing cell damage/ repair and ceasing normal replicative activities. When cell repair cannot accommodate increased DNA damage, cell cycle arrest may evolve toward a programmed cell death route (Wiman and Zhivotovsky, 2017), such as autophagy (Glick et al., 2010), necroptosis (Khoury et al., 2020) and apoptosis (Fleisher, 1997). Homeostatic regulation of growth by apoptosis has been confirmed in biliary epithelia (Bhathal and Gall, 1985). In fact, proliferative insult to rat cholangiocytes (either BDL or α-naphthyl isothiocyanate administration) has been shown to determine an apoptosis-dependent restoration of normal bile duct mass (Lesage et al., 2001). From these and other findings, apoptosis deregulation has been suggested to play an important role in determining and maintaining ductopenic cholangiopathies, such as human PBC or PSC (Celli and Que, 1998). However, in recent years, cell cycle arrest has gained attention for the possibility to give rise to a senescent cellular phenotype. This seems associated with tissue aging, as well as acute damage from pathological conditions, including those affecting the biliary system since senescent cells are generally anti-apoptotic (Childs et al., 2014).

AGING AND SENESCENCE

Aging is a complex process. Several factors contribute to this progression including genetic, mitochondrial, peptidic and paracrine components (López-Otín et al., 2013); however, at the cellular level a specific phenotype has been consistently identified in aged tissue: the senescent cell (Campisi, 2013). This phenotype is characterized by an irreversible interruption of replicative phases possibly to prevent oncogenic proliferation after cellular injury (Sager, 1991). Two other specific features belong to a senescent cell: *1)* lack of progression toward apoptosis; and *2)* development of a SASP (Coppé et al., 2008). Following the induction of SASP, senescent cells are considered to contribute to some degenerative diseases. Experiments in transgenic mice with deletion of senescent cells, demonstrated improved outcomes of neurologic, vascular and musculoskeletal degenerative processes (Campisi et al., 2019). It is important to underscore that the complex and heterogeneous SASP paracrine stimuli negatively or positively affect the microenvironment depending upon the pathophysiological setting. SASP may contribute to the prevention of cancer or even tissue repair (Campisi, 2013). In this perspective, the strong activity of SASP in wound healing seems in conflict with the reduced regenerative capability of aged tissue.

SENESCENCE IN CHOLANGIOPATHIES

Primary Biliary Cholangitis

PBC is an autoimmune chronic liver disease characterized by cholestasis and ductopenia of the interlobular bile ducts (Onofrio et al., 2019). PBC primarily affects middle-aged women who may present with abdominal discomfort, pruritus, fatigue or no symptoms, complicating its complex etiology (Onofrio et al., 2019). Diagnostic criteria for PBC include positive serum anti-mitochondrial antibodies (AMA) and chronic (~24 weeks) abnormal ALP levels or comparable liver histology analysis (Onofrio et al., 2019). Recent studies have advanced diagnosis and treatment options for PBC patients, but therapeutics targeting senescence have not been evaluated in the clinical settings (Onofrio et al., 2019). Due to increased bile duct senescence in PBC patients, understanding biliary senescence/ SASP development remains a novel strategy to understand disease progression.

Many correlative studies have evaluated the expression of senescence and SASP in human PBC samples (Sasaki et al., 2005; Sasaki et al., 2006; Sasaki et al., 2008), but mechanistic studies are scarce. Telomere shortening has been noted in the small ducts of PBC patients and is found in conjunction with expression of p16 and p21 (Sasaki et al., 2008). Another study has shown that small ducts of PBC patients highly expressed senescent markers, and this was associated with the development of non-suppurative cholangitis and the portal infiltration of inflammatory cells (Sasaki et al., 2005). Indeed, enhanced biliary senescence is a driver of worsening disease in PBC, but the cause of senescence induction is complicated. A potential cause for this increased senescence includes enhanced oxidative stress. *In vitro* work demonstrated that biliary senescence may be driven by enhanced oxidative stress as determined by H_2O_2 and nitric oxide stimulation (Sasaki et al., 2005). This theory is supported by work that found increased endoplasmic reticulum (ER) stress, which is associated with oxidative stress, in the small ducts of patients with PBC, and the *in vitro* induction of ER stress promoted senescence in cultured cholangiocytes (Sasaki et al., 2015). Enhanced cell stress is an understandable component of biliary senescence considering the large degree of immune cell-induced damage to the cholangiocytes that occurs during PBC. Additionally, understanding the impact of enhanced biliary senescence during PBC pathogenesis is relevant considering high-risk PBC patients, identified by impaired ursodeoxycholic acid (UDCA) response, have increased p21 gene and protein expression when compared to low-risk PBC patients (Hardie et al., 2016). Recent work characterized the serum proteome of PBC patients and found that patients with attenuated response to UDCA had enhanced serum levels of chemokines associated with senescence, which the authors postulate to be released from senescent cholangiocytes (Barron-Millar et al., 2021). Specifically, the serum levels of C-X-C motif chemokine ligand 11 (CXCL11) and chemokine ligand 20 (CCL20) were significantly inversely correlated with UDCA response (Barron-Millar et al., 2021). This work underlines the importance of senescence in PBC pathogenesis, but also identifies new prognostic factors to be utilized for treatment strategies (Barron-Millar et al., 2021). Additionally, others demonstrated that inducing senescence in cholangiocytes *via* oxidative stress, DNA damage and serum deprivation *in vitro* leads to a subsequent increase in secretion of various chemokines (Sasaki et al., 2010a). These senescent cholangiocytes enhanced macrophage recruitment, which was blocked using neutralizing antibodies against CCL2 and fractalkine (i.e., chemokines) (Sasaki et al., 2010a). Of relevance, CCL2 and fractalkine expression was increased in inflamed bile ducts in human PBC samples (Sasaki et al., 2010a). Moreover, senescent small ducts in PBC also express genes associated with inflammation and immune response (Sasaki et al., 2021). This work further highlights that biliary senescence induces a pro-inflammatory secretome within damaged cholangiocytes, which promotes inflammation and the recruitment of various inflammatory cells. These mechanisms are obvious drivers of a worsening prognosis, considering the association of biliary senescence with UDCA response, and so it is imperative we define these mechanisms to understand disease progression.

Aside from oxidative stress, autophagy has been implicated as a driver of cholangiocyte senescence during PBC. Expression of autophagy markers are increased in damaged small ducts in PBC patients and are co-localized with senescence marker expression (Sasaki et al., 2010b). In cultured cholangiocytes, inhibition of autophagy blocked senescence (Sasaki et al., 2010b). Autophagy markers were expressed in the ductular reactive cells of both early- and late-stage PBC patients, whereas senescent markers were predominantly found in late-stage PBC, suggesting that autophagy precedes senescence development (Sasaki et al., 2012a). Similarly, p62 sequestrome-1 (p62, involved in autophagy) aggregates are found in inflamed small ducts in PBC and are co-expressed with obligate autophagy and senescent markers (Sasaki et al., 2012b). Knockdown of p62 reduced autophagy and senescence in cultured cholangiocytes (Sasaki et al., 2012b), lending reason to a potential link between autophagy and biliary senescence in PBC initiation and progression. These studies suggest a mechanism preceding biliary senescence in PBC, which can be used as a target to block the development of biliary senescence and subsequent liver injury. *In vitro*, treatment with hydrophobic BAs reduced AE2 expression, and enhanced oxidative stress and senescence in human cholangiocytes, showing that the hepatic microenvironment may initiate biliary oxidative stress and senescence. (Hisamoto et al., 2016). Since loss of the bicarbonate umbrella, specifically through reduced AE2 expression, is a hallmark of PBC, this data is quite compelling (Arenas et al., 2019; Banales et al., 2012). In human samples, decreased expression of AE2 is correlated with increased bile duct senescence during PBC (Sasaki et al., 2018a), thus identifying that the bicarbonate umbrella may be an important component of PBC progression *via* increased senescence. As well, these studies link loss of the bicarbonate umbrella, a cholangiocyte-specific protective mechanism, with biliary senescence which is a novel and new finding. Interestingly, both the bicarbonate umbrella and SASP factor release can be utilized to identify unique biliary signatures in PBC, which may point to new mechanisms or markers. Upstream of AE2 activity is secretin/SR signaling, that is a determinant modulating the bicarbonate umbrella and bile flow (Jones et al., 2015). When looking at early-stage PBC, one study found enhanced secretin/SR expression in bile ducts of human samples and the dominant-negative TGF-β receptor II mouse model of PBC (Kennedy et al., 2019). In this murine model of early-stage PBC, treatment with a SR antagonist (Sec 5–27) reduced SR activation and subsequently decreased TGF-β1 expression, biliary senescence, and liver fibrosis (Kennedy et al., 2019). This study found elevated secretin/SR axis and subsequent TGF-β1 secretion and TGF-βR1 expression in human early-stage PBC samples compared to healthy control, insinuating a role for secretin/SR in PBC development and subsequent senescence (Kennedy et al., 2019). This work describes an upstream pathway regulating biliary senescence/SASP during PBC, and this mechanism may potentially be targeted for therapeutic use.

Underscoring our previous comments, direct targeting of senescence or other factors driving senescence may be therapeutic for PBC treatment, and this has been tested in experimental models. Expression of senescent markers (p16 and p21) and the anti-apoptotic marker, B cell lymphoma-extra-large (Bcl-xL), are enhanced in the small ducts of patients with PBC (Sasaki et al., 2020). Specifically, senescent cholangiocytes were found within the ductular reactions and corresponded with stage, hepatitis activity and inadequate response to UDCA (Sasaki et al., 2020). Lastly, the authors induced senescence in murine cholangiocytes *in vitro* and found that treatment with senolytics (AA-1331852, Navitoclax, Dasatinib and Dasatinib with Quercetin) induced apoptosis and effectively cleared senescent cholangiocytes (Sasaki et al., 2020). The polycomb group gene, Bmil downregulates p16 expression, and reduced expression of Bmil in the small ducts of PBC, and *in vitro* oxidative stress was able to repress Bmil expression in cultured cholangiocytes (Sasaki et al., 2006). Together, these findings confirm an associated theme of oxidative stress promoting senescence in PBC. Antioxidant therapies may remedy PBC-associated injury through reduced biliary senescence; however, it is imperative that we delineate the role of biliary senescence in PBC pathogenesis to define additional therapeutic options for patients. This section has highlighted the potential for antioxidant and senolytic therapies for the treatment of PBC.

Primary Sclerosing Cholangitis

PSC is an idiopathic chronic cholangiopathy characterized by increased hepatic inflammation, bridging fibrosis and progressive cholestasis (Lazaridis and LaRusso, 2015). Much like PBC, senescent cholangiocytes have been implicated in PSC progression and exacerbation of hepatic damage through paracrine secretion of inflammatory and fibrotic factors (Lazaridis and LaRusso, 2015). Therapeutic options for PSC patients are limited, with liver transplantation serving as the sole therapeutic option to improve long-term survival (Rawla and Samant, 2021). A common feature in PSC is reactive cholangiocytes, which may exhibit proliferative or senescent marker expression and increased inflammatory and fibrotic factor secretion (Lazaridis and LaRusso, 2015). The role of biliary senescence in PSC has been of rising interesting, but its exact impact on disease progression remains undefined.

Early work using primary cholangiocytes isolated from PSC patients found that these cholangiocytes highly express the senescence markers, p16 and γH2A.X, compared to normal cholangiocytes (Tabibian et al., 2014a). Similarly, another study found that cholangiocytes isolated from PSC patients and maintained in primary culture have a lower proliferative rate and high expression of SA-β-galactosidase when compared to normal cholangiocytes (Tabibian et al., 2014b). PSC cholangiocytes were also found to have increased secretion of SASP components (IL-6, IL-8, CCL2, PAI-1) compared to normal cholangiocytes, and these SASP factors induced senescence in bystander cholangiocytes as indicated by *in vitro* co-culture systems (Tabibian et al., 2014a). In this study, the induction of biliary senescence was driven by neuroblastoma RAS viral oncogene homolog (N-Ras) activation in cholangiocytes (Tabibian et al., 2014a). Others have found that cholangiocytes of PSC patients have increased expression of senescence factors as indicated by staining in liver sections (Ferreira-Gonzalez et al., 2018). Together, all of these studies suggest that biliary senescence is a key component of PSC, and similar to PBC it can confer a worsening phenotype through modulation of nearby cells. A novel murine model of inducible cholangiocyte senescence has found that upregulation of p53, through knockout of mouse double minute 2 proto-oncogene (Mdm2), leads to increased p16, p21 and γH2AX in bile ducts (Ferreira-Gonzalez et al., 2018). This work found that senescent cholangiocytes have elevated secretion of SASP factors with paracrine consequences such as increased hepatocyte senescence, exacerbated hepatic fibrosis and decreased liver regeneration (Ferreira-Gonzalez et al., 2018). Interestingly, the induction of biliary senescence in normal mice promoted portal macrophage infiltration and peribiliary fibrosis which aggravated these phenotypes when combined with DDC feeding to induce cholestasis (Ferreira-Gonzalez et al., 2018). This work demonstrates that biliary senescence alone can promote phenotypes associated with PSC, and this conclusion brings forth the question on the ability of cholangiocyte senescence to be a component of PSC etiology. In an *in vitro* model, cholangiocyte organoids (cholangoids) made from normal patient cholangiocytes that are exposed to H_2O_2 (to induce senescence, termed NHC-sen) display senescence and SASP characteristics. Further, NHC-sen cholangoids, as well as PSC cholangoids enhance macrophage recruitment compared to control (Guicciardi et al., 2018). Interestingly, isolated cholangiocytes from PSC patients have increased expression of genes associated with cell cycle arrest and senescence, as indicated by RNA-seq, and senescent cholangiocytes formed cholangoids of a smaller size that also lacked a lumen when compared to normal cholangiocytes (Jalan-Sakrikar et al., 2021). This work is supported by other findings showing that NHC-sen cells promote the proliferation of healthy cholangiocytes and monocyte migration, which was also found with plasma EVs from multidrug resistant cassette 2 knock out (*Mdr2*$^{-/-}$) mice, a genetic murine model of PSC (Al Suraih et al., 2020). The identification of increased biliary senescence in PSC is worth intensive evaluation since it is correlated with DR, fibrosis staging and other markers of severe disease in PSC patients (Cazzagon et al., 2021). Together, the above work demonstrate that biliary senescence can induce senescence of nearby cholangiocytes and drive hepatic damage associated with cholangiopathies, such as PSC.

A feature of senescent cholangiocytes is a pro-inflammatory and pro-fibrotic secretome. One study found that biliary-derived TGF-β1 promoted paracrine cholangiocyte senescence (Ferreira-Gonzalez et al., 2018) and it has been shown that TGF-β1 blocks cell cycle progression by enhancing the transcription of senescent factors such as cyclin-dependent kinase inhibitors, p21 and p27 (Datto et al., 1995). Indeed, others have found TGF-β1 promotes cholangiocyte senescence and subsequent liver fibrosis through autocrine and paracrine signaling (Wu et al., 2016). Increased biliary TGF-β1 synthesis and secretion was found to be downstream of the secretin/SR pathway, only expressed by cholangiocytes in the liver (Wu et al., 2016) thereby demonstrating a cholangiocyte-specific mechanism regulating biliary senescence in cholangiopathies. Additionally, the inhibition of secretin/SR signaling using Sec 5–27 or SR$^{-/-}$ mice reduced biliary senescence, TGF-β1 levels and liver fibrosis in models of PSC (BDL and *Mdr2*$^{-/-}$ mice) (Wu et al., 2016; Zhou et al., 2018). It is apparent that cholangiocyte-derived TGF-β1 is an important factor mediating biliary (autocrine) and liver (paracrine) damage during PSC. Aside from cholangiocytes, mast cells secrete TGF-β1 and induce biliary senescence and other markers of cholestasis (Kyritsi et al., 2021), which is an important feature considering that mast cell migration to portal areas is a key feature and damaging component of cholestasis (Wilcox et al., 1986; Tsuneyama et al., 1999; Jones et al., 2016). Mast cell farnesoid X receptor (FXR) signaling promotes biliary senescence and associated biliary and liver damage in murine models of PSC (Meadows et al., 2021). Mast cell-derived components lend to worsening phenotypes in PSC and understanding if they can be targeted to mediate damage is a topic of research currently. Stem cell factor (SCF) is another cholangiocyte secretory component, and SASP factor, found to promote senescence in models of PSC (Meadows et al., 2019). It was demonstrated that SCF Vivo-Morpholino treatment (to reduce SCF expression) significantly decreased biliary senescence, as well as DR and liver fibrosis in *Mdr2*$^{-/-}$ mice (Meadows et al., 2019). In addition, this study demonstrated enhanced serum SCF and biliary SCF expression in human PSC compared to control samples (Meadows et al., 2019). This finding is corroborated by a correlative study demonstrating aberrant biliary SCF expression in human PSC samples (Tsuneyama et al., 1999). Interestingly, cholangiocyte SCF expression correlated with increased portal infiltration of cKit (SCF receptor) positive mast cells in human PSC (Tsuneyama et al., 1999), and SCF Vivo-Morpholino reduced hepatic mast cell presence in *Mdr2*$^{-/-}$ mice (Meadows et al., 2019), insinuating that biliary senescence mediates mast cell number and activity during PSC. This work further lends to the hypothesis that cholangiocyte secreted SASP factors can modulate the microenvironment and promote damage through the recruitment of immune cells, including mast cells.

Other signaling factors have been implicated in PSC-associated biliary senescence, such as histamine signaling, as demonstrated when *Mdr2*$^{-/-}$ mice were treated with a Vivo-Morpholino targeting the H2 histamine receptor (H2HR) inhibited biliary senescence, liver inflammation and fibrogenesis (Kennedy et al., 2020). Interestingly, this study determined that H2HR inhibition selectively targets large cholangiocyte senescence through downregulation of TGF-β1 expression (Kennedy et al., 2020), which again underlines the significance of TGF-β1 signaling in cholangiocytes during cholestatic injury. Biliary heterogeneity is an important factor influencing PSC damage. Classic PSC can affect both small and large bile ducts while small-duct PSC demonstrates fibrosis and inflammation of small ducts alone (Rawla and Samant, 2021). Understanding heterogeneity of PSC senescence is important since FoxA2, a definitive endoderm marker and transcription factor, is reduced in human PSC (McDaniel et al., 2017). Previous work has also demonstrated that this factor is predominantly expressed in small mouse cholangiocytes and liver progenitor cells *in vitro* and transplant of cultured small mouse cholangiocytes enhances FoxA2 expression, reduces biliary senescence and liver fibrosis in BDL and *Mdr2*$^{-/-}$ mice (McDaniel et al., 2017). A preferential increase in large bile duct mass has been noted in *Mdr2*$^{-/-}$ mice, demonstrating that this subpopulation may be more prone to injury and thus senescent damage (Kennedy et al., 2018a). In this regard, biliary heterogeneity may be an important aspect of biliary senescence, but more studies are warranted. It is imperative that we better define biliary heterogeneity in humans, specifically in the context of disease, to understand if these pathways identified in mouse models can hold true in the clinical setting.

Aging, in the context of disease, can work hand-in-hand with senescence to perturb liver injury (Kundu et al., 2020). Aged mice show increased expression of microRNAs (miRs) associated with aging processes (miR-1a, miR-20a, miR-30e), and increased expression of these miRs correlated with increased twinfilin-1 (twf-1) levels (Maroni et al., 2019). Interestingly, twf-1 expression increased in the DDC feeding model of cholestasis and in human PSC samples, and *Twf-1*$^{-/-}$ mice subjected to DDC had reduced biliary senescence and SASP (Maroni et al., 2019). Additionally, senescence-accelerated mice (SAMP8) had increased twf-1 expression and subsequent biliary senescence/SASP (Maroni et al., 2019). However, little work on the inappropriate induction of aging processes in cholestasis, including PSC, has not been evaluated thus far. Identifying signals inducing aging pathways cholangiocytes will be an important finding for PSC studies. Interestingly, the microbiota has been implicated in biliary senescence, as well (Tabibian et al., 2016). *Mdr2*$^{-/-}$

mice housed in a germ-free facility had exacerbated biliary senescence/SASP, associated DR and liver fibrosis (Tabibian et al., 2016). This is not surprising considering the gut-liver axis is vital for physiological function. This work also demonstrates that we can target factors outside of the liver in an effort to reduce biliary senescence during PSC, and this can potentially be applied to other cholestatic injuries as well.

Since cholangiocyte senescence and SASP are related to PSC-associated biliary and liver damage, it is of interest to evaluate if blocking biliary senescence/SASP may ameliorate damage. One study treated *Mdr2*$^{-/-}$ mice with a p16 Vivo-Morpholino and found that this treatment reduced p16 expression and senescence, TGF-β1 expression and biliary secretion of SASP components (Kyritsi et al., 2020). Furthermore, p16 Vivo-Morpholino reduced DR and portal fibrosis in *Mdr2*$^{-/-}$ mice compared to controls, which was shown to be linked to reduced miR-34a/Sirtuin-1 (SIRT1) signaling (Kyritsi et al., 2020). This is relevant considering others have found SIRT1 activity to promote cholangiocyte senescence in a model of obstructive cholestasis (Jia et al., 2021). One study generated an *Mdr2*$^{-/-}$/p16$^{-/-}$ mouse, as well an *Mdr2*$^{-/-}$ mouse line crossed with the p16Ink4a apoptosis, through targeted activation of caspase (INK-ATTAC) mouse capable of selective clearance of p16-expressing cells, and found that both of these models had reduced biliary senescence and SASP, and subsequent decreased inflammation and portal fibrosis (Alsuraih et al., 2021). Additionally, the authors found that fisetin, a flavonoid that acts as a senolytic, induced similar phenotypic changes in *Mdr2*$^{-/-}$ mice, and *in vitro* selectively targeted senescent cholangiocytes (Alsuraih et al., 2021). These studies are in parallel with those in PBC by demonstrating that blocking biliary senescence may be therapeutic for the treatment of PSC. Lastly, it is known that senescent cells are resistant to apoptotic clearance as demonstrated by enhanced Bcl-xL expression in senescent cholangiocytes, as one study displayed the protective mechanism of biliary apoptosis in a model of PSC (Moncsek et al., 2018). Specifically, the clearance of senescent cholangiocytes by Bcl-xL inhibitor treatment reduced liver fibrosis and inflammatory marker expression (Moncsek et al., 2018). These studies establish the powerful impact of targeting biliary senescence for the treatment of PSC and the gaps in knowledge to be filled in with future studies.

Biliary Atresia

Biliary atresia is a devastating pediatric cholestatic and fibrogenic liver disease with a multifactorial etiology and unknown molecular mechanism of pathogenesis (Bezerra et al., 2018; Kerola et al., 2019). Early intervention with Kasai hepatic portoenterostomy, to restore bile flow, and eventual liver transplantation increases survival of biliary atresia patients (Bezerra et al., 2018). Due to its complex pathology, a major challenge with biliary atresia treatment includes therapeutic target identification for early diagnosis. Like in adult cholestatic liver diseases, biliary and hepatic progenitor cells (HPC) senescence may exacerbate liver damage; however, research on senescence/SASP factors in biliary atresia remains severely understudied (Sasaki et al., 2018b; Wu et al., 2018; Xiao et al., 2019; Winkler et al., 2021). In the following section we highlight key studies implicating biliary senescence, and SASP factors, as contributors to biliary atresia development.

Biliary atresia patients show reduced telomere length in hepatic tissues, demonstrating telomere length negatively correlates with pediatric end-stage liver disease score (Sanada et al., 2012). The stress of biliary atresia can be measured outside of the liver, implicating far reaching effects of premature liver dysfunction (Udomsinprasert et al., 2015). Peripheral leukocytes in biliary atresia patients had reduced telomere length compared to healthy control (Udomsinprasert et al., 2015). This work found that leukocyte telomere length shortened with biliary atresia progression and had positive correlation with hepatic telomere length (Udomsinprasert et al., 2015). Interestingly, this study found that in two sets of identical twins, the twin with biliary atresia presented with reduced telomere length in hepatic tissue compared with the healthy twin (Udomsinprasert et al., 2015). These data allow us to postulate that stress from exhaustive proliferation of cholangiocytes may result in biliary senescence and diminishing immune intervention in disease progression in biliary atresia patients. Genomic instability caused by shortened telomere length initiates apoptosis and senescence and provides a therapeutic avenue for biliary atresia patients upstream of senescence (López-Otín et al., 2013). Previous work demonstrated that cholangiocytes from the adeno-associated virus (AAV) murine model of biliary atresia, expressed major histocompatibility complex (MHC) I and II, but did not serve as antigen presenting cells. Instead, these cholangiocytes modulated immune response by secretion of pro-inflammatory cytokines and chemokines (tumor necrosis factor α [TNFα] and TGF-β) (Barnes et al., 2009). This study identifies that biliary immunobiology may be an important component of biliary atresia progression through the release of inflammatory mediators. While this study does not discuss biliary immune regulation in the context of senescence/SASP, it does point to a hypothesis whereby senescent cholangiocytes may have dysregulated expression of MHC components or other immune signaling factors, or vice versa, that contribute to biliary atresia.

Senescent cholangiocyte present with enhanced p16 and p21 expression, particular in DR, in PBC and PSC; however, the role of biliary senescence in pediatric cholangiopathies like biliary atresia is limited (Sasaki et al., 2018b). Biliary and HPC p16 expression was found to be elevated in biliary atresia explant livers, indicating senescence as a component of biliary atresia pathogenesis (Sasaki et al., 2018b). Biliary atresia patients undergoing Kasai portoenterostomy have increased neural cell adhesion molecule (NCAM) positive DR cells, a stemness marker expressed by HPCs in the liver, with minimal NCAM-positive bile ducts (Sasaki et al., 2018b). However, at the time of liver transplantation, these patients had elevated NCAM expression in DR and bile duct cells, implicating differentiation during disease progression. This study also found a positive correlation between bile duct p21 expression and bile duct loss in biliary atresia patients, insinuating that the NCAM-positive DR cells (suspected to be HPCs) could be attempting to resolve bile duct loss in biliary atresia patients by differentiating into bile duct epithelial cells

(Sasaki et al., 2018b). This complex study discusses HPC proliferation and differentiation into cholangiocytes in the context of DR and cholangiocytes senescence, but the signaling mechanisms are complicated and additional work is necessary.

A murine model of inducible cholangiocyte senescence shows that senescent cholangiocytes have elevated secretion of SASP factors with paracrine consequences such as increased hepatocyte senescence, exacerbated hepatic fibrosis and decreased liver regeneration (Ferreira-Gonzalez et al., 2018). In this study, inhibition of TGF-β1 reduced biliary SASP secretion and increased hepatocyte proliferation and liver function (Ferreira-Gonzalez et al., 2018). Kasai portoenterostomy may resolve some features of cholestasis and fibrosis, but in a select group of patients' fibrosis can remain following surgery (Kerola et al., 2019). In biliary atresia, TGF-β1 and decorin expression was elevated in lobular hepatocytes and fibrotic areas and correlated with liver fibrosis (Kerola et al., 2019). At 3-year follow-up, successful Kasai portoenterostomy significantly reduced hepatic TGF-β1 and connective tissue growth factor (CTGF) expression, while TGF-β2 expression was found to be increased (Kerola et al., 2019), signifying a central role for the TGF-β superfamily in promoting continued liver fibrosis after Kasai portoenterostomy. Considering that CTGF drives senescence in fibroblasts (Capparelli et al., 2012) it is reasonable to expect cholangiocyte SASP paracrine communication as central to biliary atresia progression and successfulness of Kasai portoenterostomy. Moreover, recent work found elevated levels of long non-coding RNA (lnc) H19 in serum and hepatic lysates from biliary atresia patients compared to healthy controls (Xiao et al., 2019). These H19 levels positively correlated with fibrosis in patients, marking it as a potential biomarker in disease detection. The authors also found elevated expression of fibrogenic markers, TGF-β, α-smooth muscle actin (αSMA) and ciliary localization (Cil)-1a, along with CK-7 (bipotential marker in HPC) in biliary atresia patients (Xiao et al., 2019). The isolated serum exosome analysis from biliary atresia patients revealed elevated lncH19, high mobility group AT-Hook 2 (HMGA2) and sphingosine-1-phosphate receptor 2 (S1PR2) compared to healthy controls, further implicating that hepatic fibrosis in biliary atresia could be paracrine in nature. It is plausible that these exosomes are cholangiocyte-derived and contribute to biliary atresia-associated fibrosis *via* paracrine crosstalk. While the discussed factors are not obligate SASP components, it is known that senescent and SASP cholangiocytes have an increased secretory component and could thus be a source of these pro-fibrogenic exosomes.A previous study found that *ex vivo* ductal organoids damaged with acetaminophen had induced caspase-3, apoptosis marker, and SASP factors expression, including TGF-β1, PDGF, IL-1β, IL-6, and TNF-α (Chusilp et al., 2020). This study indicates that cholangiocyte damage drives fibrotic response during biliary atresia. While fibrosis has been well established as a characteristic of biliary atresia, the crosstalk between biliary senescence and excessive fibrosis has yet to be captured. Understanding the profibrotic and prosenescent bile ducts and HPCs in biliary atresia may serve as a therapeutic target for disease attenuation in patients waiting for liver transplantation.

SENESCENCE IN FATTY LIVER DISEASES

Non-Alcoholic Fatty Liver Disease (NAFLD)/ Non-Alcoholic Steatohepatitis (NASH)

Senescence has been the focus of recent studies with respect to various metabolic conditions including NAFLD (Zhou et al., 2021). Senescence, independent of aging, can exacerbate disease phenotypes resulting in the progression of the metabolic condition. NAFLD, or the more recent term MAFLD (metabolism-associated fatty liver disease) is the direct hepatic pathological manifestation of excess lipids and fats, primarily sourced from diet (Mantovani and Dalbeni, 2020; Younossi et al., 2021). Initiation of benign steatosis escalates into infiltration of leukocytes, mast cells and development of peribiliary fibrosis with this "second hit" (Zhu et al., 2020). This phenomenon can advance to non-alcoholic steatohepatitis (NASH) and, upon persistent insults, the liver progresses to cirrhosis and potentially hepatocellular carcinoma (HCC) which warrant liver transplantation.

The role of hepatocytes has been well studied in NAFLD (Venkatesh et al., 2017; Simon et al., 2020); however, there has been increasing interest in the contribution from cholangiocytes (Mendez-Sanchez et al., 2007; Kennedy et al., 2021; Zhou et al., 2021). A study showing evidence of DR in NAFLD was performed in rats fed with choline deficient high trans-fat diet where severe hepatic injuries were identified in areas of liver section with more CK-19 positive DR as identified by immunohistochemistry (de Lima et al., 2008). Cholangiocyte damage increases with hepatic steatosis development in NAFLD and NASH patients, further indicating cholangiocyte contribution to disease development (Natarajan et al., 2014). These early studies postulate a role from cholangiocytes in NAFLD and NASH, but true contribution is still be investigated. Cholangiocytes respond to fatty acid-induced lipo-toxicity by assuming a lipo-apoptotic phenotype *in vitro* (Natarajan et al., 2014; Natarajan et al., 2017) emphasizing a critical role for bile ducts in the phenotypic manifestation of NAFLD and describing a possible mechanism contributing to DR. It was also shown that NASH patients have increased DR and bridging fibrosis, which are two main hallmarks of cholangiocyte damage widely studied in cholangiopathies (Sorrentino et al., 2005). NAFLD and end-stage NASH patients also have increased DR and senescence (Kennedy et al., 2018b). Indeed, biliary senescence may be a significant contributor to NAFLD and NASH progression, similar to the cholangiopathies discussed above.

Similar to traditional cholangiopathies mast cells have been implicated in NAFLD/NASH progression. In histidine decarboxylase knock-out (HDC KO) mice, that have loss of endogenous histamine signaling, subjected to high-fat diet (HFD) there was reduced cholangiocyte damage and senescence, indicating a role for histamine signaling in bile duct damage during NAFLD progression (Kennedy et al., 2018b). Histamine has been previously indicated to aid in regulation of food intake and body weight *via* modulation of leptin signaling (Yoshimatsu et al., 1999; Jørgensen et al., 2007). Thus, this study crucially emphasizes the contribution of senescent cholangiocyte-mediated histamine release in fatty liver disease progression (Kennedy et al., 2018b). These studies define a crucial role for histamine in worsening liver phenotypes in NAFLD and NASH, but few studies have described mast cells and their derived components. NASH patients have increased serum insulin growth factor-1 (IGF-1, SASP factor) compared to healthy controls and C57BL6J mice fed western diet (WD) secrete enhanced IGF-1, specifically from cholangiocytes (Kennedy et al., 2021). Importantly, *in vitro* studies demonstrated that inhibition of mast cell IGF-1 receptor *via* antagonist treatment decreased migration toward damaged cholangiocytes. Further, this work demonstrates that expression of SASP factors from senescent cholangiocytes induce mast cell migration that promotes microvesicular steatosis *via* microRNA 144-3p (miR-144-3p)/aldehyde hydrogenase 1A3 (ALDH1A3) signaling (Kennedy et al., 2021). In general, this work shows that senescent cholangiocytes may worsen NAFLD and NASH *via* the recruitment of immune cells, including mast cells. In an analysis of 1,022 NAFLD patient biopsies, microvesicular steatosis has been identified as an advanced phenotype and strongly, positively correlation with hepatic ballooning, higher NAFLD activity score (NAS) and advanced fibrosis (Tandra et al., 2011). NAFLD patients also exhibit elevated serum histamine, implicating a role for mast cell-histamine in micro-vesicular steatosis development. It can be surmised from these studies that cholangiocytes exhibit a dynamic response to the damaging stimuli in NAFLD/NASH and secrete factors that increase mast cell infiltration that perturb injury. Interestingly, HFD fed older mice (8 and 18 months) showed increased M1 macrophage (proinflammatory) infiltration in liver indicating the effect of cellular senescence in immune cell infiltration during NAFLD (Fontana et al., 2013). As well, this work describes the role of aging in cellular senescence, but more studies to fully understand the mechanism is warranted. Further characterization of cholangiocyte sub-population (small/large) in HFD/WD models is required to understand how biliary epithelia contribute to the damage caused during NAFLD/NASH and may also highlight important information on biliary heterogeneity in terms of senescence induction that may help to understand cholestatic disease processes better.

Alcoholic Liver Disease (ALD)

Liver pathophysiology associated with ALD is similar to NAFLD and includes severe steatosis, portal inflammation, and fibrosis ultimately leading to cirrhosis and liver failure (Yeh and Brunt, 2014). Although ALD can be differentiated from NAFLD based on etiology, aging is still an independent driving factor for the former. Previous work has shown that age was an influencing factor on the severity of liver injury, inflammation and fibrosis in mice fed with short- and long-term alcohol treatments (Ramirez et al., 2017). Further, the expression of SIRT1 was downregulated in aged animals and restoration of SIRT1 reversed the damage caused by binge alcohol feeding (Ramirez et al., 2017). The effects of alcohol on aging-related damage have been shown in Alzheimer's disease, where alcohol directly reduced telomere length, one of the major manifestations of senescence (Yamaki et al., 2019). Based on these data one would assume that ALD affects cellular senescence through its cellular toxicity. As well, these studies implicate aging in the promotion of cellular senescence. The main enzyme responsible for elimination of alcohol in humans is ALDH2, and when mutated, this enzyme increases the risk of developing alcohol-related HCC in Asian population (Matsumoto et al., 2016; Chang et al., 2017). Hepatocyte specific *Aldh2*$^{-/-}$ mice subjected to 3-h ethanol gavage showed reduced aldehyde content compared to control, suggesting a role for other hepatic cells in hepatic metabolism and clearance of alcohol (Guillot et al., 2019). Interestingly, *in vitro*, ethanol provides a dose-dependent protection against cellular senescence by activating ALDH2 in endothelial cells, thereby suggesting a pivotal role of ALDH2 in senescence (Xue et al., 2019). ALDH2 mediates anti-senescence effects during chronic ethanol challenge by activation of SIRT1/p53 pathway in human aortic endothelial cells, *in vitro* (Xue et al., 2018). siRNA mediated knockdown of ALDH2 increased senescence-associated β-galactosidase, p21 and p53 expression in human vascular endothelial cells (Nannelli et al., 2018). Small molecule activator of ALDH2, N-(1,3-benzodioxol-5-ylmethyl)-2,6-dichlorobenzamide (Alda-1), alleviates the reduced aldehyde clearance and reverse hepatic steatosis in male C57BL6J mice subjected to 8-week alcohol treatment (Zhong et al., 2015). These studies identify an interesting role of ALDH2 in blocking cellular senescence, and this factor may be an important target to inhibit biliary senescence in ALD and other cholestatic disorders. Further, inhibition of ALDH3A1 by administration of synthetic inhibitors, tetraethyl thiuram disulfide (disulfiram), diethylamino benzaldehyde, or 4-amino-4-methyl-pent-2-ynthioic acid, S-methyl ester (ampalthiol ester), reduced cellular proliferation (Muzio et al., 2012). The reduced proliferation could be due to the inhibition of ALDH3A1 since its downstream effectors/targets CCL20, G-protein coupled receptor-37 (GPR37), and DEAD-box helicase 3 Y-linked protein (DDX3Y) have been implicated in growth and differentiation (Ruzinova and Benezra, 2003; Moreb et al., 2008). ALDH3A1-siRNA treatment in lung cancer cell lines, H522 and A549, reduced proliferation *via* increased peroxisome proliferation activated receptor (PPAR) expression (Oraldi et al., 2011). Thus, expression of ALDHs might be inversely correlated with onset and progression of cellular senescence.

Increased cellular senescence and miR-34a expression has been reported in the NIAAA murine model of ALD (Wan et al., 2017). Inhibition of miR-34a by Vivo-Morpholino reduced ALT, fibrosis, senescence and pathology score in ethanol-treated mice (Wan et al., 2017). Moreover, miR-34a has been implicated in the regulation of cellular senescence of cholangiocytes and hepatic stellate cells in ALD mice (Annable et al., 2015; Wan et al., 2015). Due to the increasing incidence of biliary senescence in other liver diseases, there may be an important role in for cholangiocyte senescence and SASP in ALD progression. As well, defining a set of miRs associated with biliary senescence could be key for delineating a senescence-associated miR profile or identifying therapeutic, prognostic or diagnostic targets.

Taken together, these studies highlight a role for aldehyde metabolism and miRNA signaling in mediating liver cellular

TABLE 1 | Factors associated with cellular senescence in chronic liver disease.

Chronic liver disease	Cellular mechanism associated with senescence
Primary Biliary Cholangitis (PBC)	Telomere shortening, p16 and p21 expression Oxidative stress and ER stress Increased expression of CXCL11, CCL20, CCL2 and fractalkine Cholangiocyte autophagy including p62 signaling Loss of AE2 and the bicarbonate umbrella Enhanced secretin/SR signaling (early-stage PBC) Increased Bcl-xL (anti-apoptosis) expression Reduced Bmi1 (antioxidant) expression
Primary Sclerosing Cholangitis (PSC)	p16, p21, γH2A.X and SA-β-galactosidase expression Cholangiocyte secretion of SASP factors (IL-6, IL-8, CCL2, PAI-1) N-Ras activation in cholangiocytes Increased TGF-β1 signaling Upregulation of biliary secretin/SR signaling Mast cell-derived TGF-β1 and FXR signaling Cholangiocyte SCF secretion Increased biliary H2HR signaling Reduced biliary expression of FoxA2 Increased age-related miRs and Twf-1 signaling Enhanced miR-34a/SIRT1 activity Increased Bcl-xL (anti-apoptosis) expression
Biliary Atresia	Reduced telomere length in hepatic tissues and peripheral leukocytes Enhanced biliary MHC I and II expression, and secretion of TNFα and TGF-β p16, p21 and NCAM expression Enhanced TGF-β1, TGF-β2, decorin and CTGF expression Increased serum and hepatic H19 levels Biliary expression of TGF-β, αSMA and Cil-1a Serum exosome H19, HMGA2 and S1PR2 levels Increased caspase-3, TGF-β1, PDGF, IL-1β, IL-6, and TNF-α expression in *ex vivo* ductal organoids
Non-Alcoholic Fatty Liver Disease (NAFLD)/Non-Alcoholic Steatohepatitis (NASH)	Dysregulated histamine/leptin signaling in cholangiocytes Biliary IGF-1 secretion and mast cell miR-144-3p/ALDH1A3 signaling Age-related M1 macrophage infiltration
Alcoholic Liver Disease (ALD)	Reduced SIRT1 activity Inhibition of ALDH2 and ALDH3A1 Increased miR-34a

Table outlining the various signaling mechanisms and phenotypes associated with cellular senescence in chronic liver diseases, as discussed in the review. Senescence-associated factors and mechanisms are divided by disease, including PBC, PSC, NAFLD/NASH, and ALD.

senescence during ALD. The expression of ALDHs and miRNAs and their impact of biliary senescence on ALD is poorly understood. Further investigation is required to elucidate the role cholangiocytes, particularly senescent cholangiocytes, play in alcohol metabolism and damage progression in ALD.

FUTURE DIRECTIONS AND CONCLUSION

DR and biliary senescence/SASP are characteristic of cholangiopathies and are increasing in incidence during fatty liver disease progression and ALD, confirming biliary involvement, although mechanisms remain unclear. Biliary SASP factor secretion can increase the infiltration of mast cells and activate nearby cholangiocytes in cholestatic and NAFLD/NASH murine models, leading to increased inflammation and fibrosis. Mechanistic understanding of the role that biliary heterogeneity plays in SASP development has yet to be defined. Hepatocyte senescence drives hepatic steatosis in an age-dependent manner (Ogrodnik et al., 2017); however, further investigation into individual cell contribution to disease progression will provide novel therapeutic targets for patient treatment options. Future work should utilize cholangiocyte-specific mouse models to target biliary senescence and SASP factors to evaluate the role that these factors may play in the progression of cholangiopathies, NAFLD/NASH and ALD. As well, more studies are needed to define whether biliary senescence is an etiologic component of these liver disorders or a pathological consequence. Specifically in the context of NAFLD/NASH and ALD, that are not traditional cholangiopathies but nonetheless harbor cholestatic injury in a subset of patients, it is imperative to define which factors drive biliary damage in this setting. Understanding the mechanisms that promote biliary senescence in NAFLD/NASH and ALD is important since this injurious component can confer a worsening phenotype and poor prognosis. The recent onset of sophisticated experimental procedures, such as spatial transcriptomics and RNA sequencing, give researchers the capabilities to define the cellular niche during liver damage and can be utilized to describe biliary senescence in this setting. The power of RNA-sequencing

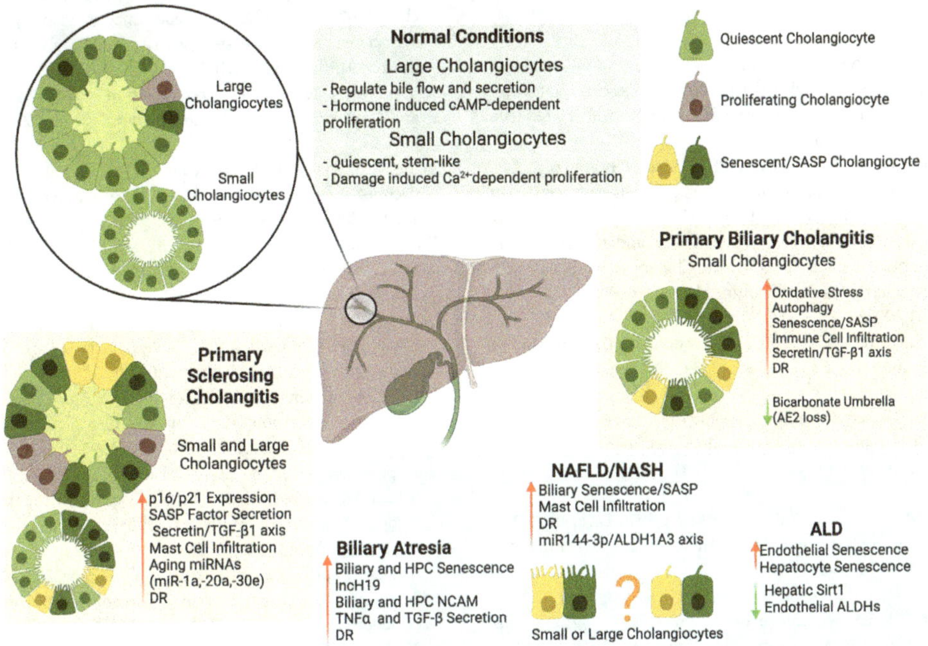

FIGURE 1 | Biliary Senescence in Liver Disease. The key findings summarized in our review indicate that biliary heterogeneity and senescence/SASP factor secretion provide a novel direction for the study and treatment of chronic liver disease. Further exploration of the mechanism behind premature cholangiocyte senescence/SASP should help clarify the role of the biliary tree in chronic liver diseases. Created with biorender.com.

can be used to evaluate the heterogeneity of biliary response to injury and induction of senescence. As well, spatial transcriptomics should be useful in defining the interaction of senescent cholangiocytes with the surrounding liver cells, and multiplex imaging assays can be used in a similar manner to define senescent cholangiocyte interaction with infiltrating immune cells. It is apparent that other experimental parameters are necessary to better define the onset of biliary senescence and the role that biliary senescence and SASP play during liver disease progression.

Biliary senescence and SASP will likely continue to gain attention in the field since cellular senescence/SASP factor secretion affects liver function and chronic liver disease progression (Meadows et al., 2019; Xiao et al., 2019; Kennedy et al., 2021). The use of senolytics may be a useful strategy to prevent senescence-associated damage in liver disease patients; however, this remains controversial. Recent work has shown that age-related NAFLD-HCC mouse models showed increased liver disease following senolytic treatment, indicating that senescence may be a consequence and not a driver of disease (Raffaele et al., 2021). Alternatively, chimeric antigen receptor (CAR) T cells can be engineered to specifically target senescent cells and were shown to ameliorate senescence-induced pathologies including hepatic fibrosis following carbon tetrachloride (CCl_4) treatment (Amor et al., 2020). As described above, some preliminary work has been performed in animal models to evaluate the use of senolytics or other factors modulating biliary senescence as therapeutic agents for liver disease, but more work is necessary. Additional work in preclinical models should be carried out to further define the usefulness of inhibiting senescence and SASP in cholangiopathies, NAFLD/NASH and ALD. While senolytics are an intuitive pharmaceutical approach for the amelioration of liver damage associated with the above disorders, there are other indirect measures by which biliary senescence/SASP can be targeted. As described above, exosomes can be implicated in liver fibrosis progression in biliary atresia, but modulation of exosomes and the utilization of this signaling mechanism as a therapeutic need to be further investigated. Additionally, targeting age-related signaling mechanisms or miRs associated with biliary senescence can be an additional route to indirectly mediate this signaling component in liver disorders. A table of the key molecules discussed in this review that regulate biliary senescence during chronic liver diseases is listed in **Table 1**.

Due to the increase of senescence in cholangiopathies and fatty liver disease, targeting senescence and SASP secretion in cholangiocytes provides a novel direction in chronic liver disease treatment and a summary of critical findings described in this review can be found in **Figure 1**. Further investigation into the mechanism for premature biliary senescence/SASP factor secretion needs to be performed before this theory can be applied to clinical practice.

AUTHOR CONTRIBUTIONS

VM = first draft, compilation, edit final draft, figure LB = first draft, edit final draft DK = first draft, edit final draft KS = first draft, edit final draft YS = literature search CW = edit final draft SC = edit final draft SG = edit final draft GA = initial concept, funding, edit final draft LK = first draft, funding, edit final draft HF = initial concept, funding, edit final draft.

REFERENCES

Al Suraih, M. S., Trussoni, C. E., Splinter, P. L., LaRusso, N. F., and O'Hara, S. P. (2020). Senescent Cholangiocytes Release Extracellular Vesicles that Alter Target Cell Phenotype via the Epidermal Growth Factor Receptor. *Liver Int.* 40, 2455–2468. doi:10.1111/liv.14569

Alpini, G., Lenzi, R., Sarkozi, L., and Tavoloni, N. (1988). Biliary Physiology in Rats with Bile Ductular Cell Hyperplasia. Evidence for a Secretory Function of Proliferated Bile Ductules. *J. Clin. Invest.* 81, 569–578. doi:10.1172/jci113355

Alsuraih, M., O'Hara, S. P., Woodrum, J. E., Pirius, N. E., and LaRusso, N. F. (2021). Genetic or Pharmacological Reduction of Cholangiocyte Senescence Improves Inflammation and Fibrosis in the Mdr2 Mouse. *JHEP Rep.* 3, 100250. doi:10.1016/j.jhepr.2021.100250

Alvaro, D., Gigliozzi, A., and Attili, A. F. (2000). Regulation and Deregulation of Cholangiocyte Proliferation. *J. Hepatol.* 33, 333–340. doi:10.1016/s0168-8278(00)80377-3

Alvaro, D., Mancino, M. G., Glaser, S., Gaudio, E., Marzioni, M., Francis, H., et al. (2007). Proliferating Cholangiocytes: A Neuroendocrine Compartment in the Diseased Liver. *Gastroenterology* 132, 415–431. doi:10.1053/j.gastro.2006.07.023

Amor, C., Feucht, J., Leibold, J., Ho, Y.-J., Zhu, C., Alonso-Curbelo, D., et al. (2020). Senolytic CAR T Cells Reverse Senescence-Associated Pathologies. *Nature* 583, 127–132. doi:10.1038/s41586-020-2403-9

Annable, T., McDaniel, K., Han, Y., Venter, J., Wu, N., Glaser, S., et al. (2015). Sa1715 Regulation of Cellular Senescence by the microRNA-34a/p53 Axis During Alcoholic Liver Injury. *Gastroenterology* 148, S1018–S1019. doi:10.1016/s0016-5085(15)33483-1

Arenas, F., Hervías, I., Sáez, E., Melero, S., Prieto, J., Parés, A., et al. (2019). Promoter Hypermethylation of the AE2/SLC4A2 Gene in PBC. *JHEP Rep.* 1, 145–153. doi:10.1016/j.jhepr.2019.05.006

Baiocchi, L., Lenci, I., Milana, M., Kennedy, L., Sato, K., Zhang, W., et al. (2021). Cyclic AMP Signaling in Biliary Proliferation: A Possible Target for Cholangiocarcinoma Treatment. *Cells* 10, 1692. doi:10.3390/cells10071692

Banales, J. M., Huebert, R. C., Karlsen, T., Strazzabosco, M., LaRusso, N. F., and Gores, G. J. (2019). Cholangiocyte Pathobiology. *Nat. Rev. Gastroenterol. Hepatol.* 16, 269–281. doi:10.1038/s41575-019-0125-y

Banales, J. M., Sáez, E., Úriz, M., Sarvide, S., Urribarri, A. D., Splinter, P., et al. (2012). Up-regulation of microRNA 506 Leads to Decreased Cl−/HCO3− Anion Exchanger 2 Expression in Biliary Epithelium of Patients with Primary Biliary Cirrhosis. *Hepatology* 56, 687–697. doi:10.1002/hep.25691

Barnes, B. H., Tucker, R. M., Wehrmann, F., Mack, D. G., Ueno, Y., and Mack, C. L. (2009). Cholangiocytes as Immune Modulators in Rotavirus-Induced Murine Biliary Atresia. *Liver Int.* 29, 1253–1261. doi:10.1111/j.1478-3231.2008.01921.x

Barron-Millar, B., Ogle, L., Mells, G., Flack, S., Badrock, J., Sandford, R., et al. (2021). The Serum Proteome and Ursodeoxycholic Acid Response in Primary Biliary Cholangitis. *Hepatology* 74, 3269–3283. doi:10.1002/hep.32011

Bezerra, J. A., Wells, R. G., Mack, C. L., Karpen, S. J., Hoofnagle, J. H., Doo, E., et al. (2018). Biliary Atresia: Clinical and Research Challenges for the Twenty-First Century. *Hepatology* 68, 1163–1173. doi:10.1002/hep.29905

Bhathal, P. S., and Gall, J. A. (1985). Deletion of Hyperplastic Biliary Epithelial Cells by Apoptosis Following Removal of the Proliferative Stimulus. *Liver* 5, 311–325. doi:10.1111/j.1600-0676.1985.tb00254.x

Blokland, K. E. C., Pouwels, S. D., Schuliga, M., Knight, D. A., and Burgess, J. K. (2020). Regulation of Cellular Senescence by Extracellular Matrix During Chronic Fibrotic Diseases. *Clin. Sci. (Lond)* 134, 2681–2706. doi:10.1042/cs20190893

Campisi, J. (2013). Aging, Cellular Senescence, and Cancer. *Annu. Rev. Physiol.* 75, 685–705. doi:10.1146/annurev-physiol-030212-183653

Campisi, J., Kapahi, P., Lithgow, G. J., Melov, S., Newman, J. C., and Verdin, E. (2019). From Discoveries in Ageing Research to Therapeutics for Healthy Ageing. *Nature* 571, 183–192. doi:10.1038/s41586-019-1365-2

Capparelli, C., Whitaker-Menezes, D., Guido, C., Balliet, R., Pestell, T. G., Howell, A., et al. (2012). CTGF Drives Autophagy, Glycolysis and Senescence in Cancer-Associated Fibroblasts via HIF1 Activation, Metabolically Promoting Tumor Growth. *Cell Cycle* 11, 2272–2284. doi:10.4161/cc.20717

Carpino, G., Cardinale, V., Folseraas, T., Overi, D., Floreani, A., Franchitto, A., et al. (2018). Hepatic Stem/Progenitor Cell Activation Differs Between Primary Sclerosing and Primary Biliary Cholangitis. *Am. J. Pathol.* 188, 627–639. doi:10.1016/j.ajpath.2017.11.010

Cazzagon, N., Sarcognato, S., Floreani, A., Corrà, G., De Martin, S., Guzzardo, V., et al. (2021). Cholangiocyte Senescence in Primary Sclerosing Cholangitis Is Associated with Disease Severity and Prognosis. *JHEP Rep.* 3, 100286. doi:10.1016/j.jhepr.2021.100286

Celli, A., and Que, F. (1998). Dysregulation of Apoptosis in the Cholangiopathies and Cholangiocarcinoma. *Semin. Liver Dis.* 18, 177–185. doi:10.1055/s-2007-1007153

Chang, J. S., Hsiao, J.-R., and Chen, C.-H. (2017). ALDH2 Polymorphism and Alcohol-Related Cancers in Asians: A Public Health Perspective. *J. Biomed. Sci.* 24, 19. doi:10.1186/s12929-017-0327-y

Chen, X. M., O'Hara, S. P., and LaRusso, N. F. (2008). The Immunobiology of Cholangiocytes. *Immunol. Cel Biol* 86, 497–505. doi:10.1038/icb.2008.37

Cheung, A. C., Lorenzo Pisarello, M. J., and LaRusso, N. F. (2018). Pathobiology of Biliary Epithelia. *Biochim. Biophys. Acta (Bba) - Mol. Basis Dis.* 1864, 1220–1231. doi:10.1016/j.bbadis.2017.06.024

Childs, B. G., Baker, D. J., Kirkland, J. L., Campisi, J., and Deursen, J. M. (2014). Senescence and Apoptosis: Dueling or Complementary Cell Fates. *EMBO Rep.* 15, 1139–1153. doi:10.15252/embr.201439245

Chusilp, S., Lee, C., Li, B., Lee, D., Yamoto, M., Ganji, N., et al. (2020). A Novel Model of Injured Liver Ductal Organoids to Investigate Cholangiocyte Apoptosis with Relevance to Biliary Atresia. *Pediatr. Surg. Int.* 36, 1471–1479. doi:10.1007/s00383-020-04765-2

Coppé, J. P., Patil, C. K., Rodier, F., Sun, Y., Muñoz, D. P., Goldstein, J., et al. (2008). Senescence-associated Secretory Phenotypes Reveal Cell-Nonautonomous Functions of Oncogenic RAS and the P53 Tumor Suppressor. *Plos Biol.* 6, 2853–2868. doi:10.1371/journal.pbio.0060301

Datto, M. B., Li, Y., Panus, J. F., Howe, D. J., Xiong, Y., and Wang, X. F. (1995). Transforming Growth Factor Beta Induces the Cyclin-dependent Kinase Inhibitor P21 Through a P53-independent Mechanism. *Proc. Natl. Acad. Sci.* 92, 5545–5549. doi:10.1073/pnas.92.12.5545

de Lima, V. M. R., Oliveira, C. P. M. S., Alves, V. A. F., Chammas, M. C., Oliveira, E. P., Stefano, J. T., et al. (2008). A Rodent Model of NASH with Cirrhosis, Oval Cell Proliferation and Hepatocellular Carcinoma. *J. Hepatol.* 49, 1055–1061. doi:10.1016/j.jhep.2008.07.024

Ferreira-Gonzalez, S., Lu, W.-Y., Raven, A., Dwyer, B., Man, T. Y., O'Duibhir, E., et al. (2018). Paracrine Cellular Senescence Exacerbates Biliary Injury and Impairs Regeneration. *Nat. Commun.* 9, 1020. doi:10.1038/s41467-018-03299-5

Fleisher, T. A. (1997). Apoptosis. *Ann. Allergy Asthma Immunol.* 78, 245–250. doi:10.1016/s1081-1206(10)63176-6

Fontana, L., Zhao, E., Amir, M., Dong, H., Tanaka, K., and Czaja, M. J. (2013). Aging Promotes the Development of Diet-Induced Murine Steatohepatitis but Not Steatosis. *Hepatology* 57, 995–1004. doi:10.1002/hep.26099

Fragoulis, A., Schenkel, J., Herzog, M., Schellenberg, T., Jahr, H., Pufe, T., et al. (2019). Nrf2 Ameliorates DDC-Induced Sclerosing Cholangitis and Biliary Fibrosis and Improves the Regenerative Capacity of the Liver. *Toxicol. Sci.* 169, 485–498. doi:10.1093/toxsci/kfz055

Franchitto, A., Onori, P., Renzi, A., Carpino, G., Mancinelli, R., Alvaro, D., et al. (2013). Recent Advances on the Mechanisms Regulating Cholangiocyte Proliferation and the Significance of the Neuroendocrine Regulation of Cholangiocyte Pathophysiology. *Ann. Transl Med.* 1, 27. doi:10.3978/j.issn.2305-5839.2012.10.03

Francis, H., Glaser, S., Demorrow, S., Gaudio, E., Ueno, Y., Venter, J., et al. (2008). Small Mouse Cholangiocytes Proliferate in Response to H1 Histamine Receptor Stimulation by Activation of the IP3/CaMK I/CREB Pathway. *Am. J. Physiology-Cell Physiol.* 295, C499–C513. doi:10.1152/ajpcell.00369.2007

Francis, H., Glaser, S., Ueno, Y., Lesage, G., Marucci, L., Benedetti, A., et al. (2004). cAMP Stimulates the Secretory and Proliferative Capacity of the Rat Intrahepatic Biliary Epithelium Through Changes in the PKA/Src/MEK/ERK1/2 Pathway. *J. Hepatol.* 41, 528–537. doi:10.1016/j.jhep.2004.06.009

Glaser, S. S., Gaudio, E., Rao, A., Pierce, L. M., Onori, P., Franchitto, A., et al. (2009). Morphological and Functional Heterogeneity of the Mouse Intrahepatic Biliary Epithelium. *Lab. Invest.* 89, 456–469. doi:10.1038/labinvest.2009.6

Glick, D., Barth, S., and Macleod, K. F. (2010). Autophagy: Cellular and Molecular Mechanisms. *J. Pathol.* 221, 3–12. doi:10.1002/path.2697

Guicciardi, M. E., Trussoni, C. E., Krishnan, A., Bronk, S. F., Lorenzo Pisarello, M. J., O'Hara, S. P., et al. (2018). Macrophages Contribute to the Pathogenesis of

Sclerosing Cholangitis in Mice. *J. Hepatol.* 69, 676–686. doi:10.1016/j.jhep.2018.05.018

Guillot, A., Ren, T., Jourdan, T., Pawlosky, R. J., Han, E., Kim, S.-J., et al. (2019). Targeting Liver Aldehyde Dehydrogenase-2 Prevents Heavy but Not Moderate Alcohol Drinking. *Proc. Natl. Acad. Sci. USA* 116, 25974–25981. doi:10.1073/pnas.1908137116

Hall, C., Sato, K., Wu, N., Zhou, T., Kyritsi, K., Meng, F., et al. (2017). Regulators of Cholangiocyte Proliferation. *Gene Expr.* 17, 155–171. doi:10.3727/105221616x692568

Han, Y., Glaser, S., Meng, F., Francis, H., Marzioni, M., McDaniel, K., et al. (2013). Recent Advances in the Morphological and Functional Heterogeneity of the Biliary Epithelium. *Exp. Biol. Med. (Maywood)* 238, 549–565. doi:10.1177/1535370213489926

Hardie, C., Green, K., Jopson, L., Millar, B., Innes, B., Pagan, S., et al. (2016). Early Molecular Stratification of High-Risk Primary Biliary Cholangitis. *EBioMedicine* 14, 65–73. doi:10.1016/j.ebiom.2016.11.021

Hisamoto, S., Shimoda, S., Harada, K., Iwasaka, S., Onohara, S., Chong, Y., et al. (2016). Hydrophobic Bile Acids Suppress Expression of AE2 in Biliary Epithelial Cells and Induce Bile Duct Inflammation in Primary Biliary Cholangitis. *J. Autoimmun.* 75, 150–160. doi:10.1016/j.jaut.2016.08.006

Jalan-Sakrikar, N., De Assuncao, T. M., Navarro-Corcuera, A., Hamdan, F. H., Loarca, L., Kirkeby, L. A., et al. (2021). Induced Pluripotent Stem Cells from Subjects with Primary Sclerosing Cholangitis Develop a Senescence Phenotype Following Biliary Differentiation. *Hepatol. Commun.* Epub ahead of print. doi:10.1002/hep4.1809

Jia, R., Yang, F., Yan, P., Ma, L., Yang, L., and Li, L. (2021). Paricalcitol Inhibits Oxidative Stress-Induced Cell Senescence of the Bile Duct Epithelium Dependent on Modulating Sirt1 Pathway in Cholestatic Mice. *Free Radic. Biol. Med.* 169, 158–168. doi:10.1016/j.freeradbiomed.2021.04.019

Jones, H., Alpini, G., and Francis, H. (2015). Bile Acid Signaling and Biliary Functions. *Acta Pharmaceutica Sinica B* 5, 123–128. doi:10.1016/j.apsb.2015.01.009

Jones, H., Hargrove, L., Kennedy, L., Meng, F., Graf-Eaton, A., Owens, J., et al. (2016). Inhibition of Mast Cell-Secreted Histamine Decreases Biliary Proliferation and Fibrosis in Primary Sclerosing Cholangitis Mdr2−/−mice. *Hepatology* 64, 1202–1216. doi:10.1002/hep.28704

Jørgensen, E. A., Knigge, U., Warberg, J., and Kjaer, A. (2007). Histamine and the Regulation of Body Weight. *Neuroendocrinology* 86, 210–214. doi:10.1159/000108341

Kanno, N., LeSage, G., Glaser, S., Alvaro, D., and Alpini, G. (2000). Functional Heterogeneity of the Intrahepatic Biliary Epithelium. *Hepatology* 31, 555–561. doi:10.1002/hep.510310302

Kennedy, L., Francis, H., Invernizzi, P., Venter, J., Wu, N., Carbone, M., et al. (2019). Secretin/secretin Receptor Signaling Mediates Biliary Damage and Liver Fibrosis in Early-stage Primary Biliary Cholangitis. *FASEB j.* 33, 10269–10279. doi:10.1096/fj.201802606r

Kennedy, L., Hargrove, L., Demieville, J., Bailey, J. M., Dar, W., Polireddy, K., et al. (2018). Knockout of L-Histidine Decarboxylase Prevents Cholangiocyte Damage and Hepatic Fibrosis in Mice Subjected to High-Fat Diet Feeding via Disrupted Histamine/Leptin Signaling. *Am. J. Pathol.* 188, 600–615. doi:10.1016/j.ajpath.2017.11.016

Kennedy, L., Hargrove, L., Demieville, J., Karstens, W., Jones, H., DeMorrow, S., et al. (2018). Blocking H1/H2 Histamine Receptors Inhibits Damage/fibrosis in Mdr2-/- Mice and Human Cholangiocarcinoma Tumorigenesis. *Hepatology* 68, 1042–1056. doi:10.1002/hep.29898

Kennedy, L., Meadows, V., Kyritsi, K., Pham, L., Kundu, D., Kulkarni, R., et al. (2020). Amelioration of Large Bile Duct Damage by Histamine-2 Receptor Vivo-Morpholino Treatment. *Am. J. Pathol.* 190, 1018–1029. doi:10.1016/j.ajpath.2020.01.013

Kennedy, L., Meadows, V., Sybenga, A., Demieville, J., Chen, L., Hargrove, L., et al. (2021). Mast Cells Promote Nonalcoholic Fatty Liver Disease Phenotypes and Microvesicular Steatosis in Mice Fed a Western Diet. *Hepatology* 74, 164–182. doi:10.1002/hep.31713

Kerola, A., Lohi, J., Heikkilä, P., Mutanen, A., Jalanko, H., and Pakarinen, M. P. (2019). Divergent Expression of Liver Transforming Growth Factor Superfamily Cytokines After Successful Portoenterostomy in Biliary Atresia. *Surgery* 165, 905–911. doi:10.1016/j.surg.2018.12.003

Khoury, M. K., Gupta, K., Franco, S. R., and Liu, B. (2020). Necroptosis in the Pathophysiology of Disease. *Am. J. Pathol.* 190, 272–285. doi:10.1016/j.ajpath.2019.10.012

Knop, J., Taborski, B., and DeMaeyer-Guignard, J. (1987). Selective Inhibition of the Generation of T Suppressor Cells of Contact Sensitivity In Vitro by Interferon. *J. Immunol.* 138, 3684–3687.

Kundu, D., Kennedy, L., Meadows, V., Baiocchi, L., Alpini, G., and Francis, H. (2020). The Dynamic Interplay Between Mast Cells, Aging/Cellular Senescence, and Liver Disease. *Gene Expr.* 20, 77–88. doi:10.3727/105221620x15960509906371

Kyritsi, K., Francis, H., Zhou, T., Ceci, L., Wu, N., Yang, Z., et al. (2020). Downregulation of P16 Decreases Biliary Damage and Liver Fibrosis in the Mdr2/ Mouse Model of Primary Sclerosing Cholangitis. *Gene Expr.* 20, 89–103. doi:10.3727/105221620x15889714507961

Kyritsi, K., Kennedy, L., Meadows, V., Hargrove, L., Demieville, J., Pham, L., et al. (2021). Mast Cells Induce Ductular Reaction Mimicking Liver Injury in Mice Through Mast Cell-Derived Transforming Growth Factor Beta 1 Signaling. *Hepatology* 73, 2397–2410. doi:10.1002/hep.31497

Lazaridis, K. N., and LaRusso, N. F. (2015). The Cholangiopathies. *Mayo Clinic Proc.* 90, 791–800. doi:10.1016/j.mayocp.2015.03.017

Lesage, G., Glaser, S., Ueno, Y., Alvaro, D., Baiocchi, L., Kanno, N., et al. (2001). Regression of Cholangiocyte Proliferation After Cessation of ANIT Feeding Is Coupled with Increased Apoptosis. *Am. J. Physiology-Gastrointestinal Liver Physiol.* 281, G182–G190. doi:10.1152/ajpgi.2001.281.1.g182

Lopes-Paciencia, S., Saint-Germain, E., Rowell, M.-C., Ruiz, A. F., Kalegari, P., and Ferbeyre, G. (2019). The Senescence-Associated Secretory Phenotype and its Regulation. *Cytokine* 117, 15–22. doi:10.1016/j.cyto.2019.01.013

López-Otín, C., Blasco, M. A., Partridge, L., Serrano, M., and Kroemer, G. (2013). The Hallmarks of Aging. *Cell* 153, 1194–1217. doi:10.1016/j.cell.2013.05.039

Mancinelli, R., Franchitto, A., Glaser, S., Meng, F., Onori, P., Demorrow, S., et al. (2013). GABA Induces the Differentiation of Small into Large Cholangiocytes by Activation of Ca2+/CaMK I-dependent Adenylyl Cyclase 8. *Hepatology* 58, 251–263. doi:10.1002/hep.26308

Mantovani, A., and Dalbeni, A. (2020). NAFLD, MAFLD and DAFLD. *Dig. Liver Dis.* 52, 1519–1520. doi:10.1016/j.dld.2020.09.013

Maroni, L., Pinto, C., Giordano, D. M., Saccomanno, S., Banales, J. M., Spallacci, D., et al. (2019). Aging-Related Expression of Twinfilin-1 Regulates Cholangiocyte Biological Response to Injury. *Hepatology* 70, 883–898. doi:10.1002/hep.30466

Matsumoto, A., Thompson, D. C., Chen, Y., Kitagawa, K., and Vasiliou, V. (2016). Roles of Defective ALDH2 Polymorphism on Liver protection and Cancer Development. *Environ. Health Prev. Med.* 21, 395–402. doi:10.1007/s12199-016-0579-2

McDaniel, K., Meng, F., Wu, N., Sato, K., Venter, J., Bernuzzi, F., et al. (2017). Forkhead Box A2 Regulates Biliary Heterogeneity and Senescence During Cholestatic Liver Injury in Mice‡. *Hepatology* 65, 544–559. doi:10.1002/hep.28831

Meadows, V., Kennedy, L., Ekser, B., Kyritsi, K., Kundu, D., Zhou, T., et al. (2021). Mast Cells Regulate Ductular Reaction and Intestinal Inflammation in Cholestasis Through Farnesoid X Receptor Signaling. *Hepatology* 74 (5), 2684–2698. doi:10.1002/hep.32028

Meadows, V., Kennedy, L., Hargrove, L., Demieville, J., Meng, F., Virani, S., et al. (2019). Downregulation of Hepatic Stem Cell Factor by Vivo-Morpholino Treatment Inhibits Mast Cell Migration and Decreases Biliary Damage/senescence and Liver Fibrosis in Mdr2−/− Mice. *Biochim. Biophys. Acta (Bba) - Mol. Basis Dis.* 1865, 165557. doi:10.1016/j.bbadis.2019.165557

Mendez-Sanchez, N., Zamora-Valdes, D., Pichardo-Bahena, R., Barredo-Prieto, B., Ponciano-Rodriguez, G., Bermejo-Martínez, L., et al. (2007). Endocannabinoid Receptor CB2 in Nonalcoholic Fatty Liver Disease. *Liver Int.* 27, 215–219. doi:10.1111/j.1478-3231.2006.01401.x

Moncsek, A., Al-Suraih, M. S., Trussoni, C. E., O'Hara, S. P., Splinter, P. L., Zuber, C., et al. (2018). Targeting Senescent Cholangiocytes and Activated Fibroblasts with B-Cell Lymphoma-Extra Large Inhibitors Ameliorates Fibrosis in Multidrug Resistance 2 Gene Knockout (Mdr2−/−) Mice. *Hepatology* 67, 247–259. doi:10.1002/hep.29464

Moreb, J. S., Baker, H. V., Chang, L.-J., Amaya, M., Lopez, M. C., Ostmark, B., et al. (2008). ALDH Isozymes Downregulation Affects Cell Growth, Cell Motility and Gene Expression in Lung Cancer Cells. *Mol. Cancer* 7, 87. doi:10.1186/1476-4598-7-87

Muzio, G., Maggiora, M., Paiuzzi, E., Oraldi, M., and Canuto, R. A. (2012). Aldehyde Dehydrogenases and Cell Proliferation. *Free Radic. Biol. Med.* 52, 735–746. doi:10.1016/j.freeradbiomed.2011.11.033

Nannelli, G., Terzuoli, E., Giorgio, V., Donnini, S., Lupetti, P., Giachetti, A., et al. (2018). ALDH2 Activity Reduces Mitochondrial Oxygen Reserve Capacity in

Endothelial Cells and Induces Senescence Properties. *Oxid Med. Cel Longev* 2018, 9765027. doi:10.1155/2018/9765027
Natarajan, S. K., Ingham, S. A., Mohr, A. M., Wehrkamp, C. J., Ray, A., Roy, S., et al. (2014). Saturated Free Fatty Acids Induce Cholangiocyte Lipoapoptosis. *Hepatology* 60, 1942–1956. doi:10.1002/hep.27175
Natarajan, S. K., Stringham, B. A., Mohr, A. M., Wehrkamp, C. J., Lu, S., Phillippi, M. A., et al. (2017). FoxO3 Increases miR-34a to Cause Palmitate-Induced Cholangiocyte Lipoapoptosis. *J. Lipid Res.* 58, 866–875. doi:10.1194/jlr.m071357
Nathanson, M. H., and Boyer, J. L. (1991). Mechanisms and Regulation of Bile Secretion. *Hepatology* 14, 551–566. doi:10.1002/hep.1840140324
Ogrodnik, M., Miwa, S., Tchkonia, T., Tiniakos, D., Wilson, C. L., Lahat, A., et al. (2017). Cellular Senescence Drives Age-dependent Hepatic Steatosis. *Nat. Commun.* 8, 15691. doi:10.1038/ncomms15691
Olynyk, J. K., Yeoh, G. C., Ramm, G. A., Clarke, S. L., Hall, P. M., Britton, R. S., et al. (1998). Gadolinium Chloride Suppresses Hepatic Oval Cell Proliferation in Rats with Biliary Obstruction. *Am. J. Pathol.* 152, 347–352.
Onofrio, F. Q., Hirschfield, G. M., and Gulamhusein, A. F. (2019). A Practical Review of Primary Biliary Cholangitis for the Gastroenterologist. *Gastroenterol. Hepatol. (N Y)* 15, 145–154.
Oraldi, M., Saracino, S., Maggiora, M., Chiaravalloti, A., Buemi, C., Martinasso, G., et al. (2011). Importance of Inverse Correlation Between ALDH3A1 and PPARγ in Tumor Cells and Tissue Regeneration. *Chemico-Biological Interactions* 191, 171–176. doi:10.1016/j.cbi.2011.01.011
Raffaele, M., Kovacovicova, K., Frohlich, J., Lo Re, O., Giallongo, S., Oben, J. A., et al. (2021). Mild Exacerbation of Obesity- and Age-dependent Liver Disease Progression by Senolytic Cocktail Dasatinib + Quercetin. *Cell Commun Signal* 19, 44. doi:10.1186/s12964-021-00731-0
Ramirez, T., Li, Y.-M., Yin, S., Xu, M.-J., Feng, D., Zhou, Z., et al. (2017). Aging Aggravates Alcoholic Liver Injury and Fibrosis in Mice by Downregulating Sirtuin 1 Expression. *J. Hepatol.* 66, 601–609. doi:10.1016/j.jhep.2016.11.004
Rao, S. G., and Jackson, J. G. (2016). SASP: Tumor Suppressor or Promoter? Yes!. *Trends Cancer* 2, 676–687. doi:10.1016/j.trecan.2016.10.001
Rawla, P., and Samant, H. (2021). *Primary Sclerosing Cholangitis*. Treasure Island, FL: StatPearls.
Ruzinova, M. B., and Benezra, R. (2003). Id Proteins in Development, Cell Cycle and Cancer. *Trends Cel Biol.* 13, 410–418. doi:10.1016/s0962-8924(03)00147-8
Sager, R. (1991). Senescence as a Mode of Tumor Suppression. *Environ. Health Perspect.* 93, 59–62. doi:10.1289/ehp.919359
Sanada, Y., Aida, J., Kawano, Y., Nakamura, K.-i., Shimomura, N., Ishikawa, N., et al. (2012). Hepatocellular Telomere Length in Biliary Atresia Measured by Q-FISH. *World J. Surg.* 36, 908–916. doi:10.1007/s00268-012-1453-z
Sasaki, M., Miyakoshi, M., Sato, Y., and Nakanuma, Y. (2012). A Possible Involvement of P62/sequestosome-1 in the Process of Biliary Epithelial Autophagy and Senescence in Primary Biliary Cirrhosis. *Liver Int.* 32, 487–499. doi:10.1111/j.1478-3231.2011.02656.x
Sasaki, M., Ikeda, H., Haga, H., Manabe, T., and Nakanuma, Y. (2005). Frequent Cellular Senescence in Small Bile Ducts in Primary Biliary Cirrhosis: A Possible Role in Bile Duct Loss. *J. Pathol.* 205, 451–459. doi:10.1002/path.1729
Sasaki, M., Ikeda, H., Sato, Y., and Nakanuma, Y. (2006). Decreased Expression of Bmi1 Is Closely Associated with Cellular Senescence in Small Bile Ducts in Primary Biliary Cirrhosis. *Am. J. Pathol.* 169, 831–845. doi:10.2353/ajpath.2006.051237
Sasaki, M., Ikeda, H., Yamaguchi, J., Nakada, S., and Nakanuma, Y. (2008). Telomere Shortening in the Damaged Small Bile Ducts in Primary Biliary Cirrhosis Reflects Ongoing Cellular Senescence. *Hepatology* 48, 186–195. doi:10.1002/hep.22348
Sasaki, M., Kuo, F.-Y., Huang, C.-C., Swanson, P. E., Chen, C.-L., Chuang, J.-H., et al. (2018). Increased Expression of Senescence-Associated Cell Cycle Regulators in the Progression of Biliary Atresia: An Immunohistochemical Study. *Histopathology* 72, 1164–1171. doi:10.1111/his.13476
Sasaki, M., Miyakoshi, M., Sato, Y., and Nakanuma, Y. (2012). Autophagy May Precede Cellular Senescence of Bile Ductular Cells in Ductular Reaction in Primary Biliary Cirrhosis. *Dig. Dis. Sci.* 57, 660–666. doi:10.1007/s10620-011-1929-y
Sasaki, M., Miyakoshi, M., Sato, Y., and Nakanuma, Y. (2010). Autophagy Mediates the Process of Cellular Senescence Characterizing Bile Duct Damages in Primary Biliary Cirrhosis. *Lab. Invest.* 90, 835–843. doi:10.1038/labinvest.2010.56
Sasaki, M., Miyakoshi, M., Sato, Y., and Nakanuma, Y. (2010). Modulation of the Microenvironment by Senescent Biliary Epithelial Cells May Be Involved in the Pathogenesis of Primary Biliary Cirrhosis. *J. Hepatol.* 53, 318–325. doi:10.1016/j.jhep.2010.03.008
Sasaki, M., Sato, Y., and Nakanuma, Y. (2018). An Impaired Biliary Bicarbonate Umbrella May Be Involved in Dysregulated Autophagy in Primary Biliary Cholangitis. *Lab. Invest.* 98, 745–754. doi:10.1038/s41374-018-0045-4
Sasaki, M., Sato, Y., and Nakanuma, Y. (2020). Increased p16INK4a-Expressing Senescent Bile Ductular Cells Are Associated with Inadequate Response to Ursodeoxycholic Acid in Primary Biliary Cholangitis. *J. Autoimmun.* 107, 102377. doi:10.1016/j.jaut.2019.102377
Sasaki, M., Sato, Y., and Nakanuma, Y. (2021). Interferon-induced Protein with Tetratricopeptide Repeats 3 May Be a Key Factor in Primary Biliary Cholangitis. *Sci. Rep.* 11, 11413. doi:10.1038/s41598-021-91016-6
Sasaki, M., Yoshimura-Miyakoshi, M., Sato, Y., and Nakanuma, Y. (2015). A Possible Involvement of Endoplasmic Reticulum Stress in Biliary Epithelial Autophagy and Senescence in Primary Biliary Cirrhosis. *J. Gastroenterol.* 50, 984–995. doi:10.1007/s00535-014-1033-0
Simon, G., Heckmann, V., Tóth, D., Pauka, D., Petrus, K., and Molnár, T. F. (2020). The Effect of Hepatic Steatosis and Fibrosis on Liver Weight and Dimensions. *Leg. Med.* 47, 101781. doi:10.1016/j.legalmed.2020.101781
Sorrentino, P., Tarantino, G., Perrella, A., Micheli, P., Perrella, O., and Conca, P. (2005). A Clinical-Morphological Study on Cholestatic Presentation of Nonalcoholic Fatty Liver Disease. *Dig. Dis. Sci.* 50, 1130–1135. doi:10.1007/s10620-005-2719-1
Tabibian, J. H., O'Hara, S. P., Splinter, P. L., Trussoni, C. E., and LaRusso, N. F. (2014). Cholangiocyte Senescence by Way of N-Ras Activation Is a Characteristic of Primary Sclerosing Cholangitis. *Hepatology* 59, 2263–2275. doi:10.1002/hep.26993
Tabibian, J. H., O'Hara, S. P., Trussoni, C. E., Tietz, P. S., Splinter, P. L., Mounajjed, T., et al. (2016). Absence of the Intestinal Microbiota Exacerbates Hepatobiliary Disease in a Murine Model of Primary Sclerosing Cholangitis. *Hepatology* 63, 185–196. doi:10.1002/hep.27927
Tabibian, J. H., Trussoni, C. E., O'Hara, S. P., Splinter, P. L., Heimbach, J. K., and LaRusso, N. F. (2014). Characterization of Cultured Cholangiocytes Isolated from Livers of Patients with Primary Sclerosing Cholangitis. *Lab. Invest.* 94, 1126–1133. doi:10.1038/labinvest.2014.94
Tandra, S., Yeh, M. M., Brunt, E. M., Vuppalanchi, R., Cummings, O. W., Ünalp-Arida, A., et al. (2011). Presence and Significance of Microvesicular Steatosis in Nonalcoholic Fatty Liver Disease. *J. Hepatol.* 55, 654–659. doi:10.1016/j.jhep.2010.11.021
Toettcher, J. E., Loewer, A., Ostheimer, G. J., Yaffe, M. B., Tidor, B., and Lahav, G. (2009). Distinct Mechanisms Act in Concert to Mediate Cell Cycle Arrest. *Pnas* 106, 785–790. doi:10.1073/pnas.0806196106
Tsuneyama, K., Kono, N., Yamashiro, M., Kouda, W., Sabit, A., Sasaki, M., et al. (1999). Aberrant Expression of Stem Cell Factor on Biliary Epithelial Cells and Peribiliary Infiltration of C-Kit-Expressing Mast Cells in Hepatolithiasis and Primary Sclerosing Cholangitis: A Possible Contribution to Bile Duct Fibrosis. *J. Pathol.* 189, 609–614. doi:10.1002/(sici)1096-9896(199912)189:4<609::aid-path474>3.0.co;2-2
Udomsinprasert, W., Poovorawan, Y., Chongsrisawat, V., Vejchapipat, P., Zhan, D., and Honsawek, S. (2015). Telomere Length in Peripheral Blood Leukocytes Is Associated with Severity of Biliary Atresia. *PLoS One* 10, e0134689. doi:10.1371/journal.pone.0134689
Venkatesh, S. K., Hennedige, T., Johnson, G. B., Hough, D. M., and Fletcher, J. G. (2017). Imaging Patterns and Focal Lesions in Fatty Liver: A Pictorial Review. *Abdom. Radiol.* 42, 1374–1392. doi:10.1007/s00261-016-1002-6
Wan, Y., Han, Y., McDaniel, K., Annable, T., Wu, N., Venter, J., et al. (2015). miR-34a Regulates Cellular Senescence in Activated Hepatic Stellate Cells During Alcohol Induced Hepatic Injury. *Gastroenterology* 148 (4), S974. doi:10.1016/s0016-5085(15)33327-8
Wan, Y., McDaniel, K., Wu, N., Ramos-Lorenzo, S., Glaser, T., Venter, J., et al. (2017). Regulation of Cellular Senescence by miR-34a in Alcoholic Liver Injury. *Am. J. Pathol.* 187, 2788–2798. doi:10.1016/j.ajpath.2017.08.027
Wilcox, J., Evill, C. A., and Sage, M. R. (1986). Effects of Intracarotid Ionic and Non-ionic Contrast Material on the Blood-Brain Barrier in a Rabbit Model. *Neuroradiology* 28, 271–274. doi:10.1007/bf00548204
Wiman, K. G., and Zhivotovsky, B. (2017). Understanding Cell Cycle and Cell Death Regulation Provides Novel Weapons Against Human Diseases. *J. Intern. Med.* 281, 483–495. doi:10.1111/joim.12609
Winkler, M., Staniczek, T., Kürschner, S. W., Schmid, C. D., Schönhaber, H., Cordero, J., et al. (2021). Endothelial GATA4 Controls Liver Fibrosis and

Regeneration by Preventing a Pathogenic Switch in Angiocrine Signaling. *J. Hepatol.* 74, 380–393. doi:10.1016/j.jhep.2020.08.033

Wu, N., Baiocchi, L., Zhou, T., Kennedy, L., Ceci, L., Meng, F., et al. (2020). Functional Role of the Secretin/Secretin Receptor Signaling During Cholestatic Liver Injury. *Hepatology* 72, 2219–2227. doi:10.1002/hep.31484

Wu, N., Meng, F., Invernizzi, P., Bernuzzi, F., Venter, J., Standeford, H., et al. (2016). The Secretin/secretin Receptor Axis Modulates Liver Fibrosis Through Changes in Transforming Growth Factor-B1 Biliary Secretion in Mice. *Hepatology* 64, 865–879. doi:10.1002/hep.28622

Wu, N., Meng, F., Zhou, T., Venter, J., Giang, T. K., Kyritsi, K., et al. (2018). The Secretin/Secretin Receptor Axis Modulates Ductular Reaction and Liver Fibrosis Through Changes in Transforming Growth Factor-B1-Mediated Biliary Senescence. *Am. J. Pathol.* 188, 2264–2280. doi:10.1016/j.ajpath.2018.06.015

Xiao, Y., Liu, R., Li, X., Gurley, E. C., Hylemon, P. B., Lu, Y., et al. (2019). Long Noncoding RNA H19 Contributes to Cholangiocyte Proliferation and Cholestatic Liver Fibrosis in Biliary Atresia. *Hepatology* 70, 1658–1673. doi:10.1002/hep.30698

Xue, L., Yang, F., Han, Z., Cui, S., Dai, S., Xu, F., et al. (2018). ALDH2 Mediates the Dose-Response Protection of Chronic Ethanol Against Endothelial Senescence Through SIRT1/p53 Pathway. *Biochem. Biophysical Res. Commun.* 504, 777–783. doi:10.1016/j.bbrc.2018.08.081

Xue, L., Zhu, W., Yang, F., Dai, S., Han, Z., Xu, F., et al. (2019). Appropriate Dose of Ethanol Exerts Anti-senescence and Anti-atherosclerosis Protective Effects by Activating ALDH2. *Biochem. Biophysical Res. Commun.* 512, 319–325. doi:10.1016/j.bbrc.2019.03.037

Yamaki, N., Matsushita, S., Hara, S., Yokoyama, A., Hishimoto, A., and Higuchi, S. (2019). Telomere Shortening in Alcohol Dependence: Roles of Alcohol and Acetaldehyde. *J. Psychiatr. Res.* 109, 27–32. doi:10.1016/j.jpsychires.2018.11.007

Yeh, M. M., and Brunt, E. M. (2014). Pathological Features of Fatty Liver Disease. *Gastroenterology* 147, 754–764. doi:10.1053/j.gastro.2014.07.056

Yoshimatsu, H., Itateyama, E., Kondou, S., Tajima, D., Himeno, K., Hidaka, S., et al. (1999). Hypothalamic Neuronal Histamine as a Target of Leptin in Feeding Behavior. *Diabetes* 48, 2286–2291. doi:10.2337/diabetes.48.12.2286

Younossi, Z. M., Rinella, M. E., Sanyal, A. J., Harrison, S. A., Brunt, E. M., Goodman, Z., et al. (2021). From NAFLD to MAFLD: Implications of a Premature Change in Terminology. *Hepatology* 73, 1194–1198. doi:10.1002/hep.31420

Zhong, W., Zhang, W., Li, Q., Xie, G., Sun, Q., Sun, X., et al. (2015). Pharmacological Activation of Aldehyde Dehydrogenase 2 by Alda-1 Reverses Alcohol-Induced Hepatic Steatosis and Cell Death in Mice. *J. Hepatol.* 62, 1375–1381. doi:10.1016/j.jhep.2014.12.022

Zhou, T., Kundu, D., Robles-Linares, J., Meadows, V., Sato, K., Baiocchi, L., et al. (2021). Feedback Signaling Between Cholangiopathies, Ductular Reaction, and Non-alcoholic Fatty Liver Disease. *Cells* 1010 (8), 2072. doi:10.3390/cells10082072

Zhou, T., Wu, N., Meng, F., Venter, J., Giang, T. K., Francis, H., et al. (2018). Knockout of Secretin Receptor Reduces Biliary Damage and Liver Fibrosis in Mdr2−/− Mice by Diminishing Senescence of Cholangiocytes. *Lab. Invest.* 98, 1449–1464. doi:10.1038/s41374-018-0093-9

Zhu, Y., Liu, R., Shen, Z., and Cai, G. (2020). Combination of Luteolin and Lycopene Effectively Protect Against the "Two-Hit" in NAFLD Through Sirt1/AMPK Signal Pathway. *Life Sci.* 256, 117990. doi:10.1016/j.lfs.2020.117990

17

Dysfunctional Immune Regulation in Autoimmune Hepatitis: From Pathogenesis to Novel Therapies

Marta Vuerich[1†], *Na Wang*[1,2,3†], *Ahmadreza Kalbasi*[1†], *Jonathon J. Graham*[1] *and Maria Serena Longhi*[1*]

[1] *Department of Anesthesia, Critical Care & Pain Medicine, Beth Israel Deaconess Medical Center, Harvard Medical School, Boston, MA, United States,* [2] *Department of Hematology, Shandong Provincial Hospital Affiliated to Shandong First Medical University, Jinan, China,* [3] *School of Medicine, Shandong University, Jinan, China*

Correspondence:
Maria Serena Longhi
mlonghi@bidmc.harvard.edu

†*These authors have contributed equally to this work and share first authorship*

Autoimmune hepatitis (AIH) is a chronic inflammatory disorder characterized by hypergammaglobulinemia, presence of serum autoantibodies and histological features of interface hepatitis. AIH therapeutic management still relies on the administration of corticosteroids, azathioprine and other immunosuppressants like calcineurin inhibitors and mycophenolate mofetil. Withdrawal of immunosuppression often results in disease relapse, and, in some cases, therapy is ineffective or associated with serious side effects. Understanding the mechanisms underlying AIH pathogenesis is therefore of paramount importance to develop more effective and well tolerated agents capable of restoring immunotolerance to liver autoantigens. Imbalance between effector and regulatory cells permits liver damage perpetuation and progression in AIH. Impaired expression and regulation of CD39, an ectoenzyme key to immunotolerance maintenance, have been reported in Tregs and effector Th17-cells derived from AIH patients. Interference with these altered immunoregulatory pathways may open new therapeutic avenues that, in addition to limiting aberrant inflammatory responses, would also reconstitute immune homeostasis. In this review, we highlight the most recent findings in AIH immunopathogenesis and discuss how these could inform and direct the development of novel therapeutic tools.

Keywords: autoimmune liver disease, Treg, Th17, ectonucleotidase, aryl hydrocarbon receptor

INTRODUCTION

Autoimmune hepatitis (AIH) was initially described as a severe form of fluctuating persistent hepatitis, associated with acneiform rashes, spider angiomas, amenorrhea and marked elevation of serum immunoglobulins (1). Subsequent studies showed that AIH occurs in individuals of all ages and, although present in both sexes, is prevalent in females (2).

AIH is diagnosed based on the presence of hypergammaglobulinemia, serum autoantibodies and histological features of interface hepatitis (3). While positivity for anti-nuclear antibody (ANA) and/or anti-smooth muscle antibody (SMA) identifies type-1 AIH (AIH-1), liver-kidney-microsomal-type-1 (LKM-1) antibodies, which specifically target the cytochrome P4502D6 (CYP2D6) liver enzyme (4), are the serological hallmarks of type-2 AIH (AIH-2) (5). Additional autoantibodies might aid in

AIH diagnosis, especially in patients negative for ANA, SMA and LKM-1 autoantibodies. Antibodies to soluble liver antigen (SLA) have been reported in 58% of AIH patients where they are often associated with severe disease (6). Anti-liver cytosol type-1 (LC1) antibodies, which target formiminotransferase cyclodeaminase (FTCD), identify AIH-2 (7), and their titer positively correlates with disease activity (8). Presence of anti-neutrophil cytoplasmic antibody (ANCA), particularly atypical p-ANCA (pANNA), might also help in AIH diagnosis, in the absence of positivity for the above-mentioned autoantibodies (9).

Interface hepatitis is present at disease presentation in 84-98% of cases (10) and is characterized by a dense mononuclear cell infiltrate eroding the limiting plate and invading the liver parenchyma (11).

In 50% of cases, AIH manifests with an insidious onset that is often associated with lethargy, malaise, arthralgia, and myalgia; 30-40% of patients present with clinical features of acute hepatitis, whereas the remaining 10-20% of cases are incidentally discovered as having elevated transaminase levels on biochemical screening (12). AIH clinical manifestations may differ, depending on the geographical location and ethnicity of the affected patients. As an example, cirrhosis is more frequent in African Americans (56-85%) than Europeans (38%) (13, 14); and when considering subjects of non-European Caucasoid ethnicity, AIH has earlier onset in African, Arabian and Asian individuals, who also show lower response to immunosuppressive treatment (13, 14). Japanese patients are reported having a later onset of the disease that in most cases improves upon treatment with immunosuppressive drugs (15).

AIH can be associated with autoimmune disorders, which can be also found in first-degree relatives in 40% of cases (16).

The aim of AIH current treatment is to control inflammation. The management of the acute phase includes the administration of prednisone or prednisolone, which is gradually decreased to lower doses, based on the decline of transaminase levels. The addition of the anti-metabolite immunosuppressant azathioprine can be considered when the transaminase levels stop decreasing on steroid treatment alone or in the presence of steroid-related side effects (17). Relapse may occur in up to 40% of cases due to low compliance or when attempting treatment withdrawal. Additional drugs have been used as steroid-saving agents with the aim of reducing steroid-related side effects, these including cyclosporine and tacrolimus (18–20) and, in difficult-to-treat-cases, mycophenolate mofetil in association with prednisone or prednisolone (21, 22). None of these treatments, however, restores immunotolerance by boosting the impaired regulatory cell compartment.

Several studies have been conducted to identify the mechanisms involved in AIH pathogenesis. It has been proposed that genetically predisposed individuals upon exposure to certain environmental conditions (23) can develop cell-mediated immune responses against liver autoantigens. The derived inflammation, permitted by defective immune regulation, progressively results in fibrosis and cirrhosis with aberrant liver re-generation. Genetic predisposition to the disease is conferred by the presence of specific genes located within the human-leukocyte-antigen (HLA) region on the short arm of chromosome 6, especially those encoding allelic variants of DQB1 and DRB1 (24, 25).

Studies on AIH pathogenesis have been furthered by the generation of animal models, developed using different strategies. In this regard, immunization of C57BL/6 female mice with a pCMV plasmid containing the N-terminal region of mouse CTLA-4 and human CYP2D6 and FTCD resulted in transaminase elevations peaking 4 and 7 months after injection (26). Additional models, obtained upon infection of mice with adenovirus Ad5 expressing human CYP2D6, supported a role for viral infection as a possible mechanism leading to tolerance breakdown and consequent development of autoimmunity (27, 28). In an additional model by Hardtke-Wolenski et al, self-limiting adenoviral infection triggered immune responses against the human FTCD in mice of NOD background and resulted in chronic AIH that was characterized by portal and lobular fibrosis (29). Other AIH models have been obtained in mice with medullary thymic epithelial cell depletion due to a conditional deletion of Traf6 expression in murine thymic epithelial cells (30); and in PD-$1^{-/-}$ mice upon neonatal thymectomy, which resulted in aberrant generation of follicular helper T-cells in the spleen (31). Overall, these studies indicate that experimental AIH may derive from different immunopathogenic routes that can be facilitated by viral infections and/or genetic predisposition, this recapitulating the human scenario.

From an immunological perspective, AIH liver damage is driven by overwhelming effector immune responses (32–35) that are not adequately controlled by suppressor/regulatory T-cells (Tregs) (36–39). Extracellular nucleotides and nucleosides are strong modulators of T-cell immunity (40). Mounting evidence links alterations of purinergic signaling with the immunological dysfunction present in autoimmune conditions (41). Both Treg and Th17-cells obtained from AIH patients express low levels and impaired activity of the immunoregulatory ectoenzyme CD39 (42, 43). We have recently reported that such dysfunction derives, at least in part, from alterations of aryl-hydrocarbon-receptor (AhR) signaling (44), suggesting that modulation of this pathway might be deployed to correct immunoregulatory defects while boosting Treg immunity in AIH.

Understanding the mechanisms underlying AIH immune dysregulation is of critical importance for developing more effective treatments. In this review, we will present and discuss the most recent experimental evidence of disrupted AhR/purinergic interactions as one of the prominent factors leading to immunotolerance breakdown in AIH. We will also review how these alterations might inform and direct towards novel therapeutic approaches that represent promising candidates for the treatment of AIH.

MECHANISMS OF LIVER DAMAGE

The mechanisms underlying the liver attack in AIH are still unclear. The autoimmune reaction is believed to be initiated by the presentation of a liver autoantigen by antigen presenting cells (APCs) to Th0 lymphocytes that upon antigen recognition become activated. There is evidence that, in AIH, HLA-class-II molecules are expressed not only on professional APCs but also on hepatocytes (45), this favoring the amplification of cellular immune responses. Following activation, Th0 lymphocytes can differentiate into Th1, Th2 or Th17-cells, this depending on the cytokines in the milieu. All these subsets are present in the hepatic inflammatory infiltrates of AIH patients (35, 46). The cytokines released by each cell subset lead to a cascade of events culminating with the maturation of B-lymphocytes into plasma-cells and consequent production of autoantibodies, which are involved in antibody-mediated-cell-cytotoxicity (47). Derived immune reactions include activation of cytotoxic T-cells with subsequent release of IL-2 and IFNγ, activation of macrophages and, importantly, upregulation of HLA-class-I and class-II molecules by hepatocytes (45). Th17-cells are also involved in AIH liver damage, by perpetrating inflammation and through induction of pro-fibrotic events (35). If this cascade of events is not opposed by effective immune regulation, perpetration of immune attack occurs with consequent progression of tissue damage.

There is evidence that the frequency of liver autoantigen-specific T-cells present in the portal infiltrate is low (33, 48); these cells could orchestrate the liver damage by favoring the recruitment of non-antigen specific lymphocytes that, in turn, carry on hepatocyte damage by producing IFNγ and other cytotoxic factors.

Following the identification of CYP2D6 as the target autoantigen of LKM-1 autoantibodies in AIH-2 (4), several investigations have been conducted to identify CYP2D6 epitopes recognized by B and T-cells. By performing a conformational epitope mapping of the CYP2D6 molecule, Ma and colleagues identified $CYP2D6_{316\text{-}327}$ as key target for autoantibodies (49). Subsequent studies performed by the same group showed that CD4 T-cell immunity in AIH-2 was polyclonal and involved multiple subsets of effectors with IFNγ, IL-4 and IL-10 producing lymphocytes targeting specific epitope regions within CYP2D6 (32). CD4-mediated immune responses were associated with liver damage, a finding also confirmed when analyzing CYP2D6-specific CD8 T-cell immunity (33). Future investigations should elucidate where autoantigen specific CD8 T-cell immune responses are initiated and perpetuated, given previous animal studies showing poor cytotoxic function and pro-inflammatory cytokine secretion in CD8 T-cells activated within the liver microenvironment (50); and additional studies showing that the spleen could modulate immune regulation as well as the intensity of hepatic inflammation (51, 52).

There is evidence that overwhelming effector cell immunity in AIH results from failure of immune regulatory mechanisms permitting the autoimmune damage to unfold and perpetuate.

Defects in regulatory cells have been studied extensively over the years, although the reasons leading to these impairments and the factors contributing to it remain still unclear.

TREG IMPAIRMENT IN AIH: THE ROLE OF CD39

A wealth of studies has provided evidence that impairment of regulatory cells plays a permissive role in the initiation and progression of autoimmune tissue damage.

Among lymphocytes with immunoregulatory/suppressive properties, $CD4^+CD25^{high}FOXP3^+$ Tregs have been those most extensively studied in the last decades. These cells play a key role in promoting and maintaining immunotolerance, by controlling effector immune responses. Tregs can be classified based on their developmental pathway. Generation of thymic Tregs (tTregs) is facilitated by intermediate affinity self-peptides/MHC interactions resulting in high intensity TCR signals (53). Peripheral Tregs (pTregs) can differentiate from T-cells in certain peripheral sites like the gut mucosa and acquire stable FOXP3 expression (54); whereas induced Tregs (iTregs) can be derived *in vitro* following Tconv exposure to suboptimal antigen stimulation in the presence of anti-inflammatory mediators (55, 56).

Tregs can suppress immune responses by different mechanisms that involve the downregulation of costimulatory molecules on APCs (57), release of cytokines like TGF-β (58), IL-10 (59) and IL-35 (60); activation of apoptosis (61), including the Galectin-9/T-cell-immunoglobulin-and-mucin-domain-3 (Tim-3) pathway (62); release of Granzymes and perforin (63); metabolic disruption *via* IL-2 deprivation from the environment (64); transfer of cyclic-adenosine-monophosphate (cAMP) to effector cells *via* gap junctions and subsequent upregulation of the inducible cAMP early repressor (65); or *via* CD39, an ectoenzyme that hydrolyzes pro-inflammatory ATP and ADP to ultimately generate immunosuppressive adenosine (40).

In vivo and *in vitro* studies have indicated that Treg impairment plays a key role in the pathogenesis of autoimmune diseases, permitting overwhelming effector cell immunity to perpetrate and perpetuate tissue damage (66–70).

Defects in suppressor lymphocytes/Tregs have been reported also in AIH and found to play an important role in permitting effectors like CD4 and CD8-cells to inflict hepatocyte damage (36–39, 71). Treg defects in AIH are multifactorial and include numerical impairment (37, 38, 72), functional defects (71, 73), high rate of immune exhaustion (74) as well as plasticity with tendency to acquire effector cell features, when exposed to or challenged with a proinflammatory stimulus (42). Subsequent investigations did not support these findings, likely as a result of differences in methodologies, patients' demographics and clinical characteristics (75, 76).

Treg numerical impairment has been shown also in mice (77, 78). In a humanized mouse model of AIH, obtained upon injection of human CYP2D6/FTCD fusion protein into HLA-$DR3^-$ or HLA-$DR3^+$ transgenic NOD recipients, Yuksel and colleagues showed that defective Tregs were associated with heightened Th1-cell immunity with HLA-$DR3^+$ mice undergoing the most severe form of the disease (78). In another study by Lapierre et al, adoptive transfer of *ex vivo* expanded $CXCR3^+$ Tregs restored peripheral tolerance to FTCD and induced AIH remission (77).

Different mechanisms might account for Treg impairment in AIH (**Figure 1**). We have shown that $CD4^+CD25^{high}$ Tregs from AIH patients display low levels of Galectin-9, contain higher frequencies of $IFN\gamma^+$ and $IL\text{-}17^+$-cells, while displaying lower proportions of $FOXP3^+$, $IL\text{-}10^+$ and $TGF\text{-}\beta^+$-cells. This impairment is associated with low expression of Tim-3,

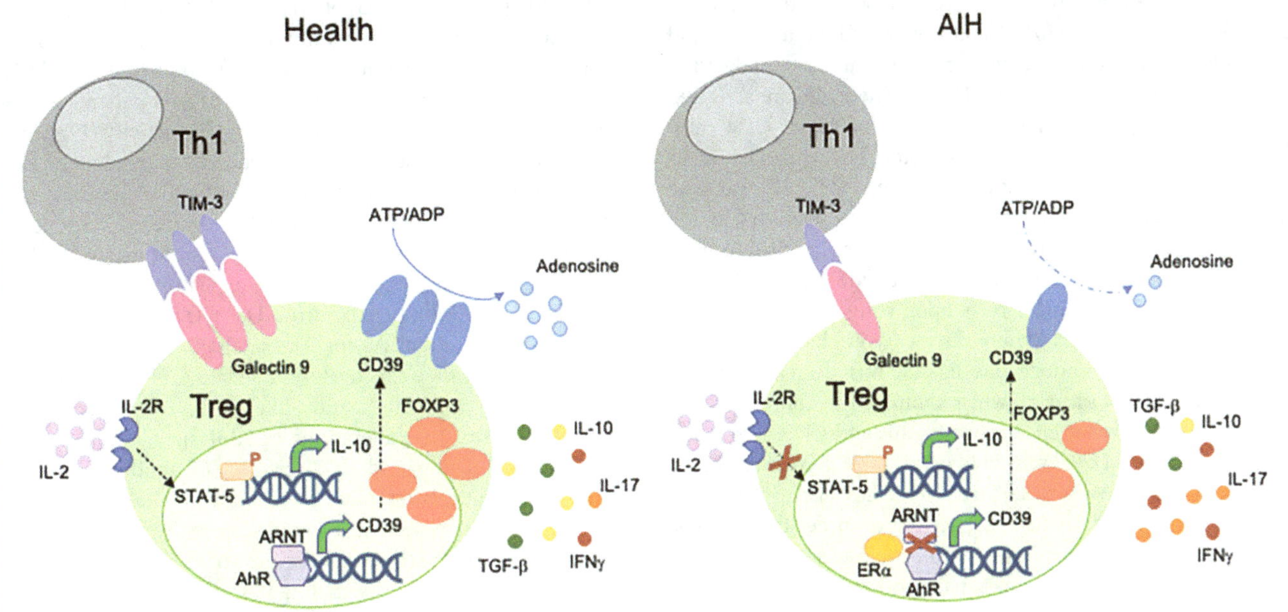

FIGURE 1 | Mechanisms of Treg impairment in AIH. Different mechanisms account for Treg impairment in AIH. Low Galectin-9 in Tregs is associated with decreased TIM-3 levels on Th1-cells. This possibly results in reduced control of the effector potential of the Th1 subset through induction of apoptosis. AIH Tregs are also defective in their response to low dose IL-2, as reflected by impaired upregulation of pSTAT-5. AIH Tregs produce low amounts of IL-10 and TGF-β, while secreting effector cytokines like IFNγ and IL-17. This indicates that, in AIH, Tregs have high tendency to acquire effector cell features. AIH Tregs also display low levels and activity of CD39, an ectoenzyme that initiates a hydrolysis cascade culminating with the generation of immunosuppressive adenosine. In health, levels of CD39 are regulated by the aryl-hydrocarbon-receptor (AhR)/aryl-hydrocarbon-receptor-nuclear-translocator (ARNT) complex. In AIH, preferential AhR binding to estrogen-receptor-alpha (Erα), an AhR non-canonical partner results in less effective upregulation of CD39 by Tregs.

the receptor of Galectin-9 on effector CD4-cells (39); this implicating that regulatory cell defects are linked with low responsiveness of T-effectors to Treg control. In a subsequent study we have reported that AIH Tregs display reduced ability to produce IL-10, this resulting in low responsiveness to low dose IL-2, as demonstrated by inability to upregulate the phosphor-signal-transducer-and-activator-of-transcription-5 (pSTAT5) (73).

In *de novo* AIH occurring after liver transplant Treg impairment was proposed to derive from high secretion of IL-12 and IL-6 by monocytes/macrophages that induced aberrant IFNγ production by Tregs impacting their function (79, 80). Blockade of TLR2 and TLR4 on monocytes resulted in reduction of IFNγ production by Tregs, further supporting the role of monocytes/macrophages in conferring Tregs proinflammatory features (79, 80).

In a mouse model of AIH, characterized by hepatocellular expression of a MHC-class II restricted immunodominant epitope of the lymphocyte choriomeningitis virus and by accumulation of CD4 T-cells specifically recognizing this epitope, Preti et al. proposed that liver damage was fostered by selective failure of peripherally induced autoreactive Tregs (81). Notably these autoreactive Tregs not only were reduced in frequency but also displayed heightened IL-17 production and reduced epigenetic demethylation (81), postulating a role for altered epigenetic regulation in Treg impairment in this model. In human AIH, *FOXP3* demethylation - a typical feature of *bona fide* Tregs - was retained in some studies (75, 79) and altered in others, where AIH derived Tregs were highly methylated (82); this indicates that further studies are needed to clearly establish the role of FOXP3 epigenetic regulation in AIH Tregs.

In subsequent studies, we have shown that Tregs obtained from the peripheral blood of AIH patients display low levels of CD39 ectoenzyme (42). In addition to displaying low CD39 levels, AIH Tregs are defective in their ectoenzymatic activity, this likely impacting their suppressive function due to lower adenosine generation (42). Impaired suppressive function of $CD39^+$ Tregs is associated with increased tendency of these cells to upregulate CD127 and producing higher levels of IL-17 and IFNγ, when exposed to anti-CD3/CD28 (42).

CD39 can be regulated at genetic, transcriptional and post-transcriptional levels. Among the factors that regulate CD39 expression at the transcriptional level, the AhR signaling plays a pivotal role. AhR is a modulator of toxin responses that also regulates effector and Treg immunity (83). AhR is activated by endogenous ligands including products of heme catabolism like unconjugated bilirubin (UCB), tryptophan metabolites, 2-(1' H-indole-3'-carbonyl)-thiazole-4-carboxylic acid methyl ester, dietary compounds like quercetin, or environmental pollutants, i.e., dioxin and benzo-*a*-pyrene. Upon binding to its ligands, AhR translocates to the cell nucleus where it forms a complex with the aryl-hydrocarbon-receptor-nuclear-translocator (ARNT), the AhR canonical partner, to regulate various genes, including cytochrome P450 enzymes, cytokines (IL-22, IL-17, IL-10), drug transporters (ABCB1, ABCC4) and CD39.

Notably, AhR activation has been demonstrated playing a role in the pathogenesis of other liver diseases, like hepatitis C, where the AhR-cytochrome P4501A1 pathway was found to favor lipid accumulation along with virus replication and assembly (84); and primary biliary cholangitis (PBC) where dioxin activated dendritic cells promoted differentiation of naïve CD4-cells, derived from PBC patients, into effector Th1 and Th17-cells (85). Importance of xenobiotics as triggers for PBC was also reported in earlier investigations (86, 87). Conversely, in the setting of experimental primary sclerosing cholangitis, administration of indole-3-carboxaldehyde could alleviate hepatic inflammation and fibrosis upon activation of the AhR-IL-22 axis (88). Further, kynurenine, a tryptophane metabolite that serves as AhR endogenous ligand, was decreased in the serum of children with AIH, when compared to controls (89).

Given the important links between AhR and CD39, we tested whether defective CD39 levels could derive from decreased AhR or ARNT expression. We found that AIH Tregs display AhR and ARNT levels comparable to Tregs derived from healthy controls; notably AIH Tregs express high levels of estrogen-receptor-alpha (Erα) (44), an AhR non-canonical partner. Further, in AIH Tregs, AhR preferentially binds to Erα rather than ARNT, this potentially resulting in less effective upregulation of CD39 upon exposure to ligands like UCB, L-kynurenine and quercetin (44). As increased Erα levels are present in patients under immunosuppression, we postulate that immunosuppressive drugs, while enabling control over inflammation, might also promote liver damage perpetuation by upregulating Erα and leading to a less effective AhR activation cascade. As silencing of Erα results in increased frequency of $CD39^+$-cells among Tregs (44), strategies potentially interfering with AhR non-canonical binding might have a role in boosting CD39 levels, by restoring AhR signaling.

There is evidence that AhR transcriptional efficiency could be regulated by factors that impact the chromatin structure (90), suggesting that AhR can undergo epigenetic regulation. Previous studies have documented global hypomethylation of CD4 T-cells in systemic lupus erythematosus, and systemic sclerosis (90, 91); it remains to be established whether these mechanisms are operative also in CD4 T cell subsets in AIH, possibly impacting AhR function and its ability to regulate downstream genes like CD39.

ABERRANT CD39 REGULATION IN AIH Th17-CELLS

Th17-cells are an effector subset that derives from CD4 lymphocytes upon exposure to IL-6 and TGF-β in mice and IL-6, IL-1β and TGF-β in humans (92). IL-23 plays an important role in the maintenance and stabilization of already differentiated Th17-cells (92). Transcription factors involved in the development of Th17-cells include RORγt, RORα and STAT-3 (92). Th17-cells can be regulated by additional factors, like AhR, which modulates CD39 and drug transporter levels (93, 94). Th17-cells have been involved in the pathogenesis of various autoimmune disorders including AIH (35).

Expression of CD39 by Th17-cells has been associated with attenuation of their pathogenic potential and acquisition of regulatory properties, as reflected by upregulation of FOXP3 and IL-10 production (93). Levels of CD39 in Th17-cells are regulated, at least in part, upon engagement of AhR by exogenous and endogenous ligands (93). Akin to Tregs, Th17-cells obtained from the peripheral blood of AIH patients express low CD39 levels and impaired ectoenzymatic activity (**Figure 2**). These defects are associated with reduced expression of A2A adenosine receptor, further confirming alterations in purinergic signaling mediators and, consequently, decreased response to adenosine. Due to lower generation of adenosine, AIH Th17-cells display impaired acquisition of regulatory properties that result in defective ability to control $CD4^+$ $CD25^-$cell proliferation and IL-17 production. As for Tregs, Th17-cells obtained from AIH patients cannot effectively upregulate CYP1A1 and CD39 when exposed to AhR ligands like UCB, L-kynurenine and quercetin, postulating alterations of AhR signaling as possible determinants of impaired CD39 levels. Differently from Tregs, however, no differences have been found in the expression of Erα. Instead, increase in the expression of hypoxia-inducible-factor-1alpha (HIF-1α), which is known to negatively regulate AhR expression (95) and signaling (94), is noted.

As discussed, the AhR signaling alterations noted in AIH impact both Treg and Th17 cell ability to upregulate CD39, this accounting for their impaired suppressive function (Tregs) and inability to acquire regulatory properties (Th17-cells). This indicates that defective immune regulation involves not only the regulatory but also the effector cell compartment. Strategies aimed at restoring alterations of AhR signaling both in Tregs and Th17-cells should be developed to guarantee a broader control over effector cell immunity in this autoimmune setting.

NEW IMMUNOTHERAPIES

Given the multiple defects underlying immunotolerance breakdown in AIH, therapeutic strategies should be developed with the aim of restoring the pool of Tregs while dampening the effector potential of these cells (**Figure 3**). Reconstitution of the Treg pool could be achieved upon adoptive transfer. In previous studies we assessed Treg ability to expand under polyclonal conditions (96). Tregs expanded from the already existing regulatory cell pool express higher FOXP3 levels and suppress effector cells more effectively (96). This strategy also resulted in *de novo* generation of Tregs from $CD4^+CD25^-$ effector lymphocytes, when using healthy controls and AIH-derived cells (96). In line with this strategy, inhibition of IL-17 was found to favor the differentiation of newly generated Tregs from $CD4^+CD25^-$ effectors (97), supporting the postulate that immune regulation could be enhanced even further when effector cells are conditioned to become suppressive. Exposure of $CD127^+CD25^+$ activated cells to TGF-β and IL-2 boosts IL-10 production and suppressive function of these cells (98). As CD39 is strictly linked with Treg ability to suppress, adoptive transfer of $CD39^{high}$ Tregs (99) would be preferable; however, since this subset is substantially impaired in AIH patients (42), strategies that enable boosting CD39 in Tregs, prior to their transfer, should be implemented. A study by Oo and colleagues showed that

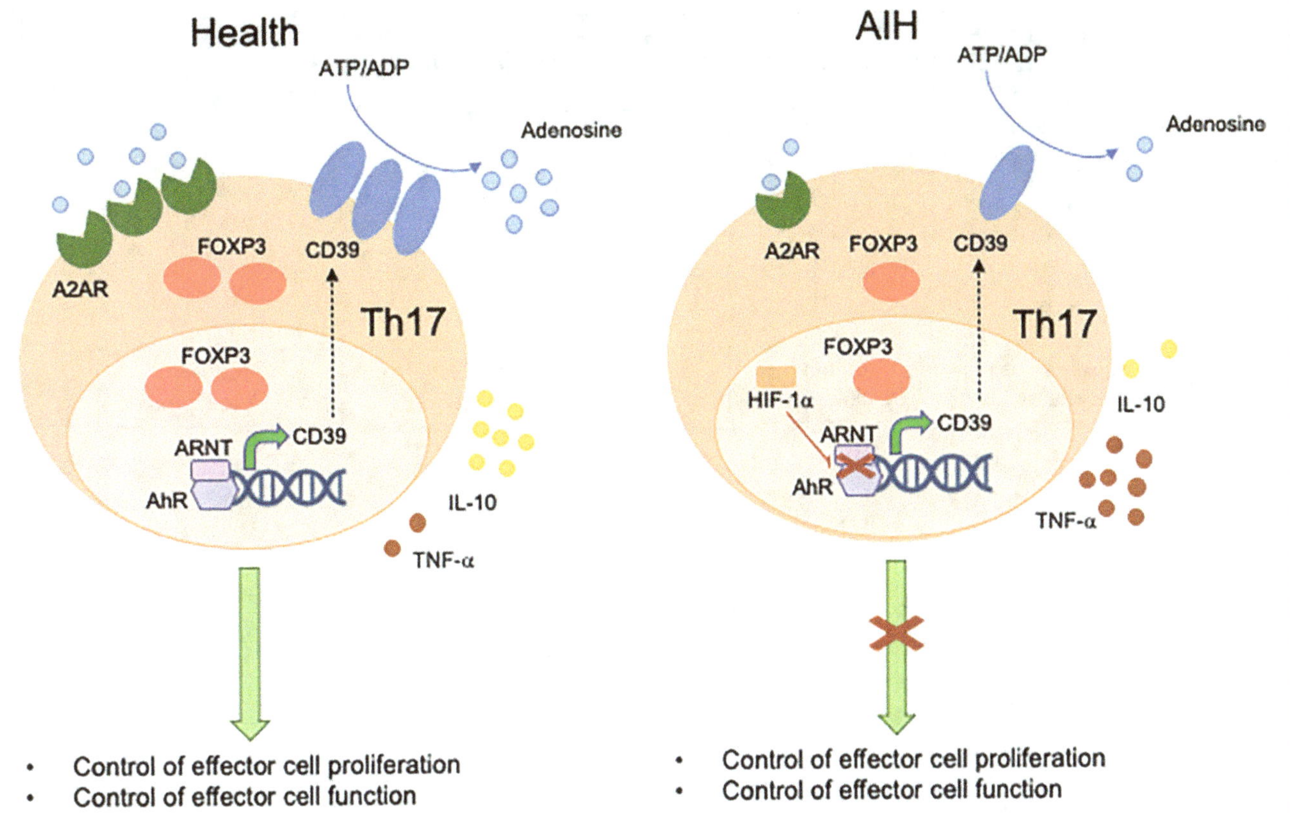

FIGURE 2 | Mechanisms of aberrant Th17-cell immunity in AIH. Expression of CD39 by Th17-cells is associated with acquisition of regulatory properties. These include increased FOXP3 expression levels, IL-10 production and control of effector cell proliferation and function. In healthy subjects, levels of CD39 in Th17-cells are regulated by the aryl-hydrocarbon-receptor (AhR)/aryl-hydrocarbon-receptor-nuclear-translocator (ARNT) complex. In AIH, Th17-cells display decreased CD39 levels and activity. This is linked, at least in part, with high levels of hypoxia-inducible-factor-1alpha (HIF-1α) that inhibits AhR levels and signaling. Th17-cells from AIH patients also display reduced levels of A2A adenosine receptor, this implicating defective response of these cells to the immunosuppressive effects of adenosine.

polyclonal Tregs, isolated from leukapheresis products, labelled with indium tropolonate and re-infused in AIH patients, homed to the liver where they were detected for up to 72 hours (100). In a murine model of AIH in the context of autoimmune-polyendocrine-syndrome-type-1, a multiorgan autoimmune condition caused by mutations of the autoimmune regulator (AIRE) gene, adoptive transfer of polyspecific Tregs was effective in treating AIH (101).

In the context of AIH-2 where the autoantigen and the CD4 and CD8 T-cell epitopes within it are known, adoptive transfer of autoantigen-specific Tregs would enable achieving a tailored and effective form of treatment to re-establish immunotolerance. In this regard, we could generate Tregs specific for HLA-DR3 and HLA-DR7 restricted CYP2D6 epitopes upon co-culture with semi-mature DCs that enable antigen presentation and promote immunotolerance induction (102). CYP2D6-Tregs suppress the proliferation and pro-inflammatory cytokine production by CD4 effectors of the same antigen specificity (102). As CYP2D6-specific Tregs showed the tendency to lose their suppressor properties when exposed to proinflammatory stimuli, treatment with retinoic acid could stabilize their phenotype and functional properties even in the presence of an inflammatory milieu (103). Effort has been made in subsequent studies to control autoantigen-specific effectors upon *in vivo* injections of peptide-major histocompatibility class-II (pMHC-II) nanomedicines with specificity for the immunodominant epitope $CYP2D6_{398\text{-}412}$ in a mouse model of AIH, obtained by infecting NOD mice with replication defective adenovirus encoding for human FTCD (104). This approach resulted in the expansion of Tr1-cells (104). Preclinical studies have provided evidence that antigen-specific Tregs deliver targeted and superior immunosuppression, when compared to other approaches, including polyclonal Tregs (105). Since generation of antigen-specific Tregs is, however, hampered by their limited ability to expand, recent studies have shown that these cells could be also obtained from polyclonal Tregs through transduction of Treg T-cell receptor or chimeric antigen receptor (CAR) (105); or, through strategies based on the CRISPR Cas9 system where an endogenous TCR can be replaced by a recombinant one (105).

In addition to cell-based therapies, the implementation of which may be limited by substantial costs, Tregs could be expanded by modifying the cytokine environment. A study by Diestelhorst et al. proposed that the marked decrease in AIH Tregs during immunosuppressive therapy might derive from

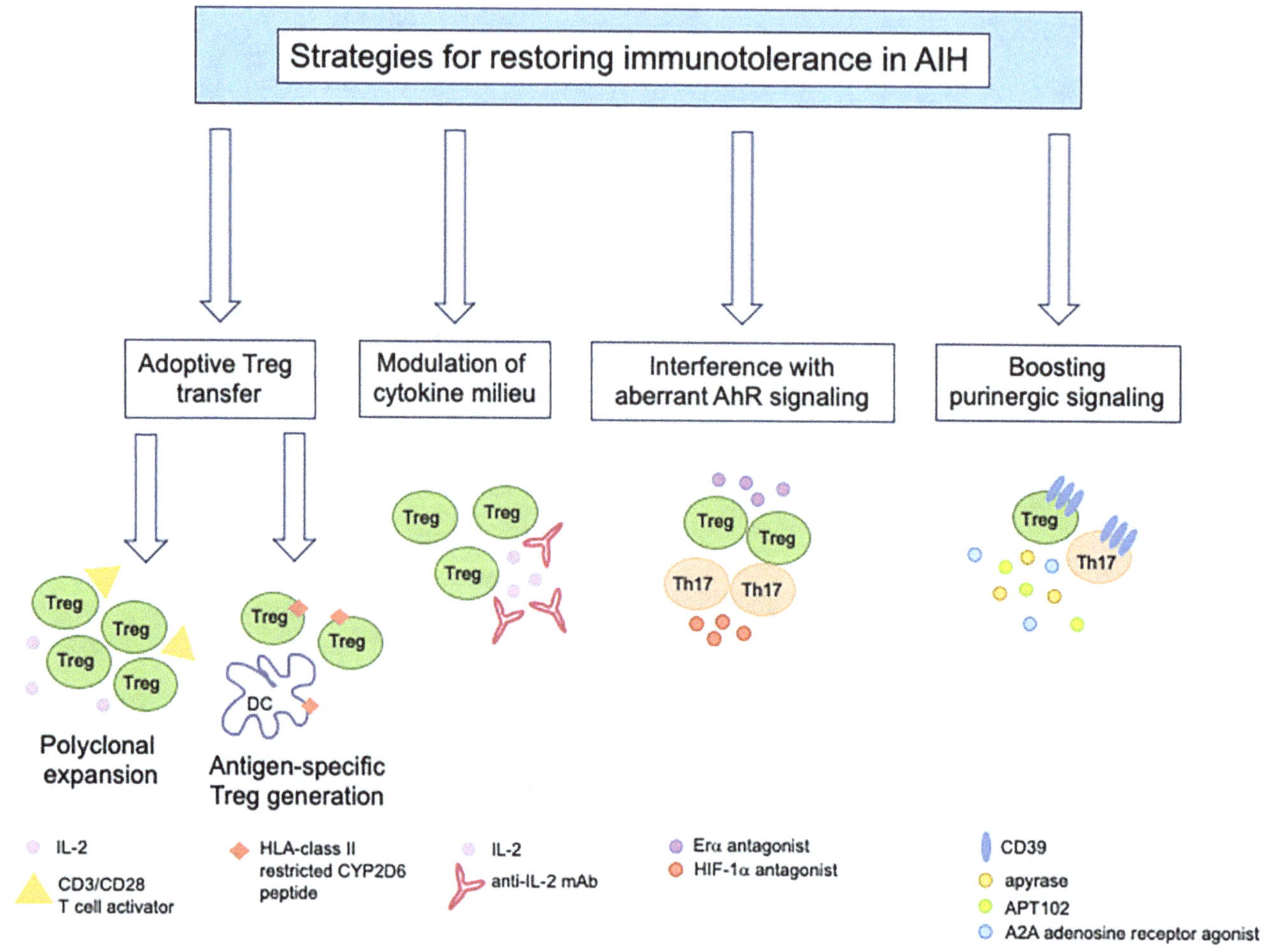

FIGURE 3 | New immunotherapies for tolerance reconstitution in AIH. Strategies that might be considered as tools to re-establish immunotolerance in AIH include: adoptive transfer of Tregs, polyclonally expanded *in vitro* in the presence of high dose IL-2 and CD3/CD28 T-cell activator or generated under antigen-specific conditions upon co-culture with semi-mature dendritic cells; modulation of the cytokine milieu by administration of low dose IL-2 or monoclonal antibody/IL-2 complex; use of Erα or HIF-1α antagonists to interfere with aberrant AhR signaling in Tregs (Erα) and Th17-cells (HIF-1α); boosting of purinergic signaling through the use of exogenous apyrase, APT102, an ADPase that was found to enhance the beneficial effects of AhR activation *in vivo* and *in vitro*, and A2A adenosine receptor agonists to amplify the immunosuppressive properties of adenosine.

decreased levels of IL-2, a cytokine key for Treg survival (106). Exposure of PBMCs from patients with autoimmune liver diseases, including AIH, to very-low-dose Proleukin, used at less than 5 IU/ml, resulted in phosphorylation of STAT-5 and increased levels of CTLA-4 and FOXP3 in the Treg subset (107). Administration of low dose IL-2 would enable *in vivo* cell reconstitution, even when the autoantigen is unknown. In a study on two AIH patients with persistent disease activity, administration of low dose IL-2 resulted in Treg expansion in both. This was evident on day 9 but returned to baseline levels on day 28 (108). Clinical response was observed in one case, suggesting that the effects of IL-2-induced Treg expansion is transient and the clinical benefit limited, at least in the small cohort studied. Additional efforts should be made to optimize and successfully implement this approach.

To prolong the half-life of IL-2 in the bloodstream, mutants have been developed to promote Treg expansion *in vivo*. Another strategy has been attempted and consists of the administration of monoclonal antibody/IL-2 complex to expand Tregs in a mouse model of colitis (109) and AIH (110). A new complex of IL-2 and anti-IL-2 monoclonal antibodies was found to stimulate Treg expansion among human T-cells *ex vivo* and in rhesus macaques *in vivo* (111).

Transient increase in the proportion of splenic Tregs was achieved in a mouse model of AIH, resulting from xenoimmunization of C57BL/6 mice with DNA coding for human liver autoantigens, after treatment with low-dose anti-CD3 antibody (112). No differences in the proportion of splenic and liver derived Tregs were noted in xenoimmunized mice subjected to anti-CD20 antibody treatment, this approach inducing AIH remission by decreasing antigen presentation (through B-cells) and help to T lymphocytes (113). Whether belimumab, an inhibitor of serum B-cell activating factor that has been recently proposed as a promising treatment option for patients with refractory AIH and advanced liver-related fibrosis, induces disease remission having also a beneficial impact on Treg frequencies, is unknow (114).

As immunoregulatory defects in AIH involve both Tregs and effector Th17-cells, future approaches targeting both cell types should be considered. Our research has shown impaired CD39 levels in both Tregs and Th17-cells obtained from the peripheral blood of AIH patients. Reduced CD39 expression is present in AIH patients during active disease and remission, suggesting an intrinsic defect of this ectoenzyme in AIH Treg and Th17 lymphocytes (42, 43). This defect derives, at least in part, from aberrant increase in the levels of Erα, an alternative AhR partner, which is upregulated in AIH Tregs; and from high expression of HIF-1α, an AhR inhibitor, which is upregulated in AIH Th17-cells. In this regard, strategies inhibiting Erα and HIF-1α may help reconstituting the altered AhR signaling in AIH, and along with this, CD39 and immunotolerance.

Alternatively, interventions that boost CD39 levels might represent an additional option to bypass the altered AhR signaling/pathway and restore immunotolerance by enhancing the levels and/or activity of this ectoenzyme.

These approaches could be based on exogenous apyrase that has ectoenzymatic activity comparable to CD39; and APT102, the extracellular domain with improved ADPase activity of human nucleoside-triphosphate-diphosphohydrolase-3, a member of the CD39 family (115). APT102 was found beneficial in enhancing the immunoregulatory properties of the AhR ligand UCB in an experimental model of colitis in mice and in promoting increased levels of immunoregulatory molecules on Tregs and Tr1-cells (115). Notably, there were no safety or toxicity concerns when APT102 treatment was protracted after resolution of colitis *in vivo* (115). Additional studies reported on the safety profile of this molecule in the vascular setting (116, 117). However, since CD39 also plays an important role in tumor development and progression (99, 118–121) and inhibition of effector immune responses against pathogens (99, 122, 123), the safety of long-term treatments aimed at restoring the levels of this ectoenzyme in the context of autoimmune diseases should be considered and carefully evaluated. A2A receptor agonists that enhance the adenosinergic signal might also have a role in restoring immunotolerance by reconstituting the purinergic milieu (41).

Strategies targeting CD39 antisense RNA, a long noncoding RNA regulating CD39 at both mRNA and protein levels, should be taken into consideration. Silencing of CD39 antisense RNA has been effective in containing disease activity in an experimental mouse model of colitis in humanized *NOD/scid/gamma* mice, reconstituted with human CD4-cells (124).

CONCLUDING REMARKS

This review has discussed the mechanisms mediating liver damage perpetuation and progression in AIH with a specific focus on the imbalance between Tregs and Th17-cells.

Numerous pathways might be involved in AIH disordered immunity. We have discussed how defects in CD39 are linked with aberrant AhR signaling in AIH-derived Tregs and Th17-cells. Standard treatment of AIH is still based on corticosteroids and azathioprine, immunosuppressive drugs that currently enable control of inflammation without, however, restoring immunotolerance and preventing progression to end-stage liver disease. Strategies targeting factors that interfere with AhR canonical pathway or directly boosting CD39 expression and activity might represent new therapeutic avenues in the treatment of AIH.

AUTHOR CONTRIBUTIONS

MV, NW, and AK wrote the manuscript. JG performed literature search. ML reviewed and edited the manuscript. All authors contributed to the article and approved the submitted version.

REFERENCES

1. Waldenstrom J. Liver, Blood Proteins and Food Proteins. *Dtsch Z Verdau Stoffwechselkr* (1952) 12(Spec No):113–21.
2. Al-Chalabi T, Underhill JA, Portmann BC, McFarlane IG, Heneghan MA. Impact of Gender on the Long-Term Outcome and Survival of Patients With Autoimmune Hepatitis. *J Hepatol* (2008) 48(1):140–7. doi: 10.1016/j.jhep.2007.08.013
3. Johnson PJ, McFarlane IG. Meeting Report: International Autoimmune Hepatitis Group. *Hepatology* (1993) 18(4):998–1005. doi: 10.1002/hep.1840180435
4. Manns MP, Johnson EF, Griffin KJ, Tan EM, Sullivan KF. Major Antigen of Liver Kidney Microsomal Autoantibodies in Idiopathic Autoimmune Hepatitis is Cytochrome P450db1. *J Clin Invest* (1989) 83(3):1066–72. doi: 10.1172/JCI113949
5. Vergani D, Alvarez F, Bianchi FB, Cancado EL, Mackay IR, Manns MP, et al. Liver Autoimmune Serology: A Consensus Statement From the Committee for Autoimmune Serology of the International Autoimmune Hepatitis Group. *J Hepatol* (2004) 41(4):677–83. doi: 10.1016/j.jhep.2004.08.002
6. Ma Y, Okamoto M, Thomas MG, Bogdanos DP, Lopes AR, Portmann B, et al. Antibodies to Conformational Epitopes of Soluble Liver Antigen Define a Severe Form of Autoimmune Liver Disease. *Hepatology* (2002) 35(3):658–64. doi: 10.1053/jhep.2002.32092
7. Muratori L, Sztul E, Muratori P, Gao Y, Ripalti A, Ponti C, et al. Distinct Epitopes on Formiminotransferase Cyclodeaminase Induce Autoimmune Liver Cytosol Antibody Type 1. *Hepatology* (2001) 34(3):494–501. doi: 10.1053/jhep.2001.27179
8. Muratori L, Cataleta M, Muratori P, Lenzi M, Bianchi FB. Liver/kidney Microsomal Antibody Type 1 and Liver Cytosol Antibody Type 1 Concentrations in Type 2 Autoimmune Hepatitis. *Gut* (1998) 42(5):721–6. doi: 10.1136/gut.42.5.721
9. Terziroli Beretta-Piccoli B, Mieli-Vergani G, Vergani D. Serology in Autoimmune Hepatitis: A Clinical-Practice Approach. *Eur J Intern Med* (2018) 48:35–43. doi: 10.1016/j.ejim.2017.10.006
10. Gleeson D, Heneghan MABritish Society of G. British Society of Gastroenterology (BSG) Guidelines for Management of Autoimmune Hepatitis. *Gut* (2011) 60(12):1611–29. doi: 10.1136/gut.2010.235259
11. Desmet VJ, Gerber M, Hoofnagle JH, Manns M, Scheuer PJ. Classification of Chronic Hepatitis: Diagnosis, Grading and Staging. *Hepatology* (1994) 19 (6):1513–20. doi: 10.1002/hep.1840190629
12. McFarlane IG. Definition and Classification of Autoimmune Hepatitis. *Semin Liver Dis* (2002) 22(4):317–24. doi: 10.1055/s-2002-35702
13. Zolfino T, Heneghan MA, Norris S, Harrison PM, Portmann BC, McFarlane IG. Characteristics of Autoimmune Hepatitis in Patients Who are Not of European Caucasoid Ethnic Origin. *Gut* (2002) 50(5):713–7. doi: 10.1136/gut.50.5.713
14. Lim KN, Casanova RL, Boyer TD, Bruno CJ. Autoimmune Hepatitis in African Americans: Presenting Features and Response to Therapy. *Am J Gastroenterol* (2001) 96(12):3390–4. doi: 10.1111/j.1572-0241.2001.05272.x

15. Takahashi A, Arinaga-Hino T, Ohira H, Torimura T, Zeniya M, Abe M, et al. Autoimmune Hepatitis in Japan: Trends in a Nationwide Survey. *J Gastroenterol* (2017) 52(5):631–40. doi: 10.1007/s00535-016-1267-0
16. Gregorio GV, Portmann B, Reid F, Donaldson PT, Doherty DG, McCartney M, et al. Autoimmune Hepatitis in Childhood: A 20-Year Experience. *Hepatology* (1997) 25(3):541–7. doi: 10.1002/hep.510250308
17. Manns MP, Czaja AJ, Gorham JD, Krawitt EL, Mieli-Vergani G, Vergani D, et al. Diagnosis and Management of Autoimmune Hepatitis. *Hepatology* (2010) 51(6):2193–213. doi: 10.1002/hep.23584
18. Alvarez F, Ciocca M, Canero-Velasco C, Ramonet M, de Davila MT, Cuarterolo M, et al. Short-Term Cyclosporine Induces a Remission of Autoimmune Hepatitis in Children. *J Hepatol* (1999) 30(2):222–7. doi: 10.1016/S0168-8278(99)80065-8
19. Cuarterolo M, Ciocca M, Velasco CC, Ramonet M, Gonzalez T, Lopez S, et al. Follow-Up of Children With Autoimmune Hepatitis Treated With Cyclosporine. *J Pediatr Gastroenterol Nutr* (2006) 43(5):635–9. doi: 10.1097/01.mpg.0000235975.75120.38
20. Van Thiel DH, Carroll P, Abu-Elmagd K, Rodriguez-Rilo H, Irish W, McMichael J, et al. Tacrolimus (FK 506), a Treatment for Primary Sclerosing Cholangitis: Results of an Open-Label Preliminary Trial. *Am J Gastroenterol* (1995) 90(3):455–9.
21. Richardson PD, James PD, Ryder SD. Mycophenolate Mofetil for Maintenance of Remission in Autoimmune Hepatitis in Patients Resistant to or Intolerant of Azathioprine. *J Hepatol* (2000) 33(3):371–5. doi: 10.1016/S0168-8278(00)80271-8
22. Aw MM, Dhawan A, Samyn M, Bargiota A, Mieli-Vergani G. Mycophenolate Mofetil as Rescue Treatment for Autoimmune Liver Disease in Children: A 5-Year Follow-Up. *J Hepatol* (2009) 51(1):156–60. doi: 10.1016/j.jhep.2009.02.024
23. Lammert C, Chalasani SN, Atkinson EJ, McCauley BM, Lazaridis KN. Environmental Risk Factors are Associated With Autoimmune Hepatitis. *Liver Int* (2021) 41(5):1162–3. doi: 10.1111/liv.14944
24. Ma Y, Su H, Yuksel M, Longhi MS, McPhail MJ, Wang P, et al. Human Leukocyte Antigen Profile Predicts Severity of Autoimmune Liver Disease in Children of European Ancestry. *Hepatology* (2021). doi: 10.1002/hep.31893
25. Djilali-Saiah I, Fakhfakh A, Louafi H, Caillat-Zucman S, Debray D, Alvarez F. HLA Class II Influences Humoral Autoimmunity in Patients With Type 2 Autoimmune Hepatitis. *J Hepatol* (2006) 45(6):844–50. doi: 10.1016/j.jhep.2006.07.034
26. Lapierre P, Djilali-Saiah I, Vitozzi S, Alvarez F. A Murine Model of Type 2 Autoimmune Hepatitis: Xenoimmunization With Human Antigens. *Hepatology* (2004) 39(4):1066–74. doi: 10.1002/hep.20109
27. Hintermann E, Ehser J, Bayer M, Pfeilschifter JM, Christen U. Mechanism of Autoimmune Hepatic Fibrogenesis Induced by an Adenovirus Encoding the Human Liver Autoantigen Cytochrome P450 2d6. *J Autoimmun* (2013) 44:49–60. doi: 10.1016/j.jaut.2013.05.001
28. Holdener M, Hintermann E, Bayer M, Rhode A, Rodrigo E, Hintereder G, et al. Breaking Tolerance to the Natural Human Liver Autoantigen Cytochrome P450 2D6 by Virus Infection. *J Exp Med* (2008) 205(6):1409–22. doi: 10.1084/jem.20071859
29. Hardtke-Wolenski M, Fischer K, Noyan F, Schlue J, Falk CS, Stahlhut M, et al. Genetic Predisposition and Environmental Danger Signals Initiate Chronic Autoimmune Hepatitis Driven by CD4+ T Cells. *Hepatology* (2013) 58(2):718–28. doi: 10.1002/hep.26380
30. Bonito AJ, Aloman C, Fiel MI, Danzl NM, Cha S, Weinstein EG, et al. Medullary Thymic Epithelial Cell Depletion Leads to Autoimmune Hepatitis. *J Clin Invest* (2013) 123(8):3510–24. doi: 10.1172/JCI65414
31. Aoki N, Kido M, Iwamoto S, Nishiura H, Maruoka R, Tanaka J, et al. Dysregulated Generation of Follicular Helper T Cells in the Spleen Triggers Fatal Autoimmune Hepatitis in Mice. *Gastroenterology* (2011) 140(4):1322–33.e1-5. doi: 10.1053/j.gastro.2011.01.002
32. Ma Y, Bogdanos DP, Hussain MJ, Underhill J, Bansal S, Longhi MS, et al. Polyclonal T-Cell Responses to Cytochrome P450IID6 are Associated With Disease Activity in Autoimmune Hepatitis Type 2. *Gastroenterology* (2006) 130(3):868–82. doi: 10.1053/j.gastro.2005.12.020
33. Longhi MS, Hussain MJ, Bogdanos DP, Quaglia A, Mieli-Vergani G, Ma Y, et al. Cytochrome P450IID6-Specific CD8 T Cell Immune Responses Mirror Disease Activity in Autoimmune Hepatitis Type 2. *Hepatology* (2007) 46 (2):472–84. doi: 10.1002/hep.21658
34. Longhi MS, Mitry RR, Samyn M, Scalori A, Hussain MJ, Quaglia A, et al. Vigorous Activation of Monocytes in Juvenile Autoimmune Liver Disease Escapes the Control of Regulatory T-Cells. *Hepatology* (2009) 50(1):130–42. doi: 10.1002/hep.22914
35. Zhao L, Tang Y, You Z, Wang Q, Liang S, Han X, et al. Interleukin-17 Contributes to the Pathogenesis of Autoimmune Hepatitis Through Inducing Hepatic Interleukin-6 Expression. *PloS One* (2011) 6(4):e18909. doi: 10.1371/journal.pone.0018909
36. Hodgson HJ, Wands JR, Isselbacher KJ. Alteration in Suppressor Cell Activity in Chronic Active Hepatitis. *Proc Natl Acad Sci USA* (1978) 75 (3):1549–53. doi: 10.1073/pnas.75.3.1549
37. Longhi MS, Ma Y, Bogdanos DP, Cheeseman P, Mieli-Vergani G, Vergani D. Impairment of CD4(+)CD25(+) Regulatory T-Cells in Autoimmune Liver Disease. *J Hepatol* (2004) 41(1):31–7. doi: 10.1016/j.jhep.2004.03.008
38. Longhi MS, Ma Y, Mitry RR, Bogdanos DP, Heneghan M, Cheeseman P, et al. Effect of CD4+ CD25+ Regulatory T-Cells on CD8 T-Cell Function in Patients With Autoimmune Hepatitis. *J Autoimmun* (2005) 25(1):63–71. doi: 10.1016/j.jaut.2005.05.001
39. Liberal R, Grant CR, Holder BS, Ma Y, Mieli-Vergani G, Vergani D, et al. The Impaired Immune Regulation of Autoimmune Hepatitis is Linked to a Defective Galectin-9/Tim-3 Pathway. *Hepatology* (2012) 56(2):677–86. doi: 10.1002/hep.25682
40. Eltzschig HK, Sitkovsky MV, Robson SC. Purinergic Signaling During Inflammation. *N Engl J Med* (2012) 367(24):2322–33. doi: 10.1056/NEJMra1205750
41. Vuerich M, Mukherjee S, Robson SC, Longhi MS. Control of Gut Inflammation by Modulation of Purinergic Signaling. *Front Immunol* (2020) 11:1882. doi: 10.3389/fimmu.2020.01882
42. Grant CR, Liberal R, Holder BS, Cardone J, Ma Y, Robson SC, et al. Dysfunctional CD39(POS) Regulatory T Cells and Aberrant Control of T-Helper Type 17 Cells in Autoimmune Hepatitis. *Hepatology* (2014) 59 (3):1007–15. doi: 10.1002/hep.26583
43. Liberal R, Grant CR, Ma Y, Csizmadia E, Jiang ZG, Heneghan MA, et al. CD39 Mediated Regulation of Th17-Cell Effector Function is Impaired in Juvenile Autoimmune Liver Disease. *J Autoimmun* (2016) 72:102–12. doi: 10.1016/j.jaut.2016.05.005
44. Vuerich M, Harshe R, Frank LA, Mukherjee S, Gromova B, Csizmadia E, et al. Altered Aryl-Hydrocarbon-Receptor Signalling Affects Regulatory and Effector Cell Immunity in Autoimmune Hepatitis. *J Hepatol* (2021) 74 (1):48–57. doi: 10.1016/j.jhep.2020.06.044
45. Lobo-Yeo A, Senaldi G, Portmann B, Mowat AP, Mieli-Vergani G, Vergani D. Class I and Class II Major Histocompatibility Complex Antigen Expression on Hepatocytes: A Study in Children With Liver Disease. *Hepatology* (1990) 12(2):224–32. doi: 10.1002/hep.1840120208
46. Senaldi G, Portmann B, Mowat AP, Mieli-Vergani G, Vergani D. Immunohistochemical Features of the Portal Tract Mononuclear Cell Infiltrate in Chronic Aggressive Hepatitis. *Arch Dis Child* (1992) 67 (12):1447–53. doi: 10.1136/adc.67.12.1447
47. Cochrane AM, Moussouros A, Thomsom AD, Eddleston AL, Williams R. Antibody-Dependent Cell-Mediated (K Cell) Cytotoxicity Against Isolated Hepatocytes in Chronic Active Hepatitis. *Lancet* (1976) 1(7957):441–4. doi: 10.1016/S0140-6736(76)91472-0
48. Mix H, Weiler-Normann C, Thimme R, Ahlenstiel G, Shin EC, Herkel J, et al. Identification of CD4 T-Cell Epitopes in Soluble Liver Antigen/Liver Pancreas Autoantigen in Autoimmune Hepatitis. *Gastroenterology* (2008) 135(6):2107–18. doi: 10.1053/j.gastro.2008.07.029
49. Ma Y, Thomas MG, Okamoto M, Bogdanos DP, Nagl S, Kerkar N, et al. Key Residues of a Major Cytochrome P4502D6 Epitope are Located on the Surface of the Molecule. *J Immunol* (2002) 169(1):277–85. doi: 10.4049/jimmunol.169.1.277
50. Holz LE, Benseler V, Vo M, McGuffog C, Van Rooijen N, McCaughan GW, et al. Naive CD8 T Cell Activation by Liver Bone Marrow-Derived Cells Leads to a "Neglected" IL-2low Bimhigh Phenotype, Poor CTL Function and Cell Death. *J Hepatol* (2012) 57(4):830–6. doi: 10.1016/j.jhep.2012.05.015
51. Kim MT, Harty JT. Splenectomy Alters Distribution and Turnover But Not Numbers or Protective Capacity of *De Novo* Generated Memory CD8 T-Cells. *Front Immunol* (2014) 5:568. doi: 10.3389/fimmu.2014.00568
52. Buitrago-Molina LE, Dywicki J, Noyan F, Trippler M, Pietrek J, Schlue J, et al. Splenectomy Prior to Experimental Induction of Autoimmune Hepatitis Promotes More Severe Hepatic Inflammation, Production of IL-17 and

Apoptosis. *Biomedicines* (2021) 9(1):58. doi: 10.3390/biomedicines9010058

53. Jordan MS, Boesteanu A, Reed AJ, Petrone AL, Holenbeck AE, Lerman MA, et al. Thymic Selection of CD4+CD25+ Regulatory T Cells Induced by an Agonist Self-Peptide. *Nat Immunol* (2001) 2(4):301–6. doi: 10.1038/86302
54. Abbas AK, Benoist C, Bluestone JA, Campbell DJ, Ghosh S, Hori S, et al. Regulatory T Cells: Recommendations to Simplify the Nomenclature. *Nat Immunol* (2013) 14(4):307–8. doi: 10.1038/ni.2554
55. Apostolou I, von Boehmer H. In Vivo Instruction of Suppressor Commitment in Naive T Cells. *J Exp Med* (2004) 199(10):1401–8. doi: 10.1084/jem.20040249
56. Kretschmer K, Apostolou I, Hawiger D, Khazaie K, Nussenzweig MC, von Boehmer H. Inducing and Expanding Regulatory T Cell Populations by Foreign Antigen. *Nat Immunol* (2005) 6(12):1219–27. doi: 10.1038/ni1265
57. Cederbom L, Hall H, Ivars F. CD4+CD25+ Regulatory T Cells Down-Regulate Co-Stimulatory Molecules on Antigen-Presenting Cells. *Eur J Immunol* (2000) 30(6):1538–43. doi: 10.1002/1521-4141(200006)30:6<1538::AID-IMMU1538>3.0.CO;2-X
58. Powrie F, Carlino J, Leach MW, Mauze S, Coffman RL. A Critical Role for Transforming Growth Factor-Beta But Not Interleukin 4 in the Suppression of T Helper Type 1-Mediated Colitis by CD45RB(low) CD4+ T Cells. *J Exp Med* (1996) 183(6):2669–74. doi: 10.1084/jem.183.6.2669
59. Asseman C, Mauze S, Leach MW, Coffman RL, Powrie F. An Essential Role for Interleukin 10 in the Function of Regulatory T Cells That Inhibit Intestinal Inflammation. *J Exp Med* (1999) 190(7):995–1004. doi: 10.1084/jem.190.7.995
60. Collison LW, Workman CJ, Kuo TT, Boyd K, Wang Y, Vignali KM, et al. The Inhibitory Cytokine IL-35 Contributes to Regulatory T-Cell Function. *Nature* (2007) 450(7169):566–9. doi: 10.1038/nature06306
61. Ren X, Ye F, Jiang Z, Chu Y, Xiong S, Wang Y. Involvement of Cellular Death in TRAIL/DR5-Dependent Suppression Induced by CD4(+)CD25(+) Regulatory T Cells. *Cell Death Differ* (2007) 14(12):2076–84. doi: 10.1038/sj.cdd.4402220
62. Kashio Y, Nakamura K, Abedin MJ, Seki M, Nishi N, Yoshida N, et al. Galectin-9 Induces Apoptosis Through the Calcium-Calpain-Caspase-1 Pathway. *J Immunol* (2003) 170(7):3631–6. doi: 10.4049/jimmunol.170.7.3631
63. Cao X, Cai SF, Fehniger TA, Song J, Collins LI, Piwnica-Worms DR, et al. Granzyme B and Perforin are Important for Regulatory T Cell-Mediated Suppression of Tumor Clearance. *Immunity* (2007) 27(4):635–46. doi: 10.1016/j.immuni.2007.08.014
64. Pandiyan P, Zheng L, Ishihara S, Reed J, Lenardo MJ. CD4+CD25+Foxp3+ Regulatory T Cells Induce Cytokine Deprivation-Mediated Apoptosis of Effector CD4+ T Cells. *Nat Immunol* (2007) 8(12):1353–62. doi: 10.1038/ni1536
65. Vaeth M, Gogishvili T, Bopp T, Klein M, Berberich-Siebelt F, Gattenloehner S, et al. Regulatory T Cells Facilitate the Nuclear Accumulation of Inducible cAMP Early Repressor (ICER) and Suppress Nuclear Factor of Activated T Cell C1 (Nfatc1). *Proc Natl Acad Sci USA* (2011) 108(6):2480–5. doi: 10.1073/pnas.1009463108
66. Lindley S, Dayan CM, Bishop A, Roep BO, Peakman M, Tree TI. Defective Suppressor Function in CD4(+)CD25(+) T-Cells From Patients With Type 1 Diabetes. *Diabetes* (2005) 54(1):92–9. doi: 10.2337/diabetes.54.1.92
67. Ehrenstein MR, Evans JG, Singh A, Moore S, Warnes G, Isenberg DA, et al. Compromised Function of Regulatory T Cells in Rheumatoid Arthritis and Reversal by Anti-TNFalpha Therapy. *J Exp Med* (2004) 200(3):277–85. doi: 10.1084/jem.20040165
68. Viglietta V, Baecher-Allan C, Weiner HL, Hafler DA. Loss of Functional Suppression by CD4+CD25+ Regulatory T Cells in Patients With Multiple Sclerosis. *J Exp Med* (2004) 199(7):971–9. doi: 10.1084/jem.20031579
69. Mao C, Wang S, Xiao Y, Xu J, Jiang Q, Jin M, et al. Impairment of Regulatory Capacity of CD4+CD25+ Regulatory T Cells Mediated by Dendritic Cell Polarization and Hyperthyroidism in Graves' Disease. *J Immunol* (2011) 186 (8):4734–43. doi: 10.4049/jimmunol.0904135
70. Sugiyama H, Gyulai R, Toichi E, Garaczi E, Shimada S, Stevens SR, et al. Dysfunctional Blood and Target Tissue CD4+CD25high Regulatory T Cells in Psoriasis: Mechanism Underlying Unrestrained Pathogenic Effector T Cell Proliferation. *J Immunol* (2005) 174(1):164–73. doi: 10.4049/jimmunol.174.1.164
71. Longhi MS, Hussain MJ, Mitry RR, Arora SK, Mieli-Vergani G, Vergani D, et al. Functional Study of CD4+CD25+ Regulatory T Cells in Health and Autoimmune Hepatitis. *J Immunol* (2006) 176(7):4484–91. doi: 10.4049/jimmunol.176.7.4484
72. Ferri S, Longhi MS, De Molo C, Lalanne C, Muratori P, Granito A, et al. A Multifaceted Imbalance of T Cells With Regulatory Function Characterizes Type 1 Autoimmune Hepatitis. *Hepatology* (2010) 52(3):999–1007. doi: 10.1002/hep.23792
73. Liberal R, Grant CR, Holder BS, Cardone J, Martinez-Llordella M, Ma Y, et al. In Autoimmune Hepatitis Type 1 or the Autoimmune Hepatitis-Sclerosing Cholangitis Variant Defective Regulatory T-Cell Responsiveness to IL-2 Results in Low IL-10 Production and Impaired Suppression. *Hepatology* (2015) 62(3):863–75. doi: 10.1002/hep.27884
74. Jeffery HC, Braitch MK, Bagnall C, Hodson J, Jeffery LE, Wawman RE, et al. Changes in Natural Killer Cells and Exhausted Memory Regulatory T Cells With Corticosteroid Therapy in Acute Autoimmune Hepatitis. *Hepatol Commun* (2018) 2(4):421–36. doi: 10.1002/hep4.1163
75. Peiseler M, Sebode M, Franke B, Wortmann F, Schwinge D, Quaas A, et al. FOXP3+ Regulatory T Cells in Autoimmune Hepatitis are Fully Functional and Not Reduced in Frequency. *J Hepatol* (2012) 57(1):125–32. doi: 10.1016/j.jhep.2012.02.029
76. Taubert R, Hardtke-Wolenski M, Noyan F, Wilms A, Baumann AK, Schlue J, et al. Intrahepatic Regulatory T Cells in Autoimmune Hepatitis are Associated With Treatment Response and Depleted With Current Therapies. *J Hepatol* (2014) 61(5):1106–14. doi: 10.1016/j.jhep.2014.05.034
77. Lapierre P, Beland K, Yang R, Alvarez F. Adoptive Transfer of Ex Vivo Expanded Regulatory T Cells in an Autoimmune Hepatitis Murine Model Restores Peripheral Tolerance. *Hepatology* (2013) 57(1):217–27. doi: 10.1002/hep.26023
78. Yuksel M, Wang Y, Tai N, Peng J, Guo J, Beland K, et al. A Novel "Humanized Mouse" Model for Autoimmune Hepatitis and the Association of Gut Microbiota With Liver Inflammation. *Hepatology* (2015) 62(5):1536–50. doi: 10.1002/hep.27998
79. Arterbery AS, Osafo-Addo A, Avitzur Y, Ciarleglio M, Deng Y, Lobritto SJ, et al. Production of Proinflammatory Cytokines by Monocytes in Liver-Transplanted Recipients With De Novo Autoimmune Hepatitis Is Enhanced and Induces TH1-Like Regulatory T Cells. *J Immunol* (2016) 196(10):4040–51. doi: 10.4049/jimmunol.1502276
80. Arterbery AS, Yao J, Ling A, Avitzur Y, Martinez M, Lobritto S, et al. Inflammasome Priming Mediated *via* Toll-Like Receptors 2 and 4, Induces Th1-Like Regulatory T Cells in De Novo Autoimmune Hepatitis. *Front Immunol* (2018) 9:1612. doi: 10.3389/fimmu.2018.01612
81. Preti M, Schlott L, Lubbering D, Krzikalla D, Muller AL, Schuran FA, et al. Failure of Thymic Deletion and Instability of Autoreactive Tregs Drive Autoimmunity in Immune-Privileged Liver. *JCI Insight* (2021) 6(6):e141462. doi: 10.1172/jci.insight.141462
82. Chen J, Liu W, Zhu W. Foxp3(+) Treg Cells Are Associated With Pathological Process of Autoimmune Hepatitis by Activating Methylation Modification in Autoimmune Hepatitis Patients. *Med Sci Monit* (2019) 25:6204–12. doi: 10.12659/MSM.915408
83. Quintana FJ, Basso AS, Iglesias AH, Korn T, Farez MF, Bettelli E, et al. Control of T(reg) and T(H)17 Cell Differentiation by the Aryl Hydrocarbon Receptor. *Nature* (2008) 453(7191):65–71. doi: 10.1038/nature06880
84. Ohashi H, Nishioka K, Nakajima S, Kim S, Suzuki R, Aizaki H, et al. The Aryl Hydrocarbon Receptor-Cytochrome P450 1A1 Pathway Controls Lipid Accumulation and Enhances the Permissiveness for Hepatitis C Virus Assembly. *J Biol Chem* (2018) 293(51):19559–71. doi: 10.1074/jbc.RA118.005033
85. She C, Wang J, Tang N, Liu Z, Xu L, Liu B. Effects of 2,3,7,8-Tetrachlorodibenzo-P-Dioxin on T Cell Differentiation in Primary Biliary Cholangitis. *BioMed Res Int* (2020) 2020:1754975. doi: 10.1155/2020/1754975
86. Probert PM, Leitch AC, Dunn MP, Meyer SK, Palmer JM, Abdelghany TM, et al. Identification of a Xenobiotic as a Potential Environmental Trigger in Primary Biliary Cholangitis. *J Hepatol* (2018) 69(5):1123–35. doi: 10.1016/j.jhep.2018.06.027
87. Selmi C, Balkwill DL, Invernizzi P, Ansari AA, Coppel RL, Podda M, et al. Patients With Primary Biliary Cirrhosis React Against a Ubiquitous Xenobiotic-Metabolizing Bacterium. *Hepatology* (2003) 38(5):1250–7. doi: 10.1053/jhep.2003.50446
88. D'Onofrio F, Renga G, Puccetti M, Pariano M, Bellet MM, Santarelli I, et al. Indole-3-Carboxaldehyde Restores Gut Mucosal Integrity and Protects From Liver Fibrosis in Murine Sclerosing Cholangitis. *Cells* (2021) 10 (7):1622. doi: 10.3390/cells10071622

89. Lytton SD, Osiecki M, Malgorzata W, Cukrowska B, Wierzbicka A, Goliszek M, et al. Tryptophan-Kynurenine Profile in Pediatric Autoimmune Hepatitis. *Immunol Res* (2019) 67(1):39–47. doi: 10.1007/s12026-019-9068-1
90. Mohammadi-Bardbori A, Akbarizadeh AR, Delju F, Rannug A. Chromatin Remodeling by Curcumin Alters Endogenous Aryl Hydrocarbon Receptor Signaling. *Chem Biol Interact* (2016) 252:19–27. doi: 10.1016/j.cbi.2016.03.037
91. Blobe GC, Schiemann WP, Lodish HF. Role of Transforming Growth Factor Beta in Human Disease. *N Engl J Med* (2000) 342(18):1350–8. doi: 10.1056/NEJM200005043421807
92. Korn T, Bettelli E, Oukka M, Kuchroo VK. IL-17 and Th17 Cells. *Annu Rev Immunol* (2009) 27:485–517. doi: 10.1146/annurev.immunol.021908.132710
93. Longhi MS, Vuerich M, Kalbasi A, Kenison JE, Yeste A, Csizmadia E, et al. Bilirubin Suppresses Th17 Immunity in Colitis by Upregulating CD39. *JCI Insight* (2017) 2(9):e92791. doi: 10.1172/jci.insight.92791
94. Xie A, Robles RJ, Mukherjee S, Zhang H, Feldbrugge L, Csizmadia E, et al. HIF-1alpha-Induced Xenobiotic Transporters Promote Th17 Responses in Crohn's Disease. *J Autoimmun* (2018) 94:122–33. doi: 10.1016/j.jaut.2018.07.022
95. Mascanfroni ID, Takenaka MC, Yeste A, Patel B, Wu Y, Kenison JE, et al. Metabolic Control of Type 1 Regulatory T Cell Differentiation by AHR and HIF1-Alpha. *Nat Med* (2015) 21(6):638–46. doi: 10.1038/nm.3868
96. Longhi MS, Meda F, Wang P, Samyn M, Mieli-Vergani G, Vergani D, et al. Expansion and *De Novo* Generation of Potentially Therapeutic Regulatory T Cells in Patients With Autoimmune Hepatitis. *Hepatology* (2008) 47(2):581–91. doi: 10.1002/hep.22071
97. Longhi MS, Liberal R, Holder B, Robson SC, Ma Y, Mieli-Vergani G, et al. Inhibition of Interleukin-17 Promotes Differentiation of CD25(-) Cells Into Stable T Regulatory Cells in Patients With Autoimmune Hepatitis. *Gastroenterology* (2012) 142(7):1526–35 e6. doi: 10.1053/j.gastro.2012.02.041
98. Liberal R, Grant CR, Yuksel M, Graham J, Kalbasi A, Ma Y, et al. Regulatory T-Cell Conditioning Endows Activated Effector T Cells With Suppressor Function in Autoimmune Hepatitis/Autoimmune Sclerosing Cholangitis. *Hepatology* (2017) 66(5):1570–84. doi: 10.1002/hep.29307
99. Zhao H, Bo C, Kang Y, Li H. What Else Can CD39 Tell Us? *Front Immunol* (2017) 8:727. doi: 10.3389/fimmu.2017.00727
100. Oo YH, Ackrill S, Cole R, Jenkins L, Anderson P, Jeffery HC, et al. Liver Homing of Clinical Grade Tregs After Therapeutic Infusion in Patients With Autoimmune Hepatitis. *JHEP Rep* (2019) 1(4):286–96. doi: 10.1016/j.jhepr.2019.08.001
101. Hardtke-Wolenski M, Taubert R, Noyan F, Sievers M, Dywicki J, Schlue J, et al. Autoimmune Hepatitis in a Murine Autoimmune Polyendocrine Syndrome Type 1 Model is Directed Against Multiple Autoantigens. *Hepatology* (2015) 61(4):1295–305. doi: 10.1002/hep.27639
102. Longhi MS, Hussain MJ, Kwok WW, Mieli-Vergani G, Ma Y, Vergani D. Autoantigen-Specific Regulatory T Cells, a Potential Tool for Immune-Tolerance Reconstitution in Type-2 Autoimmune Hepatitis. *Hepatology* (2011) 53(2):536–47. doi: 10.1002/hep.24039
103. Holder BS, Grant CR, Liberal R, Ma Y, Heneghan MA, Mieli-Vergani G, et al. Retinoic Acid Stabilizes Antigen-Specific Regulatory T-Cell Function in Autoimmune Hepatitis Type 2. *J Autoimmun* (2014) 53:26–32. doi: 10.1016/j.jaut.2014.02.001
104. Umeshappa CS, Singha S, Blanco J, Shao K, Nanjundappa RH, Yamanouchi J, et al. Suppression of a Broad Spectrum of Liver Autoimmune Pathologies by Single Peptide-MHC-Based Nanomedicines. *Nat Commun* (2019) 10 (1):2150. doi: 10.1038/s41467-019-09893-5
105. Raffin C, Vo LT, Bluestone JA. Treg Cell-Based Therapies: Challenges and Perspectives. *Nat Rev Immunol* (2020) 20(3):158–72. doi: 10.1038/s41577-019-0232-6
106. Diestelhorst J, Junge N, Schlue J, Falk CS, Manns MP, Baumann U, et al. Pediatric Autoimmune Hepatitis Shows a Disproportionate Decline of Regulatory T Cells in the Liver and of IL-2 in the Blood of Patients Undergoing Therapy. *PloS One* (2017) 12(7):e0181107. doi: 10.1371/journal.pone.0181107
107. Jeffery HC, Jeffery LE, Lutz P, Corrigan M, Webb GJ, Hirschfield GM, et al. Low-Dose Interleukin-2 Promotes STAT-5 Phosphorylation, Treg Survival and CTLA-4-Dependent Function in Autoimmune Liver Diseases. *Clin Exp Immunol* (2017) 188(3):394–411. doi: 10.1111/cei.12940
108. Lim TY, Martinez-Llordella M, Kodela E, Gray E, Heneghan MA, Sanchez-Fueyo A. Low-Dose Interleukin-2 for Refractory Autoimmune Hepatitis. *Hepatology* (2018) 68(4):1649–52. doi: 10.1002/hep.30059
109. Spangler JB, Trotta E, Tomala J, Peck A, Young TA, Savvides CS, et al. Engineering a Single-Agent Cytokine/Antibody Fusion That Selectively Expands Regulatory T Cells for Autoimmune Disease Therapy. *J Immunol* (2018) 201(7):2094–106. doi: 10.4049/jimmunol.1800578
110. Buitrago-Molina LE, Pietrek J, Noyan F, Schlue J, Manns MP, Wedemeyer H, et al. Treg-Specific IL-2 Therapy can Reestablish Intrahepatic Immune Regulation in Autoimmune Hepatitis. *J Autoimmun* (2021) 117:102591. doi: 10.1016/j.jaut.2020.102591
111. Karakus U, Sahin D, Mittl PRE, Mooij P, Koopman G, Boyman O. Receptor-Gated IL-2 Delivery by an Anti-Human IL-2 Antibody Activates Regulatory T Cells in Three Different Species. *Sci Transl Med* (2020) 12(574):eabb9283. doi: 10.1126/scitranslmed.abb9283
112. Marceau G, Yang R, Lapierre P, Beland K, Alvarez F. Low-Dose Anti-CD3 Antibody Induces Remission of Active Autoimmune Hepatitis in Xenoimmunized Mice. *Liver Int* (2015) 35(1):275–84. doi: 10.1111/liv.12498
113. Beland K, Marceau G, Labardy A, Bourbonnais S, Alvarez F. Depletion of B Cells Induces Remission of Autoimmune Hepatitis in Mice Through Reduced Antigen Presentation and Help to T Cells. *Hepatology* (2015) 62 (5):1511–23. doi: 10.1002/hep.27991
114. Arvaniti P, Giannoulis G, Gabeta S, Zachou K, Koukoulis GK, Dalekos GN. Belimumab is a Promising Third-Line Treatment Option for Refractory Autoimmune Hepatitis. *JHEP Rep* (2020) 2(4):100123. doi: 10.1016/j.jhepr.2020.100123
115. Robles RJ, Mukherjee S, Vuerich M, Xie A, Harshe R, Cowan PJ, et al. Modulation of CD39 and Exogenous APT102 Correct Immune Dysfunction in Experimental Colitis and Crohn's Disease. *J Crohns Colitis* (2020) 14 (6):818–30. doi: 10.1093/ecco-jcc/jjz182
116. Moeckel D, Jeong SS, Sun X, Broekman MJ, Nguyen A, Drosopoulos JH, et al. Optimizing Human Apyrase to Treat Arterial Thrombosis and Limit Reperfusion Injury Without Increasing Bleeding Risk. *Sci Transl Med* (2014) 6(248):248ra105. doi: 10.1126/scitranslmed.3009246
117. Ji Y, Adeola O, Strawn TL, Jeong SS, Chen R, Fay WP. Recombinant Soluble Apyrase APT102 Inhibits Thrombosis and Intimal Hyperplasia in Vein Grafts Without Adversely Affecting Hemostasis or Re-Endothelialization. *J Thromb Haemost* (2017) 15(4):814–25. doi: 10.1111/jth.13621
118. Sun X, Han L, Seth P, Bian S, Li L, Csizmadia E, et al. Disordered Purinergic Signaling and Abnormal Cellular Metabolism are Associated With Development of Liver Cancer in Cd39/ENTPD1 Null Mice. *Hepatology* (2013) 57(1):205–16. doi: 10.1002/hep.25989
119. Sun X, Wu Y, Gao W, Enjyoji K, Csizmadia E, Muller CE, et al. CD39/ENTPD1 Expression by CD4+Foxp3+ Regulatory T Cells Promotes Hepatic Metastatic Tumor Growth in Mice. *Gastroenterology* (2010) 139(3):1030–40. doi: 10.1053/j.gastro.2010.05.007
120. Allard D, Allard B, Stagg J. On the Mechanism of Anti-CD39 Immune Checkpoint Therapy. *J Immunother Cancer* (2020) 8(1):e000186. doi: 10.1136/jitc-2019-000186
121. Moesta AK, Li XY, Smyth MJ. Targeting CD39 in Cancer. *Nat Rev Immunol* (2020) 20(12):739–55. doi: 10.1038/s41577-020-0376-4
122. Gupta PK, Godec J, Wolski D, Adland E, Yates K, Pauken KE, et al. CD39 Expression Identifies Terminally Exhausted CD8+ T Cells. *PloS Pathog* (2015) 11(10):e1005177. doi: 10.1371/journal.ppat.1005177
123. Lee JS, Yilmaz O. Unfolding Role of a Danger Molecule Adenosine Signaling in Modulation of Microbial Infection and Host Cell Response. *Int J Mol Sci* (2018) 19(1):199. doi: 10.3390/ijms19010199
124. Harshe RP, Xie A, Vuerich M, Frank LA, Gromova B, Zhang H, et al. Endogenous Antisense RNA Curbs CD39 Expression in Crohn's Disease. *Nat Commun* (2020) 11(1):5894. doi: 10.1038/s41467-020-19692-y

18

Targeting Glutamine Metabolism Ameliorates Autoimmune Hepatitis *via* Inhibiting T Cell Activation and Differentiation

Qiang Yu[1†], Honghu Tu[1†], Xueyi Yin[2†], Chang Peng[3,4], Chuanyun Dou[3,4], Wenhua Yang[3], Wenbiao Wu[5], Xiaotong Guan[5], Jia Li[3,4], Hexin Yan[6], Yi Zang[2,3,5], Haowen Jiang[3*] and Qiang Xia[1,7,8*]*

[1] Department of Liver Surgery, Renji Hospital, School of Medicine, Shanghai Jiao Tong University, Shanghai, China, [2] School of Chinese Materia Medica, Nanjing University of Chinese Medicine, Nanjing, China, [3] State Key Laboratory of Drug Research, Shanghai Institute of Materia Medica, Chinese Academy of Sciences, Shanghai, China, [4] School of Pharmacy, University of Chinese Academy of Sciences, Beijing, China, [5] School of Pharmaceutical Science and Technology, Hangzhou Institute for Advanced Study, University of Chinese Academy of Sciences (UCAS), Hangzhou, China, [6] Department of Anesthesia, Renji Hospital, School of Medicine, Shanghai Jiao Tong University, Shanghai, China, [7] Shanghai Engineering Research Center of Transplantation and Immunology, Shanghai, China, [8] Shanghai Institute of Transplantation, Shanghai, China

***Correspondence:**
Qiang Xia
xiaqiang@shsmu.edu.cn
Haowen Jiang
haowenjiang@simm.ac.cn
Yi Zang
yzang@simm.ac.cn

[†]These authors have contributed equally to this work and share first authorship

Background: Autoimmune hepatitis (AIH) is mediated by a cascade of T cell-mediated events directed at liver cells and persistent inflammation within the liver can eventually result in liver cirrhosis. Targeting glutamine metabolism has an impact on T cell activation and differentiation. However, the effect of glutamine metabolism blocking upon AIH remains unknown. We use glutaminase antagonist 6-diazo-5-oxo-L-norleucine (DON) for *in vitro* assays and its prodrug 2-(2-amino-4-methylpentanamido)-DON (JHU083) for *in vivo* assays to investigate the potential therapeutic effect and molecular mechanism of glutamine metabolism blocking in an AIH murine model.

Methods: AIH mice were treated with JHU083 or vehicle before concanavalin A (ConA) administration, and disease severity was examined. Then activation and differentiation [including Th1/Th17 cells and cytotoxic T lymphocytes (CTL)] of T cells from Vehicle-WT, JHU083-AIH and Vehicle-AIH mice were tested. Furthermore, *in vitro* T cell activation and differentiation were measured using separated splenocytes stimulated with ConA with or without DON. The activation and differentiation of T cells were tested using flow cytometry, qRT-PCR and ELISA. Phosphorylation level of mammalian target of rapamycin (mTOR) and 70 kDa ribosomal protein S6 kinase (P70S6K) were examined by western blotting.

Results: JHU083 and DON significantly suppressed the activation of T cells and inhibited the differentiation of Th1/Th17 cells and CTL *in vivo* and *in vitro*. Besides, we demonstrated that glutamine metabolism blocking inhibited T cells activation and differentiation through decreasing the mRNA expression of amino acid transporter solute carrier family 7 member 5 (SLC7A5) and mitigating the activation of mTOR signaling.

Conclusions: We proved that targeting glutamine metabolism represents a potential new treatment strategy for patients with AIH and other T cell-mediated disease. Mechanistically, we demonstrated that glutamine metabolism blocking inhibits T cells activation and suppresses the differentiation of Th1/Th17 cells and CTL.

Keywords: glutamine metabolism, autoimmune hepatitis (AIH), T cells activation and differentiation, mTOR signaling, SLC7A5

INTRODUCTION

Autoimmune hepatitis (AIH) is a self-perpetuating inflammatory liver disease, and the misdiagnosis or delayed treatment of AIH can lead to liver cirrhosis, liver cancer, liver transplantation and even rapid death (1–3). AIH occurs globally in all ethnicities and affects children and adults of all ages, with a female predominance (4). It is reported that the point prevalence is up to be 10-25 per 100,000 population in the European region, and 5-25 per 100,000 population in the Asia-Pacific region (5). Although the specific pathogenesis of AIH is still unclear, it is indicated that the liver injury of AIH is mediated by a cascade of T cell-mediated events directed at liver cells and persistent inflammation within the liver can eventually result in liver cirrhosis (6).

The precise etiology and pathophysiology of AIH remains largely unknown, and lacking valid animal models for AIH research makes this situation a vicious circle. Thus, related basic research in this field is relatively limited compared with other types of hepatitis. However, some animal models can partially represent the pathogenesis of AIH, among which, intravenous injection of concanavalin A (ConA) is widely used in AIH research and this model shows the specific participation of T cells in promoting liver injury (7). ConA promotes T cells activation and differentiation into effector cells, followed by the secretion of pro-inflammatory cytokines and immune-mediated damage of liver cells caused by the cytokines and cascade reaction (8–10). The ConA-induced AIH model is considered as a valuable method for investigating the specific mechanism underlying T cell activation and differentiation in AIH.

Glutamine is a conditionally essential amino acid in rapidly proliferating cells and glutaminolysis is a very important source of energy for effector T cells (11). Glutaminase (GLS) is the first enzyme of glutaminolysis and converts glutamine to glutamate, which can be used in protein synthesis and glutathione generation (12). Early studies show that glutamine metabolism blocking not only diminishes T cells activation (13, 14), but also decreases the differentiation of T cells (15–17). 6-diazo-5-oxo-L-norleucine (DON) is a glutamine analog that competitively inhibits glutamine metabolism and suppresses the activation and differentiation of T cells (18–20). Thus, we aim to investigate the effect of glutamine metabolism blocking on ConA-induced AIH model. Despite the efficacy of DON in basic researches, its substantial peripheral toxicity has hampered its approval as a chemotherapeutic agent (21, 22). We use ethyl 2-(2-amino-4-methylpentanamido)-DON (JHU083), an orally available prodrug form of DON developed by Atsushi Kamiya and coworkers (23) to control oral bioavailability and decrease toxicity, for *in vivo* assays.

Because the mTOR signaling cascade plays a central role in the regulation of T cell activation and differentiation (24–27), blocking glutamine metabolism may affect the activation of mTOR signaling so as to influence T cells activation and differentiation. In this study, we aim to investigated whether targeting glutamine metabolism inhibits activation and differentiation of T cells and ameliorates the progression of ConA-induced AIH model.

MATERIALS AND METHODS

Animal Experimental Design

C57/BL6 mice (female, 6- to 7-week-old) were purchased from Shanghai SLAC Laboratory Animal Co (Shanghai, China). All animal procedures were performed in accordance with the Guidelines for Care and Use of Laboratory Animals of Shanghai Institute of Materia Medica (SIMM), Chinese Academy of Sciences and approved by the Institutional Animal Care and Use Committee of SIMM.

Mice were randomly divided into three groups: wild-type (WT) group (n=4, Vehicle-WT), vehicle group (Vehicle-AIH, n=6) and JHU083-treated group (JUH083-AIH, n=6). Induction of AIH was based on the treatment of mice with ConA (8mg/kg body weight (BW), C2010, Sigma-Aldrich, USA). Mice in Vehicle-WT group were treated with 5% methyl cellulose (MC) dissolved in saline by oral gavage 24h and 1h before administration of saline *via* intravenous injection. The Vehicle-AIH group received administration of 5% MC by oral 24h and 1h before ConA injection, while mice in JUH083-AIH group were treated with JHU083 (0.3mg/kg BW, HY-122218, MedChemExpress, NJ, USA) dissolved in 5% MC *via* gavage 24h and 1h before ConA treatment. Blood and liver tissues were collected from mice that were sacrificed 6h after ConA treatment. Serum alanine aminotransferase (ALT), aspartate aminotransferase (AST), lactate dehydrogenase (LDH) and alkaline phosphatase (ALP) were analyzed using an automatic biochemical analyzer (AU480, Beckman Coulter, Pasadena, CA, USA) to assess liver injury. For survival analysis, concentration of ConA was adjusted to a lethal dose (20mg/kg) and mice were under observation until 48h after ConA injection.

Histological Staining and TUNEL Assay

The tissues were fixed in 4% paraformaldehyde and embedded in paraffin. Tissue sections were prepared and stained with hematoxylin-eosin (H&E). Terminal Deoxynucleotidyl Transferase (TdT)-mediated dUTP Nick-End Labeling (TUNEL) staining was performed in paraffin-embedded liver sections using the TUNEL Kit (C1090, Beyotime, Haimen, China). Finally, the slides were scanned using a fluorescence microscope (1013688, PE Vectra3, Perkin Elmer, Waltham, MA, USA).

Isolation of Splenocytes and Cell Culture

Spleens were dissected from C57BL/6 mice and cell suspensions were prepared as following steps. Spleens were milled and centrifuged at 400g for 5 minutes. Red blood cells were lysed and splenocytes were washed with 10ml phosphate buffer solution (PBS). Cells were resuspended with complete medium (RPMI-1640 medium supplemented with 10% inactivated fetal bovine serum, 1% penicillin-streptomycin solution, 10mM 4-(2-hydroxyethyl)-1-piperazineethanesulfonic acid (HEPES), 1mM glutamine, 50μM β-mercaptoethanol and 1mM sodium pyruvate) for further culture or for cytometric assays.

T Cell Activation and Differentiation

Isolated splenocytes were activated with ConA (1.5μg/ml) with or without 2.5μM DON (HY-108357, MedChemExpress, NJ, USA). After 24h, the expression of CD69 and CD25 were analyzed by flow cytometry to evaluate the activation of CD4(+) and CD8(+) T cells. For T cell differentiation analysis, splenocytes were stimulated using ConA (1.5μg/ml) with or without DON (2.5μM). GlogiPlug (555028, BD Biosciences, USA) was added 18h after for the next 24 h of incubation. The cells were first stained with monoclonal antibodies CD4 and CD8 for 20 min at room temperature, then fixed using a Fixation/Permeabilization Solution Kit (555028, BD Biosciences, USA), and finally stained with IFN-γ, IL4, IL17 and Granzyme B antibodies. Flow cytometry analysis was conducted by flowJo_V10 software (BD Biosciences, USA). For *in vivo* T cells activation and differentiation tests, splenocytes were separated from mice in WT-Vehicle, Vehicle-AIH and JHU083-AIH group and stained with above antibodies for flow cytometry analysis. The antibodies used in the flow cytometry were as follows: CD4 (FITC, E-AB-F1097C), CD8a (PE, E-AB-F1104D), CD25 (PE-Cy5, E-AB-F1102G), CD69 (PE-Cy7, E-AB-F1187H), IL4 (PE, E-AB-F1204UD), IL17A (APC, E-AB-F1272E) were purchased from Elabscience Biotechnology (Wuhan, China), antibodies IFNγ (APC-Cy7, cat# 561479) was purchased from BD Biosciences (UK), and Granzyme B (PE-Cy7, cat# 372213) was purchased from Biolegend (San Diego, CA, USA). SLC7A5 antagonist LAT1-IN1 (HY-108540) was purchased from MedChemExpress (NJ, USA).

Enzyme Linked Immunosorbent Assay

The IFN-γ Mouse Uncoated ELISA Kit (EK280/3-48, Multi Science, China) and IL17 Mouse Uncoated ELISA Kit (EK217/2-48, Multi Science, China) were used to measure the levels of IFN-γ and IL17 in the serums of mice in Vehicle-WT, Vehicle-AIH and JHU083-AIH group and the supernatants of unstimulated splenocytes or splenocytes that were stimulated with ConA in the presence of vehicle or DON. Briefly, the serums and supernatants were collected and added to the well of corresponding microplates for 2h. After the samples were washed with wash solution, 100μL of mouse IFN-γ or IL17 conjugate was added to each well for 2h. The washing process was repeated, and 200μL of Substrate Solution was added and incubated for 30 min. Then, 50μL of Stop Solution was added to each well, and the optical density was determined within 30 min using a microplate reader (SpectraMax M5, Molecular Devices, Santa Clara, CA, USA) set to 450nm.

Western Blotting

Protein samples were homogenized with SDS loading buffer and boiled to denature the proteins. Samples with different sizes were separated by 10% SDS-polyacrylamide gel electrophoresis, and transferred to NC membranes. After blocking with 5% non-fat milk solution for 1h, membranes were incubated with β-Actin, P-mTOR, mTOR, P-P70S6K P70S6K at 4°C overnight. Then, membranes were incubated with HRP-linked anti-rabbit IgG (7074, Cell Signaling Technology, Trask Lane Danvers, MA, USA) at room temperature for 1h. Finally, the membranes were stained with ECL detection buffer (1705061, Bio-Rad, Hercules, CA, USA) and visualized using ChemiDoc system (Bio-Rad, Hercules, CA, USA). Primary antibodies including β-Actin (12620), P-mTOR (2971S), mTOR (2972S), P-P70S6K (97596), P70S6K (34475) were purchased from Cell Signaling Technology (Trask Lane Danvers, MA, USA).

Quantitative Real-Time PCR

Total RNA was extracted using TRIzol reagent (9109, TaKaRa, Dalian, China) followed by cDNA synthesis using RT Master Mix (RR036B, TaKaRa, Dalian, China). Subsequently, cDNA was used to measure the mRNA levels of IFN-γ, IL4, IL17, SLC7A5 and SLC1A5 using a Real-Time PCR System (Roche, Basel, Switzerland). β-Actin was used as the normalization control. All reactions were performed in triplicates. The relative quantifications were measured by the comparative CT method. The primer sequences used were as follows: IFN-γ: forward: CAGCAACAGCAAGGCGAAA, reverse: CTGGACCTGTGGG TTGTTGAC; IL-4: forward: CGCCATGCACGGAGATG, reverse: CGAGCTCACTCTCTGTGGTGTT; IL17: forward: AT CTGTGTCTCTGATGCTGTTGCTG, reverse: TGGAACG GTTGAGGTAGTCTGAGG; SLC7A5: forward: CTGG ATCGAGCTGCTCATC, reverse: GTTCACAGCTGTGA GGAGC; SLC1A5: forward: ATCGCACAACTAAACGGGGT, reverse: ACTGCTTCCAGGATGATGGC; β-Actin: forward: AA CAGTCCGCCTAGAAGCAC, reverse: CGTTGACATCCGTA AAGACC.

Statistical Analysis

Experimental data were expressed as the mean ± standard error of mean (SEM), and comparisons between two groups were performed using one-way ANOVA analysis. Data were analyzed using GraphPad Prism 8.0.2. Statistical significance was determined at $P < 0.05$ (*); $P < 0.01$ (**); and $P < 0.001$ (***).

RESULTS

JHU083 Attenuates ConA-Induced AIH in Mice

In order to verify the hepatoprotective effect of glutaminase antagonist JHU083 in a ConA-induced AIH model, the survival times of vehicle and JHU083 (0.3mg/kg BW) (28) treated mice in this mice model were investigated. Vehicle-AIH and JHU083-AIH mice were intravenously injected with a high dose of ConA (20mg/kg BW). Vehicle-AIH mice began to die 4h after injection and all mice died within 38h, while survival rate of JHU083-AIH mice was 70% at 24h after ConA injection and did not change after extension to 48h. On the basis of the survival curve, it was proved that JHU083 treatment greatly reduced the death rate of ConA-induced AIH mice (**Figure 1A**). Although AIH mice were ameliorated after treatment with JHU083 under the induction of

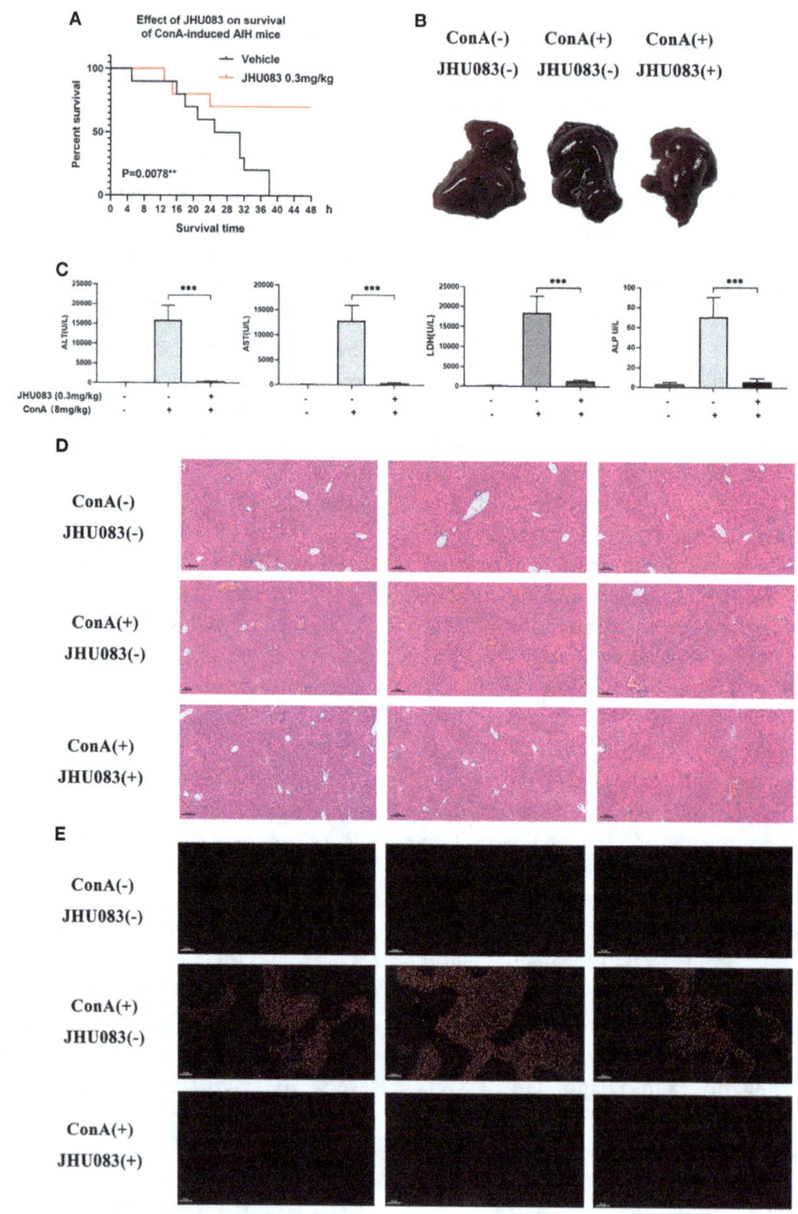

FIGURE 1 | JHU083 attenuated ConA-induced AIH. **(A)**. Survival of 20ml/kg ConA-induced autoimmune hepatitis mice gavaged with vehicle or 0.3mg/kg JHU083 24h and 1h before ConA injection. n = 10. **(B–E)** Mice of Vehicle-AIH and JHU083-AIH group were intravenously injected with 8 mg/kg ConA, and mice of Vehicle-WT group were injected with normal saline of equal volume. Mice of JHU083 group were gavaged with 0.3mg/kg JHU083 24h and 1h before ConA injection, and WT and vehicle group were treated with equal vehicle at the same time points. Representative macroscopic images of livers **(B)**, quantification of serum ALT, AST, LDH and ALP **(C)**, H&E staining **(D)** and TUNEL assay **(E)** were presented 6h after ConA injection. The scale bar for H&E staining and TUNEL assay is 100μm. Red fluorescence in TUNEL assay indicates positive signals of apoptosis. Data were expressed as means ± SEM. **P <0.01 and ***P <0.001.

20mg/kg ConA (**Supplementary Figure 1**), the pathological damages under such ConA concentration would be too severe. Therefore, we chose a non-lethal dosage instead to compare the alteration of transaminase, conditions of cells and pathological damages. Then, ConA was adjusted to a lower dose (8mg/kg), and blood and liver specimens were collected 6h post ConA injection. In JHU083-AIH group, liver congestion and necrosis were obviously mitigated in a macroscopic level (**Figure 1B**) and serum ALT, AST, LDH and ALP (**Figure 1C**) were significantly lower than mice in Vehicle-AIH group. Liver specimens were stained with H&E. At 6h after ConA administration, marked liver hyperemia and necrosis of liver cells were observed in vehicle mice rather than in JHU083 treated mice (**Figure 1D**). No pathological injury was found in Vehicle-WT mice. Apart from these, the TUNEL assay indicated that TUNEL-positive cells decreased significantly after JHU083 treatment (**Figure 1E**), indicating decreased apoptosis of liver cells. These results proved that blocking glutamine metabolism ameliorated the progression of ConA-induced AIH in mice.

JHU083 Inhibited the Activation and Differentiation of T Cells *In Vivo*

According to Ruoning Wang (29), we transplanted CFSE-labeled splenocytes into mice before ConA injection. After 6h ConA stimulation, there was no proliferation in the transplanted splenocytes (**Supplementary Figure 2**). Thus, we focused on the activation and differentiation of T cells. Given that activated effector T cells need glutamine metabolism to provide energy (11), we first measured the activation of T cells upon glutamine metabolism blocking *in vivo*. CD25 and CD69 are two markers expressed on the surface of activated T cells (30). To investigate the effect of JHU083 on the activation of T cells in AIH mice, we evaluated the activation of CD4(+) and CD8(+) T cells in spleens extracted from mice in WT-Vehicle, Vehicle-AIH and JHU083-AIH group *via* the proportions of CD25 or CD69 positive cells. Consistent with our findings on pathology, JHU083 significantly reduced percentages of activated CD4(+) and CD8(+) T cells (**Figures 2A, B**).

To further explore the effect of JHU083 on the differentiation of CD4(+) and CD8(+) T cells in AIH mice, the differentiation marker of CD4(+) (IFNγ for Th1 cells, IL4 for Th2 cells and IL17A for Th17 cells) and CD8(+) T cells (IFNγ and Granzyme B for CTLs) were evaluated using flow cytometry. We observed that the frequency of IFNγ- and IL17A-expressing CD4(+) T cells instead of IL4-expressing CD4(+) T cells were significantly lower in the spleens of JHU083-AIH mice compared to that of Vehicle-AIH mice (**Figure 3A**). Lower IFNγ and IL17 levels were presented in the serums of JHU083-AIH mice than in Vehicle-AIH mice (**Figure 3B**). Besides, the frequency of CD8(+) T cells expressing IFNγ (**Figure 3C**) or Granzyme B (**Figure 3D**) was significantly reduced after JHU083 treatment. The above outcomes indicated that blocking glutamine metabolism had negative effects on activation and differentiation of T cells *in vivo*.

DON Treatment Suppressed the Activation and Differentiation of T Cells *In Vitro*

Consistent with the results *in vivo*, ConA did not induce proliferation within 24h *in vitro* (**Supplementary Figure 3**). To evaluate the effects of blocking glutamine metabolism on T cells *in vitro*, we used DON to substitute JHU083 to investigate whether DON might suppress the activation of T cells. Splenocytes of mice were separated and cultured in RPIM 1640 medium and activated by 1.5μg/ml ConA in the presence or absence of DON (2.5μM) (**Supplementary Figure 4**). 24h after activation, splenocytes were collected and stained with CD4, CD8 and activation markers CD25 and CD69, and the

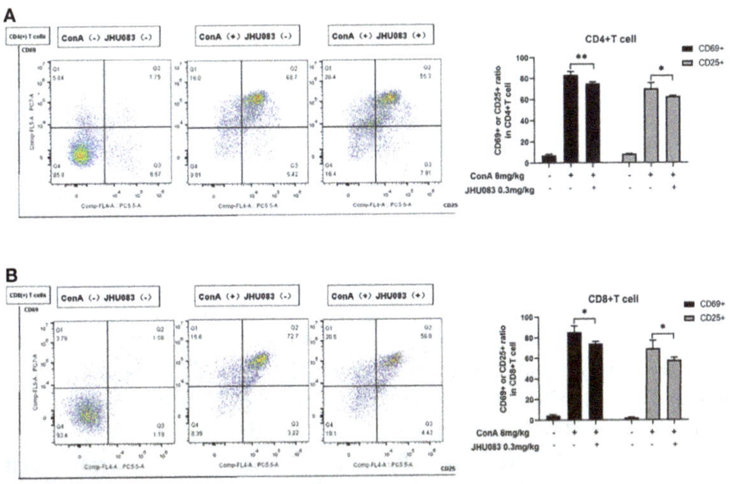

FIGURE 2 | JHU083 inhibited T cells activation *in vivo*. Mice of Vehicle-AIH and JHU083-AIH group were intravenously injected with 8ml/kg ConA, and Vehicle-WT group was injected with normal saline of equal volume. JHU083-AIH group was gavaged with 0.3mg/kg JHU083 24h and 1h before ConA injection, and mice of Vehicle-WT and Vehicle-AIH group were treated with equal vehicle at the same time points. **(A, B)** Flow cytometry was applied to analyze the expression of CD25 and CD69 of CD4(+) **(A)** and CD8(+) **(B)** T cells. Data were expressed as means ± SEM. *$P < 0.05$ and **$P < 0.01$.

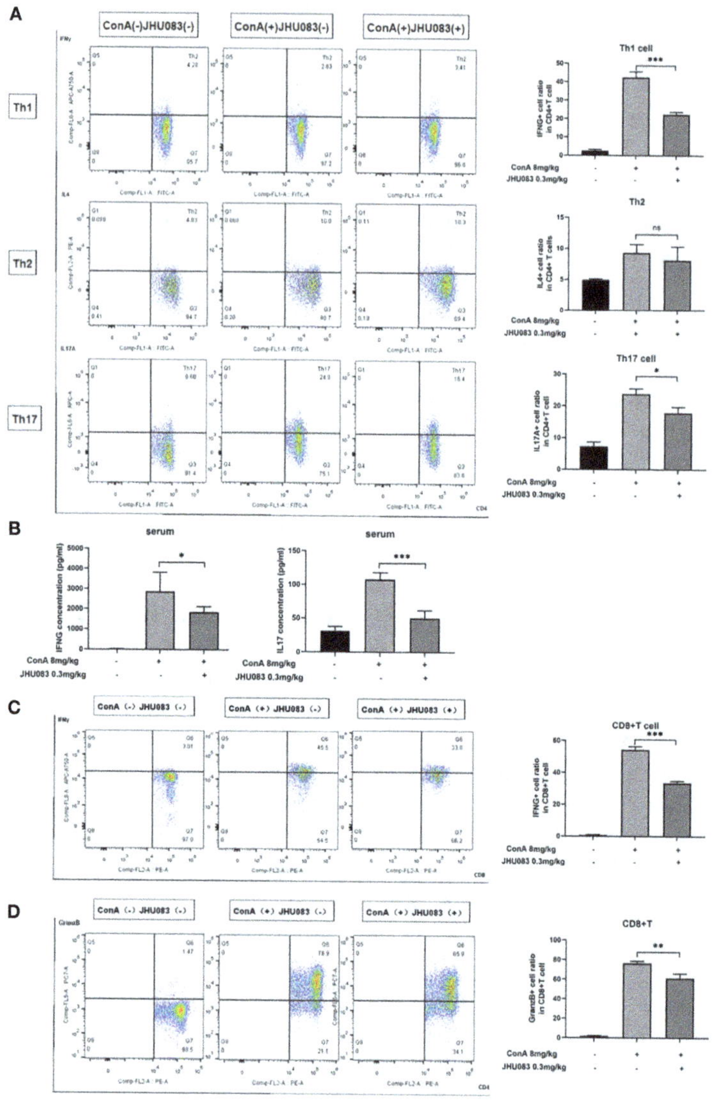

FIGURE 3 | JHU083 inhibited T cells differentiation *in vivo*. Mice of Vehicle-AIH and JHU083-AIH group were intravenously injected with 8ml/kg ConA, and Vehicle-WT group was injected with normal saline of equal volume. JHU083-AIH group was gavaged with 0.3mg/kg JHU083 24h and 1h before ConA injection, and Vehicle-WT and Vehicle-AIH group were treated with equal vehicle at the same time points. **(A)** Flow cytometry was applied to analyze the Th1 cell percentage *via* IFNγ expression, the Th2 cell percentage *via* IL4 expression, and the Th17 cell percentage *via* IL17A expression. **(B)** ELISA was applied to analyze serum IFNγ (Th1 cells) and IL17 (Th17 cells) secretions. Flow cytometry was also applied to analyze the differentiation of CD8(+) T cells into cytotoxic T lymphocytes, evidenced by secreting IFNγ **(C)** and Granzyme **(D)**. Data were expressed as means ± SEM. *$P < 0.05$, **$P < 0.01$, and ***$P < 0.001$. ns, not significant.

proportions of CD25(+) or CD69(+) cells and median fluorescence intensity (MFI) of CD25(+) or CD69(+) cells were analyzed. Although CD25 can be also expressed on regulatory T cells, we assessed the proportion of CD4+Foxp3+ Treg cells and found that DON did not affect the proportion of Treg cells (**Supplementary Figure 5**). As shown in **Figures 4A, 4B**, splenocytes treated with DON had lower expressions of CD25 and CD69 in CD4(+) and CD8(+) T cells.

To further characterize the effect of DON on the differentiation of CD4(+) and CD8(+) T cells, the above-mentioned differentiation markers of CD4(+) and CD8(+) T cells were tested. DON significantly inhibited the differentiation of Th1 and Th17 cells rather than Th2 cells (**Figure 5A**). Consistently, DON reduced mRNA expression (**Figure 5B**) and production (tested by ELISA, **Figure 5C**) of IFNγ and IL17. In addition, we proved that DON suppressed CD8(+) T cells to turn into CTL, which was evidenced by lower productions of IFNγ- (**Figure 5D**) and Granzyme B-expressing T cells (**Figure 5E**). Thus, GLS blocking played a critical role in inhibiting T cells activation and differentiation *in vitro*.

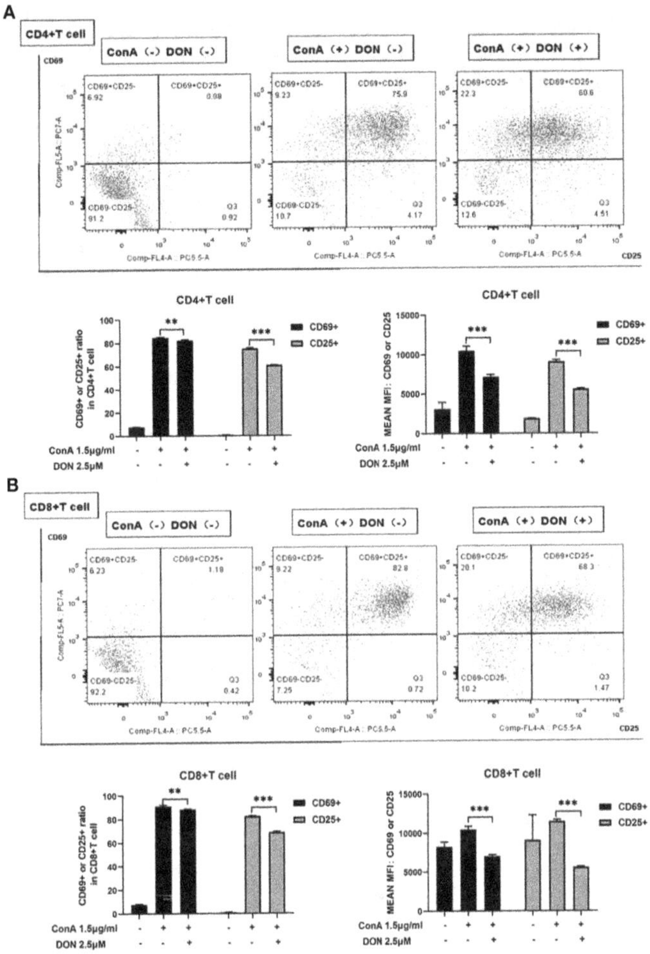

FIGURE 4 | DON treatment suppressed T cells activation *in vitro*. Freshly separated spleen cells were stimulated with 1.5mg/ml ConA with or without treating 2.5μM DON, and cells were analyzed 24h after ConA stimulation. **(A, B)** The expressions of activation markers CD25 and CD69 in CD4(+) **(A)** and CD8(+) **(B)** T cells were examined by flow cytometry. Data were expressed as means ± SEM. $^{**}P$ <0.01, and $^{***}P$ <0.001.

The Effects of Blocking Glutamine Metabolism on Activation and Differentiation of T Cells Were Mediated by mTOR Signaling and Amino Transporter SLC7A5

Mammalian target of rapamycin (mTOR) signaling is a master regulator of cell metabolism and promotes anabolic processes such as protein synthesis (31). The activation of mTOR signaling is dependent on growth factors and nutrients in cancer cells (32). For instance, leucine can promote mTOR signaling activation *via* binding to sestrin2 and arginine binds to CASTOR1 (33). Glutamine activates mTOR signaling in a RAG-dependent manner *via* glutaminolysis (34). In addition, many studies have noted that the activation and differentiation of T cell are strongly correlated with mTOR signaling (24–27). We hypothesized that blocking glutamine metabolism may affect mTOR signaling in T cells in an amino acid dependent way.

Thus, we examined the phosphorylated protein levels of mTOR signaling using proteins extracted from splenocytes that were activated by 1.5μg/ml ConA with or without treating 2.5μM DON for 24h. After activating by ConA, the protein levels of phosphorylated mTOR and 70 kDa ribosomal protein S6 kinase (P70S6K) increased sharply. But in the presence of DON, the levels of phosphorylated mTOR and P70S6K instead of their unphosphorylated proteins significantly decreased (**Figures 6A, B**).

The levels of amino acids are closely correlated with corresponding amino acid transporters. To explore how DON makes an impact on mTOR signaling, we focused on glutamine and leucine transporters because it was reported that the function of leucine and glutamine exchanger solute carrier

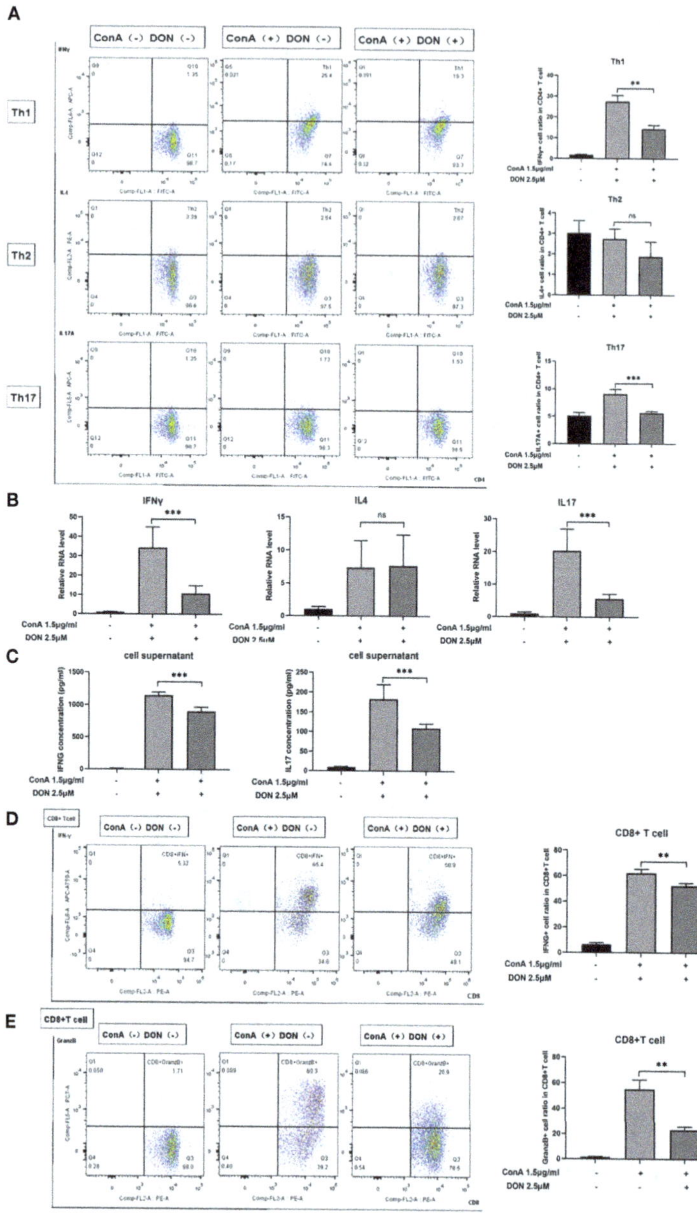

FIGURE 5 | DON treatment suppressed T cells differentiation *in vitro*. Freshly separated spleen cells were stimulated with 1.5mg/ml ConA with or without treating 2.5μM DON, and cells were analyzed 24h after ConA stimulation. **(A)** The differentiation markers of CD4+ T cells (IFNγ for Th1 cells, IL4 for Th2 cells and IL17 for Th17 cells) were detected using flowcytometry. **(B)** qRT-PCR was applied to analyze IFN-γ, IL4 and IL17 mRNA levels. **(C)** ELISA was applied to analyze supernatant IFN-γ and IL17 secretions. Flow cytometry was also applied to detect the production of activation markers of CTL, such as IFNγ **(D)** and Granzyme B **(E)**. Data were expressed as means ± SEM. $^{**}P$ <0.01 and $^{***}P$ <0.001, ns, not significant.

family 7 member 5 (SLC7A5) and glutamine transporter solute carrier family 7 member 5 (SLC1A5) affected both intracellular amino levels and activation of mTOR signaling (35–39). We discovered that DON significantly reduced the mRNA expression of SLC7A5 but had no effect on SLC1A5 (**Figure 7A**). These results suggested that SLC7A5 may play a critical part in the process of GLS inhibition to the suppression of activation of mTOR signaling. To further confirm the function of SLC7A5, we inhibited it with LAT1-IN1 (30mM) (40), the competitive antagonist of SLC7A5. After LAT1-IN1 treatment, the activation of CD4(+) and CD8(+) T cells, evidenced by the expressions of CD25 and CD69, was significantly weakened (**Figures 7B, C**). In addition, the expression levels of phosphorylated mTOR and P70S6K were inhibited by LAT1-IN1 (**Figures 7D, E**). Therefore, our findings demonstrated that GLS blocking not only suppresses T cell activation and

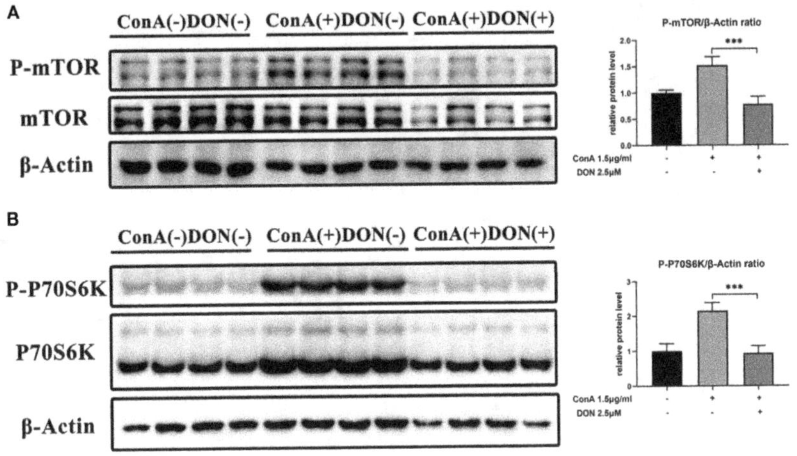

FIGURE 6 | The inhibition of activation and differentiation of T cells was mediated by mTOR signaling. Freshly separated spleen cells were stimulated with 1.5 mg/ml ConA with or without treating 2.5μM DON, and cells were collected and proteins were extracted 24h after ConA stimulation. Western blotting was applied to analyze the levels of phosphorylated mTOR **(A)** and phosphorylated P70S6K **(B)**. Data were expressed as means ± SEM. ***P <0.001.

differentiation, but also decreases mRNA expression of glutamine and leucine exchanger SLC7A5, reducing intracellular leucine level and further inhibiting activation of mTOR signaling.

DISCUSSIONS

Recent studies connecting the fields of amino acid metabolism and immunology have dramatically improved our understanding of how immune cells benefit from a metabolic reprogramming to support their activation and differentiation (41–45). The glutaminase antagonist JHU083, a prodrug of DON, has been reported to be a potential anti-inflammatory modulator to reverse experimental autoimmune encephalomyelitis through inhibiting T cells proliferation and activation (46). Another study demonstrated that GLS may have an impact on Th1 and Th17 cells differentiation (15). Emerging evidence proposed that amino acid transporters are also critical in T cell activation and differentiation (44, 45, 47). The amino acid transporter SLC7A5 is a bidirectional transporter that regulates the simultaneous transport of leucine into cells and efflux of glutamine out of cells (34) and is crucial for the activation of mTOR signalling (44, 48, 49). Notably, mTOR signaling can modulate T cells activation and differentiation (15, 48–51). Thus, we proposed a hypothesis that targeting glutamine metabolism may affect the activation and differentiation of T cell through modulating SLC7A5 and inhibiting mTOR signaling. However, it remains unknown whether targeting glutamine metabolism exerts anti-inflammatory effects on the modulation of AIH.

In this study, we evaluated the therapeutic effect of GLS antagonist JHU083 in ConA-induced AIH mice model, which was caused by a T cell-mediated autoimmune response (29). We observed a marked improvement of disease severity after treatment with JHU083. In addition, we found JHU083 or DON attenuated CD4(+) and CD8(+) T cells activation, inhibited Th1/Th17 cells and CTL differentiation *in vivo* and *in vitro*. However, the reduction of activation and differentiation of T cells may not be enough to explain the attenuation of serum transaminase and pathologic changes of livers. Blocking glutamine metabolism may also ameliorate the activation of mTOR through other mechanisms such as suppressing the production of glutathione (15) or polyamines (51), or other undiscovered mechanisms. GLS antagonist may attenuate AIH *via* other etiologies such as modulating innate immune cells as it is reported that glutamine metabolism also plays a role in innate immune cells such as macrophages (52–54). Mechanistic studies revealed that blocking glutamine metabolism lowered the mRNA expression of amino acid transporter SLC7A5, and the inhibition of SLC7A5 by LAT1-IN1 reduced the expressions of phosphorylated proteins in mTOR signaling and decreased activation of T cells. Thus, these studies showed that decreased expression of SLC7A5 mRNA, mitigated mTOR signaling and reduced activation rate of T cells and subsided Th1/Th17 cells and CTLs differentiation might be responsible for protective effect of JHU083 in AIH. We showed for the first time that JHU083 conferred protection against AIH and could be developed as novel therapeutic agent for the treatment of AIH in clinical medicine.

T cells activate and differentiate into functional subgroups need energy and metabolites, which were brought by metabolic reprogramming (51). GLS converts glutamine to glutamate to support the tricarboxylic acid cycle and redox and epigenetic reactions (15). Many researches proves that GLS antagonist inhibits the activation of T cells (15, 51, 55, 56). But it remains unclear whether it works in T cell-mediated disease models. As far as we know, our study is the first study to explore the effects of blocking glutamine metabolism on a ConA-induced T cell-mediated AIH mice model.

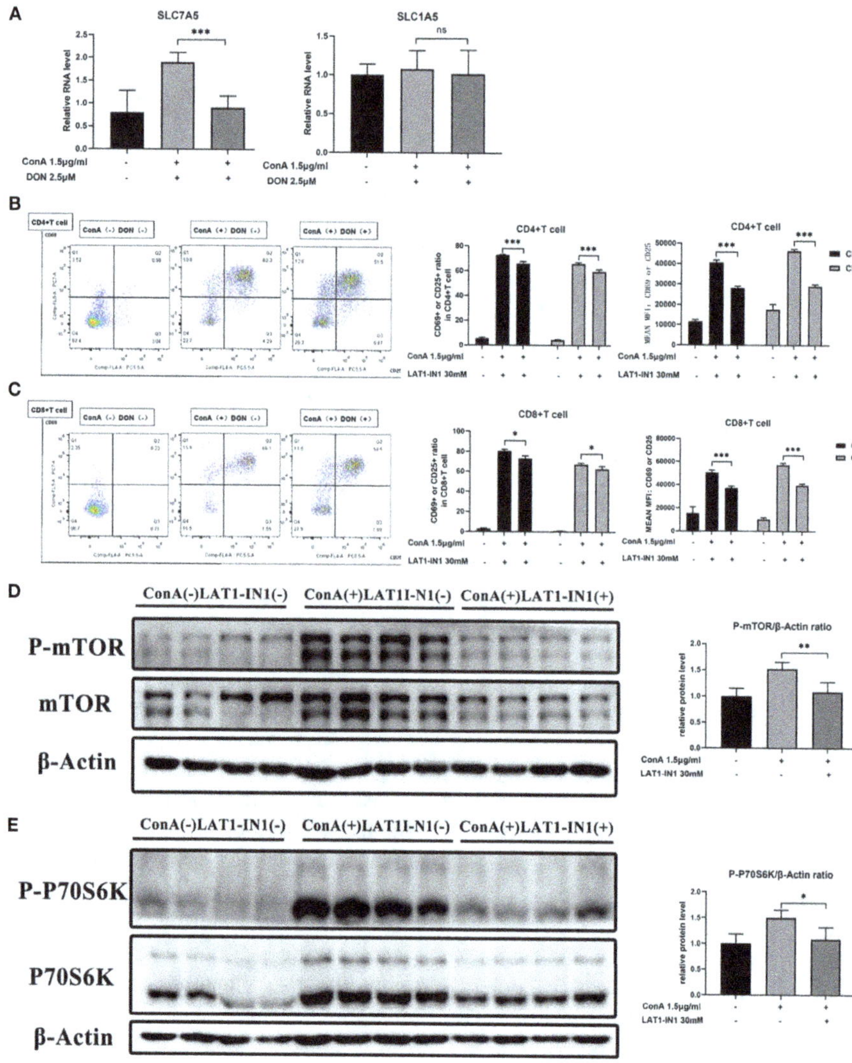

FIGURE 7 | The function of DON to mTOR signaling may be mediated by amino transporter amino transporter SLC7A5. **(A)** qRT-PCR was applied to analyze amino acid transporters SLC7A5 and SLC1A5 mRNA levels. **(B, C)** Flow cytometry was applied to analyze the degree of activation (expression of CD25 and CD69) of CD4 (+) **(B)** and CD8(+) **(C)** T cells with or without treating LAT1-IN1. The levels of phosphorylated mTOR **(D)** as well as phosphorylated P70S6K **(E)** were examined by western blotting. Data were expressed as means ± SEM. *P < 0.05, **P <0.01, and ***P <0.001. ns, not significant.

Then, we tried to find out how GLS antagonist ameliorated the inflammation and mitigated the necrosis and apoptosis of liver cells of AIH. Thus, we examined the differentiation of Th1/Th17 cells and CTL upon ConA stimulation *in vivo* and *in vitro*. One study demonstrated that GLS promotes differentiation and function of Th17 cells yet restrains Th1 cells *in vitro* (15, 17), but our results suggested that GLS antagonist significantly suppresses the differentiation of Th1/Th17 cells and CTL. Due to the fact that mTOR signaling is also strongly correlated with the activation and differentiation of T cells (15, 47–50), we tested the levels of the phosphorylated proteins in mTOR signaling and found that glutamine metabolism blocking significantly reduced the levels of phosphorylated mTOR and P70S6K. Other studies also demonstrated that GLS inhibition may inhibit the activation of mTOR signaling and differentiation of T cells through suppressing the production of polyamines (51) or glutathione (15) or downregulating Th17-promoting transcription factor, inducible cAMP early repressor (17). However, we proved that targeting glutamine metabolism may regulate the activation of mTOR signaling and inhibit the leucine-glutamine exchanger and increasing the intracellular level of leucine, as it is widely accepted that intracellular leucine level determines the activation of T cells (57–60).

Although the mice model of ConA-induced hepatitis is a well-recognized and typical tool to study AIH (9), it is acute and usually disappears after 48h and could only partially mimic the pathogenesis of AIH in the human body (61, 62). The present study was performed using mice and cellular experiments, and additional studies on human AIH are needed to verify the protective effects of blocking glutamine metabolism in the future.

Previous evidences show that blocking glutamine metabolism significantly impedes the proliferation of T cells *in vivo* (45) and *in vitro* (20, 51). Thus, GLS antagonist may be a potential drug to attenuate AIH in the human body, as human AIH is an immunoinflammatory chronic liver disease (63) and GLS inhibition may even protect liver from the damages caused by T cells. As AIH is a liver disease characterized by a T cell-mediated autoimmune response, we are provoked to investigate the effect of glutamine metabolism blocking on other T cell-mediated diseases, such as liver allograft rejection. Liver allograft rejection is caused by the recognition of non-self-donor alloantigens by recipient T cells and remains a significant cause of morbidity and graft failure in liver transplant recipients (64). The main treatment of liver allograft rejection is anti-rejection drugs such as glucocorticoids, tacrolimus, which have strong side effects (65). As we mentioned above, JHU083 is a prodrug of DON with weak side effects, and may be a promising drug to prevent or ameliorate the progression of liver allograft rejection.

In conclusion, we have demonstrated that GLS blocking reduces the activation and differentiation of T cells and disease severity in ConA-induced AIH mice, *via* reducing the mRNA expression of SLC7A5, lowering the level of intracellular leucine and further inhibiting the activation of mTOR signaling.

AUTHOR CONTRIBUTIONS

Conception and study design QY, HT, XY, YZ, HJ and QX. Acquisition of data QY, HT, XY, CP, CD, WY, WW and XG. Data analysis QY, HT, XY and CP. Data interpretation JL, HY, YZ, HJ and QX. Manuscript drafting and revising QY, HT, XY, CP, CD, WY, WW, XG, JL, HY, YZ, HJ and QX). All authors contributed to the article and approved the submitted version.

REFERENCES

1. Lohse AW, Chazouilleres O, Dalekos G, Drenth J, Heneghan M, Hofer H, et al. EASL Clinical Practice Guidelines: Autoimmune Hepatitis. *J Hepatol* (2015) 63(4):971–1004. doi: 10.1016/j.jhep.2015.06.030
2. Manns MP, Lohse AW, Vergani D. Autoimmune Hepatitis–Update 2015. *J Hepatol* (2015) 62(1 Suppl):S100–11. doi: 10.1016/j.jhep.2015.03.005
3. Montano-Loza AJ, Czaja AJ. Cell Mediators of Autoimmune Hepatitis and Their Therapeutic Implications. *Dig Dis Sci* (2015) 60(6):1528–42. doi: 10.1007/s10620-014-3473-z
4. Mieli-Vergani G, Vergani D, Czaja AJ, Manns MP, Krawitt EL, Vierling JM, et al. Autoimmune Hepatitis. *Nat Rev Dis Primers* (2018) 4:18017. doi: 10.1038/nrdp.2018.17
5. Tanaka A. Autoimmune Hepatitis: 2019 Update. *Gut Liver* (2020) 14(4):430–8. doi: 10.5009/gnl19261
6. Wang H, Zhao Y, Ren B, Qin Y, Li G, Kong D, et al. Endometrial Regenerative Cells With Galectin-9 High-Expression Attenuate Experimental Autoimmune Hepatitis. *Stem Cell Res Ther* (2021) 12(1):541. doi: 10.1186/s13287-021-02604-2
7. Heymann F, Hamesch K, Weiskirchen R, Tacke F. The Concanavalin A Model of Acute Hepatitis in Mice. *Lab Anim* (2015) 49(1 Suppl):12–20. doi: 10.1177/0023677215572841
8. Gao M, Li X, He L, Yang J, Ye X, Xiao F, et al. Diammonium Glycyrrhizinate Mitigates Liver Injury *Via* Inhibiting Proliferation Of NKT Cells And Promoting Proliferation Of Tregs. *Drug Des Devel Ther* (2019) 13:3579–89. doi: 10.2147/dddt.S220030
9. Wang HX, Liu M, Weng SY, Li JJ, Xie C, He HL, et al. Immune Mechanisms of Concanavalin A Model of Autoimmune Hepatitis. *World J Gastroenterol* (2012) 18(2):119–25. doi: 10.3748/wjg.v18.i2.119
10. Xiang M, Liu T, Tan W, Ren H, Li H, Liu J, et al. Effects of Kinsenoside, A Potential Immunosuppressive Drug for Autoimmune Hepatitis, on Dendritic Cells/CD8(+) T Cells Communication in Mice. *Hepatology* (2016) 64 (6):2135–50. doi: 10.1002/hep.28825
11. Araujo L, Khim P, Mkhikian H, Mortales CL, Demetriou M. Glycolysis and Glutaminolysis Cooperatively Control T Cell Function by Limiting Metabolite Supply to N-Glycosylation. *Elife* (2017) 6:e21330. doi: 10.7554/eLife.21330
12. Danbolt NC. Glutamate Uptake. *Prog Neurobiol* (2001) 65(1):1–105. doi: 10.1016/s0301-0082(00)00067-8
13. Byun JK, Park M, Lee S, Yun JW, Lee J, Kim JS, et al. Inhibition of Glutamine Utilization Synergizes With Immune Checkpoint Inhibitor to Promote Antitumor Immunity. *Mol Cell* (2020) 80(4):592–606.e8. doi: 10.1016/j.molcel.2020.10.015
14. Nabe S, Yamada T, Suzuki J, Toriyama K, Yasuoka T, Kuwahara M, et al. Reinforce the Antitumor Activity of CD8(+) T Cells *via* Glutamine Restriction. *Cancer Sci* (2018) 109(12):3737–50. doi: 10.1111/cas.13827
15. Johnson MO, Wolf MM, Madden MZ, Andrejeva G, Sugiura A, Contreras DC, et al. Distinct Regulation of Th17 and Th1 Cell Differentiation by Glutaminase-Dependent Metabolism. *Cell* (2018) 175(7):1780–95.e19. doi: 10.1016/j.cell.2018.10.001
16. Xia X, Cao G, Sun G, Zhu L, Tian Y, Song Y, et al. GLS1-Mediated Glutaminolysis Unbridled by MALT1 Protease Promotes Psoriasis Pathogenesis. *J Clin Invest* (2020) 130(10):5180–96. doi: 10.1172/jci129269
17. Kono M, Yoshida N, Maeda K, Tsokos GC. Transcriptional Factor ICER Promotes Glutaminolysis and the Generation of Th17 Cells. *Proc Natl Acad Sci USA* (2018) 115(10):2478–83. doi: 10.1073/pnas.1714717115
18. Nian Y, Iske J, Maenosono R, Minami K, Heinbokel T, Quante M, et al. Targeting Age-Specific Changes in CD4(+) T Cell Metabolism Ameliorates Alloimmune Responses and Prolongs Graft Survival. *Aging Cell* (2021) 20(2): e13299. doi: 10.1111/acel.13299
19. Sumbria D, Berber E, Miller L, Rouse BT. Modulating Glutamine Metabolism to Control Viral Immuno-Inflammatory Lesions. *Cell Immunol* (2021) 370:104450. doi: 10.1016/j.cellimm.2021.104450
20. Ueda Y, Saegusa J, Okano T, Sendo S, Yamada H, Nishimura K, et al. Additive Effects of Inhibiting Both mTOR and Glutamine Metabolism on the Arthritis in SKG Mice. *Sci Rep* (2019) 9(1):6374. doi: 10.1038/s41598-019-42932-1
21. Lemberg KM, Vornov JJ, Rais R, Slusher BS. We're Not "DON" Yet: Optimal Dosing and Prodrug Delivery of 6-Diazo-5-Oxo-L-Norleucine. *Mol Cancer Ther* (2018) 17(9):1824–32. doi: 10.1158/1535-7163.Mct-17-1148
22. Crosby HA, Ihnat M, Miller KE. Evaluating the Toxicity of the Analgesic Glutaminase Inhibitor 6-Diazo-5-Oxo-L-Norleucine *In Vitro* and on Rat Dermal Skin Fibroblasts. *MOJ Toxicol* (2015) 1(1):00005. doi: 10.15406/mojt.2015.01.00005
23. Zhu X, Nedelcovych MT, Thomas AG, Hasegawa Y, Moreno-Megui A, Coomer W, et al. JHU-083 Selectively Blocks Glutaminase Activity in Brain CD11b(+) Cells and Prevents Depression-Associated Behaviors Induced by Chronic Social Defeat Stress. *Neuropsychopharmacology* (2019) 44(4):683–94. doi: 10.1038/s41386-018-0177-7
24. Huang H, Long L, Zhou P, Chapman NM, Chi H. mTOR Signaling at the Crossroads of Environmental Signals and T-Cell Fate Decisions. *Immunol Rev* (2020) 295(1):15–38. doi: 10.1111/imr.12845
25. Delgoffe GM, Pollizzi KN, Waickman AT, Heikamp E, Meyers DJ, Horton MR, et al. The Kinase mTOR Regulates the Differentiation of Helper T Cells Through the Selective Activation of Signaling by Mtorc1 and Mtorc2. *Nat Immunol* (2011) 12(4):295–303. doi: 10.1038/ni.2005
26. Yang K, Shrestha S, Zeng H, Karmaus PW, Neale G, Vogel P, et al. T Cell Exit From Quiescence and Differentiation Into Th2 Cells Depend on Raptor-Mtorc1-Mediated Metabolic Reprogramming. *Immunity* (2013) 39(6):1043–56. doi: 10.1016/j.immuni.2013.09.015
27. Liu Y, Pandeswara S, Dao V, Padrón Á, Drerup JM, Lao S, et al. Biphasic Rapamycin Effects in Lymphoma and Carcinoma Treatment. *Cancer Res* (2017) 77(2):520–31. doi: 10.1158/0008-5472.Can-16-1140
28. Leone RD, Zhao L, Englert JM, Sun IM, Oh MH, Sun IH, et al. Glutamine Blockade Induces Divergent Metabolic Programs to Overcome Tumor Immune Evasion. *Science* (2019) 366(6468):1013–21. doi: 10.1126/science.aav2588

29. Wang R, Dillon CP, Shi LZ, Milasta S, Carter R, Finkelstein D, et al. The Transcription Factor Myc Controls Metabolic Reprogramming Upon T Lymphocyte Activation. *Immunity* (2011) 35(6):871–82. doi: 10.1016/j.immuni.2011.09.021
30. Sendler M, van den Brandt C, Glaubitz J, Wilden A, Golchert J, Weiss FU, et al. NLRP3 Inflammasome Regulates Development of Systemic Inflammatory Response and Compensatory Anti-Inflammatory Response Syndromes in Mice With Acute Pancreatitis. *Gastroenterology* (2020) 158 (1):253–69.e14. doi: 10.1053/j.gastro.2019.09.040
31. Saxton RA, Sabatini DM. mTOR Signaling in Growth, Metabolism, and Disease. *Cell* (2017) 168(6):960–76. doi: 10.1016/j.cell.2017.02.004
32. Mossmann D, Park S, Hall MN. mTOR Signalling and Cellular Metabolism Are Mutual Determinants in Cancer. *Nat Rev Cancer* (2018) 18(12):744–57. doi: 10.1038/s41568-018-0074-8
33. Wolfson RL, Sabatini DM. The Dawn of the Age of Amino Acid Sensors for the Mtorc1 Pathway. *Cell Metab* (2017) 26(2):301–9. doi: 10.1016/j.cmet.2017.07.001
34. Durán RV, Oppliger W, Robitaille AM, Heiserich L, Skendaj R, Gottlieb E, et al. Glutaminolysis Activates Rag-Mtorc1 Signaling. *Mol Cell* (2012) 47 (3):349–58. doi: 10.1016/j.molcel.2012.05.043
35. Nicklin P, Bergman P, Zhang B, Triantafellow E, Wang H, Nyfeler B, et al. Bidirectional Transport of Amino Acids Regulates mTOR and Autophagy. *Cell* (2009) 136(3):521–34. doi: 10.1016/j.cell.2008.11.044
36. Chen R, Zou Y, Mao D, Sun D, Gao G, Shi J, et al. The General Amino Acid Control Pathway Regulates mTOR and Autophagy During Serum/Glutamine Starvation. *J Cell Biol* (2014) 206(2):173–82. doi: 10.1083/jcb.201403009
37. Martinez RS, Salji MJ, Rushworth L, Ntala C, Rodriguez Blanco G, Hedley A, et al. SLFN5 Regulates LAT1-Mediated mTOR Activation in Castration-Resistant Prostate Cancer. *Cancer Res* (2021) 81(13):3664–78. doi: 10.1158/0008-5472.Can-20-3694
38. Elorza A, Soro-Arnáiz I, Meléndez-Rodríguez F, Rodríguez-Vaello V, Marsboom G, de Cárcer G, et al. Hif2α Acts as an Mtorc1 Activator Through the Amino Acid Carrier SLC7A5. *Mol Cell* (2012) 48(5):681–91. doi: 10.1016/j.molcel.2012.09.017
39. Cao D, Mikosz AM, Ringsby AJ, Anderson KC, Beatman EL, Koike K, et al. MicroRNA-126-3p Inhibits Angiogenic Function of Human Lung Microvascular Endothelial Cells *via* LAT1 (L-Type Amino Acid Transporter 1)-Mediated mTOR (Mammalian Target of Rapamycin) Signaling. *Arterioscler Thromb Vasc Biol* (2020) 40(5):1195–206. doi: 10.1161/atvbaha.119.313800
40. Ohshima Y, Kaira K, Yamaguchi A, Oriuchi N, Tominaga H, Nagamori S, et al. Efficacy of System L Amino Acid Transporter 1 Inhibition as a Therapeutic Target in Esophageal Squamous Cell Carcinoma. *Cancer Sci* (2016) 107(10):1499–505. doi: 10.1111/cas.13021
41. Almeida L, Lochner M, Berod L, Sparwasser T. Metabolic Pathways in T Cell Activation and Lineage Differentiation. *Semin Immunol* (2016) 28(5):514–24. doi: 10.1016/j.smim.2016.10.009
42. Buck MD, O'Sullivan D, Pearce EL. T Cell Metabolism Drives Immunity. *J Exp Med* (2015) 212(9):1345–60. doi: 10.1084/jem.20151159
43. Geiger R, Rieckmann JC, Wolf T, Basso C, Feng Y, Fuhrer T, et al. L-Arginine Modulates T Cell Metabolism and Enhances Survival and Anti-Tumor Activity. *Cell* (2016) 167(3):829–42.e13. doi: 10.1016/j.cell.2016.09.031
44. Ren W, Liu G, Yin J, Tan B, Wu G, Bazer FW, et al. Amino-Acid Transporters in T-Cell Activation and Differentiation. *Cell Death Dis* (2017) 8(3):e2655. doi: 10.1038/cddis.2016.222
45. Sinclair LV, Rolf J, Emslie E, Shi YB, Taylor PM, Cantrell DA. Control of Amino-Acid Transport by Antigen Receptors Coordinates the Metabolic Reprogramming Essential for T Cell Differentiation. *Nat Immunol* (2013) 14(5):500–8. doi: 10.1038/ni.2556
46. Hollinger KR, Smith MD, Kirby LA, Prchalova E, Alt J, Rais R, et al. Glutamine Antagonism Attenuates Physical and Cognitive Deficits in a Model of MS. *Neurol Neuroimmunol Neuroinflamm* (2019) 6(6):e609. doi: 10.1212/nxi.0000000000000609
47. Song W, Li D, Tao L, Luo Q, Chen L. Solute Carrier Transporters: The Metabolic Gatekeepers of Immune Cells. *Acta Pharm Sin B* (2020) 10(1):61–78. doi: 10.1016/j.apsb.2019.12.006
48. Liu M, Zhang J, Pinder BD, Liu Q, Wang D, Yao H, et al. WAVE2 Suppresses mTOR Activation to Maintain T Cell Homeostasis and Prevent Autoimmunity. *Science* (2021) 371(6536):eaaz4544. doi: 10.1126/science.aaz4544
49. Jin J, Kim C, Xia Q, Gould TM, Cao W, Zhang H, et al. Activation of Mtorc1 at Late Endosomes Misdirects T Cell Fate Decision in Older Individuals. *Sci Immunol* (2021) 6(60):eabg0791. doi: 10.1126/sciimmunol.abg0791
50. Deason K, Troutman TD, Jain A, Challa DK, Mandraju R, Brewer T, et al. BCAP Links IL-1R to the PI3K-mTOR Pathway and Regulates Pathogenic Th17 Cell Differentiation. *J Exp Med* (2018) 215(9):2413–28. doi: 10.1084/jem.20171810
51. Zhang J, Zhao L, Wang J, Cheng Z, Sun M, Zhao J, et al. Targeting Mechanistic Target of Rapamycin Complex 1 Restricts Proinflammatory T Cell Differentiation and Ameliorates Takayasu Arteritis. *Arthritis Rheumatol* (2020) 72(2):303–15. doi: 10.1002/art.41084
52. Liu PS, Wang H, Li X, Chao T, Teav T, Christen S, et al. α-Ketoglutarate Orchestrates Macrophage Activation Through Metabolic and Epigenetic Reprogramming. *Nat Immunol* (2017) 18(9):985–94. doi: 10.1038/ni.3796
53. Jones N, Blagih J, Zani F, Rees A, Hill DG, Jenkins BJ, et al. Fructose Reprogrammes Glutamine-Dependent Oxidative Metabolism to Support LPS-Induced Inflammation. *Nat Commun* (2021) 12(1):1209. doi: 10.1038/s41467-021-21461-4
54. Oh MH, Sun IH, Zhao L, Leone RD, Sun IM, Xu W, et al. Targeting Glutamine Metabolism Enhances Tumor-Specific Immunity by Modulating Suppressive Myeloid Cells. *J Clin Invest* (2020) 130(7):3865–84. doi: 10.1172/jci131859
55. Edwards DN, Ngwa VM, Raybuck AL, Wang S, Hwang Y, Kim LC, et al. Selective Glutamine Metabolism Inhibition in Tumor Cells Improves Antitumor T Lymphocyte Activity in Triple-Negative Breast Cancer. *J Clin Invest* (2021) 131(4):e140100. doi: 10.1172/jci140100
56. Hajjar S, Nathan N, Joseph J, Mottawea W, Ariana A, Pyatibrat S, et al. Foxo3a Tempers Excessive Glutaminolysis in Activated T Cells to Prevent Fatal Gut Inflammation in the Murine IL-10(-/-) Model of Colitis. *Cell Death Differ* (2021) 29(3):585–99. doi: 10.1038/s41418-021-00876-y
57. Beugnet A, Tee AR, Taylor PM, Proud CG. Regulation of Targets of mTOR (Mammalian Target of Rapamycin) Signalling by Intracellular Amino Acid Availability. *Biochem J* (2003) 372(Pt 2):555–66. doi: 10.1042/bj20021266
58. Ananieva EA, Powell JD, Hutson SM. Leucine Metabolism in T Cell Activation: mTOR Signaling and Beyond. *Adv Nutr* (2016) 7(4):798s–805s. doi: 10.3945/an.115.011221
59. Van Winkle LJ, Tesch JK, Shah A, Campione AL. System B0,+ Amino Acid Transport Regulates the Penetration Stage of Blastocyst Implantation With Possible Long-Term Developmental Consequences Through Adulthood. *Hum Reprod Update* (2006) 12(2):145–57. doi: 10.1093/humupd/dmi044
60. Maciolek JA, Pasternak JA, Wilson HL. Metabolism of Activated T Lymphocytes. *Curr Opin Immunol* (2014) 27:60–74. doi: 10.1016/j.coi.2014.01.006
61. Wang H, Feng X, Yan W, Tian D. Regulatory T Cells in Autoimmune Hepatitis: Unveiling Their Roles in Mouse Models and Patients. *Front Immunol* (2020) 11:575572. doi: 10.3389/fimmu.2020.575572
62. Yang J, Wang B, Zhang CF, Xu XH, Zhang MA. C(21)-Steroidal Glycoside From Cynanchum Atratum Attenuates Concanavalin A-Induced Liver Injury in Mice. *Molecules* (2019) 24(6):1087. doi: 10.3390/molecules24061087
63. Komori A. Recent Updates on the Management of Autoimmune Hepatitis. *Clin Mol Hepatol* (2021) 27(1):58–69. doi: 10.3350/cmh.2020.0189
64. Ronca V, Wootton G, Milani C, Cain O. The Immunological Basis of Liver Allograft Rejection. *Front Immunol* (2020) 11:2155. doi: 10.3389/fimmu.2020.02155
65. Encke J, Uhl W, Stremmel W, Sauer P. Immunosuppression and Modulation in Liver Transplantation. *Nephrol Dial Transplant* (2004) 19 Suppl 40:iv22–5. doi: 10.1093/ndt/gfh1037

Permissions

All chapters in this book were first published Frontiers; hereby published with permission under the Creative Commons Attribution License or equivalent. Every chapter published in this book has been scrutinized by our experts. Their significance has been extensively debated. The topics covered herein carry significant findings which will fuel the growth of the discipline. They may even be implemented as practical applications or may be referred to as a beginning point for another development.

The contributors of this book come from diverse backgrounds, making this book a truly international effort. This book will bring forth new frontiers with its revolutionizing research information and detailed analysis of the nascent developments around the world.

We would like to thank all the contributing authors for lending their expertise to make the book truly unique. They have played a crucial role in the development of this book. Without their invaluable contributions this book wouldn't have been possible. They have made vital efforts to compile up to date information on the varied aspects of this subject to make this book a valuable addition to the collection of many professionals and students.

This book was conceptualized with the vision of imparting up-to-date information and advanced data in this field. To ensure the same, a matchless editorial board was set up. Every individual on the board went through rigorous rounds of assessment to prove their worth. After which they invested a large part of their time researching and compiling the most relevant data for our readers.

The editorial board has been involved in producing this book since its inception. They have spent rigorous hours researching and exploring the diverse topics which have resulted in the successful publishing of this book. They have passed on their knowledge of decades through this book. To expedite this challenging task, the publisher supported the team at every step. A small team of assistant editors was also appointed to further simplify the editing procedure and attain best results for the readers.

Apart from the editorial board, the designing team has also invested a significant amount of their time in understanding the subject and creating the most relevant covers. They scrutinized every image to scout for the most suitable representation of the subject and create an appropriate cover for the book.

The publishing team has been an ardent support to the editorial, designing and production team. Their endless efforts to recruit the best for this project, has resulted in the accomplishment of this book. They are a veteran in the field of academics and their pool of knowledge is as vast as their experience in printing. Their expertise and guidance has proved useful at every step. Their uncompromising quality standards have made this book an exceptional effort. Their encouragement from time to time has been an inspiration for everyone.

The publisher and the editorial board hope that this book will prove to be a valuable piece of knowledge for researchers, students, practitioners and scholars across the globe.

List of Contributors

Clara I. Colino, José M. Lanao and Carmen Gutierrez-Millan
Area of Pharmacy and Pharmaceutical Technology, Department of Pharmaceutical Sciences, University of Salamanca, Salamanca, Spain
The Institute for Biomedical Research of Salamanca (IBSAL), Salamanca, Spain

Chieh-Yu Liao, Myeong Jun Song, Amy S. Mauer and Harmeet Malhi
Division of Gastroenterology and Hepatology, Mayo Clinic, Rochester, MN, United States

Yandong Gao and Alexander Revzin
Department of Physiology and Biomedical Engineering, Mayo Clinic, Rochester, MN, United States

Matti Sällberg and Anna Pasetto
Division of Clinical Microbiology, Department of Laboratory Medicine, Karolinska Institutet, Stockholm, Sweden

Alex Amoros, Carla Pitarch, Carmen Deulofeu and Marco Pavesi
European Foundation for the Study of Chronic Liver Failure, Barcelona, Spain

Tilman Sauerbruch
Department of Internal Medicine I, University of Bonn, Bonn, Germany

Jonel Trebicka
European Foundation for the Study of Chronic Liver Failure, Barcelona, Spain
Department of Internal Medicine I, University of Bonn, Bonn, Germany
Faculty of Health Sciences, University of Southern Denmark, Odense, Denmark
Department of Mechanical Biology, Institute for Bioengineering of Catalonia, Barcelona, Spain
J.W. Goethe University Hospital, Frankfurt, Germany
Department of Gastroenterology and Hepatology, Odense University Hospital, Odense, Denmark

Tania Welzel and Stefan Zeuzem
J.W. Goethe University Hospital, Frankfurt, Germany

Esther Titos and José Alcaraz-Quiles
Department of Biochemistry and Molecular Genetics, Hospital Clínic, IDIBAPS and CIBERehd, Barcelona, Spain

Joan Clària
European Foundation for the Study of Chronic Liver Failure, Barcelona, Spain
Department of Biochemistry and Molecular Genetics, Hospital Clínic, IDIBAPS and CIBERehd, Barcelona, Spain

Javier Fernandez-Gomez, Elsa Sola and Pere Ginès
Liver Unit, Hospital Clínic, IDIBAPS and CIBERehd, Barcelona, Spain

Salvatore Piano and Paolo Angeli
Unit of Internal Medicine and Hepatology, Department of Medicine, DIMED, University of Padova, Padova, Italy

Paolo Caraceni and Mauro Bernardi
Department of Medical and Surgical Sciences, University of Bologna, Bologna, Italy

Karl Oettl and Rudolf E. Stauber
Department of Gastroenterology and Hepatology, Medical University of Graz, Graz, Austria

Wim Laleman and Frederic Nevens
University Hospital Gasthuisberg, KU Leuven, Leuven, Belgium

Jane McNaughtan, Rajeshwar P. Mookerjee and Rajiv Jalan
Royal Free Hospital, London, United Kingdom

Minneke J. Coenraad
Department of Gastroenterology and Hepatology, Leiden University Medical Center, Leiden, Netherlands

Christian Steib and Alexander Gerbes
Department of Medicine II, Liver Center Munich, University Hospital LMU Munich, Munich, Germany

Rita Garcia and Rafael Bañares
Department of Digestive Diseases and CIBERehd, Facultad de Medicina, Hospital General Universitario Gregorio Marañón, Instituto de Investigación Sanitaria Gregorio Marañón, Universidad Complutense, Madrid, Spain

Thierry Gustot
Erasme Hospital, Université Libre de Bruxelles, Brussels, Belgium

Miguel A. Rodriguez Gandia and Agustin Albillos
Hospital Ramón y Cajal, Madrid, Spain

Victor Vargas
Vall'd Hebron Hospital, Barcelona, Spain

Faouzi Saliba
Hôpital Paul Brousse, Université Paris-Sud, Villejuif, France

Carlo Alessandria
Division of Gastroenterology and Hepatology, San Giovanni Battista Hospital, Torino, Italy

Andrea de Gottardi
Department of Hepatology, Inselspital, Bern, Switzerland

Heinz Zoller
Department of Hepatology and Gastroenterology, University Clinic Innsbruck, Innsbruck, Austria

Richard Moreau
European Foundation for the Study of Chronic Liver Failure, Barcelona, Spain
Inserm, U1149, Centre de Recherche sur l'Inflammation (CRI), UMRS1149, Paris, France
Université Paris Diderot-Paris 7, Département Hospitalo-Universitaire (DHU) UNITY, Paris, France
Service d'Hépatologie, Hôpital Beaujon, Assistance Publique-Hôpitaux de Paris, Paris, France
Laboratoire d'Excellence Inflamex, ComUE Sorbonne Paris Cité, Paris, France
Centre National de la Recherche Scientifique (CNRS), Paris, France

Zhao Shan
Center for Life Sciences, School of Life Sciences, Yunnan University, Kunming, China

Cynthia Ju
Department of Anesthesiology, McGovern Medical School, University of Texas Health Science Center at Houston, Houston, TX, United States

Lei Sun, Yunjuan Nie and Huiqiong He
Engineering Research Center of Cell & Therapeutic Antibody, Ministry of Education, School of Pharmacy, Shanghai Jiao Tong University, Shanghai, China

Qiong Wu, Rui Wang and Dan Zhang
Anhui Province Key Laboratory of Translational Cancer Research, Bengbu Medical College, Bengbu, China

Ni Cheng
Department of Pharmacology, University of Illinois College of Medicine, Chicago, IL, United States

Gang Wang
Jiangsu Center for the Collaboration and Innovation of Cancer Biotherapy, Cancer Institute, Xuzhou Medical University, Xuzhou, China

Feng Qian
Engineering Research Center of Cell & Therapeutic Antibody, Ministry of Education, School of Pharmacy, Shanghai Jiao Tong University, Shanghai, China
Anhui Province Key Laboratory of Translational Cancer Research, Bengbu Medical College, Bengbu, China
Jiangsu Center for the Collaboration and Innovation of Cancer Biotherapy, Cancer Institute, Xuzhou Medical University, Xuzhou, China

Richard D. Ye
Institute of Chinese Medical Sciences, University of Macau, Macau, China

Daphne van der Heide and Ruchi Bansal
Department of Biomaterials Science and Technology, Faculty of Science and Technology, Technical Medical Center, University of Twente, Enschede, Netherlands

Ralf Weiskirchen
Institute of Molecular Pathobiochemistry, Experimental Gene Therapy and Clinical Chemistry (IFMPEGKC), RWTH University Hospital Aachen, Aachen, Germany

Chris John Weston and David H. Adams
Centre for Liver and Gastrointestinal Research, Institute of Immunology and Immunotherapy, Medical School, University of Birmingham, Birmingham, United Kingdom
NIHR Birmingham Biomedical Research Centre, University Hospitals Birmingham NHS Foundation Trust and University of Birmingham, Birmingham, United Kingdom

Henning Wolfgang Zimmermann
Medical Department III, University Hospital of Aachen, Aachen, Germany

Lang Dou, Xiaomin Shi, Xiaoshun He and Yifang Gao
Organ Transplantation Center, The First Affiliated Hospital, Sun Yat-sen University, Guangzhou, China
Guangdong Provincial Key Laboratory of Organ Donation and Transplant Immunology, The First Affiliated Hospital, Sun Yat-sen University, Guangzhou, China
Guangdong Provincial International Cooperation Base of Science and Technology (Organ Transplantation), The First Affiliated Hospital, Sun Yat-sen University, Guangzhou, China

Elizabeth C. Stahl, Martin J. Haschak, Branimir Popovic and Bryan N. Brown
Department of Bioengineering, Pittsburgh Liver Research Center, McGowan Institute for Regenerative Medicine, University of Pittsburgh, Pittsburgh, PA, United States

Andrea Kristina Horst, Gisa Tiegs and Linda Diehl
Institute for Experimental Immunology and Hepatology, University Medical Center Hamburg-Eppendorf, Hamburg, Germany

Axel Périanin
Inserm, U1149, Centre de Recherche sur l'Inflammation, Paris, France
UMRS1149, Université Paris Diderot-Paris 7, Paris, France
Centre National de la Recherche Scientifique (CNRS), Paris, France

Vicente Arroyo
European Foundation for the Study of Chronic Liver Failure, Barcelona, Spain
EF Clif, EASL-CLIF Consortium and Grifols Chair, Barcelona, Spain

Maria E. Moreno-Fernandez and Michelle S. M. A. Damen
Department of Pediatrics, University of Cincinnati College of Medicine, Cincinnati, OH, United States
Division of Immunobiology, Cincinnati Children's Hospital Medical Center and the University of Cincinnati College of Medicine, Cincinnati, OH, United States

Jarren R. Oates
Department of Pediatrics, University of Cincinnati College of Medicine, Cincinnati, OH, United States
Division of Immunobiology, Cincinnati Children's Hospital Medical Center and the University of Cincinnati College of Medicine, Cincinnati, OH, United States
Immunology Graduate Program, Cincinnati Children's Hospital Medical Center and the University of Cincinnati College of Medicine, Cincinnati, OH, United States

Melanie C. McKell and Joseph E. Qualls
Department of Pediatrics, University of Cincinnati College of Medicine, Cincinnati, OH, United States
Immunology Graduate Program, Cincinnati Children's Hospital Medical Center and the University of Cincinnati College of Medicine, Cincinnati, OH, United States
Division of Infectious Diseases, Cincinnati Children's Hospital Medical Center and the University of Cincinnati College of Medicine, Cincinnati, OH, United States

George S. Deepe Jr.
Department of Medicine, University of Cincinnati College of Medicine, Cincinnati, OH, United States

Senad Divanovic
Department of Pediatrics, University of Cincinnati College of Medicine, Cincinnati, OH, United States
Division of Immunobiology, Cincinnati Children's Hospital Medical Center and the University of Cincinnati College of Medicine, Cincinnati, OH, United States
Immunology Graduate Program, Cincinnati Children's Hospital Medical Center and the University of Cincinnati College of Medicine, Cincinnati, OH, United States
Center for Inflammation and Tolerance, Cincinnati Children's Hospital Medical Center, Cincinnati, OH, United States

Camila Alvarez-Silva
Novo Nordisk Foundation Center for Basic Metabolic Research, Faculty of Health and Medical Sciences, University of Copenhagen, Copenhagen, Denmark

Robert Schierwagen and Frank E. Uschner
Department of Internal Medicine I, Goethe University Clinic Frankfurt, Frankfurt, Germany
Department of Internal Medicine I, University of Bonn, Bonn, Germany

Alessandra Pohlmann, Fernando Magdaleno and Patrick Ryan
Department of Internal Medicine I, University of Bonn, Bonn, Germany

Maria J. G. T. Vehreschild
Medical Clinic II, University Center for Infectious Diseases, University Hospital Frankfurt, Frankfurt, Germany

Joan Claria
European Foundation for the Study of Chronic Liver Failure, Barcelona, Spain

Eicke Latz
Institute of Innate Immunity, University of Bonn, Bonn, Germany
Division of Infectious Diseases and Immunology, University of Massachusetts Medical School, Worcester, MA, United States
German Center for Neurodegenerative Diseases (DZNE), Bonn, Germany
Centre for Inflammation Research, Norwegian University of Science and Technology, Trondheim, Norway

Benjamin Lelouvier
Vaiomer, Labège, France

Manimozhiyan Arumugam
Novo Nordisk Foundation Center for Basic Metabolic Research, Faculty of Health and Medical Sciences, University of Copenhagen, Copenhagen, Denmark
Department of Gastroenterology and Hepatology, Odense University Hospital, Odense, Denmark

Xiaocheng Charlie Dong
Center for Diabetes and Metabolic Diseases, Department of Biochemistry and Molecular Biology, Indiana University School of Medicine, Indianapolis, IN, United States

Vik Meadows, Debjyoti Kundu and Keisaku Sato
Hepatology and Gastroenterology, Medicine, Indiana University, Indianapolis, IN, United States

Leonardo Baiocchi
Hepatology Unit, University of Tor Vergata, Rome, Italy

Yessenia Fuentes
Clinical and Translational Sciences Institute, STEM GEHCS Program, Indiana University School of Medicine, Indianapolis, IN, United States

Chaodong Wu
Department of Nutrition, Texas A&M University, College Station, TX, United States

Sanjukta Chakraborty and Shannon Glaser
Department of Medical Physiology, Texas A&M University College of Medicine, Bryan, TX, United States

Gianfranco Alpini, Lindsey Kennedy and Heather Francis
Richard L. Roudebush VA Medical Center, Indianapolis, IN, United States

Marta Vuerich, Ahmadreza Kalbasi, Jonathon J. Graham and Maria Serena Longhi
Department of Anesthesia, Critical Care & Pain Medicine, Beth Israel Deaconess Medical Center, Harvard Medical School, Boston, MA, United States

Na Wang
Department of Anesthesia, Critical Care & Pain Medicine, Beth Israel Deaconess Medical Center, Harvard Medical School, Boston, MA, United States
Department of Hematology, Shandong Provincial Hospital Affiliated to Shandong First Medical University, Jinan, China
School of Medicine, Shandong University, Jinan, China

Qiang Yu and Honghu Tu
Department of Liver Surgery, Renji Hospital, School of Medicine, Shanghai Jiao Tong University, Shanghai, China

Xueyi Yin
School of Chinese Materia Medica, Nanjing University of Chinese Medicine, Nanjing, China

Wenhua Yang and Haowen Jiang
State Key Laboratory of Drug Research, Shanghai Institute of Materia Medica, Chinese Academy of Sciences, Shanghai, China

Chang Peng, Chuanyun Dou and Jia Li
State Key Laboratory of Drug Research, Shanghai Institute of Materia Medica, Chinese Academy of Sciences, Shanghai, China
School of Pharmacy, University of Chinese Academy of Sciences, Beijing, China

Wenbiao Wu and Xiaotong Guan
School of Pharmaceutical Science and Technology, Hangzhou Institute for Advanced Study, University of Chinese Academy of Sciences (UCAS), Hangzhou, China

Yi Zang
School of Chinese Materia Medica, Nanjing University of Chinese Medicine, Nanjing, China
State Key Laboratory of Drug Research, Shanghai Institute of Materia Medica, Chinese Academy of Sciences, Shanghai, China
School of Pharmaceutical Science and Technology, Hangzhou Institute for Advanced Study, University of Chinese Academy of Sciences (UCAS), Hangzhou, China

Hexin Yan
Department of Anesthesia, Renji Hospital, School of Medicine, Shanghai Jiao Tong University, Shanghai, China

Qiang Xia
Department of Liver Surgery, Renji Hospital, School of Medicine, Shanghai Jiao Tong University, Shanghai, China
Shanghai Engineering Research Center of Transplantation and Immunology, Shanghai, China
Shanghai Institute of Transplantation, Shanghai, China

Index

www.ingramcontent.com/pod-product-compliance
Lightning Source LLC
LaVergne TN
LVHW060058220926
848484LV00008BA/2168
9798887400365